THE EYE MANIFESTATIONS
OF INTERNAL DISEASES

THE EYE MANIFESTATIONS
OF INTERNAL DISEASES

BY

I. S. TASSMAN, M.D.

Associate Professor of Ophthalmology, Graduate School of Medicine,
University of Pennsylvania, Philadelphia; Attending Surgeon,
Wills Hospital, Philadelphia, Pa.

WITH 243 ILLUSTRATIONS
INCLUDING 24 IN COLOR

SECOND EDITION

ST. LOUIS
THE C. V. MOSBY COMPANY
1946

Published November, 1946
Reprinted February, 1947

Printed in the
United States of America

Press of
The C. V. Mosby Company
St. Louis

AFFECTIONATELY DEDICATED

TO

MY WIFE, S. S. T.

PREFACE TO THE SECOND EDITION

The reception given to the first edition of this volume has been most gratifying. The author is grateful for the way in which this effort was received
and for the many encouraging and generous reviews which were accorded the
first edition.

The purpose of the book was an attempt to bridge any existing gap between the eye manifestations and the other medical aspects of internal diseases
and thereby serve the needs of the ophthalmologist and all others engaged
either in general or specialized practice. To accomplish this, the arrangement
of the book was planned so that the desired information would be easy to find.
The text is, therefore, systematized and simple in style. It was intended to be
concise and comprehensive but not necessarily encyclopedic. Since this was
apparently accomplished, the arrangement of the material and table of contents have not been changed in any radical way in this edition. The first five
chapters again constitute a first part which provides a description of the normal structure of the eye, a general description of the causes of eye manifestations, and a brief description of the examination of the patient and of some of
the routine tests, methods, and appliances employed in examining the eye.
These are intended especially for student beginners and those who are not
experienced in ophthalmology. Two chapters are devoted to the structural
abnormalities and manifestations. Here the basic and fundamental lesions
which may involve the intrinsic structures of the eye are described individually, so that the inexperienced may also be better able to understand and
appreciate the picture of the eye manifestations that follow in the subsequent
chapters.

The second part, beginning with Chapter VI, presents the essential description of the eye manifestations of a different disease or system of diseases
in each chapter. The important features of the ocular condition are described,
together with management, differential diagnosis, treatment, and prognosis
whenever possible. A brief preliminary description of the primary or systemic
disease is included for the benefit of the student and ophthalmologist who may
not have a close contact with these conditions in his routine practice. It is
not intended to provide a detailed description of systemic diseases for intern-
ists, who already have an intimate knowledge of these diseases. Ophthalmology
is a branch of internal medicine, and in many instances the ocular manifestations appear very early in the course of a disease and are often of important
diagnostic and prognostic significance. For this reason, importance is attached
to the description of the ocular condition.

The Congenital and Hereditary Manifestations are considered in a separate chapter. In this chapter are given the ocular conditions found in the
more important hereditary and heredofamilial diseases and a description of
the congenital eye malformations and anatomical defects of development. The
eye manifestations of infections and the infectious diseases include those of all
the acute and chronic infectious diseases, with separate chapters on such important subjects as syphilis and tuberculosis. The other infections are con-
veniently grouped as Virus Infections, Fungus Infections, Ocular Parasites and

7

Parasitic Infections, and Focal Infections. A separate chapter is devoted to the eye manifestations of the more important drug and chemical intoxications.

The succeeding chapters deal with the eye manifestations of nearly every disease—from those of the cardiovascular system to the diseases affecting the bones of the skull. Although it is true that a few of the diseases included might not be considered to present any direct eye manifestations and that some of the conditions described as eye manifestations of the disease in question might not be accurately designated as such, they do nevertheless occur at times, either as accompanying factors or sequelae and complications, and are therefore included.

The descriptions of a number of new diseases have been added. A number of new illustrations have also been added and, in general, an attempt has been made to keep the material up to date. A few examples of the new additions include the descriptions of Ocular Allergy, Epidemic Keratoconjunctivitis, Hurler's Disease, Osteopetrosis, Lymphogranuloma Venereum, Bowen's Disease of the Cornea, Toxoplasmic Encephalomyelitis, and Purtscher's Disease. Many new references and new additions to the diseases previously included will also be found. An effort has also been made in this edition to enlarge on the treatment of the various conditions and to include the most recent methods and forms of treatment whenever possible. It should probably be stated here that treatment with penicillin is still in the investigative stage, and since no final reports by reliable authorities responsible for these investigations and their evaluation are available at this writing, the subject is preferably omitted. The use of penicillin in the treatment of gonorrheal ophthalmia and ocular syphilis is mentioned in the text, but otherwise the reader is, for the time being, referred to the publications of such authors in particular as Lt. Col. John E. L. Keyes (Lancet 1, March 27, 1943; Brit. M. J. 2, Nov. 20, 1943; Lancet 2, Nov. 20, 1943); E. P. Abraham et al. (Lancet 2, Aug. 16, 1941); A. Sorsby (Brit. M. J. 2, Dec. 4, 1943); C. S. Keefer et al. (J. A. M. A. 122, Aug. 28, 1943); W. P. Griffey (Arch. Ophth. 31, Feb. 1944); G. T. W. Cashell (Brit. M. J. 1, March 25, 1944); and J. V. Klauder and G. J. Dublin (to be published in Arch. Ophth.).

Standard textbooks and the recognized medical and ophthalmologic publications have been referred to again in order to obtain the latest and most authoritative knowledge of the subject under discussion. Descriptions have been borrowed from recognized authorities in the specialty of ophthalmology in particular and in the field of medicine in general. Illustrations have also been borrowed in a number of instances in order to provide as complete and accurate a description as possible.

Acknowledgment is hereby made, therefore, of my grateful appreciation to all individual authors for references and quotations from their original articles and for the use of illustrations which were borrowed. Individual credit is also given for these in the text. Acknowledgment is also gratefully made here and separately to the publishers of the various textbooks and journals referred to in compiling the subject matter and illustrations which appear in the volume.

To Dr. William Zentmayer, former Professor of Ophthalmology, Graduate School of Medicine, University of Pennsylvania, I desire to express again my appreciation for his kind interest and advice. The description of Glaucoma, which seemed to fit best in Chapter V, is based on his lecture notes to former graduate students. His earlier notes served as a beginning for my own lectures on Medical Ophthalmology and also as an inspiration for this book.

To my colleagues, The Board of Attending Surgeons at Wills Hospital, I again express my grateful appreciation for their kind cooperation in the use of clinical material for references and illustrations. I wish to express my sincere thanks to all who may have provided me with any assistance either directly or indirectly. Failure to give credit in any instance is an unintentional omission. It therefore remains only to express the hope that this book will continue to meet the need of ophthalmologists, as well as of others engaged in general or specialized practice of medicine.

I. S. T.

ACKNOWLEDGMENTS

Meakins' Practice of Medicine, ed. 2, The C. V. Mosby Co., St. Louis, was followed in general for the description of the internal diseases and illustrations credited in the text.

Chapter I, The Normal Structure of the Eye and Orbit, is based on the description by Wolff: The Anatomy of the Eye and Orbit, The Blakiston Co., Philadelphia. Acknowledgment is also made for illustrations credited in the text.

References and illustrations from Duke-Elder: Text-Book of Ophthalmology, Vols. 1, 2, and 3; Traquair: Clinical Perimetry; and Rae: Neuro-Ophthalmology, The C. V. Mosby Co., St. Louis.

Troncoso: Internal Diseases of the Eye and Atlas of Ophthalmology, F. A. Davis & Co., Philadelphia, for references and illustrations.

Fuchs (Duane): Text-Book of Ophthalmology, ed. 8, revised, J. B. Lippincott Co., Philadelphia, for references and illustrations.

Ramsay: Clinical Ophthalmology for the General Practitioner, Oxford Medical Publications, for references and illustrations.

Berens: The Eye and Its Diseases, W. B. Saunders Co., Philadelphia.

Parsons: Diseases of the Eye, The Macmillan Co., New York.

Whitby and Britton: Disorders of the Blood, ed. 4, The Blakiston Co., Philadelphia.

To the Archives of Ophthalmology, The American Journal of Ophthalmology, and Journal of the American Medical Association, and all individual authors for references to original articles and the use of illustrations which appeared in these journals. An attempt is made to give individual credit for these in the text.

CONTENTS

CHAPTER I

CHAPTER V

CHAPTER VI

CHAPTER VII

CHAPTER VIII

CHAPTER IX

COLOR PLATES

THE EYE MANIFESTATIONS
OF
INTERNAL DISEASES

CHAPTER I

NORMAL STRUCTURE OF THE EYE AND ORBIT

The Appendages of the Eye

The appendages of the eye include the eyelids, the conjunctiva, and the lacrimal apparatus.

The eyelids originate from the external skin and act as folds which are freely movable to cover and protect the eyeballs. The upper eyelid is limited superiorly by the eyebrow while the lower eyelid is merely continuous with the skin of the cheek and has no sharp lower line of limitation. Together, the upper and lower eyelids enclose a space known as the palpebral fissure; at each lateral extremity they join to form the inner and outer angles of the eye. The inner angle is known as the internal canthus and the outer is the external canthus. The outer angle forms a rather sharp point and is closely adherent to the eyeball, whereas the inner angle is rather more free and when put on a stretch, exposes a small, curved notch of skin which is known as the caruncle. In looking directly forward with the eyes open, the upper eyelid should just cover the upper margin of the cornea whereas the lower eyelid is just below the lower margin of the cornea. The upper eyelid is supplied by the levator palpebrae superioris muscle, which renders it more freely movable than the lower.

The skin covering the eyelids is about the thinnest in the human body. Being very loosely attached, it can be readily made to change or adjust its position with opening and closure of the eyelids. In older people it may be thrown into folds or wrinkles and may even overhang the lids, in marked cases. At the free border of the lid the skin is held closely adherent to the tarsus by firm connective tissue. The free border of the lids is reflected along a line to the anterior and posterior margins, between which lies a narrow surface known as the intermarginal surface.

The eyelashes or cilia spring from the anterior margins of the lids and are arranged in rows of two or three. Those of the upper lid curl upward and are more numerous, while those of the lower lid curl downward.

When the eyes are shut, the two surfaces formed by the free borders of the upper and lower lids come together in close apposition, so that any fluid formed by secretion of the meibomian glands is retained. The openings of the meibomian glands occur as a row of small puncta which lie directly in front of the posterior border of the lid margin. The cilia and meibomian glands are usually not found to the inner side of the lacrimal punctum, which is located near the medial sixth of the margin.

Eversion of the eyelids exposes to view their posterior surfaces, covered by conjunctiva, which is closely adherent to the tarsus. The tarsal plates are joined with a thin peripheral fascia known as the septum orbitale to form a fibrous layer or supporting framework for the lids. The tarsus of the upper eyelid is larger than that of the lower and is curved anteriorly. This anterior surface is separated from the fibers of the orbicularis palpebrarum muscle by loose tissue, while the posterior surface is covered by the conjunctiva. The extremities of the tarsal plates are attached to the orbital margin by fibrous ligaments known respectively as the median lateral tarsal or palpebral ligaments.

The meibomian glands are sebaceous glands which are imbedded in the dense fibrous tissue of the tarsus and extend from the attached to the free borders. They are elongated and lie parallel with each other. Their function is to lubricate the edges of the lids.

At the free margins of the lids there are found, connected with the follicles of the cilia, small sebaceous glands known as Zeis's glands. Other small sweat glands occurring near the free margin of the lids and which open into the follicles of the cilia are known as Moll's glands.

Two voluntary muscles are found in the eyelids, namely, the orbicularis palpebrarum and the levator palpebrae superioris.

The orbicularis is circular and surrounds the palpebral fissure, lying just under the skin, and is actually a flat expansion of the skin. It is the sphincter muscle of the eye and consists of two portions: (1) Palpebral or Central, (2) Orbital or Peripheral. The palpebral portion lies in the lids themselves and originates from the internal or medial palpebral ligament which is a fibrous ligament attached to the frontal process of the superior maxilla just under the skin of the inner angle of the eye. The fibers of the orbicularis cover the free border of the lids in circular arches extending across to the external canthus, uniting here in the lateral peripheral raphe. The orbital portion is the external part of the orbicularis and arises from the inner and upper margins of the orbit inside the supraorbital notch and from the lower orbital margin inside the infra-orbital foramen. The palpebral portion is employed in closing or blinking the eye and for narrowing the palpebral fissure. The orbital portion acts to draw the skin of the temples and face in toward the inner side of the orbit when the eyes are very tightly closed. It is usually brought into action by any strong effort involving the facial muscles. The orbicularis is supplied by the facial or seventh cranial nerve.

The pars lacrimalis of the orbicularis is sometimes called Horner's muscle and arises behind the lacrimal sac at the upper portion of the posterior lacrimal crest. The ciliary portion of the orbicularis is the muscle of Riolan and is continuous medially with Horner's muscle.

The levator palpebrae superioris muscle arises from the posterior or bottom of the orbit, around the optic foramen, and extends forward under the roof of the orbit, lying on the superior rectus muscle with which it is connected by fascia. It spreads out in fan shape, its tendon extending over the tarsal plate. Its action is to raise the upper eyelid and it is supplied by the oculomotor (third) nerve.

Arising from the fibers of the levator of the eyelid is a muscle named after H. Müller, which extends to the upper margin of the tarsus. A similar muscle of Müller is found below the interior rectus muscle and extends into the tarsus of the lower lid. These two muscles are made up of unstriped fibers and are supplied by the sympathetic.

The action of the levator palpebrae superioris in elevating the lid is augmented by the action of the occipitofrontalis muscle. The frontal portion of the latter muscle is inserted into the skin under the eyebrows and the fibers are in close relationship with those of the orbicularis. Here are also found the fibers of the corrugator muscle which act to assist in knitting the brows. In drawing the scalp upward and backward, the fibers of the frontalis act at the same time to elevate the upper eyelid to some extent. It is supplied by the seventh cranial nerve.

The blood supply of the eyelids comes from the superior and inferior tarsal arches, and these come from the medial and lateral palpebral branches of the ophthalmic and lacrimal arteries. The orbicularis, meibomian glands and conjunctiva are supplied by branches which extend forward from the tarsal arches. The conjunctiva and free margin of the eyelids are very vascular.

The veins of the eyelids form a dense plexus which frequently can be seen through the conjunctiva near the fornices. They are more numerous than the arteries and are wider and of larger caliber. The blood from the upper lid leaves by the superior palpebral vein which empties into the angular. The angular vein is a continuation of the frontal and continues into the facial vein. It extends from a little below the level of the eyebrow to the level of the lower margin of the orbit, when it becomes the facial. The angular vein lies with the angular artery on the nasal process of the superior maxillary bone, a little internal to the lacrimal sac. From the lower lid, some branches of the inferior palpebral vein empty into the angular, and others empty directly into the facial.

The angular, facial and ophthalmic veins have no valves. There is a free anastomosis between the ophthalmic and the facial veins, which gives to the blood from the lids and orbit a double outlet, the one intracranial, via the ophthalmic and the cavernous sinus, and the other extracranial, via the facial and the internal jugular.

There are numerous lymphatics in the eyelids which drain the skin, conjunctiva and meibomian glands. They connect with the glands in front of the ear as well as those of the parotid. As a result the latter are sometimes found to be involved in infections of the conjunctiva or eyelids.

The Conjunctiva

The conjunctiva forms a sac of thin mucous membrane lining the palpebral fissure. As it is reflected back from the posterior surface of the lids to the eyeball, it thereby acts as an attachment between the two parts, and on the eyeball itself it extends forward to the cornea.

According to its location, it is divided into three parts. The part which covers the lids is the palpebral portion. Since the greater portion of the latter covers the tarsus and is closely adherent to it, this is often called the tarsal conjunctiva. It can be exposed to view by everting the eyelid. In doing so the retrotarsal fold or fornix, which constitutes the second portion of the conjunctiva, is also exposed. This connects the palpebral or tarsal portion with the third division covering the eyeball itself and which is known as the bulbar conjunctiva.

The fornix contains small glands resembling lacrimal glands which are known as Krause's glands. It is also supplied with blood vessels and lies in folds which permit free movement of the eyeball. In severe inflammations the conjunctiva of the fornix may appear greatly swollen and chemotic.

The bulbar conjunctiva loosely covers the underlying sclera and is continuous anteriorly with the epithelium of the cornea. Being thin and elastic, the bulbar conjunctiva can be readily moved or picked up with a forceps. It is also in close relationship with the capsule of Tenon which covers the tendons of the recti muscles. The plica semilunaris is a semilunar fold at the inner angle of the eye which is formed by a crescentic reduplication of the bulbar conjunctiva. It is similar to the nictitating membranes found in animals. Just inside the semilunar fold is the caruncle, which is a small red elevation lying in a pit at the inner angle.

The blood supply of the conjunctiva comes from the palpebral branches of the nasal and lacrimal arteries of the lids and the anterior ciliary arteries. The latter travel along the course of the tendons of the recti muscles and send off anterior conjunctival vessels which by anastomosis with posterior conjunctival branches, form the pericorneal plexus and vascular arcades of the limbus. Around the limbus the conjunctival vessels are superficial while the ciliary vessels are deeper and radiate out from the margins of the cornea. Veins accompany the conjunctival arteries and empty into the palpebral and ophthalmic veins.

The Lacrimal Apparatus

The lacrimal apparatus consists of the lacrimal gland, palpebral or accessory glands, the canaliculi, the lacrimal sac, and the nasal duct.

The lacrimal gland secretes the tears which moisten and lubricate the eyeball after reaching the conjunctival sac through a number of ducts leading to the upper fornix. The gland consists of a superior or orbital portion which is located at the upper, outer angle of the orbit where it lies in a shallow depression known as the lacrimal fossa, and a smaller inferior or palpebral portion which lies just below the upper fornix at the outer angle. It can sometimes be seen here as a small mass when the upper lid is everted and the fornix is exposed to view. Krause's glands, found in the fornix, may be considered as accessories or continuations of the inferior lacrimal gland extending to the inner angle.

In size and shape the lacrimal gland resembles a small almond. Transversely, it measures about 20 mm., anteroposteriorly, about 12 mm. The inner border is almost in line with the outer edge of the superior rectus muscle. The outer border descends almost to the upper edge of the external rectus. Histologically, the lacrimal gland is of the salivary type, i.e., acinous. This similarity is of important significance, and is exemplified in Mikulicz's disease, or simultaneous noninflammatory enlargement of the head glands of this type. The excretory ducts of the superior gland are three or four in number, and pass between the lobules of the accessory gland, to empty into the outer portion of the superior fornix. The external duct is the largest and empties near the external canthus.

Separating the orbital from the palpebral glands are the tendonous expansion of the levator palpebrae superioris, Müller's nonstriated muscle, and the gland capsule. There are numerous apertures or free spaces, through which the excreting ducts and connective tissue trabeculae pass.

The punctum lacrimalis is the opening into the lacrimal passage. There is one found on the free border of the upper and lower lids close to the inner angle. They are known as the upper and lower puncta and are located on small prominences of the lids, known as the papilla lacrimalis. Each eyelid must be drawn away from the eyeball in order to bring the respective punctum into view. Each punctum leads into a canaliculus which consists of a short vertical portion and a longer horizontal portion. The canaliculi, after passing behind the caruncle, meet to empty into the lacrimal sac.

The lacrimal sac rests in the lacrimal fossa, a deeply grooved portion of the orbital surface of the lacrimal bone. It extends vertically with its upper extremity rounded and the lower extremity continuous with the nasal canal. Between the sac and the periosteum there is loose connective tissue which permits of considerable expansion. When distended, its length is about 12 mm. and its diameter 6 or 7 mm. Behind the sac is Horner's muscle, and in front of it is the inner palpebral ligament or tendo-oculi. It is therefore embraced by these two structures. The fundus reaches above the palpebral ligament.

The nasal duct extends from the lower end of the sac, to the upper part of the meatus of the nose, or that part which is just beneath the inferior turbinate bone. The bony canal is formed by the superior maxillary, the lacrimal, and the inferior turbinate bones. It is from 12 to 14 mm. long and its average diameter about 3.8 mm. At its nasal extremity the canal may be continued obliquely beneath the nasal mucous membrane. Emerging from beneath the nasal mucous membrane, the nasal opening is slitlike and protected by a mucous membrane flap. The narrowest part of the entire lacrimal canal is at the junction of the sac with the nasal duct. The lacrimal sac and the nasal duct together constitute the lacrimal canal. About one-half is sac and the other half is nasal duct.

The general direction of the lacrimal canal from above is downward, outward, and backward. A probe when inserted into the sac points toward the alae of the nose.

The arterial supply of the lacrimal gland is through the lacrimal artery, which is usually the first branch of the ophthalmic. The lacrimal canal receives blood principally through the nasal branch of the ophthalmic. The nerve supply of the lacrimal apparatus is from the ophthalmic division of the fifth which divides before reaching the orbit, into the lacrimal, nasal and frontal. The three nerves enter the orbit through the sphenoidal fissure. The lacrimal is the smallest; it runs along the upper border of the external rectus muscle and enters the lacrimal gland. The infratrochlear branch of the nasal nerve which is given off just before the latter enters the anterior internal orbital canal supplies the lacrimal sac.

The Structure of the Eyeball

The eyeball is an almost spherical globe, which is lodged in the anterior portion of the orbit. It is 24 mm. in its anteroposterior diameter, 23.5 mm. in the transverse and about 23 mm. in the vertical. Because of its shape and structure, it is considered to consist of two segments, an anterior and a posterior segment. The anterior segment is more sharply curved because of the shape of the cornea, while the posterior segment, which comprises that part from the cornea backward, is almost truly spherical.

As a whole, the eyeball consists of three coats or coverings which enclose its contents. These coats in order are: (1) The cornea and sclera: The cornea is the most anterior portion and comprises about one-sixth of the entire outer or protective covering; the sclera constitutes the remaining or posterior portion of the outer covering. The cornea is transparent, while the sclera is opaque and white. (2) The middle coat consists of the choroid, iris and ciliary body, which together are known as the uveal tract. This coat is well supplied with blood vessels and its function is the nutrition of the eye. (3) The retina, which is the inner coat of the eye, receives the visual impressions and is made up almost entirely of nerve tissue. It is also well supplied with blood vessels. The retina together with the optic nerve comprises the sensory apparatus of the eye.

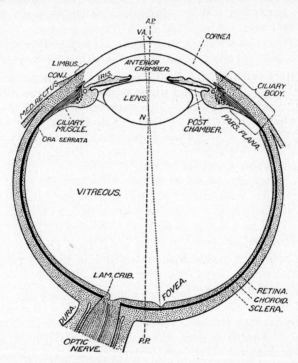

Fig. 1.—Horizontal section of the eyeball. *P.P.*, Posterior pole. *A.P.*, Anterior pole. *V.A.*, Visual axis. (After Salzmann, from Wolff: The Anatomy of the Eye and Orbit, The Blakiston Co.)

Separating the iris from the vitreous, which is enclosed in the posterior part of the eye, we find the crystalline lens. The iris divides the portion in front of the lens into two chambers, known as the anterior and posterior chambers. These two chambers contain the aqueous humor. The anterior chamber is limited in front by the posterior surface of the cornea and a small part of the sclera. Together with the iris, the ciliary body and the most anterior portion of the lens in the pupil form the posterior boundary. The angle formed at the point where the cornea, ciliary body and iris meet is called the angle of the anterior chamber.

The anterior boundary of the posterior chamber is the iris while the posterior boundary is formed by the lens and suspensory ligament. The three coats of the eye will be described first.

The Outer Coat

THE CORNEA

As has already been stated, the cornea is the most anterior structure of the eyeball. Although apparently round and occupying the front and center of the eyeball, it is actually slightly elliptical when viewed from in front, since the horizontal diameter measures 12 mm. as compared with 11 mm. for the vertical diameter. It is transparent and slightly thicker at its edge than in the center. Its radius of curvature is slightly greater on the posterior surface than on the anterior, the average of which is about 7.5 mm. This radius of curvature is greater than that for the rest of the eyeball, which accounts for the greater anteroposterior diameter of the latter. The sclera, coming from behind, encloses more of the anterior surface of the cornea than the posterior, with the result that the cornea fits snugly into the sclera, with which it is continuous. The manner in which the cornea fits into the sclera is often compared to the fit of a watch crystal. It is the degree and kind of curvature of the cornea which is greatly responsible for the presence of astigmatism in the eye.

The structure of the cornea is made up of five layers: (1) An anterior layer of stratified epithelium which is really an anterior continuation of the conjunctiva. It consists of a number of layers of cells including round, cylindrical and flat cells. (2) An anterior elastic layer known as Bowman's membrane is the next. This is sharply separated from the epithelium and forms the outer section of the stroma. (3) The substantia propria or stroma of the cornea. This is made up of a number of transparent lamella consisting of fibers or fibrils which are piled upon one another in the form of bundles. These are held together by a kind of cement. Two varieties of cells are found between the lamella. These are the fixed cells and the wandering cells. The first are connective tissue cells which in appearance resemble bone corpuscles and consist of a nucleus and branches which join with those of other cells. The wandering cells are considered important in inflammatory conditions of the cornea, where they increase greatly in number. (4) Descemet's membrane. This is the posterior elastic membrane of the cornea and is very resistant to irritants. It differs from Bowman's membrane in that it is sharply differentiated from the stroma of the cornea, and when injured by any process it can be regenerated. (5) The endothelial layer is the most posterior epithelial layer of the cornea and consists of a single layer of flat cells lining the inner surface of Descemet's membrane.

There are no blood vessels normally found in the cornea itself, but at its margins there is a network of marginal loops coming from the anterior ciliary vessels.

The cornea is abundantly supplied with nerve fibers which come partly from the ciliary nerves and partly from those of the surrounding conjunctiva. The cornea is therefore very sensitive and responds immediately to the slightest irritation or presence of the most minute foreign particles.

The Sclera

The sclera is the tough, opaque portion of the outer coat, comprising that part posterior to the cornea. In its posterior portion it is about 1 mm. in thickness becoming thinner anteriorly, but again slightly thicker in its most anterior part because of attachment of the muscle tendons. At this point its fibrils unite with the cornea without any sharp line of demarcation. Covering the sclera is a loose connective tissue known as episcleral tissue which connects anteriorly with the conjunctiva. This episcleral tissue contains numerous blood vessels, but the sclera itself has very few except for those which pass over it into the eye itself. The sclera becomes much thinner at the posterior pole of the eye and here it becomes the lamina cribrosa which is its weakest point. The fibers of the optic nerve pass through the lamina cribrosa, at which point they show the effects of pressure in an inflammatory condition. At a point a little to the inner side of the posterior pole, there is an aperture where the optic nerve pierces the sclera.

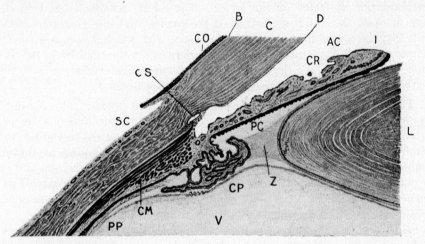

Fig. 2.—The region of the angle of the anterior chamber. *AC*, Anterior chamber. *B*, Bowman's membrane. *C*, Cornea. *CM*, Ciliary muscle. *CO*, Conjunctiva. *CP*, Ciliary processes. *CR*, Iris crypts. *CS*, Canal of Schlemm. *D*, Descemet's membrane. *I*, Iris. *L*, Lens. *PC*, Posterior chamber. *PP*, Pars plana of ciliary body. *SC*, Sclera. *V*, Vitreous. *Z*, Zonule of Zinn. (From Duke-Elder: Text-Book of Ophthalmology, The C. V. Mosby Co.)

The Sclerocorneal Margin.—The structural elements of the cornea and sclera are histologically almost identical, but the cornea is transparent whereas the sclera is densely opaque. Since the two structures are directly continuous with each other, the point at which this takes place is known as the sclerocorneal junction. This forms an important zone of the eyeball within which the cornea, sclera, iris and ciliary body all meet, and which contains in its posterior portion the venous channel known as Schlemm's canal. The exterior and posterior scleral processes mark, in their terminations, the corneal margin at its anterior and posterior surfaces. The external corneal margin is considerably in advance of its posterior margin which corresponds with the root of the iris.

Schlemm's Canal is a circular channel surrounding the limbus of the cornea, close to the angle of the anterior chamber. It lies within the posterior scleral process and is marked by its anterior border. Its lumen is elliptical and measures about 0.3 mm. in its long diameter and 0.05 mm. in its shorter diameter.

The pectinate ligament and the meridional fibers of the ciliary muscle are in close relationship internally. Schlemm's canal is in direct communication with the anterior ciliary veins, and through the spaces of Fontana, it stands in close relationship with the anterior chamber.

The Uveal Tract (Middle Coat)

THE CHOROID

The middle coat of the eye which, as already stated, consists of the choroid, iris and ciliary body, is the vascular coat. These three structures are commonly called the uveal tract. The choroid is thin and comprises the most posterior part of the uveal tract. It is brown in color and lies between the retina and sclera. Its outer surface is slightly rough, while its interior is somewhat smoother.

The choroid contains many blood vessels which are apparently arranged in layers, with the largest vessels on the scleral surface and the smallest in the retinal layer. These smaller vessels are the choriocapillaris which nourish the retina. The choroidal vessels can commonly be seen on examination with the ophthalmoscope.

The choroid is more loosely attached at the posterior pole of the eye where the vessels enter from the sclera. The vascular part of the choroid is covered on its outer side by the suprachoroid and on its inner side by the lamina-vitrea, both of which are nonvascular. With the exception of the latter two, all the other layers of the choroid contain pigment, which accounts for its color. There is also a layer of veins which are separated by intervascular spaces and which are surrounded by perivascular lymphatics where they pass through the sclera. All the layers of the choroid continue on anteriorly into the ciliary body, while the choriocapillaris terminates at the ora-serrata.

THE IRIS

The iris is the most anterior portion of the uveal tract or middle coat of the eye. It is round and thin, with a pupillary opening in the center. The ability of the iris to change its form under various conditions of light also changes the size of the pupil and thereby regulates the amount of light which enters the eye. At its peripheral border, the iris arises from the ciliary body, from which it extends out over the lens, so that its free or smaller circle glides freely over the anterior capsule of the lens which gives it a support. If the lens has been removed from an eye or if it should be displaced from its normal position, any movement of the eyeball will cause a vibration or tremulous movement of the iris, which is known as iridodonesis. The pupillary border may, when the lens is absent, recede so that the iris plane becomes vertical, and the anterior chamber deeper. Or, the plane of the pupillary border may be posterior to that of the ciliary body; the iris is then saucer-shaped.

The average thickness of the iris is 0.4 mm. Changes in its surface, breadth and thickness take place during alterations in the width of the pupil.

On its anterior surface the iris contains numerous elevations which ordinarily stand out clearly and are well defined, but in pathologic conditions of the iris they are blurred and difficult to distinguish. As a result it is important to be able to recognize their appearance in the course of any examination. The small blood vessels which lie in the stroma of the iris and extend from the ciliary to the pupillary margin produce ridges which extend radially and cause these markings. The ridges interlace with a circular ridge of the iris which divides the latter into two zones; one zone outside of the small circle of the iris, while the other lies inside the small circle and along the pupillary margin. Small pitlike depressions or crypts are found in its surface near the small circle of the iris. Other small openings are also found in the periphery of the anterior surface near its root. The latter are scarcely ever visible, however. A narrow fringe of black pigment surrounds the pupillary margin of the iris.

The structure of the iris based on Wolff's description follows: It consists from before backwards of five layers.

1. The anterior epithelium, which consists of flat cells resembling the endothelium of serous membranes. Although they are continuous with those on the posterior surface of the cornea at the angle of the anterior chamber, their structure is different.

2. The anterior limiting membrane, which is really a condensation of the anterior part of the stroma, consists mainly of pigment cells which resemble those of the stroma and also some collagenous fibrilla and nerve endings. It contains no blood vessels. In the blue iris the anterior limiting membrane is thin and contains few pigment cells. In the brown iris it is densely pigmented and thick. In this way it determines the color of the iris.

3. The stroma is loose and consists of connective tissue which contains pigment cells and which includes the following structures: (a) the sphincter pupillae muscle, (b) vessels and nerves of the iris, (c) the pigment cells.

The sphincter pupillae is made up of a flat bar of unstriped muscle fibers 1 mm. broad, forming a ring around the pupillary margin near the posterior surface. With its contraction the pupil is constricted, and the edge of the pigment is pulled onto the anterior surface of the iris. It receives branches from the third cranial nerve by way of the short ciliaries. The sphincter muscle is held firmly to the surrounding structure by vessels and bundles of connective tissue.

The vessels for the most part run radially which gives rise to the ridges seen on the anterior surface and they form the bulk of the iris. They change their shape with the change in size of the pupil. They arise from the long and anterior ciliary arteries.

The pigment cells are small and have an oval nucleus and several processes which unite to form a plexus. They cover the vessels and nerves. The pigment is composed of both fine and coarse granules which are paler than those of the choroid. Round pigment cells without processes, the so-called clump cells, are found near the sphincter pupillae and rarely near the ciliary border. Their pigment, which consists of round dark granules, resembles that of the cells on the posterior surface of the iris from which they are derived.

4. The posterior membrane (Bruch) is a thin layer which lies between the stroma and pigment layer. Within this membrane, or closely associated posteriorly, are the radially disposed fibers which constitute the dilator pupillae muscle. The dilator fibers mingle with the circular fibers of sphincter of the iris close to the edge of the pupil. It also sends out several other spurs accompanied by pigment and continues along into the ciliary body. The contraction

of this muscle dilates the pupil by drawing the pupillary margin toward its root. It is supplied by the ciliary nerves from the sympathetic.

5. The posterior epithelium is made up of two layers of cells which are highly pigmented and difficult to distinguish except in the albinotic eye. The anterior layer is made up of flat spindle cells while the posterior layer consists of large polyhedral or cubicle cells with rather small round nuclei. The processes of the spindle cells are dilator fibers. Pigment granules are dark brown and are either round or rod-shaped. The pigment epithelium curls over the pupillary margin after lining the back of the iris and produces the black fringe over the pupillary margin. In the tearing away of a posterior synechia the posterior layer at the back of the iris adheres to the lens and the anterior remains attached to the posterior membrane.

In newborn children the iris has a deep blue color; there is little pigment in the stroma, which is thin; and the posterior pigment layer can be seen. With oncoming age the stroma thickens and if the pigmentation does not increase, the iris retains a light blue color, but if a corresponding increase occurs in the amount of pigmentation in the stroma, the iris becomes darker in color. Occasionally this change takes place only in certain sections of the iris so that a brown section may be found with the remainder of the iris light in color. There may also be found a difference in the color of the iris in each eye, and when present this condition is known as heterochromia. It can therefore be seen that the color of the iris depends on the amount of pigment in the individual, and as a consequence the iris is always darker in the darker races.

The Blood Vessels of the Iris.—The arteries of the iris are derived from the long posterior ciliary and the anterior ciliary arteries, which are branches of the ophthalmic, given off close to where the latter artery lies below the optic nerve. A circular anastomosis is formed within the ciliary region, just beyond the root of the iris. This is the *circulus arteriosus iridis major,* from which the iridial branches are given off and extend radially toward the pupillary margin. Within the sphincter zone a second circular anastomosis is formed known as the *circulus arteriosus iridis minor*. The latter lies near the anterior surface of the iris, giving off three sets of branches, one to the sphincter muscle, one to the posterior portion of the stroma layer, and one for distribution within the anterior boundary layer.

The veins follow the general course of the arteries and finally empty into the venal vorticosae.

The Nerves of the Iris.—These are motor, sensory and vasomotor in character. Both medullated and nonmedullated fibers are represented. They are derived from the ciliary plexus, formed by branches of the ciliary nerves in the ciliary body. The iris plexus becomes denser as it approaches the sphincter muscle. The pale nonmedullated fibers apparently belong to the sympathetic, and those which pass backward toward the dilator muscle, presumably innervate these fibers. Others are vasomotor. Of the medullated fibers, some are sensory and distributed over the anterior surface of the iris, and others are motor, passing to the sphincter muscle.

THE CILIARY BODY

The ciliary body is attached at its anterior border to the sclera behind Schlemm's canal. Posteriorly it unites with the sclera so that a clear separation between the two can only be distinguished on its inner surface. In an antero-posterior section of the eye the ciliary would be found to begin at the ora-serrata. The ciliary muscle is found on its outer surface which is attached to the sclera. The color of the ciliary body is black; that of the choroid from which it arises being brown. The ciliary processes are about seventy in number and arise from the anterior margin of the black zone. They are lighter in color and very prominent. The depressions between the apices of the ciliary processes are deeply pigmented. The ciliary processes belong to the part of the ciliary body known as the corona ciliaris, while the posterior portion, which is smooth and uniformly black, is the pars plana or orbiculus ciliaris.

The ciliary muscle fibers are arranged in bundles which form a reticulum, with connective tissue and chromatophores found between. The fibers of the ciliary muscle are divided into meridional, radial and circular portions. The meridional and radial are known as Brucke's portion while the circular is known as Müller's. The vascular layer of the ciliary body is on the inner side of the ciliary muscle and is comprised of numerous blood vessels which are found in a connective tissue stroma filled with chromatophores. There are also numerous vessels in the ciliary processes so that the corona is the most vascular portion of the eyeball. The lamina vitrea of the ciliary body is a hemogeneous body on the inner surface of the vascular layer of the ciliary processes. This is followed by a layer of highly pigmented cells known as the pigment epithelium and then a layer of cylindrical or cubicle cells which are nonpigmented. The latter two layers comprise the pars ciliaris retinae.

THE RETINA

The retina is a thin membrane which constitutes the innermost coat of the eye. It is normally transparent and has a purplish-red color due to the visual purple contained in the rods. It is of interest that the latter is destroyed by intense light and this occurs after death, with the result that the retina becomes opaque and also loses its color.

At the inner side of the posterior pole of the eye is the point where the head of the optic nerve enters the retina. This is called the optic disc or papilla of the optic nerve. This is also the point of entry of the central artery and the central vein of the retina. In the center of the optic nerve head is the physiologic excavation or cuplike depression. No ophthalmoscopic examination of the eye can be complete without a detailed examination of the optic nerve head and the retina. Although it is called a papilla, the nerve head is normally flat and its margins should be distinctly outlined from the rest of the retina.

At a point located exactly at the posterior pole of the eye is the macula lutea. It has a faint yellow color because of which it is sometimes called the "yellow spot" and in its center is the point of most acute vision, a slight depression known as the fovea centralis.

The retina is intimately connected with the choroid in two places, one at the head of the optic nerve and the other anteriorly at the ora-serrata. This is the line representing the boundary between the choroid and ciliary body and which extends forward farther on the nasal side and above than on the temporal side and below. Actually, however, the retina is continuous beyond this point by reason of its pigment layer of epithelium.

A series of ten layers constitute the structure of the retina; these are from without inward as follows:

1. The layer of pigment epithelium is the outermost layer and is composed of flat hexagonal cells sending fine projections in-between the rods and cones. The pigment is composed of fine granules in the outer part of the cell. The granules in the processes are spindle or rod shaped.

2. Layer of rods and cones, which is the sensitive part of the retina and is composed of the visual cells of the retina. The cells are bipolar with a peripheral process which corresponds to the sensory ending of a somatic nerve. A rod consists of an outer and an inner segment and contains the visual purple. The latter, however, is absent in the rods located in an area of about 4 mm. around the ora-serrata and also around the fovea centralis, where the rods are absent. The cones are also made up of two segments and their shape varies in different parts of the retina. The nutrition of the visual cells is obtained from the choriocapillaris.

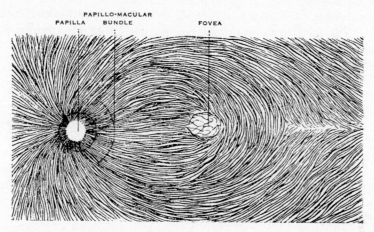

Fig. 3.—Papillomacular bundle, nerve fiber layer. (From Poirier, after Dogiel and Greef.—Wolff: The Anatomy of the Eye and Orbit, The Blakiston Co.)

3. The external limiting membrane is a thin membrane with openings for the passage of rod and cone fibers going to the outer molecular layer. It is formed by the fibers of Müller.

4. The outer nuclear layer is made up principally of rod and cone nuclei or granules. The granules are several layers deep and become thin at the outer side of the disc and thickest near the center of the fovea. In the center of the fovea, however, the layer practically disappears.

5. The outer molecular layer is composed of two parts, the one being the processes of horizontal cells and the other, fibers of Müller. This layer is also thickest at the macula and practically disappears at the fovea.

6. The inner nuclear layer, which consists principally of rod and cone bipolar cells and the nuclei of fibers of Müller. This layer becomes thin as it approaches the fovea where it, too, disappears.

7. The internal plexiform or internal molecular layer, made up principally of interlaced bipolar cell axones and ganglion cell dendrones, distal cell processes, fibers of Müller, and a few nuclei. This layer is also absent at the fovea centralis.

8. The layer of ganglion cells which are multipolar, resembling those of the central nervous system. These cells are generally large and vary greatly in shape and size. The axis cylinder protrudes from the inner and then passes into the nerve fiber layer. Dendrites are given off from the other sides and extend into the inner molecular layer. A number of layers of ganglion cells are found around the macula but decrease as they approach the fovea and here disappear. In other parts of the retina they occur in a single row, with the exception of the temporal side of the disc where they are present in two layers. In this layer are also fibers of Müller and neuroglia.

9. The nerve fiber layer or stratum opticum, which is made up principally of axones of the ganglion cells. These become continuous with the optic nerve by passing through the lamina cribrosa. The nerve fibers in this layer are arranged in bundles running parallel with the surface of the retina and the fibers all converge toward the optic nerve head. The fibers on the inner side of the disc are straight and uninterrupted, while most of those on the outer side must travel around the macula either above or below and thereby form a kind of raphe. The fibers connecting the macula itself with the disc are known as the papillomacular bundle, in which region the nerve layer is thinnest. This is also one of the most important parts of the nerve fiber layer. The thickest portion of the layer is around the margin of the optic nerve head. The nerve fiber layer also becomes thinner out in the periphery.

10. The internal limiting membrane bounds the retina internally and the vitreous externally. It is a thin hyaline membrane formed by the approximation of the fibers of Müller base to base.

Since the nerve fiber layer is the only one found at the optic nerve head, vision is not present when light strikes at this point, which accounts for the area in the retina known as the blind spot. At the fovea, however, the vision is most acute since this spot is the most sensitive to visual impressions. This area is most easily affected by trauma and disease.

The blood supply of the retina is obtained principally from the central retinal artery. In the outer portion the rods and cones and the outer nuclear layer receive their nourishment mostly from the choriocapillaris. The central retinal artery passes along the dural sheath of the optic nerve and with the vein crosses the subarachnoid space to enter the nerve surrounded by pial covering. It then passes up to the center of the nerve with the vein on the temporal side and then pierces the lamina cribrosa to enter the eye.

At the inner side of the excavation of the disc it branches into a superior and inferior artery and each of these divides into nasal and temporal branches. Most of the retinal vessels are located in the nerve fiber layer of the retina and some in the ganglion cell layer. These vessels in the retina are an individual system and do not anastomose with any other system. The macular region of the retina receives small twiglike branches from the superior and inferior temporal vessels, but no blood vessels are found in the fovea. An occasional cilioretinal artery is present extending from the outer edge of the disc to the macula, which area it supplies. Such an artery arises as a branch from an anastomosis from the posterior ciliary arteries. It is significant clinically that flame-shaped hemorrhages, as seen on examination with the ophthalmoscope, are located in the nerve fiber layer, their shape being determined by the structure of this layer,

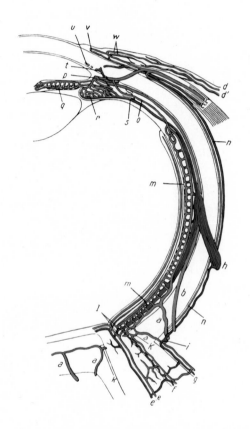

Fig. 4.—Schematic representation of the vascular system of the eye. *a*, Short posterior ciliary arteries. *b*, Long posterior ciliary arteries. *cc′*, Anterior ciliary artery and vein. *dd′*, Posterior conjunctival artery and vein. *ee′*, Central retinal artery and vein. *f, g*, Vessels of inner and outer sheaths of the nerve. *h*, Vena vorticosa. *i*, Short posterior ciliary vein. *k*, Branch of short posterior ciliary artery to optic nerve. *l*, Anastamoses of choroidal vessels with those of optic nerve. *m*, Choriocapillaris. *n*, Episcleral branches. *o*, Recurrent choroidal artery. *p*, Circulus arteriosus iridis major. *q*, Vessels of the iris. *r*, Ciliary process. *s*, Branch of vena vorticosa from ciliary muscle. *t*, Branch of anterior ciliary vein from ciliary muscle. *u*, Canal of Schlemm. *v*, Limbal network. *w*, Anterior conjunctival artery and vein. (From Duke-Elder: Text-Book of Ophthalmology.)

whereas small round punctate hemorrhages, such as those which are seen to occur in diabetes, are located in the deeper layers of the retina. Occlusion of the central retinal artery causes sudden blindness.

The retinal veins accompany the arteries and the central retinal vein is formed at the level of the lamina cribrosa from the superior and inferior retinal veins. The central vein most often empties directly into the cavernous sinus, but occasionally may open into the superior or inferior ophthalmic veins.

There is some lymph circulation between various parts of the retina but no true lymph vessels. The perivascular sheaths carry lymph which is conveyed into the lymph spaces of the optic nerve through the lamina cribrosa.

Optic Nerve

That portion of the optic nerve which is viewed by the examiner with the ophthalmoscope is the head of the optic nerve and is commonly called the optic disc. This is really the presentation of the intraocular portion of the nerve which is located inside the sclera. The portion of nerve between the eyeball and the optic foramen is considered as the orbital portion and that between the optic foramen and the chiasm as the intracranial portion. In order that the nerve can leave the eye it must go through the choroid and the sclera as has been previously stated. This occurs at a point just inside the posterior pole of the eye, and in leaving the sclera it passes through a small foramen or sclerotic-choroidal canal called the foramen sclera. This is accomplished by the external portion of the sclera being reflected back on the optic nerve to form its outer sheath, while the inner portion stretches over the foramen like a diaphragm and contains a number of small openings to permit separate fiber bundles of the optic nerve to pass through it. It can be seen from this, therefore, that there is no actual opening into the sclera for the passage of the optic nerve into the orbit, but rather a kind of diaphragm formation containing small perforations called the lamina cribrosa.

In the normal eye the lamina cribrosa stretches straight across the optic nerve, but its appearance and position are altered in pathologic conditions, particularly in glaucoma. In the latter condition the increased intraocular tension causes its recession with a deepening of the excavation. Since the optic nerve in the lamina cribrosa lies between tight fibrous layers, it is readily constricted at this point, when swelling takes place.

In the eyeball the fibers connecting the optic nerve with the macula, and which are known as the papillomacular bundle, are perhaps of greatest importance from a physiologic standpoint, since each nerve fiber connects with a separate terminal in the macula from which individual impressions are conveyed to the brain. The fibers which pass through the lamina cribrosa are transparent since they are nonmedullated; they become opaque, however, behind the lamina, where they take on a medullated sheath. The intraorbital portion of the nerve is therefore somewhat broader than the part contained in the sclera.

The central vessels of the optic nerve, namely, the central retinal artery and central retinal vein, are found in the anterior part of the orbital portion of the nerve, entering on the lower and inner side about 10 mm. behind the eyeball. At the nerve head they ascend over the inner side of the excavation, where they divide into the retinal vessels. The pink color of the optic disc is somewhat more pronounced on the inner side of the physiologic cup than on the outer because of the increased capillarity on this side. The inner edge of the optic disc is also slightly more blurred than the outer in the normal eye.

A dark ring produced by a heaping of pigment epithelium is commonly seen around the margins of the optic disc in the normal eye. This is known as the scleral or choroidal ring.

Between the eyeball and the optic foramen where it leaves the orbit, the optic nerve is just elastic enough to permit the normal amount of movement of the eyeball itself. When stretched, however, at this point it serves to fix the eyeball in place and prevents its freedom of movement. Such a condition might occur where the eyeball protrudes markedly forward, as in a case of exophthalmos. In the orbit the optic nerve is composed of a great many fibers and some connective tissue. The connective tissue lies between the bundles of fibers, which run parallel and form a septum or framework above the course of the nerve. Spaces for the conveyance of lymph are found between the bundles in the septa.

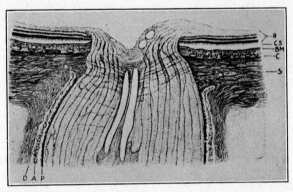

Fig. 5.—Longitudinal section through the optic nerve. R, Retina. CS, Space (normally potential) between retina and pigment epithelium. BM, Bruch's membrane, the dark line above which is the pigment epithelium. C, Choroid. S, Sclera. D, Dura. A, Arachnoid. P, Pia. (From Duke-Elder: Text-Book of Ophthalmology.)

The sheaths of the optic nerve are derived from the pia, arachnoid and dura of the brain. The pia is the inner sheath close to the trunk of the nerve. Bands of connective tissue forming septa pass with blood vessels from the pia into the nerve itself. The dura forms the external sheath and loosely surrounds the nerve, being much thicker than the inner sheath. This results in an intervaginal space remaining between the two. The arachnoid is the middle sheath and is closely attached to the dural while at the same time it is connected by means of connective tissue to the inner sheath. The intervaginal space is divided into a subdural and subarachnoid space. These are lined with endothelium and considered as lymph spaces that communicate with the cerebral subdural and subarachnoid spaces.

The optic nerve passes through the optic foramen from the orbit to enter the cranium. It is accompanied in the optic canal by the ophthalmic artery, which lies on the inner side of the nerve. From here to the chiasm it is surrounded by the pial sheath only. At the chiasm the two nerves cross and their fibers decussate, forming the optic tracts after they leave the chiasm. From here they travel backward, becoming farther apart as they proceed to the primary optic centers. These are constituted principally by the external geniculate body, the anterior corpus quadrigeminum and the optic thalamus. From here they go on to the oculomotor nucleus and to the cortex.

The chiasmal portion of the optic nerve is commonly affected in tumors occurring in this region. It lies here in an oblique position over the pituitary fossa behind and above the optic groove of the sphenoid bone. In most instances it has been known to lie over the fossa so that a part of the latter is seen in front of it.

The Crystalline Lens

Within the eyeball itself is the crystalline lens which is located between the iris and the vitreous. It is a transparent elastic body measuring about 8 to 9 mm. in its lateral diameter and about 5 mm. in its anteroposterior diameter. It has an anterior and a posterior curved surface giving it the shape of a double convex body. Because of its structure, the lens is capable of changing its shape by increasing and decreasing its convexity, and therefore its anterior and posterior diameter, during the act of accommodation of the eye. In this way it enables the eye of young people to see clearly for distant and near objects. This plasticity or ability of the lens to increase its convexity in accommodation decreases with oncoming age and hardening, so that the eye of the average individual is reduced to the stage of presbyopia at the age of about forty-five years.

The pupil is just in front and at the center of the anterior aspect of the lens, while the posterior surface of the iris rests upon the lens capsule. The posterior chamber and ciliary processes are also just in front of the anterior surface. Adjacent to the ciliary processes is the equator of the lens which is a rough border receiving the zonular fibers.

The posterior surface of the lens is considered by some to rest in a slight excavation in the hyaloid membrane in front of the vitreous.

Enveloping the lens itself is the transparent elastic and homogenous membrane known as the capsule of the lens. The anterior capsule is somewhat thicker than the posterior portion. The capsule is also somewhat thicker where it joins the zonular fibers. Rupture of this capsule because of trauma or injury results in opacity of the lens structure and escape of the lens substance into the anterior chamber.

The anterior capsule is covered by a single layer of cells which comprises the epithelium of the lens. These anterior epithelial cells become arranged in rows at the equator, after which they become elongated and are changed into lens fibers. These fibers are arranged in the form of lamellated radiations so that opacities occurring in the lens in most cases also appear to be striated or radiating in their appearance.

The lens fibers are held closely together by a cement-like or amorphous substance. They consist of long six-sided prismatic fibers and radiate from the anterior to the posterior pole of the lens. At the posterior pole they form a stellate figure in the shape of a ''Y'' which can often be seen in the normal eye under the proper illumination.

The nucleus or central portion of the lens is somewhat harder than the cortex, which is the outer portion of the lens. In early age the entire lens is soft, becoming harder with oncoming age. The color of the lens also changes somewhat from youth to older age, taking on a dark yellowish tinge as time

goes on. With oncoming cataract, the nucleus becomes sclerosed in many instances and the entire lens loses its plasticity.

The suspensory ligament of the lens is known as the zonule of Zinn which
is made up of a number of fine homogeneous fibers which originate on the inner
surface of the ciliary body, whence they leave at the apices of the ciliary processes
and are suspended over the edge of the lens. Some go to the equator, while
others go both anteriorly and posteriorly to attach themselves to the lens capsule.
A cross section of that portion between the fibers and equator of the lens would
reveal a triangular space which is connected with the posterior chamber and is
known as the canal of Petit.

The Vitreous

The posterior cavity of the eyeball behind the lens is occupied by a
gelatinous mass, which is colorless and transparent and is known as the vitreous.
In front it is said to contain a slight excavation for the reception of the posterior
surface of the lens. This is known as the fossa patellaris. On its sides the
vitreous is in apposition with the ciliary body and the retina. It is not, however, directly adherent to the retina itself. The vitreous contains no blood vessels, but the hyaloid canal, which contains the hyaloid artery in the fetus, sometimes runs through its center from the fossa patellaris anteriorly to the front of
the nerve head posteriorly. This canal or remnant of hyaloid can often be seen,
when present, on examination with the ophthalmoscope.

The Structure of the Orbit

The orbit is a bony cavity whose shape is that of a quadrilateral pyramid
with its base forward at the anterior aperture and the apex posteriorly at the
optic foramen. The inner walls of the two orbits are almost parallel to each
other, but the temporal walls diverge from each other and become further
separated as they come forward.

The roof of the orbit is formed in front by the orbital plate of the frontal
bone and behind by the lesser wing of the sphenoid. It has a somewhat triangular shape and is concave anteriorly. It contains a fossa for the lacrimal gland
which is located behind the external angle of the frontal bone. It also contains
a small depression for the pulley of the superior oblique muscle which is close
to the internal angle. The orbital roof is thin and can easily be fractured as a
result of direct traumatism. It sometimes contains ethmoidal cells and a portion
of the frontal sinus, which runs from the external angle back to the optic
foramen. Just above the roof are the meninges of the frontal lobe of the brain
and the frontal nerve is in contact with the periorbita. The levator palpebrae is
below the nerve and below this is the superior rectus. The supraorbital artery
extends along its anterior portion. The supraorbital or sphenoidal fissure is
located between the roof and lateral wall of the orbit, formed by the lesser
and greater wing of the sphenoid. It is the largest communication between
the orbit and the middle cranial fossa. Passing through the sphenoidal fissure
are the superior and inferior divisions of the third nerve, the nasociliary nerve,
and the sixth nerve.

The nasal or inner wall of the orbit is somewhat rough and is made up from
anterior to posterior by the frontal process of the superior maxillary, the
lacrimal bone, the os planum of the ethmoid and a small portion of the sphenoid.

This is the thinnest wall of the orbit and since the greater portion of it is made up by the os planum or lamina papyracea (paper plate), it can be easily seen why orbital infections are commonly caused by an ethmoiditis. The internal rectus muscle extends along this inner wall, while the superior oblique is in the angle between it and the roof. The nasociliary nerve and termination of the ophthalmic artery are between these two muscles. The lacrimal sac with its fascia lies just anterior to the nasal wall. The attachment of Horner's muscle, the septum orbitale and the check ligament of the internal rectus muscle are just behind this wall.

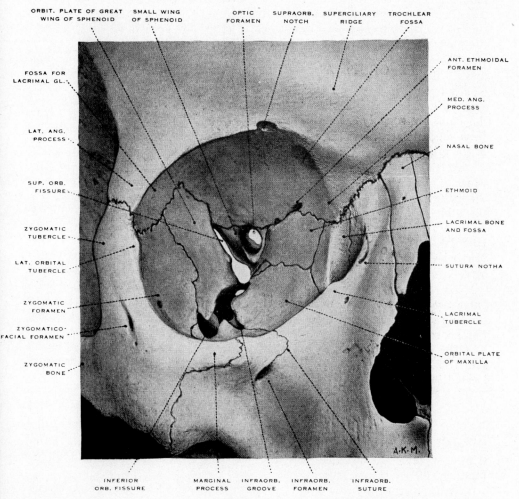

ORBIT. PLATE OF GREAT WING OF SPHENOID   SMALL WING OF SPHENOID   OPTIC FORAMEN   SUPRAORB. NOTCH   SUPERCILIARY RIDGE   TROCHLEAR FOSSA

FOSSA FOR LACRIMAL GL.

ANT. ETHMOIDAL FORAMEN

MED. ANG. PROCESS

LAT. ANG. PROCESS

NASAL BONE

SUP. ORB. FISSURE

ETHMOID

ZYGOMATIC TUBERCLE

LACRIMAL BONE AND FOSSA

LAT. ORBITAL TUBERCLE

SUTURA NOTHA

ZYGOMATIC FORAMEN

ZYGOMATICO-FACIAL FORAMEN

LACRIMAL TUBERCLE

ZYGOMATIC BONE

ORBITAL PLATE OF MAXILLA

INFERIOR ORB. FISSURE   MARGINAL PROCESS   INFRAORB. GROOVE   INFRAORB. FORAMEN   INFRAORB. SUTURE

Fig. 6.—The orbit from in front. (From Wolff: The Anatomy of the Eye and Orbit, The Blakiston Co.)

The floor of the orbit is somewhat triangular in shape and similar to that of the roof. It is formed by the orbital plate of the superior maxillary bone, which comprises its major portion, the malar bone and the orbital surface of the palatal bone.

The antrum of Highmore is just inferior to the floor of the orbit and is separated from it by a very thin layer of bone; as a result large growths in the antrum may protrude through the floor into the orbit and cause displacement of the eyeball. Infection from the ethmoid may also extend through the floor posteriorly into the orbit. At the apex, the inferior rectus lies in contact posteriorly, but is separated from it anteriorly by the inferior oblique. The latter muscle extends outward, upward and backward near the floor. In the infraorbital canal are found the infraorbital nerve and vessels. The inferior orbital fissure lies between the floor of the orbit and the external wall and forms a communication between the orbit and the sphenoid, maxillary, and the zygomatic fossa. It also conducts the second division of the fifth nerve, branches from the sphenopalatine ganglion, the zygomatic nerve, and a communication between the pterygoid plexus and the inferior ophthalmic vein.

The outer wall of the orbit resembles a triangle in shape with its base anterior. This is probably the strongest wall of the orbit and is formed principally by the orbital surface of the great wing of the sphenoid behind, and the zygomatic process of the malar bone in front. The most posterior portion of the outer wall is somewhat thinner and weaker where it separates the orbit from the temporal fossa. The external rectus muscle lies on the external wall in the orbit with the lacrimal nerve and artery above.

At the posterior or apex of the orbit is the optic foramen or optic canal which is formed by two roots of the lesser wing of the sphenoid. It is cone shaped, with the small circle of the cone posterior, and extends from the apex of the orbit to the middle cranial fossa. It transmits the optic nerve with the dura, arachnoid, and pial coverings, the ophthalmic artery lying below and lateral to the nerve, and a few branches from the sympathetic. It is in close proximity on its medial surface to the sphenoidal air sinus and sometimes to a posterior ethmoidal air cell from which it is separated by a thin plate of bone.

The superior margin of the orbit is prominent and at the junction of its outer two-thirds with its inner third is the supraorbital notch which transmits the supraorbital nerve. This margin overhangs the eyeball and acts as a protection above.

The inferior margin of the eyeball is not prominent, but is covered by the skin from the lower lid which serves to conceal it. The infraorbital foramen is located just at its inner third and about 4 mm. below the margin.

The Extraocular Muscles

The extrinsic muscles of the eye are the external muscles which control the position and movement of the eyeball and are distinguished from the intrinsic or internal unstriped muscles composed of the sphincter and dilator pupillae and the ciliary muscle.

There are six extrinsic muscles, sometimes described as three pairs, in each eye. These are the superior and inferior recti muscles, the external and internal (medial) recti, and the superior and inferior oblique muscles.

The superior and inferior recti, together with the external and medial recti, all arise at the apex of the orbit from around the rim of the optic foramen. Their directions are divergent as they extend forward and as a result they form a muscular conelike space which has its small opening or circumference behind at the optic foramen, while the larger circle at the base is formed anteriorly by the eyeball. The longest of the extrinsic muscles is the superior rectus, the shortest is the inferior rectus; the medial rectus is longer than the external. The superior and medial recti are closely attached behind to the sheath of the optic nerve. Because of this fact, movements of the eyeball are sometimes accompanied by pain in inflammatory conditions of the nerve.

The recti muscles all follow the wall of the orbit in a course forward to be inserted by their tendons into the sclera. Each one has its point of insertion at a different distance from the cornea.

THE SUPERIOR RECTUS MUSCLE

The superior rectus muscle, which has its origin from the sheath of the optic nerve just above and outside the optic foramen, is inserted into the sclera by the widest tendon (10.8 mm.), at a point 7.7 mm. from the cornea. It is separated from the roof of the orbit by the levator muscle and the frontal nerve, which are in relation with it above. It is separated below by orbital fat from the optic nerve behind, and the ophthalmic artery. The reflected tendon of the superior oblique muscle, in reaching its point of insertion anteriorly, passes between the superior rectus and the globe. The ophthalmic artery and nasal nerve are also found internally between the superior rectus and the internal rectus and superior oblique. The lacrimal artery and nerve are located externally between the superior rectus and the external rectus muscles.

The action of the superior rectus muscle is to draw the eye upward and inward, while at the same time it rotates the eye inward on its anteroposterior axis. It also has an auxiliary action in assisting the levator to elevate the upper eyelid. The nerve supply of the superior rectus comes from the superior division of the third cranial or oculomotor nerve.

THE INFERIOR RECTUS MUSCLE

The inferior rectus muscle arises from just below the optic foramen behind and passes forward and slightly outward to be inserted into the sclera by a tendon about 5.5 mm. long and 9.8 mm. wide at the point of insertion, which is located about 6.5 mm. from the cornea. By an expansion of its sheath to the lower lid, it forms an attachment with the latter. Its action is to make the eye look down and in, while at the same time it rotates the eye outward on its anteroposterior axis. The nerve supply is from the inferior division of the oculomotor. The latter lies above the muscle and it is also separated from the optic nerve above and behind by orbital fat. In front of its external border is the nerve to the inferior oblique. The floor of the orbit is just below the muscle, which is in contact behind with the orbital portion of the palate bone and in front with the superior maxillary from which it is separated by orbital fat. Below the muscle is also found the canal containing the infraorbital vessels and nerve. Its sheath becomes united with that of the inferior oblique which also crosses it below.

THE INTERNAL OR MEDIAL RECTUS MUSCLE

The internal or medial rectus muscle is one of the strongest of the extraocular muscles and arises from the inner and inferior margin of the optic foramen, and from the optic sheath. After following a forward course along the inner wall of the orbit, it is inserted into the sclera 5.5 mm. from the cornea.

The action of the internal rectus is to turn the eye inward in the act of adduction which is performed by the two internal recti muscles acting together. It lies below the superior oblique muscle with the ophthalmic artery and the nasal nerve lying between the two. The floor of the orbit lies below while on the inner side is orbital fat separating it from the lamina papyracea of the ethmoid bone, and on its outer side it is bordered by orbital fat. It is supplied by the inferior division of the third or oculomotor nerve.

THE EXTERNAL RECTUS MUSCLE

The external rectus muscle has its origin by two heads, which are curved and attached around the sphenoidal fissure. It follows a course anteriorly along the outer wall of the orbit to be inserted into the sclera at a point 6.9 mm. from the cornea. At its point of origin the muscle is in close proximity to the upper and lower divisions of the third nerve, nasociliary nerve, the sixth nerve and a branch from the sympathetic nerve. The fourth nerve, frontal nerve and lacrimal nerves together with the recurrent lacrimal artery and superior ophthalmic vein are found above the origin of the muscle. More anteriorly along the course of the external rectus are found the lacrimal artery and nerve, while anterior and above is the lacrimal gland. The floor of the orbit and the tendon of the inferior oblique in front lie below the muscle. The ciliary ganglion and ophthalmic artery lie between the external rectus and the optic nerve in the posterior part of the orbit on the inner wall. The external rectus is supplied by the sixth cranial or the abducens nerve.

THE SUPERIOR OBLIQUE MUSCLE

The superior oblique muscle is somewhat peculiar, in that it is very long and thin and follows a changing course and shape. Its tendon at the point of origin is narrow and comes from the upper and inner border of the optic foramen. The narrow, round muscle then goes forward along the upper and inner angle of the orbit to a point on the under surface of the frontal bone a few millimeters behind the orbit margin. Here it passes through what is called a pulley which is formed by fibrous tissue, encircling it and attached to the bone. On passing through this pulley, the muscle changes its shape and course, turning almost sharply downward, outward and backward. It passes through the capsule of Tenon and under the superior rectus muscle. On the outer side of the eye it becomes fan shaped and attached in an oblique line in the upper posterior quadrant. Because of the nature of its insertion, it acts to draw the eyeball downward, in spite of the fact that most of the belly of the muscle lies superior. In depressing the eyeball it causes it at the same time to rotate inward on its anteroposterior axis. In causing the eyeball to look downward, it acts in this respect in association with the inferior rectus muscle.

The superior oblique muscle is separated from the upper and inner wall of the orbit by a layer of orbital fat. The internal rectus muscle lies below it and the ophthalmic artery and the nasal nerve are found between them. It is innervated by the fourth cranial or trochlear nerve.

THE INFERIOR OBLIQUE MUSCLE

The inferior oblique muscle is also peculiar in that it arises from the front part of the orbit. Its tendon is round and comes from a point on the orbital portion of the superior maxilla just external to the opening of the nasolacrimal duct. In passing backward it makes a sharp curve between the floor of the orbit and the inferior rectus, after which it passes upward, under the external rectus and is inserted below the horizontal plane of the eyeball, into the posterior and outer portion. In spite of the fact that it originates below the eyeball, the nature of its insertion causes the eye to look upward while at the same time it rotates the anteroposterior axis outward. In elevating the eye, its action takes place in conjunction with the similar action of the superior rectus muscle.

The nerve supply of the inferior oblique comes from the inferior division of the third or oculomotor nerve.

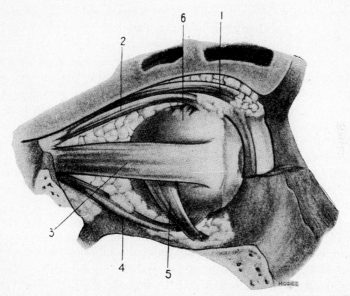

Fig. 7.—The extrinsic muscles of the eye. *1*, Levator palpebrae superioris. *2*, Superior rectus. *3*, Lateral rectus. *4*, Inferior rectus. *5*, Inferior oblique. *6*, Superior oblique. (From Duke-Elder: Text-Book of Ophthalmology.)

The Capsule of Tenon

The capsule of Tenon is a thin fascia which surrounds the eyeball, through which the tendons of the extraocular muscles must pass before they are inserted into the sclera. This passage is accomplished by an enveloping of the tendon, or a reflection of the capsule over the tendon. In this way they are connected or adherent to Tenon's capsule. From this connection of the muscles with the capsule, prolongations or expansions are also sent to the various parts of the bony orbit. As a result, the eyeball is held in place and the actions of the muscles are limited. In other words, these continuations of the fascia serve as check ligaments. The prolongation from the superior rectus muscle goes to the levator palpebrae, and as a result the upper eyelid is elevated whenever the eyeball is elevated by the action of the superior rectus.

A similar action takes place with the lower eyelid, which is lowered when the inferior rectus muscle acts to depress the eyeball, because prolongations of fascia connect the under surface of the inferior rectus with the tarsal plate and the orbicularis.

In exposing the muscles to view, it is necessary to incise and separate Tenon's capsule anteriorly. It envelops the eyeball from the cornea anteriorly to the optic nerve posteriorly.

It can be seen from the action of these individual muscles that movement of the eyeballs in a vertical axis is accomplished principally by the superior and inferior recti. Since the action of these muscles, however, is supplemented by the action of the two obliques, *straight upward rotation* would be produced by the combined action of the superior rectus and inferior oblique, the outward rotation of the latter overcoming the slight inward rotation caused by the superior rectus.

In *looking straight down,* the movement is produced by the combined action of the inferior rectus and superior oblique, since the outward action of the latter overcomes the inward rotation of the former.

When the eye is turned out, the recti muscles are concerned in raising and lowering the eyeball, whereas the obliques are concerned in upward and downward rotation when the eye is turned in.

Adduction or movement of the eyes inward is accomplished principally by the action of the internal recti muscles, but on extreme adduction the superior and inferior recti are also concerned.

Abduction or outward rotation of the eyes is produced principally by the external recti muscles which may also be affected by the oblique muscles. Straight outward rotation, however, is produced by the external rectus while rotation straight inward is produced by the internal rectus.

Upward and inward rotation of the eyeball is produced principally by the action of the superior rectus, internal rectus and inferior oblique. The inferior oblique controls the internal action of the superior rectus.

Upward and outward rotation of the eyeball is produced by the action of the superior rectus, external rectus and the inferior oblique. In this movement of the eyeball, the inferior oblique acts as a control over the inward rotation of the superior rectus.

Downward and inward rotation of the eyeball is produced by the combined actions of the inferior rectus, internal rectus, and the superior oblique.

Downward and outward rotation of the eyeball is produced by the combined actions of the inferior rectus, external rectus, and superior oblique. The outward rotation produced by the superior oblique overcomes the inward rotary action of the inferior rectus muscle.

In studying the movements of the eyeball it is necessary to remember that: In looking up and out the upper half of the vertical axis of the eyeball is turned outward, whereas in looking up and in, it is turned inward toward the nose. In looking down and out, the lower part of the vertical axis of the eyeball is directed outward while in looking down and in, it is directed inward toward the nose. The actions of the superior and inferior oblique muscles should not be confused because of the way they are named. The superior oblique acts to draw the eyeball downward while the action of the inferior oblique is to raise the eyeball upward. However, the superior and inferior recti are also concerned in raising and lowering the eyeball, respectively, but in looking up and out the inferior oblique is mostly concerned, while in looking up and in, the superior rectus is principally concerned. Likewise, in looking down and out, the principal action is that of the superior oblique, while in looking down and in the principal action is that of the inferior rectus.

The movements of the two eyes normally function as one because of the association in corresponding action between the muscles of the two eyes. Where a muscle of one eye has a definite action in producing a certain movement of the eye, there is an antagonistic muscle in the opposite eye whose action produces the opposite result in that eye. At the same time the corresponding muscle of the opposite eye is stimulated to the same action as that of its fellow in the first eye, which results in the associated movements of the two eyes.

Therefore, the two eyes are turned upward while the visual axes are parallel, by two sets of muscles which produce this movement in the two eyes simultaneously, and in the same way they are turned down by the simultaneous action of two sets of depressor muscles.

The lateral movements with visual axes parallel are produced by the simultaneous action of the right internal rectus and left external rectus in turning the eyes both to the left, while the simultaneous action of the left internal rectus and right external rectus turn the eyes both to the right.

Internal rotation of both eyes together results in the act of convergence, the position of the eyes necessary in near work. This movement is produced by the joint action of the internal rectus of each eye.

The Motor Nerves of the Orbit

The motor nerves of the orbit consist of the third or oculomotor, the fourth or trochlear nerve, and the sixth or abducens nerve. Together they supply all the extrinsic muscles of the eye and the levator palpebrae superioris.

THE THIRD OR OCULOMOTOR NERVE

The third or oculomotor nerve is a large nerve most of whose fibers are motor. Its nucleus is in the floor of the aqueduct of Sylvius below the superior corpus quadrigeminum. The nerve arises principally from the oculomotor sulcus on the inner side of the cerebral peduncle. It also has a small portion which arises from the front part of the crus cerebri. It is here in close relationship to the posterior cerebral artery and its posterior portion is close to the upper margin of the pons.

Its intracranial portion is surrounded by pia and follows a downward and forward course in close relationship to the posterior cerebral and superior cerebellar arteries. Between the free and attached margins of the tentorium cerebelli, it pierces the dura lateral to the posterior clinoid process of the sphenoid bone and enters the cavernous sinus on its lateral wall. Here it receives communications from the first division of the fifth and the sympathetic. The first and second divisions of the fifth, as well as the fourth nerve, sixth nerve and internal carotid artery lie in close relationship. It enters the orbit through the superior orbital fissure and annulus of Zinn and divides into two divisions, the superior or smaller division and inferior or larger division. The superior division passes upward over the optic nerve and supplies the superior rectus and the levator palpebral superioris. The inferior division supplies the internal rectus, the inferior rectus, and the inferior oblique after passing under the optic nerve. It also sends a short branch to the ciliary ganglion which supplies the sphincter pupillae and the ciliary muscle.

It can be seen from the above that all the extrinsic muscles of the eye with the exception of the external rectus and superior oblique are supplied by the oculomotor nerve. In addition it also supplies the sphincter pupillae and the ciliary muscle. The superior rectus and levator palpebrae superioris are supplied by the superior branch while the internal rectus, inferior rectus, inferior oblique and the ciliary ganglion are supplied by the inferior branch.

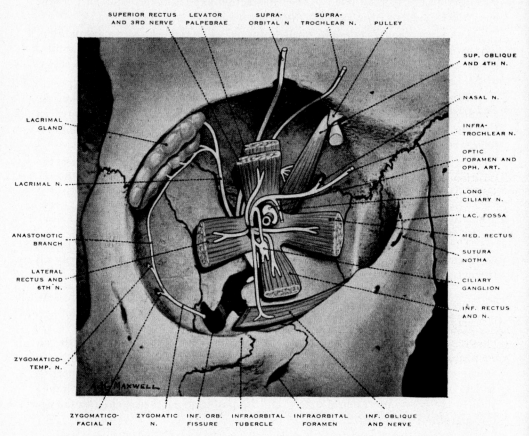

Fig. 8.—The orbital nerves from in front. (From Wolff: The Anatomy of the Eye and Orbit, The Blakiston Co.)

Paralysis of the oculomotor nerve may be total or partial and results in restriction of movement of the structures supplied. In total paralysis all branches of the third nerve will be affected with the result that there will be a complete ptosis of the upper lid on the affected side. All of the extraocular muscles except the external rectus and the superior oblique will be paralyzed. The eye will therefore be drawn strongly outward and slightly downward.

The pupil will be dilated and fixed because of a paralysis of the sphincter pupillae. The ciliary muscle will also be found to be paralyzed, with inability of the eye to accommodate for near objects. Printed matter will appear blurred when an attempt is made to read. Because of the paralysis, the affected muscles lose their tone and fail to retract the eyeball back into the orbit, so that a slight degree of proptosis may be present.

When the sphincter of the iris and ciliary muscle alone is paralyzed as a result of paralysis of the third nerve, the condition is a partial paralysis and is seen in tabes, cerebral syphilis and paresis. This is known as ophthalmoplegia interna. A partial paralysis of the third nerve may also affect only the extra-ocular muscles.

Since the third nerve in its course is in close relationship to the posterior cerebral, superior cerebellar, internal carotid and basilar arteries, aneurysm of any of these may cause pressure on the nerve.

THE TROCHLEAR OR FOURTH NERVE

The trochlear (fourth cranial nerve) supplies the superior oblique muscle. The nucleus is posterior to the third nerve nucleus and is a continuation of the base of the anterior horn of the spinal column. From the posterior aspect of the cerebral peduncle, the fibers pass downward and pass out in the superior medullary velum. In the posterior cranial fossa the nerve lies between the superior cerebellar peduncle and the cerebral peduncle. At the upper border of the pons it runs forward between the posterior cerebral and superior cerebellar arteries. Behind the third nerve and the posterior clinoid process it passes through the dura below the free margin of the tentorium cerebelli. It lies in the cavernous sinus along the lateral wall. The fourth nerve enters the orbit through the sphenoidal fissure, crosses the superior rectus to supply the superior oblique muscle.

When the fourth nerve is paralyzed, it results in an impairment in the action of the superior oblique muscle. The eye on the affected side is therefore found to be limited principally in downward and outward rotation. Moreover, the patient has diplopia when the eyes are rotated in downward rotation.

THE ABDUCENS OR SIXTH CRANIAL NERVE

The sixth cranial nerve supplies the external rectus muscle. Its nucleus lies close to the midline of the pons under the floor of the fourth ventricle. It runs along the whole length of the pons with some fibers passing through the pyramid.

After following a course upward, forward and outward in the posterior cranial fossa, the nerve passes through the dura opposite the dorsum sella of the sphenoid. It then crosses the inferior petrosal sinus and passes vertically behind the apex of the petrous portion of the temporal bone where it bends forward at an acute angle in a groove between the apex and the posterior clinoid processes. On entering the cavernous sinus it is in association with the internal carotid artery. The third, fourth, and first and second divisions of the fifth nerve are found in the lateral wall of the sinus. The abducens enters the orbit through the sphenoidal fissure within the annulus of Zinn. It then passes on to enter the external rectus muscle.

Any lesion of the sixth nerve results in impairment of function of the external rectus muscle. This is characterized by limitation of outward rotation of the eyeball on the affected side. A common site for injury to the sixth nerve is at the apex of the petrous portion of the temporal bone. At this point it makes almost a right angle turn in its course. Any swelling of the apex of the bone here or fracture of the skull may result in pressure on the nerve at this point. Gradenigo's syndrome is a paralysis of the sixth nerve at the tip of the petrous portion of the temporal bone, which occurs in purulent middle ear disease. It is usually accompanied by pain in the face on the affected side.

Abducens paralysis may also occur as a congenital condition and also in some infectious diseases, syphilis, and diabetes.

The Sensory Nerves of the Orbit

THE TRIGEMINAL OR FIFTH NERVE

The trigeminal or fifth nerve has two portions, being composed of a sensory root and a motor root which arise above the middle of the pons. The sensory ganglion of the fifth nerve is known as the semilunar or Gasserian ganglion. It is a crescent-shaped structure which lies in a fossa near the tip of the petrous portion of the temporal bone between the two layers of dura. The middle meningeal artery passes through the foramen spinosum on the outer side of the ganglion. The third, fourth and sixth nerves, internal carotid artery and cavernous sinus are located on the inner side.

The fifth nerve gives off three branches or divisions as follows:

1. The first or ophthalmic nerve
2. The second or maxillary nerve
3. The third or mandibular nerve

The ophthalmic nerve divides into three branches just before entering the orbit through the superior orbital fissure. These branches are the lacrimal, frontal and nasociliary nerves. The lacrimal nerve after entering the orbit passes along the lateral wall together with the lacrimal artery to reach the lacrimal gland. Here it supplies fibers to the gland itself and also sends branches to anastomose with the zygomatic nerve. It also sends branches to the skin and conjunctiva of the upper and lower eyelids.

The frontal nerve enters the orbit through the sphenoidal fissure after arising from the ophthalmic in the cavernous sinus. In the middle of the orbit it divides into the supraorbital and the supratrochlear branches. The supraorbital branch leaves the orbit by way of the supraorbital notch or foramen, accompanied by the supraorbital artery. It passes up over the forehead and scalp to the occipital bone while sending small branches to the orbicularis and the frontal sinus. The supratrochlear nerve is smaller and passes out of the orbit near the trochlea where it sends a communication to the infratrochlear nerve. It supplies the skin of the lower forehead, and the conjunctiva and skin of the middle of the upper lid.

The nasociliary leaves the lateral wall of the cavernous sinus and passes through the superior orbital fissure in the annulus of Zinn to enter the orbit. After passing between the superior oblique and internal rectus muscles it leaves the orbit through the anterior ethmoidal foramen. It then sends branches to the anterior ethmoidal cells and the frontal sinus, after which it enters the anterior cranial fossa. From here it passes down through the nasal fissure at the side of the cribriform plate of the ethmoid to reach the nasal cavity. Here it supplies branches to the cavity of the nose, the septum and the skin of the lower part of the nose.

The branches given off by the nasociliary nerve are, (a) the long or sensory root of the ciliary ganglion. This passes along the outside of the optic nerve to the upper posterior portion of the ganglion. (b) The long ciliary nerves which are two in number and which go to the eyeball to supply the iris, cornea, ciliary muscle and dilator of the pupil with sensory fibers. (c) The infratrochlear nerve which communicates with the supratrochlear nerve and then supplies branches to the skin, conjunctiva, canaliculi, caruncle and the lacrimal sac. (d) A posterior ethmoidal nerve (Krause-Luschka) which is not always present. This enters the posterior ethmoidal foramen to supply the posterior ethmoidal and sphenoidal cells.

The maxillary nerve or second division of the fifth comes off from the Gasserian ganglion and passes through the foramen rotundum from the middle cranial fossa. It enters the orbit through the inferior orbital fissure where it is known as the infraorbital nerve. Passing through the infraorbital foramen it divides into the inferior palpebral, nasal and labial branches which supply the same areas of the skin. The maxillary also gives off anterior and posterior superior alveolar or dental branches as well as several sphenopalatine branches to the sphenopalatine or Meckel's ganglion. A zygomatic branch or temporomalar nerve enters into the orbit through the inferior orbital fissure and divides into two branches after communicating with the lacrimal nerve. These are the zygomatic-temporal branch which passes through the canal in the zygomatic bone to go to the skin on the side of the forehead and the zygomatic-facial branch which goes to the skin of the cheek after passing through the zygomatic canal. These two branches communicate with the facial nerve.

The mandibular nerve or third division of the fifth consists of two portions: the sensory root, which arises from the Gasserian ganglion, and the motor portion, which is the motor part of the trigeminal. Since this nerve has very little application here, further discussion will not be necessary. The two ganglia already mentioned in connection with the orbital nerves will require some brief consideration. These are: (1) the ciliary ganglion, (2) the sphenopalatine ganglion.

The ciliary ganglion consists of a small flat body the size of a pinhead and located in loose, fatty tissue at the apex of the orbit between the optic nerve and the external rectus muscle in front of the annulus of Zinn. Its two principal types of cells are multipolar cells which comprise the greatest number and are ganglion cells of the autonomic system. The other type is bipolar cells of the sensory cerebrospinal variety. The ganglion acts as a center for the sensory and autonomic nerve control of the eye and is supplied by a motor, sensory and sympathetic route. The motor portion comes from the branch of the third nerve to the inferior oblique and contains the fibers of a parasympathetic variety which go to the sphincter of the iris and the ciliary muscle. The sensory portion comes from the nasociliary branch of the ophthalmic division of the trigeminal and sends sensory fibers to the cornea, iris and ciliary body. The sympathetic comes from the sympathetic plexus in the cavernous sinus and may be present alone or together with the sensory portion. It sends vasomotor fibers to the eyeball.

The short ciliary nerves are six to eight in number branching from the anterior pole of the ganglion. These divide into twelve to twenty short ciliary nerves which run above and below the optic nerve and go through the sclera where the optic nerve leaves the globe. They send sensory motor and sympathetic fibers to the eyeball. The nerve of Tiedemann also comes off from the short ciliary nerves and goes to the retina with the central artery.

The ciliary ganglion is not always constant and may be entirely absent or there may be several accessory ganglia. Further, certain roots may be absent or multiple.

The sphenopalatine or Meckel's ganglion is a small triangular-shaped body with a motor, sensory and sympathetic root, located in the upper part of the pterygopalatine fossa, close to the sphenopalatine foramen. The motor root comes from the geniculate ganglion of the facial nerve through the great superficial petrosal nerve. The sensory consists of twigs coming from the sphenopalatine branches of the maxillary nerve. The sympathetic comes from the carotid plexus by way of the deep petrosal nerve. The two petrosal nerves join in the foramen lacerum to form the Vidian nerve, and the latter enters the ganglion as a motor and sympathetic root. The cells of the ganglion are considered to belong to the autonomic variety and its functions to the involuntary system which is concerned with the supply of smooth muscles, glands and vasomotor functions.

It sends branches to the orbital periosteum, muscle of Müller, the ciliary ganglion, sheath of the optic nerve, lacrimal gland, sphenoidal sinus and posterior ethmoidal cells.

The Facial or Seventh Nerve

The nucleus of the seventh nerve is located in the pons. Fibers run back and then upward inside the sixth nerve nucleus to the floor of the fourth ventricle. They bend around the sixth nerve nucleus and pass along inside the spinal root of the fifth, leaving the brain lateral to the sixth nerve. It leaves the skull through the stylomastoid foramen and gives off a number of branches. The temporal branches supply the orbicularis muscle. This nerve is sometimes involved in association with affections of the sixth nerve.

Blood Vessels of the Orbit

The arteries of the orbit come principally from the ophthalmic artery which is derived from the internal carotid.

The ophthalmic artery comes off from the carotid where the latter leaves the cavernous sinus. It follows a rather tortuous course forward and outward under the optic nerve and then goes to the inner side of the nerve as it approaches the optic foramen. Here it pierces the sheath of the nerve and enters the orbit where it is found in the muscle cone in company with the ciliary ganglion, the external rectus and the optic nerve. It passes above the nerve under the superior rectus muscle with the nasociliary nerve to the inner wall of the orbit.

Then after running forward between the superior oblique and internal rectus, to the upper, inner angle, it divides into two terminal branches, a nasal and frontal artery.

The branches of the ophthalmic artery are as follows:

1. The central artery of the retina which is a small branch given off near the optic foramen and pierces the optic nerve about 10 mm. behind the globe. It is covered by pia and approaches the lamina cribrosa where it enters the globe. It sends small branches to the nerve fiber layer of the retina.

2. The lacrimal artery which arises from the ophthalmic artery close to the optic foramen and lateral to the optic nerve. It proceeds forward along the lateral wall of the orbit and at the upper margin of the external rectus muscle to the lacrimal gland. After passing through the latter it gives off several branches which supply the upper and lower eyelids principally. It also gives off a recurrent meningeal branch which passes back out of the orbit through the superior orbital fissure.

3. Muscular branches which include two main trunks, one to supply the superior rectus, the levator palpebrae, and the superior oblique, and the other to the inferior rectus, internal rectus and the inferior oblique. These muscular branches also give off the anterior ciliary arteries which run along the tendons to the eyeball and anastomose finally with the long posterior ciliaries at the anterior part of the ciliary body.

4. The posterior ciliary arteries which arise as two trunks and divide into twelve to fifteen branches. These pierce the sclera around the optic nerve and one group known as the short posterior ciliary arteries is distributed to the choroid for the uveal tract. The other group is composed of two branches known as the long posterior ciliary artery which goes forward to the ciliary body where they anastomose with the anterior ciliary arteries and form the plexus of arteries supplying the iris as described previously.

5. The supraorbital artery which leaves the ophthalmic artery after it has crossed the optic nerve and goes forward to the inner side of the superior rectus and then under the roof of the orbit. Together with the supraorbital nerve it passes through the supraorbital foramen and up under the frontalis to the scalp. It supplies the superior rectus, the levator, upper eyelid, periorbital and diploe of the roof of the orbit.

6. The posterior ethmoidal artery is a small artery which passes through the posterior ethmoidal foramen after supplying the mucous membrane of the posterior ethmoidal cells.

7. The anterior ethmoidal artery branches from the ophthalmic between the internal rectus and superior oblique and passes through the superior orbital fissure.

8. Medial palpebral branches which are the superior and inferior and supply the upper and lower eyelids and send small branches to the lacrimal sac.

9. An anterior meningeal artery which is a small branch passing out into the anterior cranial fossa.

10. The frontal artery which is a terminal branch of the ophthalmic and leaves the orbit by going through the septum orbitali at the upper inner angle together with the supratrochlear nerve. It supplies the inner part of the forehead and scalp.

11. The nasal artery which is the other terminal branch and leaves the orbit through the septum orbitali above the medial palpebral ligament. It unites with the angular artery and the terminal branches of the facial artery. It supplies the lacrimal sac and the skin around the upper part of the nose.

The Veins of the Orbit

The veins of the orbit and their tributaries form three principal drainage systems: one formed by the superior and inferior ophthalmic veins which drain into the cavernous sinus; another formed by anastomoses between the ophthalmic veins with the angular vein and veins of the face and nose; a third, with the pterygoid plexus.

The Superior Ophthalmic Vein

The superior ophthalmic vein is formed by the junction of the supraorbital vein and the angular veins of the face at the upper, inner angle of the orbit along the side of the nose. It runs backward with the ophthalmic artery and leaves the orbit through the superior orbital fissure to enter the cavernous sinus. The superior ophthalmic vein has many tributaries which correspond to the branches of the artery and they include large branches from the nose and the two superior venae vorticosae. Sometimes the latter joins the lacrimal veins first and enters the cavernous sinus separately.

The Inferior Ophthalmic Vein

The inferior ophthalmic vein is formed as a network on the floor of the orbit where it receives tributaries from the inferior rectus, inferior oblique, lacrimal sac and the two inferior venae vorticosae. It either joins with the superior ophthalmic vein to enter the cavernous sinus or it may do so alone. It also communicates with pterygoid and the facial vein. The pterygoid plexus which lies in the pterygoid fossae communicates with the cavernous sinus.

The angular vein is formed by the communication of the supraorbital and frontal veins, at the inner and upper angle of the orbit alongside the nose. It communicates with the superior ophthalmic and facial veins. It runs along the outside of the nose and crosses the medial palpebral ligament on the nasal side where it lies just under the skin and passes through the orbicularis.

The Central Retinal Vein

The central retinal vein may join the superior or inferior ophthalmic vein, or it may empty into the cavernous sinus alone. In either case it has been shown by Sesemann to send an anastomotic branch to the superior ophthalmic vein. This serves to maintain the venous flow to a certain extent and prevent pressure from stasis in cavernous sinus thrombosis.

The Cavernous Sinus

This is a venous sinus formed in the cranial cavity by a splitting of the dura on the side of the sphenoid bone at the superior orbital fissure and runs to the apex of the petrous portion of the temporal bone. It contains the carotid artery and the sixth nerve. The third, fourth, and two divisions of the fifth are also found in the lateral wall, while at the anterior end the fourth nerve crosses above the third. The Gasserian ganglion lies in contact with the lateral wall. It becomes confluent with the basilar sinus and also the superior and inferior petrosal sinuses. By means of the latter it leads into the transverse sinus and internal jugular vein. The two cavernous sinuses communicate by means of the anterior and posterior transverse sinuses. It communicates with the pterygoid and veins of the face by branches received through the foramen ovale, foramen lacerum, and the foramen rotundum. It empties into the jugular vein through the carotid canal.

Because of the anastomoses of the veins described, which drain into the cavernous sinus, the latter may become readily involved as the result of infections about the nose and face.

Reference

Wolff: The Anatomy of the Eye and Orbit, P. Blakiston's Son & Co., Philadelphia, 1936.

CHAPTER II

THE GENERAL CAUSES OF EYE MANIFESTATIONS

Before describing in detail the manifestations of internal diseases as they occur in the eye, it will probably be well to consider first, in general, some of the causes which can produce lesions in the ocular tissues, and also the manner in which these lesions occur.

The general causes might be considered in several different ways, but they will be enumerated here principally according to the nature of the etiologic factor. That is, according to the kind of agent or influence producing the ocular manifestation and whether the effect is produced on the eye alone, in simultaneous association with lesions elsewhere or following the manifestations in other organs of the body. In certain instances the eye might be the only organ affected by an injurious agent or influence, although other organs or parts could be affected either separately or primarily by the same causative factor. The ocular condition can therefore occur as either a primary or a secondary manifestation. In the latter instance, a primary source is located in some structure or organ of the body outside of the eye.

Although not occurring strictly within the scope of this text, there are also several external causes which should be briefly considered. These comprise certain physical agents and trauma arising outside of the body and which may affect the eye directly and often independently of other organs.

In many cases it is almost impossible to classify accurately the ocular condition according to a general cause and definitely to attribute certain manifestations to a particular one. In such instances it is occasionally found, for example, that a congenital malformation might be due either to a defect in embryologic development or to a possible intrauterine inflammation occurring before birth.

In some cases, the presence of a brain lesion or an intracranial tumor might produce eye manifestations because of either direct or indirect pressure on some part of the optic tract or visual pathway. Such a condition would be considered as a mechanical cause. Another illustration of the presence of an ocular condition due to a mechanical cause is seen in the exophthalmos produced by an overgrowth or thickening of the bones of the orbit occurring in Paget's disease.

Although there are a few instances where it is difficult to classify a condition accurately with regard to the manner of production, the principal causes of eye manifestations can be considered in general to include:

1. Congenital and hereditary causes
2. Infections and infectious diseases
3. Degenerations and diseases of other organs
4. Mechanical causes

Congenital and Hereditary Causes

CONGENITAL MALFORMATIONS

In this group may be included those factors which are present before birth, and which by their very nature constitute a defect which prevents the normal anatomic development of the organ. As a result, therefore, a malformation or an anomaly of some structure of the eye is found at the time of birth or shortly after. This can be illustrated by the presence of colobomas in the lids, iris, choroid or optic nerves.

Interstitial keratitis in a child is an example of an ocular condition caused by congenital syphilis. Some of the congenital anomalies, such as those affecting the choroid and macula, have been described as the result of inflammations and again as developmental defects resulting from other causes.

In some cases a malformation is produced by pressure of other structures on the eye in the course of its development in utero. Although mechanical in the nature of production, the influence is present before birth and may produce malformations of the lids, such as congenital ptosis, congenital malformations of the bones of the orbit with accompanying changes in the optic nerve, microphthalmos and anophthalmos. In the latter condition there may be present nothing more than a mere rudimentary eye or in other instances a slightly larger but still an underdeveloped eye. In a child with such an eye, the socket and orbit may also be found to be underdeveloped and this also fails to mature normally after birth because of failure of growth of the eyeball. The fissure of the eye may be narrowed in all its dimensions and as a result, some form of surgical correction is later necessary.

In another group of cases, the remains of fetal structures are found to be present in the eye after birth. Among these may be included: retained pupillary membranes, which usually occur as fine, dark and often hairlike strands extending across the pupil from one margin to the other. A persistent hyaloid membrane may be seen in the eye of an individual as the result of a failure of the membrane to regress with the disappearance of the artery itself before birth. Such a membrane can occasionally be seen with the ophthalmoscope to extend from the posterior surface of the lens back to the optic nerve head.

Hereditary and Familial Influences.—In some cases, the malformation which affects the ocular structure is part of a general impairment of the individual, and although it is the only sign of abnormality to be found at birth, the defects in other parts may become manifest during the period of growth. These conditions are the result of some basic impairment which prevents the normal development of the structures.

Albinism is another condition occurring in varying degrees as the result of probable lack of certain elements necessary for the normal development of the organ before birth.

Certain tumors of the eye are present at birth which develop and are recognized some time later. These may be due to malformations of development which might be recognized at the time of birth such as nevi and angiomas. Others are discovered somewhat later in life, although they are hereditary and familial in origin. These may also be accompanied by manifestations in other organs in addition to the manifestation present in the eye.

Certain weaknesses or tendencies to disease may be present in individuals as the result of heredity. Such inherited weakness may manifest itself in the eyes in the form of a predisposition to certain diseases as glaucoma, strabismus, myopia and also as a sensitivity in those suffering with spring catarrh and hay fever. Heredity is also considered to be a prominent factor in accounting for the presence in the eye of such diseases as retinitis pigmentosa and a form of congenital optic atrophy known as Leber's disease. In some instances, the defects are considered to be familial and may occur in more than one member of the same family and in succeeding generations of the family. Sometimes they are transmitted through the male and at other times through the female side of the family. Such defects occurring in the lens manifest themselves as opacities in the form of congenital cataracts. Many such cases are recorded in which the condition was present in different members of the same family and in various numbers of preceding generations of the family.

Ocular Allergy.—The importance of allergy as a factor in the causation of ocular conditions has increased enormously in recent years. There are many clinical conditions affecting the eyes which are today considered as allergic manifestations. Most persons in whom these occur are said to have an inherited allergic tendency or predisposition. The biochemical and physiologic condition of these individuals is in the proper state for development of a hypersensitivity to certain allergens when the eyes are exposed to the irritant either by direct contact or through systemic absorption.

These patients will usually give a history of other members of their immediate family being hypersensitive also. They are often subject to regular headaches, hay fever, asthma and other respiratory manifestations, vasomotor disturbances, evidences of instability of the autonomic nervous system, and an increased eosinophilia.

In a comprehensive review of the subject of *Allergies in Ophthalmology,* Lemoine[1] states that dysfunction of the suprarenal gland must also play an important part in the disturbed sodium-potassium-water balance and edema of the shock organ tissues in allergic manifestations. The anterior pituitary, thyroid, and gonads are also said to be involved. Other factors occasionally responsible are emotional strain, psychic disturbances, improper diet, and insufficient physical exercise.

Almost any of the ocular tissues may present allergic manifestations. In the eyelids, the skin may show allergic manifestations which are more marked than those found in any other of the cutaneous surfaces. One of the commonest symptoms complained of is itching of the lids. This is often accompanied by redness, burning, and puffiness. Various drugs and chemicals such as atropine, mercury, and eserine are often responsible. Certain cosmetic preparations such as nail polish, face powders, face and hand lotions, and eyelash and eyebrow dyes are also common causes. Another group of offenders includes feathers, cat fur, fur coats, horsehair and even spectacle frames in rare instances. Of course, foods and pollens should always be considered. In some of these cases, the only symptoms complained of may be a marked puffiness of the eyelids on one or both sides. In others, the irritation may be so severe as to present a marked dermatitis.

Allergy of the conjunctiva is often more marked. It is usually caused by the same agents and occurs often in association with the lid involvement. The conjunctival manifestations are usually (1) redness, chemosis of the bulbar conjunctiva, and sometimes hypertrophy of the follicles in the acute form;

(2) a form of chronic conjunctivitis; and (3) vernal conjunctivitis or vernal catarrh. Congestion, lacrimation, and photophobia are common symptoms. Photophobia is a prominent manifestation in a number of these cases, although this sensitivity is due mostly to light rather than to pollens or other irritants. I have seen patients with photophobia benefited greatly by the use of light absorptive lenses. In the chronic or even subacute forms of conjunctivitis, the redness of the lid margins and bulbar conjunctiva as well as the itching is often quite troublesome. The chronic cases usually recur regularly in the summer months for an indefinite period. There may be periods of remission with absence of the more annoying symptoms, but the itching and moderate redness of the lid margins are nearly always present. Many of these cases are associated with a rhinologic condition or moderate involvement of the sinuses producing a bacterial antigen. Others are due to pollens or air-borne plant and animal allergens, but very often more than one causative agent is present.

Vernal conjunctivitis or vernal catarrh is generally considered to be an allergic manifestation of the eyes (see page 109). The eyes are often found to be allergic to pollens which are most prevalent at the time the condition is active. Phlyctenular conjunctivitis is also regarded sometimes as an allergic manifestation.

The cornea is commonly considered to be sensitive to tuberculoprotein. This may be manifested by the presence of phlyctenular keratoconjunctivitis and phlyctenular keratitis. Bacterial toxins and foods are less commonly the causative agents in these cases. In cases of interstitial keratitis, which is an ocular manifestation of congenital syphilis, the corneal tissue has at times been said to be sensitized. Sometimes ulcers of the cornea are due to a sensitivity. Such ulcers may be superficial and vary in size, occurring even as small as pin points. They can be very troublesome, however. Keratoconjunctivitis is frequently caused also by contact with certain drugs, foods, and cosmetics.

A large number of cases of inflammation of the uveal tract, especially cases of uveitis and choroiditis, have been considered to be allergic in origin and due to toxins of the tubercle bacillus. The pigment of the uveal tract which is absorbed from an injured eye may produce an involvement of the other eye in the form of sympathetic ophthalmia because of an allergic reaction to the pigment.

Sensitivity to lens protein has been considered to occur in some patients with iritis and iridocyclitis of varying degree following cataract operations or traumatic rupture of the lens capsule. Positive skin reactions to lens protein have been demonstrated in these patients.

The retina and optic nerve have occasionally been said to reveal allergic manifestations in the form of retinitis, detachment of the retina, and optic neuritis, but such cases are probably very rare.

Infections

INFECTIOUS DISEASES

Under this heading are included principally those localized infections, inflammations and diseases of an infectious nature which act as a primary source of infection for the structures of the eye. Either the causative micro-organisms or their toxins reach the eye where they produce a secondary infection or inflammatory process.

In some of the acute infectious diseases, the eye becomes involved as the result of a metastatic inflammation which may be localized in any one or more of its structures. Paralysis of the extraocular muscles also may result from the presence of toxic conditions which act upon the ocular nerve concerned. Ocular palsies may occur as the result of a focus of infection elsewhere. Infective processes which are present in the nasal sinuses, teeth or tonsils may lead to metastatic inflammations in the eye and occasionally to extraocular muscle palsies. Ophthalmoplegia, either acute or subacute, may be the result of infective agents occurring in diphtheria, measles, septicemia, thyphus fever, influenza and other diseases of an infectious nature. Such inflammatory conditions in the eye are metastatic and endogenous in origin. Some of the metastatic inflammations affecting the eye may not occur for some time after the primary affection. Primary disease may be in a state of quiescence, but can still serve as the cause of an active inflammation in the eye. Syphilis and tuberculosis are responsible for occurrence of many ocular manifestations, but the patient may not be otherwise seriously affected by the disease.

Occasionally, the eye is the seat of the primary infection, in which case it is of ectogenous origin. The external structures comprising the eyelids, conjunctiva and cornea are directly exposed to infection and injury from outside the body. Moreover, such external physical causes as excessive heat, light, x-rays, ultraviolet, foreign bodies, and chemicals may produce severe injuries and inflammations when brought in contact with the eye. However, since these are not manifestations of any systemic disease they will receive only brief mention here. It will suffice to state that burns of the skin of the lids and burns of the cornea may be caused by exposure to excessive heat. Glass-blowers' cataract can be caused by excessive exposure to infrared rays. Prolonged exposure to very strong artificial light or direct sunlight may cause temporary scotomas or even more permanent interference with the vision due to inflammation of the retina. The latter condition has been known to occur in people who watched an eclipse of the sun without using smoked glasses. Marked congestion and irritation of the conjunctiva and even retinitis may result from prolonged exposure to the rays of a sun lamp without the use of goggles. The same condition may occur in the eyes of acetylene welders who are exposed directly to the rays produced by an acetylene torch. Infections may be caused in the interior of the eye by foreign bodies which have perforated one of the external structures.

The skin of the lids and the conjunctiva are commonly the seat of micro-organisms such as *Staphylococcus albus* and the *Bacillus xerosis,* either of which, under certain conditions, may be the cause of an inflammation.

Acute catarrhal conjunctivitis can be caused by the Koch-Weeks bacillus and the bacillus of Morax-Axenfeld. Conjunctivitis is also the result of infection by the Klebs-Löffler bacillus, the *Staphylococcus aureus, Micrococcus catarrhalis,* pneumococci and streptococci. The gonococcus may infect the eye either by contamination from an outside source, as a complication from infection in another part (endogenous), or as ophthalmia neonatorum in a newborn infant to whom it is transmitted from the vaginal discharge of the mother either before or at the time of its passage through the birth canal. Before birth, the infection would probably take place by passage through the membranes. The interior of the eyeball is infected only after perforation has taken place through the cornea. The cornea can be the seat of a primary process or it may be affected secondary to an inflammation of the conjunctiva, or from some other source.

Purulent Metastatic Infection.—Endogenous infection may occur in the eye either as a purulent or as a nonpurulent condition. Purulent infections are produced by pathogenic microorganisms which are conveyed into the smaller vessels of the eye from other organs or parts. The common causes are streptococci, pneumococci and such diseases as meningitis, influenza and typhoid fever. In some conditions, only a certain structure of the eye may become involved, the resulting infection being only of moderate degree which will eventually recover. In others, because of the virulence of the invading organism and a lowered resistance on the part of the patient, the entire eyeball may become involved by the infection, which will result in panophthalmitis and total loss of the eye. This can occur in pneumococcal meningitis and as the result of embolic infection in typhoid fever.

Infection of the eyeball may occur because of the presence of an active purulent infection elsewhere as in the teeth, tonsils, sinuses or other parts.

Nonpurulent Metastatic Infection.—Nonpurulent infections of endogenous variety frequently occur in the infectious diseases of a chronic nature, such as tuberculosis, syphilis, gonorrhea, rheumatic affections and others. These conditions may produce inflammation of various types and degrees in the different structures of the eye, more especially the iris, ciliary body, and choroid. Syphilitic iritis and iridocyclitis, tuberculous iritis, choroiditis or uveitis are examples. It is not definitely known in any individual case whether the condition results from the presence of the bacteria themselves in the ocular tissue or from the effect of their toxins. In tuberculous choroiditis, in the absence of demonstrable tubercle bacilli or tubercles, Eggston[2] and others ascribed the condition to an allergic reaction to the tuberculoprotein which is present. Occasionally, nodules, which are considered to be tubercles, are seen on the iris or in the choroid and lead to a definite diagnosis of tuberculous iritis or choroiditis. Such cases have been diagnosed, however, in the absence of tubercles, by Von Michel[3] in 1930 and at about the same time by Verhoeff[4] in this country.

Tubercles when seen on the iris usually occur on either the ciliary or pupillary borders, since here are found the anastomoses of small vessels to which the tubercle bacillus is conveyed from the primary site. According to Adler and Meyer[5] who reviewed the subject of tuberculous lesions of the uveal tract, these lesions vary in their course and appearance according to the number and virulence of the infecting organisms, the state of the body immunity and the degree of allergy to tuberculoprotein. They also stated that tuberculous uveitis is always secondary to a primary lesion elsewhere and develops only when the tuberculous nodule elsewhere breaks down in the secondary stage, and the bacilli enter the blood stream. As a result, a metastasis takes place to the uveal tract where the bacilli are carried by the circulation. It is rare that they are carried by the lymphatics or that the ocular lesion occurs as the result of extension or spreading along adjacent structures.

The involvement of any certain part does not necessarily depend on the vascularity of that particular structure. The nonvascular cornea is often the seat of the affection in the eye and it is possible that the bacteria or their toxins have at least a selective effect for certain parts. A case of metastatic syphilitic corneal abscess was reported by Klien[6] in which the most probable mode of infection was explained as metastasis of spirochetes into the iris and cornea.

Klauder,[7] who has contributed much to the study of ocular syphilis, stressed principally such factors as strains of the spirochete, tissue predisposition, trauma, immunologic response and others in the localization of the lesion in the eye. Particularly, with reference to tissue predisposition, he stated that this is intimately concerned with the question of strains of the *Spirochaeta pallida*, and that although the problems of resistance and predisposition of tissues as well as localization of the spirochete are complex and not completely understood, the cornea is conspicuous for its predisposition in both congenital and acquired syphilis.

Trauma is an important factor in determining the localization of syphilis in the cornea in the form of interstitial keratitis. The cornea is probably more commonly affected in this way than any other structure of the eye, although syphilitic iridocyclitis may occur occasionally after ocular operations. Either of these conditions may become activated by injury or operative trauma to the eyeball.

Degenerations and Diseases of Other Organs

The disorders and diseases which occur in many organs of the body may be either accompanied or followed by manifestations of the disease in the eye. A consideration of this group draws attention to several general etiologic factors which cannot always be specifically identified and separated, but which, in spite of certain apparent differences in their nature, are intimately related in their ultimate effect. The influence of these factors in the production of eye manifestations must therefore be explained in several ways.

Degenerative Conditions.—First, they may act in the nature of a degenerative process in the organ primarily affected, with an accompanying or a secondary degeneration affecting the structures of the eye. The latter is caused by a diminished nutrition as the result of interference with the blood supply to the organ. Or it might be part of a degenerative process which is taking place in other similar structures at the same time. Such degenerative diseases may affect the nervous system with accompanying degenerative changes in some structure of the eye, such as the retina.

Oncoming senility with general sclerosis and gradual impairment of the nutrition is accompanied by degenerative changes in the eye. In older people, as a result of senile degeneration, the skin of the lids may become wrinkled, thin and more darkly pigmented because of changes in the cell structure and accumulation of pigment. Degenerative changes in the number and structure of the epithelial cells of the cornea may lead to atrophy of the corneal epithelium. Hyaline changes may take place in the epithelial cells of the conjunctiva which lead to the formation of pinguecula. Arcus senilis may occur with oncoming age and is characterized by the presence of an opaque, grayish-white circle around the circumference of the cornea, which has been attributed to a fatty degeneration of the substantia propria. Tay's choroiditis or choroiditis guttata senilis is an example of a senile change characterized by the presence of small, oval, yellowish-white areas which arrange themselves in the retina around the macula, as the result of a colloid or hyaline degeneration.

Sclerosis of the lens of the eye usually accompanies a generalized sclerosis. Usually in middle life, a loss of the power of accommodation of the eye becomes manifest. The condition which is known as presbyopia results because of the loss of plasticity of the lens in the presence of the oncoming sclerosis. The eye therefore is no longer able to adapt itself to changes from distant to near vision. The increased hardening of the nucleus of the lens in still older people is accompanied by a change in color to a dark amber and in very pronounced cases to a deep red color.

When the general nutrition of an individual is deficient for a long period of time, such as that which is occasioned by a lack of dietary essentials, certain degenerative changes may affect the conjunctival and corneal epithelium, such as has been described in xerosis and xerophthalmia or in keratomalacia in infants. In xerophthalmia, for example, night blindness is described as a characteristic symptom and is attributed to the absence of vitamin A in the diet of the individual. As a result of its absence or deficiency in the retina, the visual purple which is destroyed by intense light, fails to regenerate. Another result of the same deficiency is a keratinization of the epithelium of the cornea and conjunctiva.

Circulatory and Metabolic Diseases.—Secondly, the ocular changes may result from an interference to the blood supply, because of the pathology present in other organs or from a generalized pathology primarily affecting the blood vessels themselves. Very frequently both of these conditions exist in the same individual. As the result of alterations in the structure and function of an organ, certain deleterious products may be produced in the system which act in the nature of a toxin or chemical irritant, either directly to the tissues of the eye or to the general vascular system. With the latter, changes take place in the blood vessels, the nutrition of the eye is subsequently diminished and degenerative changes in its various structures will ultimately take place.

In some diseases, the alterations and changes which take place in the constituents and composition of the blood will cause an impairment of nutrition and accompanying degenerative changes in the eye.

Whether the decrease in the blood supply is due to changes in blood vessels themselves or to chemical changes and toxins liberated in the course of disease of some other organ, the ultimate result is a degeneration followed by atrophy in the various eye structures affected. In some diseases of the kidneys, in diabetes or other metabolic diseases, in arteriosclerosis and vascular hypertension occurring either alone or in combination, pathologic changes may occur in the eye which can affect principally the retinal vessels and the retinal tissue. The resulting pathology which was formerly designated as a "retinitis" is really a form of degeneration rather than an inflammation and has therefore been recently described more accurately as a "retinosis" (Troncoso). These changes are usually characterized by the presence of hemorrhages, edema and patches of exudate in the retinal tissue.

Glandular Dysfunction.—The character of the eye manifestations often leads to the recognition and identity of the disease in a primary organ and the relationship between the two conditions may in many instances depend on an altered chemical action. This is illustrated by the alterations which occur in the function of some of the endocrine glands, characterized by marked variations in the amount of their secretions. For example, as a result of hypersecretion of the thyroid gland, important evidences may be found in the eye. Disturbances in function of the parathyroid glands may cause changes in the optic nerve and opacities in the lens. Diseases of the pituitary gland may also cause certain changes which will manifest themselves principally in the optic nerve and retina. Glandular alterations may occur at times as part of a physiologic process, such as the enlargement of the pituitary which takes place during pregnancy and which may be accompanied by manifestations in the eye without other signs of disease. Although this is usually considered as a physiologic process, it is, however, also felt by some that toxins are formed which act as the direct causative factor.

There are, therefore, three principal explanations to be given for the ocular manifestations produced in the course of the primary diseases mentioned thus far. All of these have to do in some way with a gradual reduction of the blood supply and impairment of the nutrition, resulting in a degenerative process in the eye. First, that they are of vascular origin and due primarily to changes in the vessel walls and to generalized hypertension. Second, that they are due to the toxic chemical action on the retinal tissue and the vessels by certain products of degeneration produced as the result of disease in another organ. Third, that a disturbance of metabolism with a breaking down of cellular elements and the production of toxins takes place simultaneously in the primary organ, the vascular system and the retina.

Sudden Loss of Blood Supply.—In the disorders and diseases discussed thus far, the eye manifestations were produced principally because of an interference with the blood supply which was incomplete and gradual in its course. In several diseases, however, a sudden and complete interference with the blood supply may occur as the result of a sudden occlusion of the central retinal artery or vein or one of their branches. In endocarditis and valvular heart disease, usually associated with generalized vascular hypertension, an embolus may be carried to the central artery by the circulation, and becoming lodged there, can cause sudden and complete blindness. A sudden anemia is produced with an absence of blood in the larger arteries, while the smaller arteries cannot be seen when the eye is examined with the ophthalmoscope. The optic nerve head as a result, becomes white and atrophic. In such an occlusion the appearance of the macula is characterized by what is commonly described as the ''cherry-red spot.'' In the presence of generalized vascular disease, renal disease or syphilis, the occlusion may be the result of a thrombosis. In many instances it is difficult to determine whether the obstruction is actually due to an embolus or thrombus and the opinions of most authors are not in full agreement in this regard. According to Troncoso, embolism is the most probable cause when valvular disease of the heart and endocarditis are present in young people, while obliterative endarteritis is more liable to occur in older patients.

When an embolus lodges in one of the branches of the central artery, it will cause only interference with function in that part of the retina supplied by the branch. The visual interference resulting will be partial and characterized by a scotoma or defect in the visual field which corresponds to the area supplied by the vessel which is occluded.

Thrombosis of the central vein may occur with the sudden appearance of large and numerous hemorrhages throughout the retina, in such diseases as syphilis, generalized arteriosclerosis, diabetes and nephritis. Here also, the thrombosis may occur in a smaller branch of the central vein, with an interference to the vision corresponding to the area affected.

Changes in the vasculature can also be produced with lesions occurring in the eyes as the result of indirect traumatism or traumatism to some other part of the body. Blows to the front or side of the head may cause fracture of the skull or bones of the orbit resulting in severe hemorrhage into the orbit with displacement of the eyeball, interference with rotation of the eyeball, and impairment of vision. A severe blow to the orbit may even cause hemorrhage within the eyeball.

Severe trauma to other parts of the body may also produce lesions in the eye. This is illustrated in Purtscher's disease, where hemorrhages occur in the retina of the eye as the result of severe injury to the chest. (See Purtscher's disease.)

Mechanical Causes

The mechanical causes are concerned principally in those conditions which produce pressure, either directly or indirectly, on the eyeball itself or some structure of the eye such as the optic nerve or one of the other nerves supplying the eye. The most common of such conditions are intracranial tumors, hemorrhages and aneurysms. As a result, such evidences as displacement of the eyeball, extraocular muscle palsies, swelling, edema and choking of the optic nerve head, hemorrhages and edema in the retina may all be found in various instances. The type of the eye manifestation present will depend mainly on the part of the eye or visual pathway affected by the pressure of the primary lesion. A rather frequent occurrence is a tumor growth in the region of the sella with pressure from the tumor on the optic chiasm, which is manifested, among other things, by more or less typical changes in the visual fields.

Other tumors not of pituitary origin, such as gumma and metastatic carcinoma, may produce hypopituitarism, which may be followed by manifestations in the optic nerve. In those conditions in which an increase in the intracranial tension occurs, a mechanical pressure is produced on the optic nerve from an accumulation of lymph in the intervaginal space of the optic nerve, manifested by choked disc. Papilledema occurs in about 80 per cent of the intracranial tumors. Intracranial cysts may also cause eye manifestations as the result of pressure.

Optic atrophy may occur from pressure on the nerve in the optic canal. In these conditions there takes place a gradual thickening of the bones of the orbit which results in a narrowing of the optic canal, sufficient to cause pressure on the nerve. Bony tumor growths around the optic canal may also cause a narrowing with pressure which will manifest itself by changes in the optic nerve. Leontiasis ossea and Paget's disease could be considered as examples of the above-mentioned conditions.

A tumor growth, encapsulated abscess or a very large hemorrhage in the orbit may cause pressure as well as traction on the eyeball. In such cases, the eyeball is usually displaced from its normal position, and in marked cases, hemorrhages in the retina and vitreous and detachment of the retina may result. Secondary tumors in and about the eyeball may occur as the result of metastasis from some other organ.

Paralysis of almost any or all of the extraocular muscles may occur as the result of pressure applied either directly or indirectly on the affected nerve at some point in its course. Tumors of the pons may cause ocular paralysis in this manner. Hemorrhages and tumors in the brain may cause a total ophthalmoplegia by reason of the pressure exerted. These conditions manifest themselves by an inability of the eye to rotate in the direction of the affected muscle or muscles.

The pressure which is exerted on the sixth nerve by a swelling or abscess at the apex of the petrous portion of the temporal bone will manifest itself by a paralysis of the external rectus muscle on the affected side, and an inability of the eye to rotate outward. (See also Malignancy of bones of the orbit.)

Nuclear lesions, because of pressure, may cause conjugate lateral paralysis and loss of power of rotation to one side. Midbrain tumors may cause paralysis of upward vertical movements of the eyes and cerebral lesions may cause lateral paralysis.

References

1. Lemoine, Albert N.: Allergies in Ophthalmology, Arch. Ophth. 28: 79-92, 1942.
2. Eggston, A. A.: The Use of Tuberculin in Diagnosis and Treatment in Ophthalmology, Arch. Ophth. 8: 671, No. 5, November, 1932.
3. Von Michel, in Schieck, F., and Bruckner, A.: Kurzes Handbuch der Ophthalmologie, Berlin, Julius Springer 5: 28, 1930.
4. Verhoeff, F. H.: Acute Tuberculous Iritis: Microscopic Examination of the Eye Showing This Condition, Tr. Sect. Ophth. A. M. A. 1930, p. 21.
5. Adler, Francis Heed, and Meyer, George R.: Tuberculous Lesions of the Uveal Tract, Arch. Ophth. 18: 275, No. 2, August, 1937.
6. Klien, Bertha A.: Acute Metastatic Syphilitic Corneal Abscess: A Clinical and Histopathologic Study, Arch. Ophth. 14: 612, No. 4, October, 1935.
7. Klauder, Joseph V.: Ocular Syphilis. II. Factors Influencing the Localization of Syphilis, Arch. Ophth. 7: 268, No. 2, February, 1932.

CHAPTER III

THE EXAMINATION OF THE PATIENT

General Inspection

The methods for collecting diagnostic evidence of disease in the eyes should not differ greatly from those employed in other conditions, and should actually commence the moment the patient is presented to view. In a general preliminary inspection, a knowledge can be obtained which might prove useful, by observing such conditions as:

1. The position of the patient, whether standing, sitting, or confined to bed. Any rotation or inclination of the head not the result of habit, and new to the individual, might at once suggest an effort to avoid diplopia, compensation for paralysis of an eye muscle, a rheumatic condition, or an affection of the neck muscles. The first two conditions are voluntary, the latter involuntary, and the difference is quite apparent. This is an important observation because patients who have in this way learned to correct an existing diplopia due to a muscle paralysis, may fail to mention the fact that at times they see double, especially when looking in certain directions.

When a patient has photophobia, he attempts to avoid light. In mild cases, this may cause only a wrinkling of the forehead or knitting of the eyebrows, whereas in more severe cases, he looks directly downward flexing the head on the chest. In contrast to this, those who have been blind for a long time usually hold the head upright or turn the face upward as if seeking for light. Those who have recently lost all or nearly all vision are likely to look downward, either because of mental depression, or in order to watch their footsteps as much as possible.

In standing and sitting postures, any swaying from side to side and equilibrium should be observed for indications of vertigo. Face twitching, blinking of eyelids, tremors, and tics should be noted. Signs of paralysis agitans and Parkinsonian disease should be noted.

In observing a patient confined to bed, conditions of great weakness, discomfort, pain, embarrassed breathing should all be noted. Abdominal pain might necessitate both legs being drawn up in an effort to relieve the abdominal tension. The position of opisthotonos is characteristic of such conditions as strychnine poisoning, tetanus, hysteria and epilepsy. Rigidity and contraction of the posterior neck muscles are characteristic of meningitis and may cause a retraction of the head. Dyspnea may force the patient to sit upright, with the body supported by the hands, and the arms forward to throw back the shoulders. Lateral decubitus may suggest the presence of a chest affection causing pain on breathing. A lateral position with all joints flexed and the patient "curled up" is found in hepatic, renal and intestinal colic; also in cerebellar disease, and in cerebral irritation following brain concussion.

2. The various movements of the body and of the extremities should be noted since departures from the normal are caused by pain. Certain restrictions in movement may point directly to some focus or disorder. Tremors of the head

and of the extremities are characteristic of such diseases as paralysis agitans, disseminated sclerosis, hysteria, senility, chronic alcoholism, or conditions caused by other excesses. Tremors of the eyeballs and nystagmus especially should be noted. These are all readily detected on inspection, but may be quite easily overlooked if this part of the examination is neglected.

3. The gait of a patient may give notice of the existence of some serious disorder of the nervous system. Examples can be observed in such conditions as tabes dorsalis, spastic paralysis, hemiplegia, paralysis agitans, cerebellar tumor, or any brain tumor or abscess.

The ataxic gait is characterized by separated or spread legs, sudden high raising of the foot with forward propulsion, uncertainty and wavering of the extremity while in the air, and a quick forcible planting of the foot with the heel down first. The head is a little forward, and the eyes fixed on the ground in order to aid in equilibrium.

With cerebellar ataxia, or with vertigo, there is swaying of the body and reeling; ordinary alcoholic intoxication can illustrate such a gait. The eyes are fixed on the ground, the face expressing considerable anxiety. True vertigo resulting from brain disease is more intense than visual vertigo from diplopia.

The spastic gait is characterized by rigidity. The legs are adducted even to crossing, the arms are flexed, and the feet are dragged. There is not the same need for fixing the ground with the eyes, and often, owing to tilting of the pelvis, a better balance is obtained by holding the head erect.

4. Evidence of pain should be looked for and its presence noted. The patient usually makes an effort to protect a painful part. The hand will often be found covering as nearly as possible the seat of pain. The face is very expressive, and few can control the facial muscles so as not to betray suffering. Pain in the eye causes a patient first to narrow the palpebral fissure of the affected eye, and if more severe, both fissures may be narrowed. In very exteme cases, one or both eyes may be closed, and greater protection may be obtained by the further aid of the frontalis and corrugator muscles, and the hand pressed against the closed eye. Headache may cause the same appearance, particularly that of frowning or lowering the eyebrows.

5. The facies and facial appearance, as already described, may indicate the presence of pain in the eyes or head. In addition, however, a great many diseases may present a physiognomy which is at once peculiar and expressive. A glance at the face is often quite sufficient to put the clinician's train of thought in harmony with the patient's condition. Emaciation is promptly revealed in the face; the flush of fever, the puffiness of the eyelids significant of cardiac and renal disease, the cachexia of malignant disease, the dull and lusterless eyes of stupor and apathy, the brilliant eyes of exalted states of the nervous system, the blue lips due to disturbances of venous circulation, jaundice, unilateral facial immobility with obliteration of the normal creases and furrows from facial paralysis, and many other alterations in the facial appearance may present themselves for interpretation.

The face in myxedema, acromegaly, hyperthyroidism, and in certain forms of mental disease, is characteristic. Any enlargement and separation of the central facial bones proptosing and spreading the eyes, gives the patient an unmistakable appearance. The proptosed eyeballs, widened palpebral fissures, anxious expression and nervous appearance seen in Grave's disease, often point at once to the diagnosis on primary inspection.

General inspection may reveal signs of stigmas. Anatomic stigmas are manifested by asymmetry of the face and cranium, unusual configuration of the skull, high narrow forehead, large projecting jaws, narrow palpebral fissure, disordered ocular muscles, irregularly curved cornea and keratoconus, nystagmus, misshaped and irregular teeth, highly arched fauces, malformation of the palate, deformities of the extremities and genital organs, and too much or too little hair. Physiologic stigmas also noticeable are tremor, hypersensitiveness or hyposensitiveness of the special senses, defective speech, and diminished endurance of emotional and nervous strain.

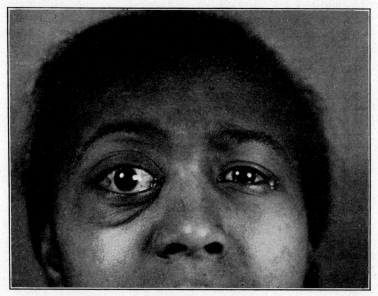

Fig. 9.—Exophthalmos. Note the more marked protrusion of the right eye with widened palpebral fissure and anxious expression of the patient. (I. S. Tassman, Wills Hospital.)

6. The speech and manner of speech are altered in certain diseases and conditions and may afford collateral evidence of processes also affecting the eye. Paralysis of the tongue, soft palate and facial muscles causes an indistinct and imperfect speech affecting mostly certain letters. Diphtheria, bulbar or pseudobulbar paralysis, or amyotrophic lateral sclerosis may be the cause. In general paresis of the insane the speech is slow, the words slurred, and the lips and tongue are tremulous. The patient with paralysis agitans hesitates at the beginning of the sentence, and finishes in a rapid expulsive manner. The voice is high and fretful.

A scanning speech is characteristic of disseminated sclerosis; with nystagmus, weakness of the legs, and increased knee jerks, it is of great significance. It is also found in Friedreich's ataxia. Each word is spoken slowly and each syllable is accentuated.

Finally, some idea of the patient's temperament should be formed. The value attached to certain symptoms and the way in which certain symptoms are stressed by a patient is greatly influenced and determined by the temperament.

Some patients may complain of great pain which would be only lightly mentioned by others. The nervous temperament is characterized by marked sensitiveness of the nervous system to slight impressions. The phlegmatic temperament on the other hand is characterized by diminished sensibility to pain, slow psychic reaction and want of energy. A neurasthenic individual might present himself for examination with a long list of symptoms all enumerated in detail on a sheet of paper.

Other temperaments may exhibit marked irritability, strong passions, and active voluntary muscles; persistent sullenness or dullness may indicate a melancholic temperament. A sanguine temperament may show irritability, liability to nervous exhaustion, and sudden change of mood.

Having obtained the information available by a general inspection of the patient while observing principally the features thus far presented, a careful history should now be obtained after which a more detailed examination of the eyes can be made.

History and Case Record

An accurate history and record of the case is of great importance in ophthalmology as in other branches of medicine. Many of the functional tests are made with instruments of precision and can be repeated subsequently under similar conditions, thus giving results, comparison of which is of great value.

The history and status of the case should contain all the information which can have any bearing, direct or indirect, upon the case, but need not contain an array of facts unrelated to the condition under consideration. It should be practiced with the aim of having each history complete and individual for the case at hand. The questions should be systematic and direct, each one calling for desired information, and not of useless import. They should not be suggestive in nature, so that a patient might feel that a certain answer is expected. The physician must employ skill in questioning as well as in interpreting the answer, particularly with reference to such important symptoms as photophobia, diplopia, headache and vertigo. A good history can be obtained quickly and at the same time accurately.

Printed question forms on cards covering every phase of the patient's routine are used by some, especially in hospitals and institutions, but such methods, although they might prove useful in certain forms of practice, tend to lose their individuality and lessen the chance for eliciting the essential characteristics of the particular case. The routine questions which are asked in every case can be recorded in blank form.

The name, address, age, color, social state (married or single), occupation, visual acuity, state of the accommodation of the eye are fundamentals that are required in all cases and should be at the beginning of every record. After this, a record should be made to meet all the requirements of the individual case. A definite plan, of course, should be followed, and this should start with the present condition or the nature of the chief complaint. The patient should be asked directly what it is that caused him to come for examination. The time of onset, the location, mode of commencement, progress or extension and change in character of the first symptoms should all be noted. If the vision was found to be impaired or poor, "When was it first noticed? Did it fail rapidly or slowly?" When headache is complained of, as it frequently is, the locality, frequency, duration, time of occurrence, and whether or not it is influenced by use of the eyes, are all factors of importance in determining the relationship of the headache.

The patient should be questioned concerning the behavior of the eyes in near work; that is, whether or not words and letters blur or run together, whether the eyes tire quickly, whether or not they are painful. Sometimes a patient volunteers certain information and complains of disturbances such as "seeing double." A statement of this kind should be more closely investigated, since it would indicate the presence of a diplopia. Many people make this statement, however, when they actually mean that certain objects, principally words and letters, blur or have a blurred edge or extra fringe. It is necessary, therefore, whenever a patient speaks of "seeing double," to ask in return, "Do you see actually two objects when you look at any single thing?" It is often found that this is not what was meant by the statement. Photophobia is another complaint which is sometimes confusing. This is particularly true with regard to the degree or severity. Many patients state that they are unable to withstand the light. This might refer to ordinary daylight, the light to which they are exposed in their employment, or to very strong sunlight, such as might be encountered on a beach or while on the water. Vertigo and dizziness are other complaints often presented which require the interpretation of the examiner after further questioning. For example, many patients neglect to state that the vertigo or dizziness occurs only in bending over or stooping; others are affected any time, even while lying in bed. Occurring at such periods, vertigo could scarcely be of ocular origin primarily. This complaint, however, is often associated with headache and is noticed principally while riding in a vehicle, such as an automobile or train. In these cases, the complaint could be due to ocular disturbances, so that it is of importance to ascertain a knowledge of the time and place of onset of such complaints.

Lacrimation, the presence of secretion or discharge which agglutinates the lids, and any other inflammatory or other ocular trouble should all be recorded.

In recording time, exact dates should always be noted, and names of days of the week are avoided since they are meaningless at a later date. Certain abbreviations are practical and are in general use. O. D. (oculus dextra, right eye); O. S. (oculus sinistra, left eye); O_2, both eyes; O. U., either eye; V., vision; Ac., accommodation; A. C., anterior chamber; med., media, are all examples of those in common use.

The patient is then questioned concerning the general health, especially with regard to such conditions as rheumatism, cardiac or circulatory diseases, gastrointestinal disturbances, nervous affections, tuberculosis, syphilis, other infectious diseases, and any illness from which the patient recently recovered. They should be questioned with regard to vascular hypertension, renal disease and diabetes, in particular.

The diseases of childhood should be noted in some cases, generally with a view to excluding those which immunize.

The menstrual function may play an important role in eye diseases, either directly or indirectly through the nervous system. Its advent, its fulfillment and its termination in the menopause are marked by more or less profound impressions upon the nervous system, and disturbance of balance. A record of these phenomena must, therefore, enter into the histories of a large number of female patients.

Personal habits should receive attention, and the use of tobacco, alcohol (beer, wine, whiskey), drugs and opiates, either occasionally or habitually, should be determined in certain cases. The history of excess of all kinds is generally obtained gradually and without apparent intent, after having gained the confidence of the patient.

The occupation of the patient is of great importance in relation to the condition complained of. Those who are employed daily in performing close work, such as clerks, students, teachers, bank tellers, secretaries, printers, writers, and others, may complain of symptoms which are directly caused by the use of the eyes. The exact nature of the work performed by the patient must often be elicited. Many are inclined to generalize when questioned concerning their employment. Paint workers, acetylene welders, furnace workers, those who are in daily contact with chemicals and drugs, may all suffer with conditions affecting the eyes. In other instances, certain systemic diseases of occupational origin may be present, with complications in the ocular structures.

Any change or progress of the condition should be recorded under the date of each subsequent visit or examination of the patient. A record should be kept of all medicines and treatment prescribed and these can be underlined. Consultations and recommendations should be noted, and the termination or final disposition of the case should be recorded.

Routine Examination of the Eyes

The subjective examination of the eye consists principally in determining the state of the visual function and the ability of the eye to see. The visual function is complicated and depends on the ability of the eye to receive and transmit light to the brain where its reception is interpreted as an impression. It is, therefore, necessary first for the eye to be able to distinguish and appreciate various intensities of light. This function is known as the *light sense*. Secondly, the ability to distinguish form is necessary in order to recognize objects. This function is known as the *form sense*. Finally, it is necessary that the eye have the ability to recognize and distinguish color. This is known as the *color sense*.

Light which enters the normal eye is transmitted back to a point of focus on the fovea of the retina. The ability to obtain a clear focus or image on the retina depends in great part on the state of the *refractive system* or, as it is sometimes called, the *dioptric apparatus* of the eye. This system is composed of the cornea, aqueous humor, lens and vitreous humor. For an eye to have good vision it is, therefore, necessary that the refractive system be normal in order that an image may be clearly focused on the retina. An object is seen as clearly as the image which is formed.

The retina is not sensitive to light to the same extent in all portions. The visual acuity, therefore, varies in different parts of the retina. The fovea centralis of the macular region is the most sensitive part of the retina, and that part in which visual acuity is greatest. Outside of the macula, the visual acuity decreases. The farther out in the periphery of the retina, the lower the visual acuity becomes. The vision obtained at the macula is known as *central* or *direct* vision, while that which is obtained outside of the macula is known as *peripheral* or *indirect* vision. The extent to which the eye has the ability to see to all sides, above and below, while in a position fixed straight ahead, is known as the field of vision. This represents or indicates the total extent to which the retina is stimulated by light to produce an impression while the eye is fixed in a position straight forward.

The ordinary determination of the vision or visual acuity of the eye by the use of the Snellen test letters at a definite distance indicates the amount or degree of central vision. The method for determining the extent and character of the peripheral or indirect vision is known as perimetry and is sometimes spoken of as the visual field test. The light sense of the eye is tested by the use of an instrument which, in principle, is a photometer. The examination includes the determination of the threshold, or "light minimum," and the determination of the least perceptible difference in light intensity which is the "light difference."

In the subjective examination of the eyes, it is well to follow a definite routine of procedure. The first step, therefore, in such procedure, after completing and recording the history of the case, should be the test of the visual acuity and determination of the amount of central vision.

To Test the Visual Acuity.—For this purpose, the Snellen test card is commonly used. It consists of rows of letters or figures so constructed that each letter subtends an angle of five minutes at a distance of six meters from the normal eye. There is usually one larger letter at the top of every card with letters or figures of progressively smaller size in each succeeding row down the card. The reason for this is that each row should be read by a normal eye at a certain definite distance. This distance is often designated on the card at the end of each row. To test the vision, the patient is seated comfortably and directly in front of the test card which is usually on the opposite wall of the room at a distance of six meters or twenty feet. The vision is tested both with and without the patient's glasses. The right eye is usually tested first by holding a card or cover over the left eye and asking the patient to read aloud the letters or figures on the card from above downward as far as he can. The left eye is then tested in the same manner after covering the right eye. This may be followed by the patient reading the card with both eyes uncovered. In recording the result, the right eye is designated as O. D. (Ocula Dextra), and the left eye is O. S. (Ocula Sinistra). Both eyes together are designated as O_2; O. U. is used for either eye. The visual acuity is recorded by a fraction, the numerator of which represents the distance at which the vision is tested, and the denominator represents the line or row of letters the patient is able to read at that distance. For example: if the test is being made at a distance of six meters or twenty feet and the patient can read only the largest letter on the card which should normally be seen at six meters or twenty feet, then the visual acuity of this eye should be recorded as 6/60 in the metric system, or otherwise 20/20. If the patient at a distance of six meters or twenty feet can read the line designated for the normal eye at this distance, the visual acuity is recorded as 6/6 or 20/20. If a shorter distance is being used for the test as, for example, fifteen feet, and the patient can read the line of letters designated for the normal eye at fifteen feet, the visual acuity is recorded as 15/15 for this eye. In other words, the test card may be at any distance from the patient and the vision will be recorded by a fraction, the numerator indicating the distance and the denominator the line or row of letters read by the patient at that distance. Examples of the record of the visual acuity of a patient for distance would be:

O. D. 6/6:   O. S. 6/15 (Metric system)
O. D. 15/20: O. S. 15/15 (English system)

If the patient wears glasses, this should be followed by a record of the visual acuity with glasses, as:

O. D. 6/15   O. D. 6/9
O. S. 6/12   c.c.   O. S. 6/6

Another example: O. D. 20/40   O. D. 20/20
O. S. 20/30   c.c.   O. S. 20/20

(c.c. is an abbreviation for "cum correction" or "with glasses.")

If the patient is unable to read the largest figure on the card at the distance tested, the card is brought closer to the patient, or the patient is instructed to approach the card until he is able to see only the largest letter. The vision is then recorded in terms of that distance. For example, if it should be necessary for the patient to approach to the distance of two meters from the card in order to be able to see the largest letter or figure on the top row, then the visual acuity is recorded as 2/60 in the eye tested. When the vision is found to be so poor that it cannot be tested with the card, an attempt is made to have the patient count the number of fingers held up by the examiner in front of the eye. If, for instance, the greatest distance at which the fingers can be correctly counted is ten inches from the eye, the visual acuity is recorded as: "Fingers at 10 in." or "F. 10 in." If the vision in an eye is not sufficient for this, it is tested by moving the hand in front of the eye. On recognizing the movement of the hand, the record is made as: "Hand Movements" or "H.M." Should only light perception be present in an eye, it is recorded as: "L.P." When even this is absent, the eye is blind and is recorded as such by the word "nil."

If only light perception is present in an eye, the ability to project light should then be tested. This is done by asking the patient to cover the opposite eye with a handkerchief. The eye to be tested is directed straight ahead. The examiner takes a position in front of the patient in a dark room, and holding a small flashlight, directs the light into the patient's eye from five directions, i.e., above, below, right, left and in front. The patient is asked to point to the direction from which the light is flashed while looking straight ahead. If the replies are correct, the light projection of the eye tested is recorded as good in all directions. This would indicate the probable healthy condition of the retina and eye grounds. Should the response be incorrect after several repeated tests, the light projection is recorded as faulty in the directions indicated. This would suggest the possible presence of some pathology in the retina or other portion of the interior of the eye, and it is important to determine this before operating on an eye with mature cataract.

When an eye has no light perception, it is considered to be blind. In such a case there is an absence of visual function. Amaurosis and amblyopia are terms employed to indicate blindness, especially with reference to function, but actually imply a symptom of some pathologic process which has destroyed the vision.

In order to test the near vision of the patient, the Jaeger or Snellen test types are employed. These contain printed lines of various sized type, each to be read normally at a certain distance in front of the eye. On the Jaeger card the sizes of the type are indicated as J. No. 1 to J. No. 6. The patient is tested with the smallest size type he can read. This is brought close to the eye until it blurs. If this should be at a distance of 30 cm., it is recorded as such. It is then withdrawn from the eye until a distance is reached where it is read best, continuing farther until it again becomes blurred. This is done both with and without the patient wearing his glasses, recording the result as: J. No. 1: 30 cm. to 55 cm. Since each size of type employed should be read normally at a certain distance, the visual acuity for near distance may also be stated as a fraction. Thus, if the patient can read at 33 cm. the type which should normally be read at 50 cm., the vision is recorded for near as $\dfrac{33\,0.3}{50\,0.5}$ or M.

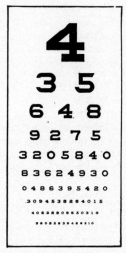

Fig. 10.—Snellen test card for distant vision. (Courtesy of Street, Linder, and Propert, Philadelphia.)

For children below school age who are unable to read, cards may be used with pictures of animals, boats, stars and other illustrations which might be recognized by the patient. These figures are constructed in the same manner as the letters and numbers on other cards, but it is much more difficult to make them clear enough to be readily recognized by a child of this age in order to prove an accurate test of visual acuity.

Another card which is useful for adults who are unable to read and may also be employed with small children, is an illiterate card which consists of a series of the letter E. The horizontal lines or prongs of the E point in different directions, and the patient is asked to point the fingers of his hand in the same direction in which he can see the prongs of the E point. The result is then recorded in the same manner as with the card bearing letters or numbers.

No. 1.

The eye is the organ of vision, and resembles a photographer's camera in its construction. The iris is the diaphragm, with a pupillary opening in the center, which adjusts itself to the amount of light by dilating or contracting. Like the camera, the vitreous chamber is darkened inside by the pigmented layer of the choroid. The retina, or nervous layer, is the sensitive plate of the camera, and receives the impression or image of the object. The crystalline lens is so adjusted by the aid of the ciliary muscle as to bring the light to a focus   0.37

No. 2.

on the retina. In order to accomplish its function successfully all the media of the eye must be transparent. These media are from before backwards the cornea, the aqueous humor, the crystalline lens, and the vitreous humor. Any haziness of one or more of these media will, of course, interfere with the visual function. The first essential, then, of perfect vision is an absolute transparency of all the media, and the second is an accurate focusing of the rays of light on   0.50

No. 3.

the retina through the adjustment of the crystalline lens. These impressions when received upon the retina are gathered up and concentrated, as it were, in the optic nerve through which they are carried to the brain. In short-sighted persons the eye-ball is too long, and the light rays come to a focus in   0.62

No. 4.

front of the retina, while in far-sighted persons the eye-ball is too short, and the focal point, therefore, falls behind the retina. In either case a blurred image is received upon the retina. In order to   0.75

No. 6.

overcome this blurring, and thus correct the optical defect, the eye unconsciously makes an effort by which the ciliary muscle acts on the lens. This effort explains why eye-strain may   0.87

No. 8.

cause pain and discomfort. An optical correction for the refractive error is found in spectacle lenses. In near-sightedness a   1.00

No. 10.

concave spherical lens will cause the focal point to recede until it falls directly on the retina;   1.50

No. 12.

while in far-sightedness   2.00

Fig. 11.—Jaeger test card for near vision. (Courtesy of Street, Linder, and Propert, Philadelphia.)

The Light Sense

The determination of the light sense can be accomplished in a general way by reducing the illumination of the room while the patient observes a letter on the test card. The result is compared with that noted by the examiner. In this way a general idea of the dark adaptation may be obtained.

A number of different photometers are now obtainable, however, with which the dark adaptation can be more accurately estimated. The oldest of these is Förster's photometer. Nearly all have a means for controlling the size of the pupil, since variations in the latter under different conditions of light would affect the result. It should be remembered also that exposure to strong light prior to testing the dark adaptation alters the result, since more of the visual purple is destroyed by such exposure than by ordinary room light. Förster's photometer was a rectangular box about 13 inches long, 10 inches wide, and 6 or 7 inches high. The inside was black. Two openings were mounted at the end where the eyes to be examined are placed. The light source was at another opening alongside of these. Most of the modern photometers are of simple construction, having an opening for the eyes to be examined, test objects to be observed by the patient, a controlled light source, and a resultant record of the test. Readings in the form of a graph are obtained of the dark adaptation of the eyes examined, for certain definite periods of time.

Although the macula is the retinal area of greatest visual acuity, the light sense is less acute here than in the surrounding retina, with weak illumination. For example, when a very dim star is fixed directly with the eye, it often cannot be seen, but when a closely adjacent brighter star is looked at directly, the first dim star comes into view. This phenomenon is explained by the fact that the fovea is not capable of adapting itself for a very weak illumination—as is the rest of the retina—because the fovea contains only cones and no rods, and is, therefore, without the visual purple which is considered necessary for dark adaptation.

Hemeralopia or night blindness causes a reduction in the visual acuity with oncoming darkness. This is observed clinically in a number of diseases which affect principally the retina and the optic nerve. Retinitis pigmentosa is an outstanding example. Such an impairment is found also in avitaminosis A, which may result in xerophthalmia. In this condition, hemeralopia is a characteristic finding. Prolonged exposure to strong light, diseases of the liver with jaundice, and some cases of high myopia are also, at times, characterized by hemeralopia.

The Color Sense

A disturbance of the color sense is usually considered as color blindness. This is an impairment which may be either congenital or acquired. Congenital color blindness is described in the chapter dealing with congenital conditions of the eye. Acquired color blindness sometimes occurs in certain diseases of the eye in which the optic nerve, retina, and the sensory apparatus, especially, are affected.

Perception of color is affected in nearly all individuals by the degree of illumination. The ability to recognize color is always lessened with decreased illumination, and in the dark it is almost impossible for the normal eye to perceive color.

Color blindness may be total or partial, the latter form being more common. The greater number of these cases belong to the group of red-green blindness which may show many variations. Some show only a mild manifestation of the impairment, while in others it is more pronounced. In many instances, the patient is not aware of his color defect until it is brought to his attention in the course of an examination of the eyes. The visual acuity in these cases is otherwise unaffected. When the patient is aware of the deficiency, he is, in many instances, able to overcome the handicap to a certain degree by training. Most of the time, however, they refrain from discussing or making statements concerning color. In certain occupations, since it is important that the color sense be normal, a test of the eyes for color blindness is a requirement.

Tests for Color Blindness.—A number of color tests have been devised most of which are intended to determine the ability to detect and separate various shades of colors, as well as the ability to distinguish the primary or pure colors.

The yarn test is a standard test in common use. It was originally devised by Holmgren and later modified by others. It consists of a number of shades of standard colored yarn. Red-green blindness can be determined readily by this test, as well as difficulty in recognizing the various shades.

The Ishihara test consists of a book of cards or plates each of which shows a confusion of small dots or blocks of various colors which surround a figure. For example, a 5 is formed in the center by the grouping of similar-colored blocks. An individual who is color blind will have difficulty, or will be unable to distinguish the figure in the confusion of colors on the card.

Other similar tests are Stilling's test and Green's test. Nagel's test consists of a series of cards each of which shows a ring of colors. Some of these present different shades of one color, while others show several different colors. The patient must select the card with one color, and match those showing various shades of the same color.

Lantern tests are also employed. The lantern is made of glass of various colors and variations of color for the patient to distinguish.

In testing a patient for color blindness, it is well to employ several different tests rather than to depend on the results obtained from one. Moreover, the tests should be repeated several times in order to obtain an accurate determinaion.

Perimetry and Peripheral Vision

Perimetry is the measure of the extent of the visual field, and the visual acuity throughout its entire area. This also includes scotometry, which deals with isolated areas of depressed vision within the field.

The visual field may be defined as a projection outward of all retinal points at which visual sensation can be initiated. Its outline would be nearly circular were it not for the prominence of brow, nose, and cheek, which restrict it on the upper, inner, and lower aspects. These reductions depend on the individual variation of the features. A vertical line running through the center of fixation divides the field into a larger temporal and a smaller nasal half.

The extent of the field varies within certain limits with the intensity of the stimulus employed. Using a 3 mm. white object on a perimeter, with a 330 mm. radius, that is, an object subtending an angle of about 5°, the average extent of the field is found to be about 95° outward, 75° downward, 60° inward and 60° upward. Using larger objects, the field can even be pushed to about 107° outward.

The acuity of vision is least at the periphery of the field, and becomes gradually greater up to about 10° from the visual axis where it increases rapidly to the maximum at a point corresponding to the center of the fovea. The area 10° about the point of visual axis or central vision is called the pericentral visual area. The point corresponding to the visual axis is called the fixation point.

There is a normal blind spot in the visual field corresponding to the projection of the optic disc. It is vertically oval in shape. Its center is situated about 15.5° to the temporal side of the fixation point, and 1.5° below the horizontal meridian. It is 5.5° in width, and 7.5° in length. This area is totally blind, and is surrounded by an amblyopic area for white of about 1°.

The Examination of the Visual Field.—This is ordinarily made on a perimeter by using graduated test objects in much the same way as the central vision is tested with letters of graduated size. The size of the test object is measured by the angle its diameter makes at the nodal point of the eye. Another way is to express as a fraction the diameter of the test object over the distance at which it is used in testing. If O equals the diameter of the test object, and R the distance the test object is from the eye (the latter corresponds to the radius of the field), then O/R equals the angular size of the test object. To convert this into degrees, multiply $O/R \times 180/\pi$.

Since the extent of the field depends on the amount of the stimulus employed, then by varying the diameter of the test object from the widest which would give the greatest extent of the field, to one so small that it can only be seen at the fixation point, a graphic record of the field may thus be constructed. Charting the field in this way is known as a quantitative perimetry. The outline for each test object is known as an isopter. Each isopter is designated by the visual angle subtended at the nodal point of the eye. This, explained above, is expressed as a fraction, O/R. Thus, the field for 3/330 is the field obtained by using a 3 mm. test object at a distance of 330 mm. from the eye. To convert this into degrees of angular measurement, multiply 3/330 by $180/\pi$.

The color fields also vary with the size of the test object; a colored object of the same size as a white one produces a smaller field. The largest color field is obtained with a blue test object; the field for red color is slightly smaller, and that for green is the smallest.

The binocular field is the field obtained when both eyes are fixed upon the same point. It is about 210° horizontally, and about 150° vertically. The nasal part of each field overlaps the other to the extent of about 65°. Thus, the center portion of about 130° is seen with both eyes. The outer part, which is not overlapped, is equal to about 40°, and has only uniocular vision. This is called the temporal crescent.

Clinical Examination.—Clinically, the visual field may be examined by three methods: (1) the confrontation method, (2) perimetry, (3) campimetry.

The confrontation method is very crude, but is useful as a rough preliminary test. The observer simply compares the patient's field of vision with his own by the following procedure: the patient and examiner are seated about 1 M. apart and facing each other. One of the patient's eyes is occluded. The examiner closes the eye opposite the covered eye of the patient. Each fixes on the open eye of the other. A test object is brought from the periphery on the side of the open eye in the plane midway between. The observer notes the point at which it comes into the field of the patient and compares it with the point at which it comes into his own field. He thereby may obtain an idea of the gross extent of the patient's field.

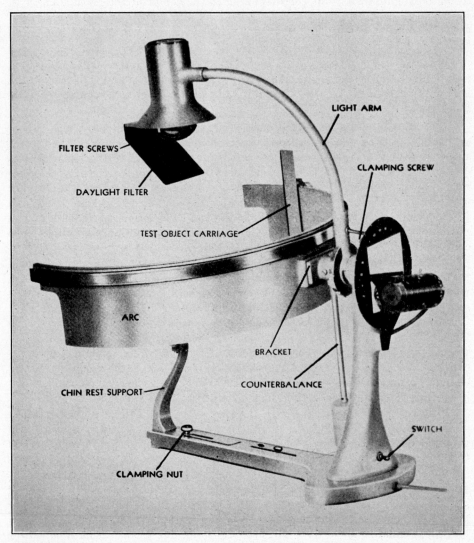

Fig. 12.—Perimeter (B & L). (Courtesy of Street, Linder, and Propert, Philadelphia.)

Examination With the Perimeter.—More accurate measurement of the visual field is obtained by using the perimeter. This consists of a 200° arc which has a radius of 330 or 333 mm. The arc itself is piveted at its center to a stand, so that it can be freely rotated in any meridian. It, therefore, will describe a hemisphere rotation at its point of attachment. The arc is marked by degrees at 10° intervals beginning from its center and reading both ways toward the periphery. At the center of the arc, there is usually a fixation point or object, light in color, and about 5 mm. in diameter.

The test objects employed are small discs which vary in diameter from 1 to 70 mm., and are of different colors, including white, blue, red, and green.

The patient is seated at one end of the perimeter with chin supported on a chin rest in such a manner that the eye to be examined is opposite the fixation point in the center of the arc and at a distance equal or corresponding to its radius. The eye which is not being examined should be covered, and the patient instructed to look steadily at the fixation point with the eye under examination. While in this position, the examiner, who stands at the side, introduces the test object at the outer extremity of the arc, and gradually carries it inward toward the center, until it is noticed by the patient in his field. This point is then noted on a chart which gives a graphic record of the field for the size and color of the object used. The procedure is carried out in eight to twelve meridians of the field.

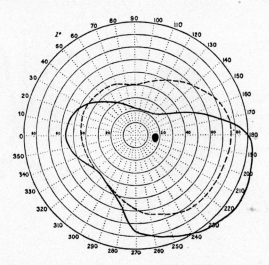

Fig. 13.—The relative field for 5/330, showing reduction due to a large nose and drooping upper lid. Broken line shows field for 1/330 with lid raised. (From Traquair: An Introduction to Clinical Perimetry, The C. V. Mosby Co.)

The Screen Campimeter, or Tangent Plane.—The area of the field 25° from the fixation point is most accurately examined on a plane at a longer distance, thus giving a projection on a larger scale. The screen or campimeter is a large square of black cloth 2 M. wide with a fixation object at the center. The patient faces the screen, preferably 2 M. away, looking directly at the fixation object, the chin supported on a rest.

This arrangement produces an angle of 27° from the fixation point to the edge of the screen with the eye and includes the central area to this extent projected to a flat surface.

The best way to use the screen is to mark off the blind spot first, using a 30 or a 40 mm. white test object, and working from its center to the periphery. The field is then examined with a 1 or a 2 mm. object moved from the periphery to the fixation point in eight to twelve meridians.

The findings are transferred to a chart by a tangent scale which could have been marked on the screen. A field should not be pronounced normal unless at least three white isopters are plotted. 3/330, 1/330, 1/2,000, or 2/2,000 are the ones generally used; and one or two colored ones, 5/330, 10/2,000, or 5/2,000 would be very acceptable.

Alterations in the Visual Field.—Defects in the field are characterized by alterations in: 1, Position; 2, Shape; 3, Size; 4, Intensity; 5, Uniformity; 6, Margins; 7, Quality; and 8, Behavior and Course.

Field changes may be divided into contractures and scotomas.

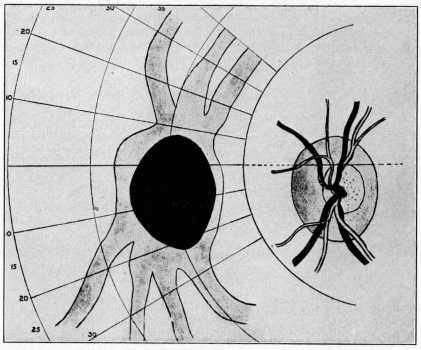

Fig. 14.—The normal blind spot (left) and the disc projected (right). (From Traquair: An Introduction to Clinical Perimetry.)

Contractures in the field are to be considered either as a depression of visual acuity in the entire field with consequent loss of the weakest part, namely, the periphery and the edges of the blind spot, or as an erosion of the edges, per se. The latter is rare, if, indeed, it does occur.

Contractures may be divided into: (A) concentric contraction; here we have reduction in size without much alteration in shape. The so-called tubular field is a special form of concentric contraction. Its character suggests functional origin. (B) Local contraction. In this type, only one part of the field, including the periphery, is affected.

An important form is the sector defect. A sector defect is defined by two radii of the field and the included periphery. Hemianopia and quadrantanopia would then come under this type.

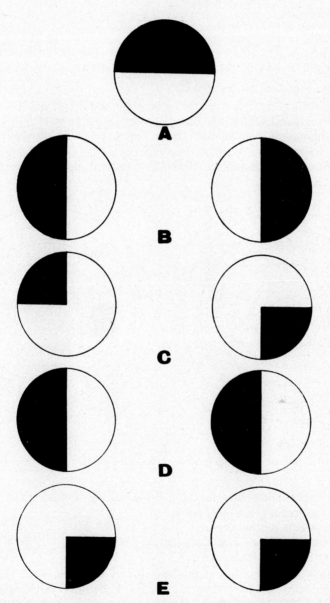

Fig. 15.—Types of hemianopia (diagrammatic). *A*, Horizontal or altitudinal. *B*, Bitemporal. *C*, Bitemporal crossed quadrant. *D*, Homonymous. *E*, Homonymous lower quadrant. (From Traquair: An Introduction to Clinical Perimetry.)

Taking hemianopia to illustrate the various kinds of sector defects based upon positions in the field, we have

1. Affecting one eye (one field)
    a. right or left temporal hemianopia
    b. right or left nasal hemianopia
    c. right or left superior horizontal hemianopia
    d. right or left inferior horizontal hemianopia

2. Affecting both eyes (two fields)
    a. right or left homonymous hemianopia nasal half of one field and the temporal half of the other (optic tract involved)
    b. bitemporal hemianopia (both temporal fields affected) (chiasmal lesion)
    c. Binasal hemianopia. Probably bilateral independent subchiasmal lesion.

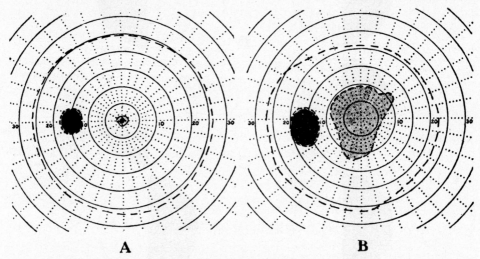

A   **B**

Fig. 16.—*A,* Normal central field with minute central scotoma; *B,* central scotoma for 1/2000 white. (From Traquair: An Introduction to Clinical Perimetry.)

The quadrantanopias affecting both fields may be homonymous, bitemporal, or binasal, inferior, superior, or crossed.

Irregular sector defects occur in diverse forms. Many have the apex at the blind spot and exhibit one boundary on the nasal horizontal meridian. These are nerve fiber bundle defects.

Scotomas.—A scotoma is a patch-like loss of vision in the field.

There are two kinds: that visible as a definite dark spot, positive scotoma, which is due to an opacity anterior to the retina, and negative scotoma, which is recognized as a gap in the visual field. For example, the physiologic blind spot is a negative scotoma.

Scotomas may assume various sizes and shapes.

1. Peripheral
2. Central—Fixation involved
3. Paracentral—Fixation and adjacent areas are involved

4. Pericentral—Adjacent area involved, fixation spared
    a. supracentral
    b. infracentral
    c. temporocentral
    d. nasocentral
5. Centrocecal—Includes central fixation and blind spot. (Papillomacular area involved.)

Examination of the Extraocular Muscles and Position of the Eye

When the gaze is directed off in the distance, the normal position of the visual axes of the two eyes should be parallel. Any deviation from this normal position is caused by an abnormal function or action of one or more of the extraocular muscles. This can be illustrated by an ordinary case of monocular convergent strabismus in which one of the eyes is directed straight ahead while the visual axis of the opposite eye turns in. Another illustration is the inability of one eye to rotate outward beyond a certain point because of a paresis of the sixth nerve on that side. This occurs in a number of infectious diseases, and also as a congenital condition. This is also true of the third nerve which supplies the extraocular muscles with the exception of the external rectus and superior oblique. The next step in the routine examination of the eye should, therefore, be tests of the extraocular muscles to determine any impairment of their function. This, if present, would prevent the possibility of normal function of the two eyes, especially in regard to single binocular vision. Impairment, such as paralysis, might also indicate the presence of intracranial lesions, retrobulbar lesions and others.

When the extraocular muscles are in a state of normal balance, the condition is known as orthophoria, and the visual axes of the two eyes are parallel. When an actual deviation of one or both eyes is present, the condition is obvious and can be observed on inspection. This is designated as heterotropia. In many cases, however, the eyes have only a tendency to deviate, since a normal balance between the ocular muscles does not exist. This condition known as heterophoria is not obvious on ordinary inspection and must be tested for when its presence is suspected.

Test of the Ocular Rotations and Excursions.—Have the patient fix with each eye separately and then with both eyes on the examiner's finger. Direct the patient to hold the head motionless, and to follow the finger as it is moved in all directions. The limitation of movement in any direction can then be noted. Also, whether an eye fixes directly on the finger or to one or the other side of it.

Examination of the Corneal Images.—A light is held by the examiner in front of the patient's eyes and the position of the corneal reflection of the light is noted in each eye. Ordinarily, when the eyes are parallel, the reflection on the cornea of each eye should be identical in position. When one eye deviates, however, the reflection of the light in the cornea of this eye will differ in its position from that of the other eye. This test does not afford an exact estimate of the extent of deviation.

Test for Deviation.—*The Screen Test.*—While the patient looks directly at an object held about 33 cm. in front of the eyes, the examiner quickly moves a card from one eye to the other of the patient while noting if any deviation of either eye is present when the card is removed. If neither eye deviates when this is done, the condition is noted as orthophoria. If either eye turns in under the cover and moves out to fix when the card is shifted to the opposite eye, the condition is revealed as esophoria. If either deviates outward under the card and moves in to fix on shifting the card to the opposite eye, exophoria is denoted. The degree of esophoria present can be measured by placing a prism of sufficient power with its base out in front of each eye to reverse this movement. One degree less than the strength of such a prism will measure the extent of deviation. In exophoria the same procedure is followed using the prisms with the bases in. If, on uncovering either eye, there was a movement downward, the condition is hyperphoria. This can be measured by a prism of sufficient strength to stop the movement placed in front of the opposite side with the base down.

The Parallax Test.—Another test is to cover one eye with a card while the other remains uncovered and fixed upon an object, such as a small light, at a distance of six meters. The card is shifted from one eye to the other, and the patient is asked whether or not the object observed appears to move. If so, he sees one image after the other. If the object moves to the right when the right eye is uncovered, the patient has esophoria with a homonymous diplopia (image of right eye was on the right of the image of left eye). If the object appeared to move to the left, the condition is exophoria with a crossed diplopia (image of right eye to the left of the image of the left eye). If the object appears to move down, right hyperphoria is indicated; if up, left hyperphoria. The strength of a prism placed before the eyes with its base in a direction to stop the movement of the object observed, will measure the amount of the parallax present. For example, if a homonymous parallax is overcome by a $10^\triangle$ prism base out in front of the eye, the amount of esophoria is equal to $10^\triangle$.

Additional methods for testing the ocular muscle balance by using the Maddox rod and phorometer, can be found in any textbook on refraction and muscles, covering this subject in detail.

Test for Convergence—Near Point.—The nearest point on which the eyes can be converged with an effort is called the convergence near point. This can be determined by moving a small object, such as a small light or pencil point, up to the eyes while the patient observes it as close as possible. The nearest point at which he can do this can be measured, and will indicate the near point. At the same time, the examiner may observe whether or not the two eyes converge equally and to the same extent. In cases of convergence weakness, especially of one eye, this eye can be seen to lag.

Test for Diplopia.—The diplopia is dependent on the deviation, which determines its character and extent. A muscle paralysis that causes deviation inward will show a homonymous diplopia, while that causing a deviation outward is characterized by a crossed diplopia. A vertical deviation is associated with a vertical diplopia. The diplopia increases according to the extent of the deviation of the affected muscle, consequently, the greater the deviation, the greater is the separation between the images of the two eyes.

If the diplopia is found to be principally lateral, it increases when looking to the right or to the left; the paralysis must affect a lateral rotator. A right rotator is affected if the diplopia increases to the right. This would indicate either the right external rectus or left internal rectus. If it increases to the left, it points to a left rotator, either the left external rectus or the right internal rectus.

If the diplopia is homonymous, the external is paralyzed; if crossed, it is the internal. When the diplopia is principally vertical and increases quickly when looking up, an elevator is paralyzed. This will be a right-hand elevator, either the right superior rectus or left superior oblique, if the vertical diplopia increases mostly in looking up and to the right. If it increases looking up and to the left, the paralyzed muscle is a left-hand elevator, either the left superior rectus or the right inferior oblique. The higher image belongs to the paralyzed eye, for example, in paralysis of the right superior rectus and right superior oblique, the image of the right eye is higher.

If the vertical diplopia increases quickly in looking down, a depressor muscle is paralyzed. This would indicate a right-hand depressor, the right inferior rectus and left superior oblique, if the vertical diplopia increased principally in looking down to the right. If it increases mostly in looking down and to the left, a left-hand depressor, the left inferior rectus, and right superior oblique are paralyzed. The lower image belongs to the eye which is paralyzed.

The image of the paralyzed eye always lies on the side toward which the diplopia increases. The field of double vision is measured on a tangent screen or curtain, one side of which is black. The patient is placed in a position facing the black side of the screen at a distance of ¾ M. The eyes of the patient are directed to a pin in the center of the curtain, and on the same level a red glass is placed before the right eye of the patient. The examiner then moves a small electric light across the curtain in six cardinal directions, that is, directly to the right, directly to the left, up and to the right, up and to the left, down to the right, and down to the left. The points where diplopia occurs in each direction are noted by inserting a pin in the curtain, when the patient indicates that he sees two lights—one red and one white. The red light belongs to the right eye, and the white light to the left eye. A black pin is placed in the curtain at the position of the examiner's electric light, and a light colored pin at the position of the other image. The second is the false image, and if this is red, it indicates that the left eye is fixing. If it is white, the right eye is fixing. The position of the pins will disclose the degree of separation of the two images. The plot formed by the pins on the curtain shows the limits of the field of single vision, and the amount and the kind of diplopia which can be read on a diagram laid out on the back of the curtain. This can then be transferred to a card which is marked with a similar diagram, and can be kept as a permanent record.

CHAPTER IV

STRUCTURAL ABNORMALITIES AND MANIFESTATIONS

Examination of the Eyelids

Inspection is the means for examination of the eyelids and the conjunctival sac. The principal points on the eyelids to be noted are the condition of the margins and the cutaneous surfaces, the length and width of the palpebral fissures, the condition of the internal and external canthi, the lashes, the caruncle, and the puncta lacrimali.

The skin of the lids should be thin, delicate, and freely movable. It is somewhat darker than the skin elsewhere. In infancy and early childhood, the skin surface of the lid is smooth and rounded out due to the presence of fat. This disappears in later life, so that the skin which is now less elastic, is thrown into folds. The creasing and folding of the skin increases usually with advancing age.

At the base of the upper lid is a deep furrow where the skin passes under the overhanging brow. This furrow may deepen with age either from an increase of fat in the brow tissues, or from absorption of the orbital fat, and a recession of the palpebral base line. The furrow is more or less obliterated when the lids are closed. The furrow is also obliterated when the lid is swollen, as from edema or inflammation. The lower lid, which is continuous with the cheek, has only a slight line of demarcation which is produced by a few creases corresponding to the position of the lower orbital margin. When the lower lid is swollen or edematous, the lower boundary line becomes accentuated. The lid margins are transitional between the skin surface anteriorly and the mucous membrane surface posteriorly. The exact dividing line is a rather well-marked angular ridge immediately back of the lashes.

Abnormalities of the Eyelids

Ankyloblepharon.—The lid margins may be united throughout their entire length (congenital ankyloblepharon) or at one of several points by connecting bands (partial ankyloblepharon). Ankyloblepharon at the outer canthus reduces the normal length of the palpebral fissure simulating blepharophimosis. (See congenital anomalies of the lids.)

Blepharophimosis.—The palpebral fissure is shortened at the outer canthus by the encroachment of a vertical fold of skin. If this fold is obliterated by stretching the skin beyond the canthus, the lid margins are found to be normal and not adherent. This differentiates the condition from ankyloblepharon. It is very often an acquired condition and may be caused by chronic conjunctival inflammations and long continued lacrimation and blepharophimosis. The constant moisture around the outer canthus may result in eczema.

Entropion.—A turning inward of the entire lid margin toward the eyeball. As a result, the lashes are brought into contact with the eyeball and are crowded into the conjunctival sac, causing a constant wetting and matted appearance. The condition may be either spastic (muscular) or cicatricial (organic).

Spastic entropion is due to an overaction of those fibers of the orbicularis muscle which lie next to the lid margin. It almost always affects the lower lid. It may be caused by irritation due to conjunctivitis, keratitis, loose skin, or it may occasionally occur after the application of a bandage for several days as after cataract operation. It may also occur after removal of the eyeball, or in enophthalmos when the normal relationship between the lid and its supporting structures is disturbed.

Cicatricial entropion results from disease or injury of the tarsal and conjunctival portions of the lid. The most frequent cause is trachoma which has progressed to the late stage in which the conjunctiva and tarsus are destroyed as such, and in large part replaced by connective tissue and contracting scars. It may also result from cicatrization following burns, incised wounds, severe destructive inflammations, such as diphtheritic conjunctivitis.

As a result of the cilia being turned against the cornea and bulbar conjunctiva, it may cause injection and lacrimation; the corneal epithelium may become thickened and denuded, which may be followed by ulceration and vascularization. As the result of constant irritation from the tears the margins of the lids become reddened and eczematous. The cilia become a constant source of irritation, and the patient always complains of a sensation of a foreign body irritating the eye.

On examination the lid can be seen to be turned in and when entropion is complete, the margin of the lid is hidden from view. With a spastic entropion the conjunctiva will show no scarring and nothing more than perhaps a slight thickening and injection from the irritation present. When the skin of the lid is drawn downward, it will spring back into its original position when released, only to turn in again as soon as the patient winks or moves the eye.

Ectropion is the condition occurring in eversion of the lid from the eyeball. It may be either spastic, paralytic, senile, or cicatricial. It nearly always affects the lower lid, but the spastic and cicatricial varieties may also affect the upper lid.

In spastic ectropion, there is an excessive power given in some instances to the fibers of the orbicularis muscle lying next to the orbital zone of the lids. Thickening of the conjunctiva from prolonged conjunctivitis, protrusion of the eyeball, and pressure from cysts or tumors forcing the lids forward may act as mechanical contributing factors. Sometimes in children suffering with disease of the conjunctiva or cornea which is attended with blepharospasm, an acute temporary blepharospasm can be produced when the lids are everted for the purpose of examination or treatment. The tarsal plate being reversed, is held in this position by spasm of the orbicularis muscle.

Paralytic ectropion occurs in the lower lid as a result of facial paralysis involving the orbicularis muscle. Being deprived of its innervation it becomes relaxed and fails to remain in contact with the eyeball. It falls away so that the lacrimal punctum also loses its close adherence to the eyeball, resulting in interference with normal drainage of the tears.

Senile ectropion occurs in aged people as the result of a loss of muscle tone in the orbicularis. The muscle then becomes relaxed and fails to maintain its normal position. It affects only the lower lid and may result in chronic conjunctivitis and blepharitis.

Cicatricial ectropion is usually the result of an injury or of a destructive inflammatory process. It may affect either lid. The most common causes are burns and lacerated wounds resulting in cicatrices which may draw the lid away from the eyeball.

On examination, the lid in ectropion will be seen to be drawn away from the eyeball and retracted. As a result the lacrimal punctum is no longer in contact with the eyeball and in addition to interference with normal tear drainage, there may be signs of redness, thickening of the lid, an inflamed and eczematous condition of the lid margin. As a result of exposure, the bulbar conjunctiva may become thickened and reddened resulting in a chronic conjunctivitis. The cornea also may show signs of a keratitis resulting from exposure because of imperfect closure of the lid.

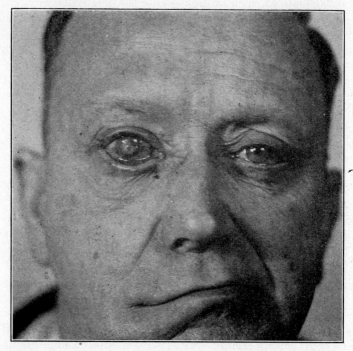

Fig. 17.—Paralytic ectropion. Note the paralysis of right side of face with sagging of right lower eyelid. (I. S. Tassman, Wills Hospital.)

Trichiasis.—When the lashes are turned inward and remain in contact with the eyeball, the condition is known as trichiasis. Although the cilia are inverted, the lid margin retains its normal position. Trichiasis may be either partial, when only part of the cilia are inverted, or total, when all of the cilia are directed inward. The cilia themselves are usually irregular and broken. The condition usually occurs as a result of trachoma or old cases of blepharitis. The symptoms result from direct irritation and are photophobia, lacrimation, and the feeling of the presence of a foreign body. The bulbar conjunctiva becomes thickened, the corneal epithelium thickens, blood vessels form under the epithelium causing the condition known as pannus, and the cornea may ulcerate. Very often the offending cilia producing these complications are overlooked because of an incomplete examination. Those cilia near the inner canthus are very fine and sometimes can be seen only with the aid of a loupe.

Distichiasis is a condition in which a supplementary or extra row of cilia is present and is also directed inward to irritate the eyeball. Such a double row of cilia is usually acquired although it may be congenital. The lashes of the inner or second row are shorter and finer than those of the normal row. The constant irritation occurring in distichiasis results in practically the same symptoms as those occurring in entropion and trichiasis. The bulbar conjunctiva becomes injected and thickened; there is a constant sensation of a foreign body being present; excessive lacrimation and photophobia are disturbing and a gradual narrowing of the palpebral fissure may take place.

Epicanthus is a bilateral and symmetrical condition of the eyelids, in which a vertical fold of skin passes downward from the inner extremity of the brow to the inner extremity of the lower lid at its junction with the side of the nose. This is always a congenital condition and is described in that chapter.

The Skin of the Eyelids.—The skin of the eyelids and adnexa may be affected by a great variety of conditions and pathologic processes. It is particularly exposed and sensitive to the heat and cold and to many irritations and traumatisms from without. It may become stretched and broken by conditions which exist beneath it, such as subcutaneous tumors and collections of fluids. Alterations in the secretions affecting the several kinds and various glands may greatly affect the pathology of the skin, as may also bacteriologic and parasitic infections. Degeneration of the skin is a physiologic condition in old age and is characterized by thinning of the corium and an increase in pigment. It may also play a pathologic role.

The skin of the eyelids may be affected by a number of dermatologic lesions, either primary or secondary. The primary lesions may include macula, papules, tubercles, wheals, tumors, vesicles, blebs, and pustules.

The secondary lesions result from more or less complete subsidence of a pathologic process, or they may result from a mechanical injury, such as a laceration or an insect bite. Among the secondary lesions affecting the skin of the eyelids are:

Hypertrophy or thickening, which results from the imperfect involution of inflammatory exudates.

Cicatrices or scars, resulting from complete healing of an inflammatory infiltration which has been of sufficient intensity to destroy a part of the corium.

Pigmentation which may result from almost any primary lesion.

Excoriations resulting from rupture of vesicles or pustules.

Ulcers remaining after inflammatory destruction of the deeper tissues.

Fissures which are a variety of ulceration representing a tear in the pathologically changed skin.

Scales which may result from the subsidence of macules or papules, also from the drying of exudate on the skin surface, following the rupture of vesicles and scabs, sebaceous material. Scab formation may occur with any of the other conditions.

Swelling and edema of the eyelids occur frequently. One or both eyes may be involved as the result of local inflammation or secondary to a circulatory disturbance.   Usually swelling will yield to finger pressure which produces pitting.   Edema and redness of the lids may occur on one side as a result of sinus disease.   Circulatory disturbances may cause an edema of the eyelids which is more pronounced at certain times, depending principally on the position of the patient.   Allergy and sensitivity may cause edema of the eyelids and it may also occur in some of the acute infectious diseases.   Depending upon the extent and severity of the swelling and edema, there will be a corresponding amount of interference with the action of the eyelid, so that in marked cases, the eye may be completely closed.   In such cases the skin of the lids is very tense and firm, and in the presence of inflammation, may be hot and tender to the touch.   As the edema subsides, the skin becomes more loose and wrinkled.   In extreme cases of swelling and edema it will be impossible to part the lids for examination of the eyeball.   It is, therefore, necessary to employ a lid retractor or an instrument known as a Desmarres elevator, which after being slightly moistened can be gently inserted between the margins of the two lids and slowly drawn up or down, thereby exposing the eyeball to view.

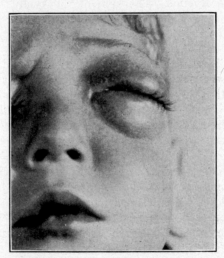

Fig. 18.—Swelling and edema with closure of the eyelids.   (From Dr. J. S. Shipman Clinic, Wills Hospital.)

Herpes may occur on the eyelids and is characterized by a collection of small vesicles, which may be accompanied by swelling and redness around the lesion.   These may occur in some of the febrile conditions and infections.   They may produce considerable itching and burning.

Hordeolum occurs very frequently on the eyelids as the result of suppuration in the glands of the lid.   When Zeis's glands are affected, it results in external hordeolum while suppuration of the meibomian glands of the tarsus causes what is known as hordeolum interna.   The latter is less common but more difficult to correct because of the dense and tough nature of the tarsus.   In order to be exposed to view, it is necessary for the examiner to evert the eyelid.

These hordeola or styes are very often located close to or at the margin of the lid.   They may be accompanied by considerable swelling and edema of the surrounding eyelid.   They are very tender to the touch, especially over a small, circumscribed area near the center. A small, white, or yellowish-white spot will appear at this point in a day or so, which is the focus at which the pus collects. Usually the collection reaches a stage where it automatically ruptures. They usually occur in children and young people, particularly in those who are undernourished. They may also occur in association with uncorrected refracted errors.

Sometimes, when seen early, the hordeolum can be cleared up by removal of the cilia which can be seen to extend from the tip of the swelling. In other cases the application of heat will serve to soften the swelling and lead to an evacuation of the pus. This is usually found to be caused by the staphylococcus. When the condition does not respond otherwise, it is necessary to incise and curette the infection. A mild antiseptic wash, such as boric acid or metaphen solution, can be prescribed, after which the condition will gradually subside and disappear. In some patients hordeola may occur multiple or they may be recurrent. In these some underlying factor, such as chronic constipation, anemia, poor nutrition, refractive errors, some irregularities of glandular function or menstruation may be present and should be looked for.

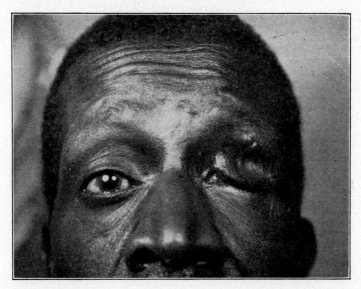

Fig. 19.—Cicatrix of the eyelid. (I. S. Tassman, Wills Hospital.)

Chalazion is the result of a chronic or long-standing infection of the meibomian glands which results in a small, slowly growing tumor or swelling in the lid. It is more common in the upper lid although the lower lid is also frequently affected. Usually it is not accompanied by redness, soreness, or other external signs of inflammation and it rarely causes pain. The patient is conscious of its presence, however, and when it reaches sufficient size it feels heavy, interferes with the action of the eyelid and appears unsightly. Occasionally several may be present at the same time. On palpation the chalazion can be felt under the finger as a small, hard swelling. It may reach a size where it can almost be grasped between the thumb and forefinger. In the larger ones the skin of the lid fits tightly over the swelling. Chalazia usually extend deeply in the lid and may project through to the tarsal plate. Here they are closely adherent especially when they are of long duration.

Their treatment consists in surgical removal, by incision over the swelling and a clean dissection, if possible, with excision of the entire sac.

Blepharitis Marginalis.—A subacute or chronic inflammation of the margins of the eyelids affecting the cilia and glands. It usually occurs in one of two forms, namely, squamous blepharitis and ulcerative blepharitis. In the squamous type the skin around the margins of the lids is covered with fine, white, flaky scales which can be easily removed, or wiped off with an applicator. The skin at the edge of the lid is also slightly reddened. The cilia are usually broken off with removal of the scales but will later regenerate, since the follicles are not destroyed. In some cases the margins of the lid become moist from a secretion which usually collects and hardens into small crusts producing a seborrheic condition around the base of the cilia.

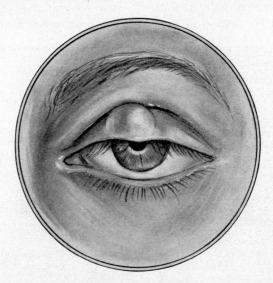

Fig. 20.—Chalazion of the upper eyelid.

When the crusts are removed, in some cases an ulceration is present at the base. This occurs in the ulcerative blepharitis; suppuration of the follicles and sebaceous glands takes place and pus can be found when the cilia are removed. Ulceration results from the suppuration and with healing, scar formation occurs with destruction of the hair follicles. In long-standing cases the cilia are found to be short and matted together. Many of the eyelashes are destroyed and they may be present only in small patches. The edges of the lids are always reddened and later become thickened and heavy. Trichiasis may result and with change in the position of the punctum, epiphora and lacrimation will occur.

The condition is very common among children and young people, especially in those who may also be suffering with other disturbances of secretion, assimilation, nutrition, and anemia. Many young women with pale skin and in an apparently undernourished condition will be found to be affected with blepharitis. In addition, exposure to certain irritating external influences may tend to aggravate the condition. Fumes and smoke, loss of sleep, and continued exposure to strong light may be contributing factors. The condition may be accompanied by other affections such as hordeolum, conjunctivitis and phlyctenules of the conjunctiva.

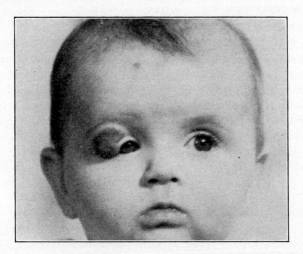

Fig. 21.—Hemangioma of eyelid in a baby aged 4 months. (I S. Tassman, Willis Hospital.)

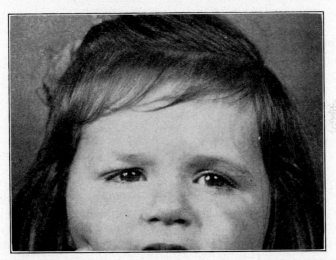

Fig. 22.—Photograph of same patient shown in Fig. 21 two years later. Hemangioma completely removed. (I. S. Tassman, Willis Hospital.)

Blepharitis is treated by both local and general means. In spite of all treatment, however, the condition, especially when of long standing, is very obstinate and does not respond well except for temporary remissions. Occasionally, it may run its course and cease to be troublesome after full development of the individual, but these instances are rare. The efforts of treatment in nearly all cases should be directed in general toward building up and improving the physical condition of the patient, and if possible, toward correcting any underlying disorder. The nutrition of the patient should be improved by a satisfactory diet. In many instances improper food or excessive use of certain kinds of food, such as sweets, candy, pies, pastry, and so forth, should be eliminated. Fresh air, sunlight, and good hygienic conditions are essential. Cod-liver oil should be prescribed and other internal medication including tonics should be employed. Errors of refraction, when present, as they often are, should be properly and regularly corrected. The eyelids should be cleansed regularly morning and night with a warm solution of boric acid or plain warm water. The scales and crusts should be removed from the edges of the lids. This can be done by using a small cotton applicator tightly packed, the tip containing a small amount of boric ointment. This should always be done before retiring at night. Ammoniated mercury ointment, 1 per cent, and yellow oxide of mercury ointment, 1 per cent, are commonly prescribed for local use, but these may only prove of very temporary benefit in cleansing the lid of scales. Broken and inverted cilia should be removed with a pair of forceps and the surrounding skin area should be kept dry and free of any secretion. The local use of 5 per cent sulfathiazole ointment has recently been found to be very effective.

Tumors and Cysts of Eyelids.—The eyelids may be the seat of either malignant or benign tumors and cysts. Carcinoma, beginning as a papule, may occur on the edges of the lid resulting in ulcers which are at first small, and later spread gradually destroying the structure of the lid and surrounding tissues. Sarcoma may occur in the form of pigmented melanosarcoma. Epithelioma is not uncommon, as well as chancre and chancroid of the eyelid. Any ulceration should be examined closely and studied carefully, employing all means available before a diagnosis of the condition is made.

Angiomas may be present in the eyelids as well as other varieties of tumors, such as fibromas, lipomas, adenomas of the glands, and lymphomas.

Examination of the Lacrimal Apparatus

Examination of the lacrimal apparatus is made principally by inspection and palpation. In suspected cases of obstruction, lacrimal probes and lacrimal syringes are employed. The superior lacrimal gland is ordinarily concealed within the orbit which prevents inspection, but when enlarged, as in inflammation, abscess, or tumor, it may be seen to present behind the base of the lid beneath the orbital margin and displace the eyeball. Since the lacrimal gland is the only structure occupying the upper, outer angle of the orbit, this condition is very characteristic. On the other hand, the palpebral or accessory glands are more easily inspected by everting the upper lid and rolling out the fornix. The normal superior gland can be reached by deep palpation under the orbital margin through the base of the lid. It is located with less difficulty when enlarged, inflamed, or painful. The accessory glands can be palpated through the upper lid at its base, or directly, when exposed through the conjunctiva of the fornix.

In the examination of the lacrimal apparatus the points to be determined are the position of the puncta lacrimali, whether or not they are patent, the condition of the lacrimal sac, and the condition of the nasal duct. The openings of the canaliculi at the puncta should normally be in contact with the bulbar conjunctiva. Guided by capillarity, the tears can then normally enter the canaliculi. Their position can be determined, therefore, by direct inspection, on drawing the inner third of the lid margin gently away from the eyeball and then permitting it to return to its original position.

The lacrimal sac should normally transmit the ocular secretions, and when obstructed, these secretions are retained instead of flowing into the inferior meatus of the nose, and the sac becomes distended. This may produce a rounded swelling just below the inner canthus of the eye which is known as a mucocele. When pressure is made over such a swelling, the contents of the sac may be forced slowly downward through a partially obstructed nasal duct, or may return through the canaliculi into the conjunctival sac. In dacryocystitis pressure over this area will also cause pus to flow from the canaliculus above.

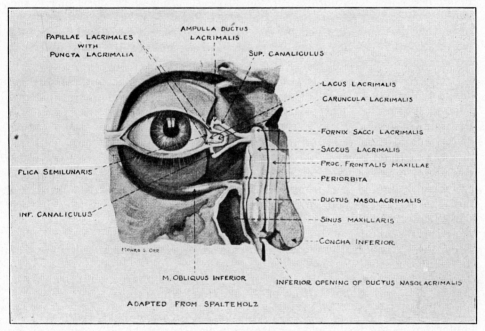

Fig. 23.—Anatomy of the tear passages adapted from Spalteholz. (From Ramsay: Clinical Ophthalmology for the General Practitioner, Oxford Medical Publications.)

The lacrimal sac and lower portion of the lacrimal canal, or the nasal duct, can be explored especially for obstruction by the use of probes. The most common probes in use are known as Bowman's probes. These are cylindrical in shape, and are made in about eight sizes. They are flexible but firm. Passing a probe through the lacrimal canal should be performed with great care, although some guarded force may be required in the proper direction. The probe should be curved to correspond to the probable course in its passage. The lid is drawn outward thereby putting tension on the canaliculus and leading a straight line into the sac. The tip of the probe is then introduced into the canaliculus, being directed horizontally, until it reaches the wall of the nose with which it comes in contact. The direction of the probe is then changed after withdrawing it very slightly, by swinging the distal end upward through a vertical arc, so that it is now held vertically. This movement will at the same time draw the edge of the lids inward. The probe is then in position to be passed down through the nasal duct into the nose. From this point on, the guiding hand must retain control of the probe which is pushed downward steadily but slowly and guardedly. Lack of care in this respect might lead to forcing a false passage. The probe is then guided downward, backward, and slightly outward into the canal, or until it meets an obstruction. The presence of such an obstruction is transmitted to the guiding hand. In carrying out this procedure, it is necessary to begin by introducing the smallest probe, and, in many instances, it is necessary to dilate the punctum first with a very fine pointed dilator. In other instances, it might be found necessary to slit the canaliculus with a canaliculus knife. This was done more commonly in the past than at the present time, and is rarely found necessary. Withdrawal of the probe should also be done slowly and quietly. When a probe is properly inserted, it will feel locked, and when the projecting portion is grasped by the examiner, it cannot be rocked freely in a lateral direction. When a smaller probe has been successfully introduced, it is withdrawn and probes of larger size are used.

The lacrimal syringe is also employed in diagnosis to determine whether or not the canal is patent. This will afford an even better knowledge than the passage of a probe. The passage of the fluid through the lacrimal canal will determine how rapidly and freely this occurs and may also indicate the condition of the mucous membrane and the amount of infection present, if any.

The lacrimal syringe consists of the usual style barrel and plunger. The tips are of different sizes and forms. The barrel is filled with a solution such as normal saline or mercurophen. The tip is inserted into the canalicus, and then the barrel is fitted in. Having accomplished this, the plunger is very slowly and gradually pressed forward into the barrel. In cases of marked obstruction, the solution is forced back and regurgitates through the canaliculus, filling the conjunctival sac. When patent, however, the patient will state that the solution reaches the nose.

Abnormalities of the Lacrimal Apparatus

Occlusion.—Both the puncta and the canaliculi may be contracted or obliterated as the result of injury to their membranes, which would result in an interference with normal drainage of the tears. The canaliculus or canaliculi may also become occluded because of the presence of foreign bodies and concretions. Small masses of fungi occurring in streptothricosis and in sporotrichosis may form the obstruction.

Eversion of the puncta is sometimes found in early ectropion which also prevents the normal drainage of tears.

Epiphora.—Epiphora is a very common symptom which is caused by either increase in secretion or an interference with the drainage of the tears. It is characterized by a more or less constant "watering" of the eyes, and therefore gives rise at times to the term, "watery eye." It is caused by exposure to irritants, such as cold air, intense smoke, foreign bodies on the eyeball, inflammations of the eye and nose, and irritation of the first and second branches of the trigeminus. Any of the conditions which would prevent the normal conduction of tears into the nose result in epiphora. The symptom is often complained of by older people, in whom there can be found no specific cause. This is usually aggravated by exposure to cold weather. In some instances epiphora might be caused by abnormal irritability of the nasal mucous membrane.

Abnormalities of the Lacrimal Gland.—The lacrimal gland may suffer from an inflammatory condition which may occur principally with mumps. The condition is known as dacryadenitis and may cause a suppurative condition of the gland which terminates either in eventual resolution or in other cases abscess formation and the discharge of pus. The treatment of dacryadenitis is mainly symptomatic and depends on whether or not suppuration is present and the extent and degree of the same.

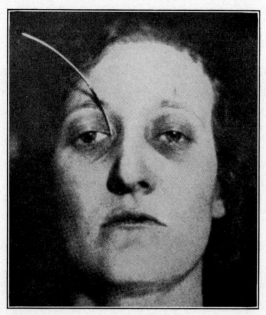

Fig. 24.—Patient with probe through the opening of the tear sac. (From Goar: Arch. Ophth. November, 1931.)

Mikulicz's Disease.—Under Mikulicz's disease are included all cases of symmetric bilateral noninflammatory enlargement of the lacrimal glands, with accompanying enlargement of the salivary glands, especially the parotid. According to Leucutia and Price[1] the swelling of these glands occurs without involvement of the lymphatic system and without alteration of the blood. Those cases in which enlargements of the lacrimal and salivary glands are manifestations of some well-defined disease, such as leucemia, tuberculosis, syphilis, lymphosarcoma, Hodgkin's disease, and uveoparotid fever, should be included under the term Mikulicz's syndrome. They stated that Mikulicz's disease should not be considered an "aleucemic stage" of leucemia because with the former the average duration of life is considerably longer, and the radiosensitivity of the lymphocytic infiltration is definitely less in Mikulicz's disease than in the more malignant and less differentiated lymphatic proliferations in leucemia.

The symptoms are swelling and drooping of the lids with marked narrowing of the palpebral fissure. Sclerosis and destruction of the gland have been said to occur with cessation of the lacrimal secretion.

Leucutia and Price treated Mikulicz's disease by radiation therapy employing divided doses, from 15 to 50 per cent of an erythema dose, spread over a long period, rather than one single massive dose. The cases which they grouped as Mikulicz's syndrome require a technique which should conform to the routine procedure of irradiation employed in the particular entity which is associated.

Tumors.—The lacrimal gland may be involved by tumor growths which result in its enlargement and accompanying pressure symptoms. These tumors include adenoma, carcinoma, myoma, and cylindroma. They are considered mostly to be mixed tumors.

The treatment of tumors of the lacrimal gland is surgical removal. Since most of the growths are superficial, this can be accomplished with little difficulty by an incision parallel with the upper inner margin of the orbit.

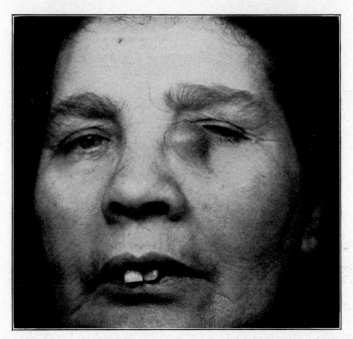

Fig. 25.—Dacryocystitis with acute lacrimal abscess.

Dacryocystitis.—Inflammation of the lacrimal sac is known as dacryocystitis. It is usually due to an interference with the drainage of tears through the tear sac with consequent damming back of the tears. An obstruction in the sac should always be looked for and attempt made to inject saline solution into the canaliculus to determine whether or not it runs into the nose. In mild cases the only symptom may be epiphora without distention of the sac. In advanced cases distention of the sac may occur, with suppuration. When moderate pressure is made over the region of the sac at the inner angle of the eye, pus can be expressed from the puncta on the affected side.

The immediate cause of the obstruction which results in an inflammation of the sac and dacryocystitis is often difficult to determine. It may result from the presence of inflammation in the nasal mucous membrane or from obstruction in the nose caused by polyps. It may also result from cicatricial contraction following ulceration occurring in syphilis and tuberculosis. In the latter condition the infection can also be transmitted from the conjunctival sac.

The disease usually runs a chronic course over a long period of time. The sac becomes distended with pus in advanced cases. The condition is always aggravated by smoke, air, and other irritants. In some cases the distention extends up under the skin of the nose and ruptures through the sac. A superficial abscess may form with redness, tenderness, and chemosis of the skin of the eyelid. This is accompanied by pain and in some cases, an elevation in temperature. With perforation, the pus is discharged. This is followed by relief from pain and swelling, but a lacrimal fistula results. The latter may eventually heal with the possibility of a recurrence of the dacryocystitis.

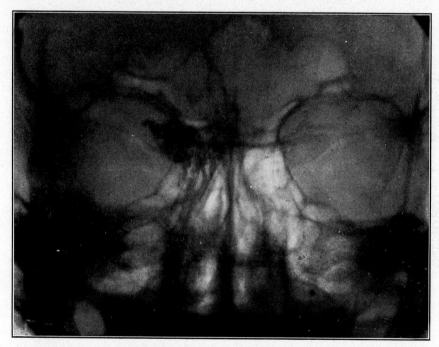

Fig. 26.—Lipiodol injection of a lacrimal sac in a dacryocystitis. (Spaeth.)

The treatment of dacryocystitis is symptomatic and surgical. The former is directed toward the relief of the constriction and clearing up the infection by use of antiseptic solutions injected into the sac. In advanced cases which have failed to yield to the nonoperative treatment with sounds and irrigation, surgical removal of the infected sac is indicated.

Examination of the Conjunctival Sac

In order to examine the palpebral conjunctiva, and that of the upper and lower fornix or cul-de-sac, it is necessary to evert the lids. This must always be done. Eversion of the lower lid is a very simple procedure; it is necessary only to place a finger on the lid near the middle and just below the lower border of the tarsus. The patient is told to look upward while the lid is drawn downward. This causes the tarsus to reverse and the lid to evert. The greater the rotation of the eyeball upward, the better the fornix rolls into view. It is sometimes necessary to manipulate the examining finger, in order to get it under the fornix and push it up.

Eversion of the upper lid is more difficult and should be practiced in order to avoid pain and irritation to the eyeball. It is necessary when the upper lid is being everted, for the eyeball to be rotated far downward. This requires the cooperation of the patient, since it is impossible to turn the upper lid when the eyeball is rolled upward, without using great force and causing pain and discomfort to the patient.

The examiner should face the patient and place the finger tips of his left hand on the patient's forehead, leaving the thumb to swing free. The patient is then told to *look down,* and no attempt should be made to proceed further until the eyes are so rotated. The tip of the thumb of the left hand is then placed on the lid and the skin of the lid drawn a little upward. This causes a slight eversion of the lid margin, and by maintaining this condition for a few moments, and insisting upon continued downward rotation, the spasm of the orbicularis which frequently ensues as soon as the lids are touched, relaxes. At this point the right hand is brought into service. The edge of the lid including the lashes is now grasped gently between the thumb and forefinger of the right hand. The lid is drawn a little downward and away from the eyeball, and is held fixed in this position. The thumb of the left hand then pushes directly downward all of the lid tissues lying above the upper border of the tarsus. The tarsus, owing to its firmness, then snaps over the thumb of the left hand and reverses. The important points in the manipulation are not to seize the lashes alone with the right hand, but to grasp the edge of the lid including the lashes, and not to attempt to turn the edge of the lid up over the thumb as a fulcrum, but to hold the lid margin away from the eyeball and push the upper tarsal border behind it. If the lashes alone are held, it may cause pain, and if any upward motion or traction is made at the lid margin, the patient is apt to turn the eyeball up also. The duty of the thumb of the left hand is first to press gently on the eyeball and thus aid the patient in maintaining downward rotation; then to slip the skin up a little and explore the margin; and finally at the proper moment, to carry all underlying tissues downward. In performing the latter movement, the firm but light pressure on the eyeball is not disagreeable to the patient, and aids in the downward rotation. It is not necessary to use a pencil, matchstick, or other instrument instead of the thumb, since this may prove a hindrance, and should the patient draw away just at the critical moment, he cannot be followed as readily as when the hand of the examiner is resting on the forehead. Employing the procedure described, the head of the patient can be controlled and the upper lid is everted without difficulty and without annoyance to the patient.

The upper lid thus everted exposes only the tarsal conjunctiva. For exposure of the fornix, further manipulation is necessary. Before this is done however, the tarsal conjunctiva should be inspected by the examiner to note its color, whether or not its surface is smooth or contains any elevations, irregularities, scars, signs of discharge, or foreign body. The latter when present might be very small and the examination should be made in good light; an ordinary hand flashlight for direct illumination can be employed, or any good office lamp might provide the illumination.

In order to expose the fornix to view, the margin of the everted lid can be pushed firmly upward toward the brow with the thumb of the right hand, then the eyeball is rotated strongly downward and the thumb of the left hand is placed against the lower lid and pushed gently against the eyeball. In this way the fornix can in most cases be made to roll completely outward.

Great difficulty is sometimes experienced in everting old trachomatous eyelids. These are often short, the tarsal plate having been destroyed, and the lashes gone. This leaves a smooth rounded margin which cannot be seized between the thumb and forefinger. Such lids can be better turned with one hand. The thumb is placed against the lower margin of the lower lid with the nail extending out, and the forefinger draws the lid downward so that it rides up on the thumb. The thumb is then passed under the lid, and with a quick turn the lid is held between the thumb and finger, after which it can be everted.

When the patient is a young child, it may be necessary to place the head with the face turned upward between the knees of the examiner, while a nurse or assistant holds the arms of the patient. The lids can then be everted as described above, and the conjunctival sac examined. It might be helpful in some instances to instill one drop of a 4 per cent solution of cocaine into the conjunctival sac before attempting to evert the lid. This might tend to relieve any spasm which is present.

Abnormalities of the Conjunctiva

The conjunctiva may be the seat of a large variety of lesions, either of a primary nature, or secondary to some inflammation or disease elsewhere. All of the lesions discussed can be observed on examination by direct inspection and with direct illumination.

Papillae or small, rounded elevations may be seen on the tarsal conjunctiva. In vernal conjunctivitis or spring catarrh, such elevations occur in large numbers and cover the entire tarsal conjunctiva of the lid, giving it a typical cobblestone appearance. In follicular conjunctivitis elevated follicles are seen on the tarsal and palpebral conjunctiva. They resemble very much the elevations occurring in vernal conjunctivitis in some instances, but are smaller in size, and give the conjunctiva a velvety appearance. Both of these conditions can usually be observed on eversion of the lids. They cause considerable irritation to the eyeball and are accompanied by photophobia and lacrimation.

Scars.—These may be found on the under surface of the upper lid especially, and are common in cases of long-standing trachoma and severe burns. They usually appear as white or grayish-white patches, more or less circumscribed in certain areas of the tarsal conjunctiva.

Hyperemia.—Congestion or injection of the conjunctival vessels is a common finding in nearly all cases of irritation or inflammation. A small foreign body lodged on the eyeball for a very short time might cause considerable injection of the bulbar conjunctiva. In many instances the injection is general throughout the conjunctiva, while in others, it is confined to those vessels around the limbus of the cornea. The latter is designated as pericorneal or circumcorneal injection and is characteristic in iritis and iridocyclitis. It is usually slightly darker than that occurring in the periphery.

Edema and Chemosis occur very frequently as the result of irritation and early inflammation. They are characterized by a flabby swelling of the membrane which might be seen to protrude between the eyelids in very marked cases. They occur in nearly all forms of conjunctivitis, trauma, insect bites, as a result of sinus disease, and occasionally as the result of pressure from orbital growths.

Hemorrhage usually occurs under the conjunctiva and is known as sub-conjunctival hemorrhage. It can be readily recognized on inspection by a more or less circumscribed area of blood in and under the conjunctival membrane. The appearance is unmistakable. It is usually caused by trauma, foreign bodies striking the conjunctiva, and rupture of small conjunctival vessels from excessive strain.

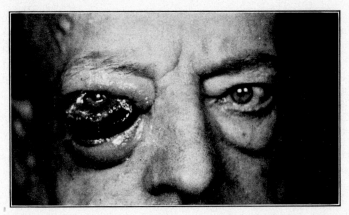

Fig. 28.—Chemosis of the conjunctiva. (Clinic of Dr. W. J. Harrison, Wills Hospital.)

Vesicles may occur in the conjunctiva as herpes in which they are usually found in the bulbar portion. They are not common but might be found with some febrile conditions and infectious diseases. Vesicles in the form of bullae occur in the fornix and bulbar conjunctiva in pemphigus. This is a more serious disease which might affect the conjunctiva, and in which these vesicles or bullae ulcerate and later cause cicatrization with a drying of the conjunctiva. The condition is very chronic and usually terminates in the loss of sight and shrinking of the eyeball.

Pinguecula are small, rounded and slightly raised areas which are usually yellowish in color and occur in the conjunctiva just outside or near the limbus of the cornea. They represent a thickening of the conjunctiva and are said to be caused by exposure to air and wind. No other specific cause is known.

Symblepharon.—Bands of connective tissue which result usually from burns of the conjunctiva. Occasionally they follow severe lacerations or other injuries. They may be single or multiple in number and are scars which connect the conjunctiva of the upper or lower lids with the bulbar conjunctiva. They can be readily seen on inspection when the eyelids are separated.

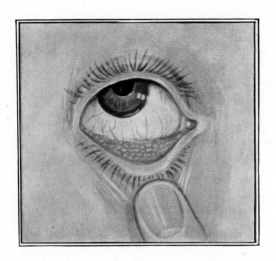

Fig. 27.—Follicular conjunctivitis.

Pterygium.—A band of mucous membrane, triangular in shape, occurring in the bulbar conjunctiva just outside or inside of the cornea. The apex of the triangle extends toward and over the limbus of the cornea. They usually occur singly, but sometimes one may be found on each side of the cornea. Occasionally, pterygia may be accompanied by irritation and redness. When they encroach on the cornea, greater irritation follows which may lead to interference with the vision, and when the cornea is affected, they are classed as a form of degeneration. The exact cause is not known, but exposure to wind and air is believed to be the chief factor.

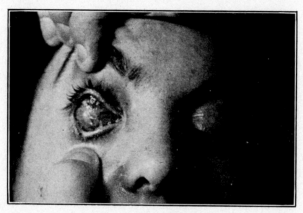

Fig. 29.—Symblepharon following chemical burn, right eye. (I. S. Tassman, Wills Hospital.)

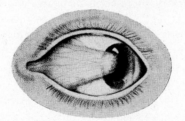

Fig. 30.—Pterygium. (From Duke-Elder: Text-Book of Ophthalmology.)

Xerosis.—Triangular or wedge-shaped white patches or spots which occur in the bulbar conjunctiva on each side of the cornea. They may be small and round and usually are found in conjunction with xerophthalmia resulting from a deficiency of vitamin A in the diet. As a rule, the larger areas are covered with a fine, loose network which resembles seafoam in appearance, and are generally accompanied by other symptoms of xerophthalmia, such as night blindness.

Ulcers occur, as a rule, in the tarsal conjunctiva in cases of tuberculosis which is either primary or secondary. They usually begin as small areas of granulation, reddish in tint, with a rather broad, yellowish base. These areas spread slowly and are chronic in nature despite any form of treatment employed. Around the ulcer may be found small, gray nodules which project outward extending the area. In severe cases the entire thickness of the lid may become involved. When portions of the tissue are removed and examined in the laboratory, the presence of the tubercle bacillus can be demonstrated. These ulcers occur more commonly in the lower lid and affect young people. When they do show signs of yielding to treatment, they are apt to recur. When such ulcers extend from the skin over to the conjunctiva of the lid, they are known as lupus of the conjunctiva.

Conjunctivitis.—Any inflammation of the conjunctiva is characterized as a conjunctivitis. It occurs in many different forms for various reasons. A very troublesome form of conjunctivitis often occurs as an allergic manifestation. (See Ocular allergy.) Almost all affections of the external eye cause an irritation of the conjunctiva resulting in a conjunctivitis. The causes of this condition may originate outside of the body, within the eye, or elsewhere in the body. Each may produce a conjunctivitis which has its own peculiar characteristics. In the first group are those external influences, such as excessive light, heat, chemicals, foreign bodies, bacteria, infective viruses, and others which might produce an inflammatory condition of the conjunctiva. Some of these conditions may be only a temporary, catarrhal affection which may clear up with mild treatment in a short time. Others, such as those caused by bacteria, may take on a purulent nature and persist for a longer period of time. A few forms of conjunctivitis are believed to be due to virus infection. These may occur in the conjunctiva alone, or in association with disease of other organs. Trachoma is a form of chronic conjunctivitis which illustrates the first variety, while variola is a disease in which the ocular affection is associated with dermatologic lesions.

Conjunctivitis occurs in some form in nearly all of the acute and chronic infectious diseases, prominent among which are diphtheria, gonorrhea, syphilis, tuberculosis, and many others. In some of these it may occur as a primary condition, while in others it is a manifestation of the internal disease and may be present at the same time as the primary affection or occur as a sequela of the disease.

An epidemic form of acute conjunctivitis associated with preauricular adenopathy and deep punctate corneal infiltrates is known as epidemic keratoconjunctivitis. The corneal infiltration is usually observed when the acute symptoms of the conjunctivitis subside. The conjunctivitis is very sudden in onset and is accompanied by pain and a sensation of a foreign body in the eye. There is considerable lacrimation and the edema, which is quite marked, involves the bulbar conjunctiva especially. The conjunctival vessels are hyperemic and the patient may complain of burning, itching and pain on rotation of the eyes. Later, follicles occur in the conjunctiva, especially in the lower lids and fornices. Considerable papillary hypertrophy and hyperemia occur between the follicles. Lymphadenopathy may be marked at this time, and upper respiratory symptoms may also be present.

The acute symptoms usually subside about the sixth day or a little later in some cases. At about this time, a pseudomembrane develops, usually on the lower lid but also at times on the upper. This is then followed somewhat later by the presence of keratitic precipitates. This condition will be described in greater detail later under the corneal manifestations. It is said to be caused by a filtrable virus which has been isolated from conjunctival scrapings. It has recently occurred in epidemic form throughout most of the United States. (See Epidemic keratoconjunctivitis.)

The treatment of conjunctivitis depends on the causative agent and varies according to the type of manifestation. In the simple catarrhal variety local treatment with a mild eyewash and protection from light may be all that is required. In more severe cases and in the purulent form, more active treatment with antiseptic solutions, applications to the conjunctival sac, and frequent flushing are necessary. Treatment of the primary disease is administered at the same time.

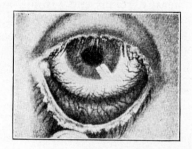
Acute mucopurulent

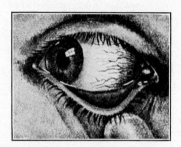
Angular conjunctivitis

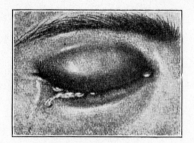
Purulent (gonococcal)

Fig. 31.—Varieties of conjunctivitis. (From Duke-Elder: Text-Book of Ophthalmology.)

In the treatment of allergic forms of conjunctivitis it is necessary first to remove the patient from the conditions or surroundings which expose him to the allergen responsible. Or it may suffice, if possible, to remove or eliminate the agents which have been found to produce the allergic condition. Wherever possible, in suspected cases especially, a complete examination by an allergist should be obtained.

Thygeson,[2] in describing the mechanism of production of conjunctival inflammation, discusses:

1. Bacteria, which produce the condition by the chemical action of toxic products which are liberated. The bacteria may proliferate superficially on the surface of the conjunctiva (e.g., Morax-Axenfeld); they may proliferate on the living epithelial cells (e.g., conjunctivitis due to Koch-Weeks bacillus); they may proliferate beneath the epithelium (e.g., gonorrheal endogenous conjunctivitis).

2. Viruses: these are also supposed to liberate toxins although this is not definitely established. They probably multiply only in the living cells and some in the epithelium (e.g., virus of trachoma and of inclusion conjunctivitis).

3. Allergy: this form of conjunctivitis is thought to arise from injury to the conjunctival cells by an antigen-antibody reaction occurring on or in those by which the antibody has been fixed. (See Ocular allergy.)

In discussing the treatment of conjunctivitis, he included such therapeutic agents as antiseptics; chemotherapeutic agents as ethyl hydrocupreine hydrochloride (specific for pneumococcus); zinc sulfate (specific for Morax-Axenfeld bacillus); sulfanilamide; nonspecific protein and fever therapy; immunologic agents and procedures (vaccine therapy, toxins and toxoids, antibacterial serums, tuberculin); physical therapy (cold, heat, ultraviolet, radium, x-ray, massage); astringents (silver, zinc, copper, alum, tannic acid); vasoconstrictors (epinephrine hydrochloride 1:1000, ephedrine 3 per cent).

The following table by Thygeson summarizes the treatment for some forms of chronic conjunctivitis:

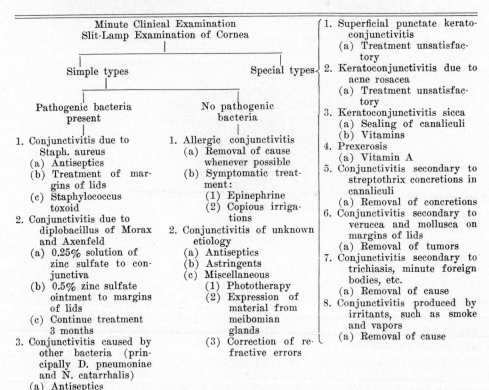

Inclusion conjunctivitis is a virus disease sometimes called inclusion blennorrhea and also swimming pool conjunctivitis because it sometimes occurs among swimmers in epidemic form. It occurs most commonly among newborn infants in the form of an acute papillary conjunctivitis. Occasionally adults are affected in the form of an acute or subacute follicular conjunctivitis. It is caused by a filtrable virus similar to that which occurs in trachoma. It is localized in the conjunctival epithelium and involves only the underlying tissue by infiltration of the soluble toxic products which are liberated. The small inclusion bodies of the virus stain blue with Giemsa stain, while the large ones stain bluish red. They are morphologically indistinguishable from those of trachoma. Infection with inclusion conjunctivitis is similar to that of trachoma also because it confers no permanent immunity. The incubation period of the disease is about five to ten days, in which respect it also resembles trachoma. In the latter disease, however, the follicular and papillary reactions are followed by pannus and cicatrization, whereas these are absent in inclusion conjunctivitis. The condition is fairly common in Negroes and usually involves the lower fornices and tarsus.

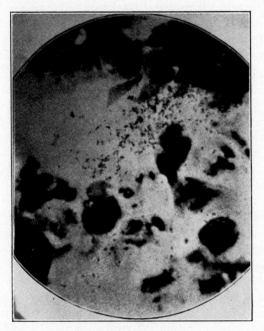

Fig. 32.—Elementary bodies of trachoma (Giemsa stain; ×1500). (From Thygeson: Arch. Ophth., February, 1943.)

The treatment is also similar to that of early trachoma since it responds to the use of sulfanilamide. In infants, sulfathiazole ointment can be employed, while in adults, sulfanilamide both locally and orally can be given. The inclusion bodies disappear after about three days of treatment but therapy should be continued for approximately a week.

Trachoma is a chronic form of conjunctivitis affecting both eyes and is now generally believed to be caused by an infectious virus. This virus of trachoma is very similar in morphology to that of inclusion conjunctivitis. The nature and identity of the filtrable virus of trachoma were revealed by the work of several different investigators, especially that of Thygeson[3] in recent years. He described the elementary bodies of trachoma as being similar to those of the Rickettsiae described earlier by Prowasek and, later, others. The virus bodies of trachoma were found to stain well with Giemsa and similar dyes but to stain faintly, if at all, with the ordinary stains. Infection with trachoma in human beings or monkeys does not confer permanent immunity. The virus has a strict localization for the conjunctival and corneal epithelium. Secondary effects such as subepithelial infiltration, necrosis and cicatrization are undoubtedly the result of soluble products liberated in the epithelium. The virus of trachoma could not be cultivated in tissue culture or in the yolk sac or chorioallantois of the developing chick embryo. Efforts to grow the virus on human conjunctival and corneal epithelium have failed. It has been claimed in one or two instances that Rickettsia-like organisms were identified in the epithelial tissues of trachoma, but Thygeson's investigations failed to confirm this. He concluded that the trachoma virus as well as the viruses of inclusion conjunctivitis, psittacosis and lymphogranuloma venereum form a transitional group of atypical viruses between the typical large viruses and the Rickettsiae.

Diagnosis is almost impossible in the early stage. The first symptoms are practically the same as those found in any form of conjunctivitis, namely, lacrimation, irritation and photophobia. There is usually very little or no purulent secretion. A general thickening and hypertrophy of the tarsal conjunctiva take place. The upper lid is usually more severely affected. Small follicles can be seen on the tarsal conjunctiva, and microscopic examination may, at this time, reveal the presence of inclusion bodies. Later, the follicles, which are deep seated, increase in size, giving the everted lid a granular appearance. The hypertrophy continues with papilla formation on the tarsal conjunctiva, which gives the latter an irregular, rough surface. The vessels of the tarsal conjunctiva cannot be seen as growth of the papillae increases. This period of hypertrophy and infiltration finally subsides with a regression and eventual disappearance of papillae and follicles. This is followed by scar formation which, in the later stages, is white in color. A late complication of trachoma is the occurrence of pannus at the upper portion of the cornea. This begins as a roughness of the corneal epithelium at the limbus and is succeeded by the extension of small superficial blood vessels from the limbus down over the cornea. This vascularization of the cornea may progress as long as the disease continues to affect the conjunctiva. The vision is decreased corresponding in amount to the degree of pannus. Ulceration of the cornea may also occur at the same time. This may be accompanied by a mild iritis. Healing of the corneal ulcers also leads to increased loss of vision.

With the healing of trachoma and scar formation on the tarsal surfaces of the lids, a gradual contraction takes place over a period of time. Shrinking of the tarsus causes the lid to become inverted gradually and the cilia to come in contact with the eyeball causing trichiasis. This is followed by a continuous irritation of the eyeball, with additional pain, and sometimes further ulceration of the cornea. The upper lid is affected to a greater extent than the lower, and in this stage of the condition it is very difficult to evert for examination. In some cases, an added infection takes place in the late stage which may result in panophthalmitis and loss of the eye. In most of the cases of trachoma the vision remains seriously impaired, or the patient becomes blind as the result of mixed infection or other complications.

Trachoma must be differentiated from folliculosis of the conjunctiva, and in some instances from vernal conjunctivitis (spring catarrh). Folliculosis may be characterized by the occurrence of catarrhal inflammation and small follicles arranged in lines or blocks, found commonly in children. The follicles may increase in size, and with the added inflammation present, the condition sometimes resembles trachoma. This may subside, however, with disappearance of the follicles in a comparatively short time. In other instances the follicles become large and are found irregularly over the conjunctiva. An actual hypertrophy of the tarsal conjunctiva, however, is absent. These follicles may be very large and thick in the posterior cul-de-sac and can be clearly seen when the fornix of the upper lid is presented to view. The conjunctiva of the tarsus between follicles in folliculosis is usually normal, while in trachoma the tarsal conjunctiva is deeply infiltrated.

Vernal conjunctivitis can be differentiated from trachoma usually by the time of onset and its seasonal incidence. Moreover, the itching in vernal conjunctivitis is often a characteristic subjective symptom. On examination, a stringy material is usually found in the cul-de-sac which is tenacious and tends to recur on removal. This condition is sometimes found in patients who suffer from hay fever and asthma and is considered by some to be a form of allergy.

Inclusion bodies are not ordinarily present in vernal conjunctivitis. In discussing the question of inclusion bodies in Beren's *The Eye and Its Diseases*, Lindner[4] points out the fact that inclusion bodies and "free initial bodies," which are the same as those occurring in trachoma, are found in inclusion blenorrhea of the newborn.

Inclusion conjunctivitis greatly resembles trachoma both clinically and in the nature of the identity of the causative inclusion bodies. However, the inclusion conjunctivitis virus does not lead to cicatrization and pannus formation as in trachoma. Trachoma also commonly involves the conjunctiva and fornices of the upper lids, while inclusion conjunctivitis occurs in the lower. The latter has been found to occur more commonly in Negroes, while trachoma is more common among Europeans. Both inclusion conjunctivitis and trachoma respond well to treatment with sulfanilamide.

Treatment.—Various local applications are employed including silver nitrate (2 per cent) applied to the everted eyelids, and the copper sulfate stick also applied deeply to the tarsal surface of the everted eyelids. Both of these are followed by irrigation with normal saline solution. The local treatment must be continued for a long period of time until the condition clears up. In the later stage when the follicles are very large, they can be removed by the use of forceps such as Knapp's roller forceps. This consists of rolling the lids between the forceps and can usually be performed with a local anesthetic. In cases which do not respond otherwise, removal of the tarsus of the upper lid relieves the condition but results in a deformity of the lid.

Pannus cannot be relieved by any direct treatment, but peritomy may serve to limit its further progress by severing the vessels from the cornea. Ulceration of the cornea requires the instillation of atropine sulfate (1 per cent) once or twice daily, and the occasional application of warm compresses. Sulfanilamide has been used in trachoma with considerable success. Loe[5] reported its use in a series of over 140 cases with rapid improvement of subjective and objective symptoms in a very few days after treatment was begun. Some of his cases were discharged, apparently cured, after several treatments with sulfanilamide covering a period of about ten days.

Cysts and Tumors.—Conjunctival cysts may be due to several causes, the commonest probably being a dilation of the lymph spaces. This may lead to the formation of small cysts on the bulbar conjunctiva, which resemble a lymphangiectasis. Single cysts of the bulbar conjunctiva may also occur. Traumatic cysts result from the implantation of epithelium below the conjunctiva which degenerates and leaves a space filled with fluid. Such cysts may also be of nontraumatic origin, and result from chronic inflammatory conditions. Glandular retention cysts also occur as the result of obstruction of the ducts of the meibomian glands by infiltration and cicatricial contraction in some inflammations.

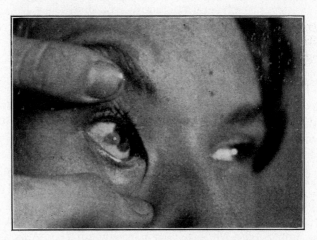

Fig. 33.—Cyst of the conjunctiva. (Clinic of Dr. Carroll Mullen, Wills Hospital.)

Tumors of the conjunctiva also include several varieties. Granulomas of the conjunctiva often occur after wounds and operations. They are also present in some of the inflammatory diseases of the conjunctiva caused by the fungus infections.

Papillomas of the conjunctiva usually are found at the inner angle and in the fornices. In a few instances they may occur at the limbus and become malignant.

Fibromas may be hard or soft and usually occur in the sockets. They are polypoid and can often be removed.

Dermoids are yellowish growths, usually found on or near the limbus of the cornea. They are usually congenital and can, as a rule, be removed without difficulty.

Epithelioma commonly occurs at the limbus or at the edge of the lids. It may spread over the surface of the conjunctiva and penetrate the globe.

Sarcoma of the conjunctiva rarely occurs. It is usually pigmented and is found at the limbus in older people. It may be round or spindle-celled in variety. On removal it tends to recur and may metastasize. The prognosis is grave.

Examination of the Cornea

The methods employed for examination of the cornea include principally:

Inspection of the cornea with the unaided eye;

Inspection under direct illumination;

Inspection under focal illumination with magnification (biomicroscopy);

Keratometry. A study of the curvature of the corneal surfaces.

In addition to the methods which depend on the use of reflected light, examination by transmitted light is useful in determining the presence of opacities.

Determination of the sensitivity of the cornea is important in many conditions, particularly in disease of the central nervous system. This is usually tested directly by touching the cornea with a thin wisp of cotton and noting the response. Normally, the cornea is very sensitive and any foreign material brought in contact will produce a rapid closure of the eyelid.

In order to determine whether or not the epithelium is denuded, which may happen after foreign bodies, burns, or ulcers, a drop of fluorescein, 2 per cent, to which a little sodium bicarbonate is added for alkalinity, is instilled into the conjunctival sac, and the patient is told to close the eye for a minute or two. This can be preceded by the instillation of a drop of a local anesthetic, such as pontocain or phenacaine. The lids are then again separated and flushed with normal saline solution. The excess of fluorescein which has a glittering greenish-gold color is thereby washed away, while the area of cornea which is denuded of epithelium is covered with a brilliant green fluorescent stain. The remainder of the cornea with the healthy epithelium intact normally presents the appearance of a brilliant convex mirror with a high luster. Small upright images of external objects are found in the corneal surface, and any imperfections will disturb the regular reflection of light at these points. These may be directly observed and detected as defects in the surface which should be perfectly uniform. Causing as they do an irregular light reflection, the images formed are distorted. The patient can be placed in a position facing a window, so that the corneal image of the window sash is seen by the examiner. With a rectilinear object, such as a window sash, it is not difficult to detect any distortion. In examining the corneal surface for imperfections, such as foreign bodies or faint opacities, the eye must be directed toward a strong light and should be rotated by the patient in various directions. By so rotating the eye, certain positions are found in which the reflex disturbance is apparent. Thus, very small and faint nebulae frequently fail to be observed when viewed directly, but when viewed obliquely, they are more readily detected.

Direct illumination from an ordinary electric bulb or from a small hand flashlight may supply the source of light for routine inspection of the cornea and its superficial surface in particular. This can be employed for examination of the stain after foreign bodies, or for the detection of foreign bodies or vascularization, and to obtain a general idea of the nature of the curvature of the anterior surface.

The reflected light of the ophthalmoscope and retinoscope, particularly when directed into the eye from a distance of one-half meter, will clearly reveal the presence of faint opacities or nebulae in the cornea.

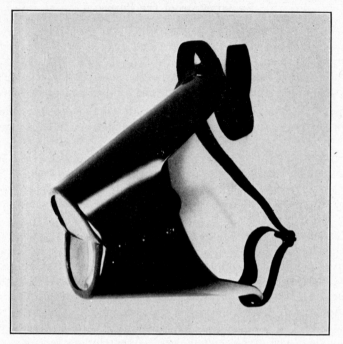

Fig. 34.—Berger loupe for magnification of external eye. (Courtesy of Street, Linder, and Propert, Philadelphia.)

Focal or oblique illumination is an important and useful method of examining the cornea and anterior segment of the eyeball. It should be employed in the routine examination of every case. This consists in concentrating the light upon the structure under examination by means of a double convex lens of about 14-16 D power. The best source of light is an ordinary electric bulb in a darkened room. Ordinary daylight or direct sunlight also affords good illumination. The cornea, anterior chamber, the iris and the lens can be thereby illuminated and even a tumor or large opacity in the vitreous close to the lens, or a detached retina directly behind the lens, can often be seen to advantage. The lens employed for this purpose should be about 6 cm. in diameter and may be set in a metallic ring either with or without a handle. It is then held between the thumb and forefinger of the examiner's hand at the focal distance from the eye to be examined. The source of artificial light should be at a distance of about 50 cm. in front of the patient. Care must be taken to avoid having the light too close, since this will prevent bringing the rays to a focus on the eye. The examiner should stand in front and just to the side of the patient, so that an unobstructed view of the cornea can be obtained. The back of the hand holding the condensing lens is held toward the light with the lens in a plane at right angles to the rays to be directed to the cornea. The lens is then brought up to and withdrawn from the eye until the focus of light coincides with the structure under examination. A uniformly illuminated view of the anterior eyeball is best obtained by focusing the light far back in the eye, these structures thus intercepting the rays before they come to a focus. The detailed examination consists in focusing first in the corneal epithelium, and then successively through the cornea and the anterior chamber, onto the anterior surface of the iris, and then through the pupil and the lens. By shifting the lens from side to side, and up and down, and by also having the patient when necessary move the eyeball as directed, every portion of these structures illuminated can be critically examined. The obliquity of the light must be varied according to the depth of desired penetration. Thus for the examination of the lens, especially in its deeper layers, the light must be made to enter almost vertically. Of course, dilatation of the pupil is necessary if the more peripheral portions of the lens are to be illuminated.

The value of focal illumination can be greatly enhanced by magnifying the illuminated structure. This is perhaps best obtained by the use of the so-called "corneal loupe." A number of different loupes for this purpose can be had, such as the Berger loupe or binocular magnifier.

Slit Lamp Examination (Biomicroscopy)

Examination of the eye with the slit lamp provides a means for illumination which has proved to be one of the most useful aids in diagnosis. Because of the magnification provided by this means, it is possible to study the structures, at least of the anterior segment of the eye, in minute detail. For the same reason, this method is sometimes known as biomicroscopy. It amplifies the clinical observations and provides a detailed picture of the changes affecting the structure which is otherwise not obtainable. As a result, it also affords an excellent opportunity to study the progress of a lesion, so that it is possible from day to day to determine with a greater degree of accuracy the extent to which a tissue is involved.

The instrument employed for this purpose is known as the slit lamp. It was first employed by Gullstrand in 1911, but it has since been modified and improved a number of times. In its present form, the slit lamp employs a system of illumination which can provide a narrow beam of light for the examination of a small optical section. Several makes of slit lamp are obtainable, the more universally used being the one made by Zeiss and that made by Bausch and Laumb. The new Poser slit lamp (B. & L.) provides a binocular microscope, with 10 x wide field eyepieces, turret mount with low power (55 mm.) and high power (40 mm.) paired objectives. The microscope and illuminating system are mounted on vertical revolving arms which can be rotated around the eye to be examined.

Types of Illumination.—Several methods of illumination are employed with the slit lamp, each of which is useful for certain purposes in the course of examination.

For a general examination of the cornea, iris, and anterior or posterior surfaces of the lens, a broad beam of light can be directed into the eye from

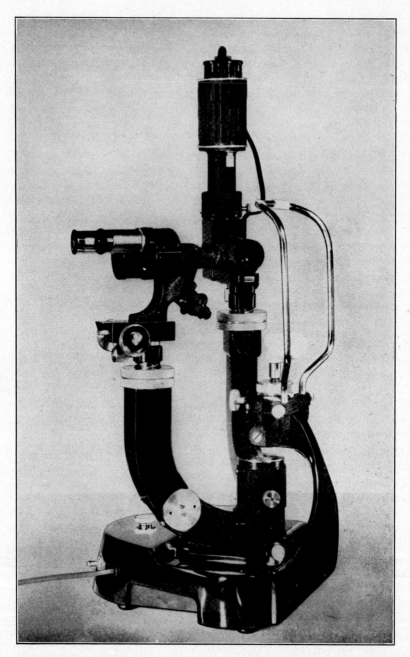

Fig. 35.—B & L poser slit lamp. (Courtesy of Street, Linder, and Propert, Philadelphia.)

a rather wide angle. This will provide diffuse illumination for a routine examination of these structures. For a more detailed examination, the following methods are employed:

1. Direct Illumination (Focal). This provides a cross section of the structure to be observed through a rectangular area of illumination, which is directed into the eye obliquely. The structures thus included in the rectangular area or shaft of light can then be focused and directly observed with the microscope of the instrument. In the normal eye, several zones of optical discontinuity are distinguished, due to variations in the amount of diffuse reflection. Very small opacities and slight differences in refractivity of the media which could not be otherwise distinguished can be made out. This method of direct illumination with a narrow beam is probably the most useful in a general examination.

2. Retro-illumination or transillumination is the method by which the structure to be examined is illuminated from behind. The light is therefore directed on a structure posterior, so that the illumination is reflected forward from the latter. For example, the light would be directed to the iris or lens in order to examine the cornea in this manner. The iris also would be examined by light directed to the lens. This method is employed for the examination of small details and the study of droplets, vacuoles, faint deposits, and slight pigment changes and holes in the iris.

3. Specular reflection was introduced by Vogt and utilizes an area which acts as a mirror produced by the reflection of light from the irregular surface. Certain zones or areas can, therefore, be mirrored and become visible, revealing extremely minute changes. The anterior and posterior corneal surfaces, the anterior and posterior lens surfaces, and the nucleus of the lens can be studied in detail in this way.

The depth and localization by stereopsis of small objects in the structure are also possible by means of slit lamp examination. The thickness of different parts of the cornea can be studied, and the exact location and depth of a wound or a foreign body can be determined.

Procedure.—The patient is seated in front of the microscope of the slit lamp with the chin supported on a chin rest and forehead pressed against a head-bar. The microscope is placed in position in front of the eye and the arm of the slit lamp is adjusted so that, with the light turned on, the beam is directed on the cornea at its limbus. The examiner adjusts his own eyes to the ocular of the microscope and then moves the beam of light onto the cornea with one hand, while he focuses the fine adjustment at the same time. The cornea, iris, lens, and vitreous are usually examined in the order named. To examine the structures with direct focal illumination, the patient is instructed to look directly at the microscope. For specular illumination, he is directed to look between the beam and the microscope.

The conjunctiva can be examined ordinarily by diffuse illumination with a large field. The cornea is examined by means of a broad beam providing a rectangular prism of light. The anterior part of the rectangle reveals the anterior surface of the cornea and the posterior part, the posterior surface. Narrowing the beam produces a section, so that two bright lines are formed, one of which is the reflection from the epithelial surface, and the other from

Bowman's membrane, the space between corresponding to the epithelium. The various surfaces and stroma of the cornea can be observed, and in this way also, infiltrations, inflammations, opacities, and various forms of keratitis can be studied. If the lens is opaque, the light can be reflected from it or from the iris by transillumination and more minute changes can be observed. By this means, vacuoles, bullae, edema of the epithelium, and other fine lesions can be studied. The endothelial cells on the posterior surface of the cornea can be examined by specular reflection.

The aqueous should ordinarily be optically nearly clear and is examined with a narrow beam of intensified light. Fine colloid particles produce what is known as an "aqueous flare," which can be seen with dispersion of a spot of light. A turbid aqueous may be observed as an early sign of sympathetic uveitis and is indicative of the presence of cells or debris, exudation, and pigment granules.

The surface of the iris can be examined by direct illumination. The pupillary reactions to the direct light can be studied and, at the same time, the mobility of the iris can also be observed. Indirect illumination permits observation of hemorrhages and growths. With retro-illumination, as already stated, the light can be directed to the lens, which will permit observation of holes and other fine details on the posterior surface.

The lens can be examined by all forms of illumination with the slit lamp. Direct illumination with a narrow beam reveals the zones of discontinuity. The anterior and posterior limiting bands are reflected from the anterior and posterior capsule. The clear space between is bounded by another bright line, which is the subcapsular line. The cortex of the lens and the various parts of the nucleus are indicated by bright bands which follow behind this. The Y sutures can be observed in the band illuminating the fetal nucleus. Opacities and other abnormalities in any part of the lens structure can be observed and localized on examination with the broad beam and in the optical section obtained on direct illumination. The shiny appearance of shagreen produced by reflection of numerous irregularities on the anterior and posterior capsule can be examined with specular reflection. Other fine details, such as vacuoles, membranes, and deposits can also be examined with retro-illumination or reflection of the light from the posterior surface.

With sufficient illumination the slit lamp can reveal the condition of the anterior vitreous and the body of the vitreous. The latter can be observed for remnants of hyaloid artery, opacities, blood, and crystals.

Ophthalmoscopy

The present-day method of ophthalmoscopy, dates back to the time of Helmholtz, who in 1851 developed this means for illuminating and examining the fundus of the eye. Since that time, the development of the ophthalmoscope has progressed by stages, so that at the present time a number of different models are obtainable for this purpose. It is not necessary to describe here details in the construction and the optical principles involved, but the latter are nearly the same in all.

There are practically two types of hand ophthalmoscopes, the first being the older reflecting instrument of Loring and the other, a more modern self-illuminating or electric ophthalmoscope which is in common use today. As the name implies, the Loring instrument requires the use of an outside source of light, which is usually supplied by a frosted electric globe with a "bull's eye" opening, on a wall bracket. The electric ophthalmoscope eliminates the need for an outside source of light since it includes a small electric globe at the top of the handle, the current for which is obtained either by batteries which are inclosed within the handle or by means of a rheostat. A popular model in common use at the present time is the May ophthalmoscope, which is constructed by Bausch and Lomb. This contains a reflecting prism and a condenser which affords a clear illumination of the area observed. Other models in common use are the Morton ophthalmoscope and the De Zeng ophthalmoscope. In these a condensing lens above the lamp also collects the rays into a beam of light just before entering the eye. The electric ophthalmoscope has distinct advantages for the direct method of examination but is probably not as satisfactory as the Loring instrument for indirect examination.

Every ophthalmoscope has an upper portion or head which contains a series of lenses, both convex and concave, which range in power from 0 to 20 diopters, plus and minus. The plus lenses are usually designated by white markings while the minus are red. In the Loring scope there are not as many, and they range here from 0 to plus and minus 7 diopters. These are arranged on a disc which can be rotated by the finger of the examiner in order to clearly focus the illuminated area observed through an aperture provided for this purpose.

The direct method of ophthalmoscopy is the one originally devised by Helmholtz and which is employed satisfactorily with the electric ophthalmoscope. The magnification of the fundus is produced by the cornea and lens of the patient's eye. When the refraction of the latter is normal, the rays which emerge from an illuminated point on the retina are parallel, and completely fill the pupil of the examiner on entering it. With the examiner's eye in a normal refractive state, these parallel rays can be seen as a red reflection in the patient's pupil. The examiner can approach the eye of the patient very closely and obtain an image of the illuminated area, while he observes a particular structure through the aperture, and in cases of high hyperopia or myopia a clear image of the patient's fundus can be obtained at a greater distance.

The ideal condition for ophthalmoscopic examination is for the eye of the patient and that of the examiner to be in a normal refractive state. In cases of high hyperopia it is necessary for the examiner to use the convex lenses of the ophthalmoscope in order to obtain a clear image, while in myopia the concave lenses of required power are necessary to focus the illuminated area clearly. In this way it is also possible to estimate the refractive condition of the patient's eye, since the strongest convex lens with which a clear image is obtained will approximately measure the hyperopia in the patient's eye, while the weakest concave lens on the ophthalmoscope with which a clear image is obtained, measures approximately the amount of myopia. The eye of the examiner should be emmetropic and his accommodation relaxed.

Ophthalmoscopic examination is usually made in a dark room, and with the patient's pupil of sufficient size to permit a satisfactory view of the interior of the eye. When the latter is too small for this purpose, it is necessary to instill a weak mydriatic. This should be avoided, however, in cases with any suspicion whatever of the presence of glaucoma. The safest drugs for this purpose are probably euphthalmine, 2 to 5 per cent, paredrine, 1 to 5 per cent, homatropine, 1 to 2 per cent. The instillation of one drop of any of these drugs should be sufficient to enlarge the pupil after a lapse of about fifteen minutes. On completion of the examination, especially in older people, it is well to instill a drop of pilocarpine 2 per cent, or eserine $\frac{1}{4}$ per cent, in order to counteract the effect of the mydriatic employed.

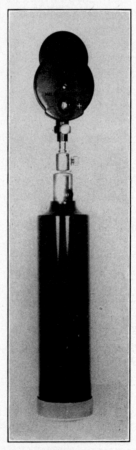

Fig. 36.—B & L May ophthalmoscope. (Courtesy of Street, Linder, and Propert, Philadelphia.)

Procedure.—

In using the direct method with any ophthalmoscope, the patient is usually seated in a chair in a darkened room, while the examiner is on the side and facing the patient. In order to examine the right eye, the ophthalmoscope is held in the right hand with the aperture in front of the right eye. The left hand and the left eye are used to examine the left eye of the patient and the position of the examiner is on the left side. The patient is instructed to look directly ahead into distance or at the wall at the opposite side of the room.

With the Loring ophthalmoscope, it is necessary to direct the light into the eye by tilting the mirror in the direction of the light source and to be at a distance of about 20 cm. to obtain the fundus reflex. While approaching the eye this reflex must be held in view through the aperture of the ophthalmoscope. This sometimes proves difficult and the pupillary reflex is lost. This difficulty is overcome, however, with the electric ophthalmoscope, since the illumination does not have to be reflected by a tilted mirror from an outside source of light and the examination can be started at a closer distance to the eye. A convex lens of higher power, such as plus 8, 10, or 20 diopters, is employed first to examine the media (cornea, lens, and vitreous) at a distance of about 10 cm. When this observation has been made, the observer slowly moves forward toward the patient, always directing the illumination into the pupil. As he does so he also rotates the disc of the ophthalmoscope with the index finger until the lens appears in front of the aperture which provides a clear image of the fundus. One of the first things to come into view is probably one or two of the retinal vessels. These should then be followed along their course until they approach the optic disc. The latter should then be examined carefully, with especial reference to its margins, color and character of the excavation. When these have been studied, the ophthalmoscope should be rotated slightly from side to side and up and down in order to observe the periphery of the fundus and the condition of the retinal vessels. The examination should never be considered complete until the macula and all the details have been studied. When the patient is looking directly forward, the optic disc is generally presented to view. In order to observe the macula, the patient should be directed to look a little to the side corresponding to the eye being examined, i.e., to the right in the case of the right eye and to the left side in examination of the left eye. Difficulties are sometimes encountered, especially by the inexperienced, in obtaining a satisfactory view in cases of very high hyperopia or myopia. Although it might prove a little more awkward, the latter can often be seen more clearly when the patient wears his correction.

The indirect method of ophthalmoscopy also offers certain advantages in examination, chief of which is the large field which can be observed in this way. This method requires the use of an additional lens with a power of about 13 diopters. This is placed at its focal distance (7.9 cm.) in front of the eye, and held in one hand of the examiner who is now seated directly in front and about 40 cm. from the patient's eye. The light is directed by the reflecting ophthalmoscope through the objective lens held by the examiner and then into the pupil examined. The refraction of the examiner should be corrected and his accommodation relaxed. The patient is instructed to look just alongside of the examiner's ear corresponding to the eye under examination, i.e., alongside the right ear if the right eye is being examined and the left ear if the left eye is being examined. This should bring the optic disc into view. With this as a landmark, the rest of the fundus can be observed by slow and careful manipulation of the ophthalmoscope and objective lens. This method is more difficult than the direct one and requires considerable practice to prove useful.

Keratometry.—This has for its purpose the measurement of the anterior curvature of the cornea. The corneal surfaces are not spherical and of equal curvature, but are ellipsoidal. The radius of curvature of the anterior corneal surface in an emmetropic eye varies from about 7 mm. to 8.5 mm. The posterior surface has a somewhat shorter radius of curvature, thus giving the cornea a meniscus form, thinner at the center than at the circumference. Corneal astigmatism represents the difference between the meridian of greatest and that of least curvature, which two meridians are at right angles to each other.

The radius of curvature of the principal meridians of the cornea can be accurately measured with the ophthalmometer. The principle upon which this instrument is constructed is that the image of an object of a certain size reflected from the convex surface at a fixed distance becomes smaller as the radius of curvature of the reflecting surface becomes shorter. The objects are in the instrument and are called ''mires.'' The reflecting surface is the cornea. The images are magnified by an eyepiece (an ocular), so that they can be readily observed.

The patient is seated on one side of the instrument facing the telescope and with his chin on a chin rest and forehead placed against a headrest. The eye not being examined is covered. The examiner adjusts the eyepiece in order to get the clearest image on the cornea of the patient. The images of the mires are then focused on the center of the cornea. The bisecting lines on the mires are now brought into continuity with the edges of the mires just touching. This is done by rotating the telescope, and sliding the step mire along the arc to, or from, the rectangular mire which is fixed. Having found this position which is the primary position, one of the principal meridians is obtained, and the reading is taken from the position of the indicator on the disc or dial of the instrument. Two readings can be taken, the one giving the radius of curvature and the other the refractive power in diopters. Having completed this, the telescope is now rotated through 90 degrees. The mires are now readjusted, so that they just touch in this meridian, and have their central lines continuous. The reading is again taken from the scale or dial of the instrument, both for the radius of curvature in this meridian and the refractive power. The difference between the refractive powers obtained in the two meridians represents the amount of corneal astigmatism present. In addition to determining the radius of curvature and refractive power of the two principal meridians of the cornea, the ophthalmometer is useful in revealing the presence of irregular astigmatism or conical cornea at a glance. It is impossible, in such cases, to find any position in which the bisecting lines on the mires are continuous. There is, furthermore, distortion of the mires.

Placido's disc may be employed to determine the regularity of the anterior corneal surface. This is a flat, circular metal disc, 23 cm. in diameter, with a series of concentric black and white alternate hand-painted circles on one surface. A small aperture is in the center. These circles are reflected on to the cornea to be examined while the examiner observes the image through the aperture of the disc. If the cornea is spherical, the image appears unaltered, and the black and white lines appear circular. If the cornea is astigmatic, the concentric circles are distorted. In regular astigmatism they become elliptical; in irregular astigmatism, broken and irregular. The long axis of the ellipse corresponds to the corneal meridian of least curvature or longest radius.

Abnormalities of the Cornea

The cornea may be affected by a large variety of lesions which are found to be present in certain diseases and under certain conditions, such as in inflammation of the surrounding or adjacent structures, and as the result of direct trauma or pressure. Although it is well protected from external injury by the covering and action of the eyelid, it is nevertheless not uncommon for the cornea to sustain an injury such as abrasion of the superficial epithelial surface, or a laceration produced by an accidental brushing from a small branch of a twig, from the edge of a newspaper, fingernail, or a foreign body lodging on the cornea. If the trauma is slight, the only lesion produced will be an abrasion or a laceration, which at worst has removed the superficial layer of epithelium. With care and proper treatment this will heal, leaving no ill effects. Foreign bodies which are lodged on the cornea and have not penetrated into the stroma will also cause a removal of a corresponding amount of superficial epithelium. This will also heal without subsequent ulceration and scarring, when properly managed and treated.

Edema of the Cornea.—This may occur from a number of causes including inflammation, degeneration, increased intraocular tension, trauma, and sometimes from unknown causes. On inspection by direct examination the cornea is found to be dull and hazy with an uneven surface. A more detailed examination can be made with the slit lamp, which reveals a bedewing of the corneal epithelium. When the surface contour is disturbed, the anterior zone of specular reflection is not as well defined, and the light is reflected irregularly from a number of very small prominences. With retro-illumination, the light being reflected from the iris, the cornea will be seen to have lost its natural luster and small, separate droplets occur in the epithelium which are surrounded by a dark ring. These droplets, by their coalescence, may become vesicles or bullae. A general relucency may take place in the substance of the cornea and folds may be found in Descemet's membrane. The endothelium may also reveal a bedewing, as seen best by retro-illumination. Edema of the cornea will occur in most of the inflammatory conditions. It is one of the earliest manifestations of interstitial keratitis, and of inflammation of the uveal tract. It may occur in various localized conditions of the cornea, such as in degenerations. In cases of increased intraocular tension the corneal epithelium shows an irregular surface, a loss of luster, and becomes dull and vesicular.

Vesicles.—These are produced by an elevation of the epithelium from Bowman's membrane by a limpid fluid. They are usually very small and occur individually or in numbers. They may be formed by the coalescence of the small droplets occurring in edema. When vesicles are larger in size, they are usually described as bullae. Vesicles may occur in the cornea in many of the inflammatory conditions affecting the eye, in degenerative and neuroparalytic conditions of the cornea, and as the result of burns, trauma, or operation. They may also occur in various forms of keratitis occurring in certain nervous conditions and others of unknown origin. The appearance of vesicles in the cornea is accompanied often by lacrimation, photophobia, and injection around the cornea.

Herpes.—The appearance of small vesicles on the cornea which is accompanied by marked signs of irritation takes place in a number of febrile conditions, especially affections of the upper respiratory tract, such as influenza, pneumonia, bronchitis, and a few other fevers. (See Virus diseases.) These vesicles are usually small and arranged in groups. They are similar to those which may be found in the skin of the face in the same diseases. Rupture of the small vesicles occurs with subsequent healing and no residual scarring. In a few instances, however, ulceration may follow, especially of the dendritic variety (see Dendritic ulcer).

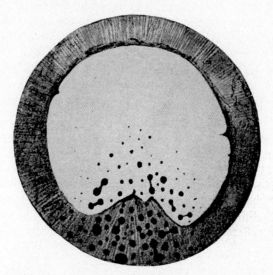

Fig. 37.—Keratitic precipitates in triangular distribution. (From Holmes Spicer: Brit. J. Ophth.) (Duke-Elder.)

Precipitates.—These usually are found to occur on the posterior surface of the cornea as the result of some inflammatory process. They may be very insignificant in size, so that they can be easily overlooked, or they may be so large that they can be readily seen by direct or oblique illumination. In all cases, however, they should be examined in detail with the slit lamp. They are said to be deposited on the posterior surface because of materials which float in the anterior chamber and because of convection current said to be present in the anterior chamber. Usually the deposits assume a triangular formation, ordinarily in the lower half of the cornea. This is often found in iridocyclitis. In rare instances, the deposits group themselves in a long fusiform spindle arrangement on the posterior surface, which has been described as *Krukenberg's spindle.*

In uveitis, deposits are found on Descemet's membrane, to which is given the name of *descemetitis.* In other instances their presence has been designated as *keratitis punctata,* and they are often spoken of as *K. P.* In tuberculosis, the deposits are large and swollen, and are described as "mutton-fat deposits." *Plastic exudates,* or precipitations, may be deposited as a mass on the back of the cornea in severe cases of iridocyclitis.

In most cases the deposition of the precipitates is preceded by edema with bedewing of the endothelium. The droplets can be seen in the endothelium by retro-illumination with the slit lamp, if examined early. Later on, collections of leucocytes, fibrin and, occasionally, granules of pigment are found. Edematous fluid may be seen more anteriorly, with posterior swelling and relucency. As the inflammatory condition subsides, some of the precipitates may become absorbed, or they may disappear completely. In other instances they may change their form and appearance as they become old, pallor, thinning and crenated edges appearing, with fibrin and particles persisting for a long time.

Punctate spots occur in the superficial cornea in *superficial punctate keratitis* as the result of infiltration. The condition is usually associated with a preliminary conjunctivitis, photophobia, and lacrimation. The spots may be either round or irregular and may assume various shapes (disc-shaped, pointed, angular, or ring). They may be present in large numbers and are scattered, so that the condition is spoken of sometimes as superficial disseminated keratitis. They may be found in the deeper epithelium, but more commonly in the superficial layers of the substantia propria. The overlying epithelium may be smooth but raised slightly. When the acute condition subsides, the spots gradually disappear, leaving no scars or impairment of vision.

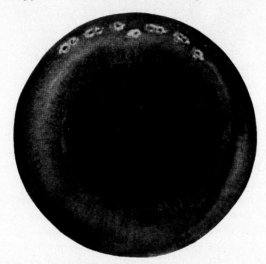

Fig. 38.—Herpetic ulcers of the cornea. (From Berliner: Arch. Ophth., September, 1933.)

Disc-shaped infiltrates occurring in the superficial layers of the substantia propria, the appearance of which resembles superficial punctate keratitis, was described by Dimmer, in 1905, as *nummular keratitis*. The condition is usually unilateral, is slow in development, and is considered to be occupational. It is seen mostly in young people who are land workers, and occurs mostly in the late summer. The cause is not known, but it has been considered to be due to some animal or vegetable virus. This condition also starts with a conjunctivitis and is accompanied by signs of irritation, such as lacrimation and photophobia. A number of disc-shaped opacities can be seen on examination, under Bowman's membrane. They are usually central, but sometimes near the limbus. They vary in size and consist of a number of very small dots. The epithelium is at first raised over the discs, but becomes flat, and a dense area develops around which is a gray halo. This later disappears, the disc becomes sharply outlined and is depressed in the center with the formation of a facet. This gives a characteristic appearance. The condition may be present for months while changing its appearance. When the lesions occur near the limbus, they may heal with resultant vascularization. Gradually, over a period of years, the lesions will disappear.

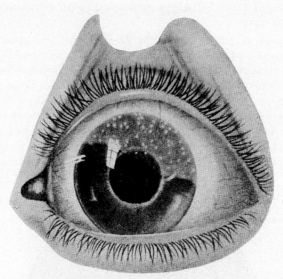

Fig. 39.—Superficial punctate keratitis of leprosy. (From King: Brit. J. Ophth.) (Duke-Elder.)

Ulcers of the cornea are either primary or secondary. Primary ulcers occur principally as the result of trauma, such as abrasions, foreign bodies, burns, and wounds, while others occur as marginal ulcers, mainly in elderly people and without any discoverable cause. Traumatic ulcers may be found also as the result of constant and repeated mechanical irritation of pressure from the presence of scars, growths on the lids, ingrown lashes, and inverted cilia. The marginal ulcers occurring in older people without any specific causes may be part of, or manifestation of, a general debilitated condition. These primary ulcers occur usually without suppuration. Such ulcers which show signs of healing readily are found to be mild in their course, and superficial; the edges are rather well circumscribed, and the cornea beyond the limits of the ulcer is found to be clear. No signs of infiltration of the surrounding cornea are seen. In addition, the floor of the ulcer, if any, is shallow and smooth. Progressive ulcers are accompanied by more severe signs of inflammation. There is always an area of infiltration around the edge of the ulcer, so that the cornea immediately adjacent is found to be cloudy. The floor of the ulcer may be covered and irregular, and there is a tendency to perforation of the cornea at the site of the ulcer.

Secondary ulcers of the cornea are usually due to a primary affection elsewhere, such as in the conjunctiva. These may occur as simple catarrhal ulcers, which are crescentic in shape and follow or accompany a catarrhal conjunctivitis. They are nearly always located at the margin of the cornea.

They usually run a rather mild course and do not tend to extension. Several such crescentic ulcers may be present at the same time, however, and by their contiguity, they will almost completely surround the circumference of the cornea, causing an annular ulcer. In the early stage, however, a crescentic ulcer will appear only as a collection of small gray dots at the margin of the cornea. These will, in a few days, however, become more pronounced, more numerous, and confluent, resulting, thereby, in a crescentic ulcer. On healing, there remains a slight arclike opacity resembling arcus senilis.

Ulcers may also occur near the corneal margin as the result of trachoma. A more severe form of ulcer, however, may occur in the cornea as the result of gonorrheal infection of the conjunctiva. These are very purulent and extensive and tend to perforation. The ulcers occurring as the result of metastatic gonorrheal infection are much milder in their course.

Phlyctenular conjunctivitis may be accompanied by small, superficial ulcers of the cornea, found usually at the margins. These ulcers, although small, may have deep depressions and extend deeply into the cornea, rather than in a lateral direction.

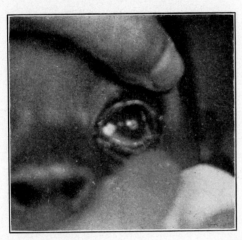

Fig. 40.—Central corneal opacity following ulcer. (Clinic of Dr. Frank Parker, Wills Hospital.)

Almost any ulcer of the cornea may be accompanied by signs of irritation, such as photophobia, lacrimation, and pain. In some instances the irritation is so great that it is very difficult to separate the eyelids in the course of examination and treatment. When an ulcer perforates, the iris may be seen to be prolapsed through the perforation.

Mooren's Ulcer *(Ulcus Rodens)* is a superficial ulcer which is found at the margin of the cornea, usually above. It has an undermined margin which is separated from the adjacent cornea by a cloudy area. It is accompanied by marked inflammation. On healing after a time, the ulcer becomes covered with vessels which extend in from the limbus. It shows a great tendency to relapse with a return of active irritation and further extension. After a time the greater part of the cornea may be involved with a corresponding interference with the vision. The condition occurs mostly in older people and may affect one or both eyes.

Ulcus Serpens is a severe ulceration of the cornea to which is often applied the name of hypopyon ulcer, or hypopyon keratitis. Since the pneumococcus has been so frequently found in the presence of ulcus serpens, it has also been called the pneumococcus ulcer of the cornea. In some instances a typical ulcus serpens may exist without the pneumococcus, and such microorganisms as the streptococcus, *Bacillus pyocyaneus,* as well as others, may be present. They are to be found in a number of the acute infectious diseases, such as measles, scarlet fever, smallpox, and others. The most frequent cause of ulcus serpens, however, is probably trauma. Even though an ulcer of this sort appears rather spontaneously in the cornea, in all probability there was a previous injury or abrasion, however slight (Fuchs). The injury may be only a slight denuding or rubbing off of corneal epithelium, produced by some rough material. Sometimes the abrasion produced by the branch of a twig

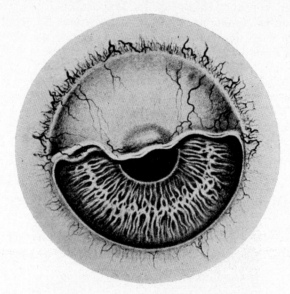

Fig. 41.—Mooren's ulcer, advanced stage. (From Duke-Elder: Text-Book of Ophthalmology.)

or a fine splinter of wood may cause the injury. The lesion is then secondarily infected, usually by microorganisms already present in the eye, and ulcus serpens results. The floor of the ulcer becomes gray and clouded with a very cloudy rim surrounding the area. In the first week this is usually disc-shaped, and later takes on a grayish appearance which occupies the center of the cornea. The clear portion of the cornea becomes invaded by grayish extensions from the central area and is somewhat cloudy. The area becomes depressed, and the edges may or may not be affected to the same extent. At the same time a hypopyon is present and is one of the chief characteristics of the condition. This consists of pus which is rather thick and does not especially change its position with change in the position of the patient's head. Later it takes on the appearance of a heavy exudate which adheres to the posterior surface of the cornea, or invades some of the deep cornea itself, and is sometimes regarded as a posterior corneal abscess. The anterior portion of the cornea occupied by the ulcer continues to break down with progression of the ulcer, until almost the entire cornea is involved. The anterior chamber may also become filled with pus, and panophthalmitis can result. If the ulcer should heal, the vision of the patient is definitely impaired in the involved eye. In cases with perforation of the cornea as the result of deep ulceration, a dense, white scar in the cornea will remain.

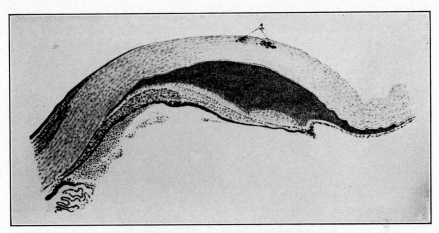

Fig. 42.—Ulcus serpens with hypopyon produced by toxins from colonies of bacteria, *a*, which reached the anterior chamber. (From Samuels: Arch. Ophth., January, 1932.)

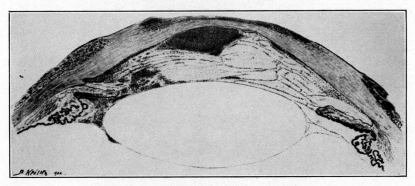

Fig. 43.—Ulcus serpens, with a dense collection of leucocytes on posterior surface of Descemet's membrane, opposite the progressive border of ulcer. The stroma is not infiltrated. (From Samuels: Arch. Ophth., January, 1932.)

Dendritic Ulcer.—More properly termed dendritic keratitis which is a herpetic manifestation of a virus infection. The lesion is a zig-zag, linear opacity with several branches or twigs, usually found in the center of the cornea. In the early stages these branches are very narrow with a kind of protuberance on the end. Later, they widen and coalesce to form an irregular shallow ulcer. On inspection they will be found at first to stain lightly with fluorescein and, on examination with the slit lamp, they are observed in the epithelium in relation with the terminal branches of the corneal nerves. Inflammatory infiltration may be seen faintly in the superficial layers of the stroma. The shape of the lesion is caused by the outward projection of the original epithelial foci. Irritation, photophobia, a sensation of a foreign body, and lacrimation of the eye usually accompany the condition. On healing, a faint grayish macula may remain which gradually thins out and eventually disappears. In other instances, however, the condition may become purulent, with the further development of an infiltrating ulcer and possible hypopyon. Dendritic ulcer or keratitis is a common eye manifestation of malaria, and in some of the acute infectious diseases and those affecting the upper respiratory tract. (See Virus infections.)

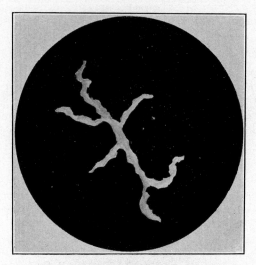

Fig. 44.—Dendritic keratitis.

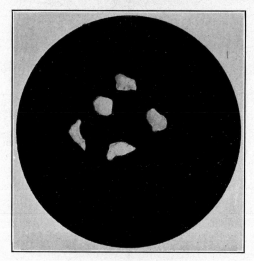

Fig. 45.—Herpes corneae.

The treatment of this form of keratitis is varied in its kind and results. Most of the patients are usually in a poor general physical condition. The removal of all possible foci of infection and general treatment of the patient are important. Quinine has been used to a great extent in treating these patients and vitamin therapy is also employed, as well as sulfanilamide, vaccines, autoserums and a variety of other measures, none of which have been found to be generally effectual.

Local treatment consists in cauterization of the corneal epithelium involved with iodine, trichloracetic acid or other agents. The use of atropine in the affected eye should be continued throughout the course of the keratitis.

Phlyctenules.—A phlyctenule is very commonly found directly on the limbus of the cornea, although they occasionally occur just inside the limbus. They usually affect the epithelium since they are part of the picture seen in phlyctenular conjunctivitis. The phlyctenule on the cornea is identical in nature with that found on the conjunctiva. When the phlyctenule becomes infected, it may result in superficial ulceration. In ordinary cases, however, they become absorbed with no destruction of the epithelium. When ulceration occurs, its surface is covered with leucocytes which give the phlyctenule a yellowish appearance. Otherwise, they appear as small nodules with a gray color, readily seen on ordinary inspection. They may occur singly, or several may be seen around the limbus of the cornea. These may coalesce and, on breaking down, will result in a marginal ulcer. Prolonged infiltration of the cornea results in the appearance of superficial vessels around the limbus. Perforation of the cornea rarely occurs.

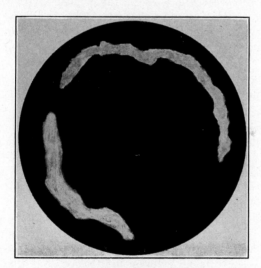

Fig. 46.—Marginal ring ulcer.

Vascularization.—The cornea normally is not supplied with blood vessels, but in most of the inflammatory processes, the very small vessels around the limbus became distended, leading to the presence of pericorneal injection. In pathologic processes involving the cornea, small new vessels will invade the latter. They proceed inward from the limbus, usually toward the active lesion. These vessels in a recent condition are very small and are difficult to see with the unaided eye. They can be readily seen and studied, however, on examination with the slit lamp. In many cases they can be seen with focal illumination. They are best examined by retro-illumination when they stand out as dark red streaks. In some instances they are clearly visible with the ordinary illumination of the slit lamp and may be of fair size and number. They occur at the same level with the lesion in the cornea, so that they will indicate the depth at which the latter occurs. Superficial vessels around the limbus of the cornea are commonly seen with phlyctenules, in superficial keratitis, and other forms of keratitis, as the result of irritation of the cornea from trichiasis and as the result of trachoma.

Pannus is the vascularization of the cornea which occurs in infiltrative processes. A new formation of vascular tissue spreads down from the limbus toward the center of the cornea. This part of the cornea is rough and covered with a number of projections, together with a grayish mass superficially located and covered by many vessels. These arise from the conjunctival vessels and pass over the limbus onto the cornea. On arriving within the area of pannus, they branch out in a latticelike formation. Pannus occurs most commonly at the upper limbus and the vision is only interfered with when the vascular area reaches or encroaches on the pupil. When superficial, it is localized between Bowman's membrane, and the epithelium which is raised up. With recovery from the pannus, the epithelium resumes its normal position in proximity to Bowman's membrane. However, if pannus penetrates Bowman's membrane, or is present over a long period of time, the latter is destroyed. In some cases a sclerosis takes place, with the formation of a dense white tissue containing a few vessels. This is similar in appearance to a dense scar following ulceration, except that it is more superficial. Pannus is seen most commonly in such diseases as trachoma, leprosy, phlyctenular keratitis, and as a degenerative condition of the cornea.

Opacities.—The opacities affecting the cornea can be divided into two general groups, viz., those that result from noninflammatory causes, such as contusions, injury, or pressure, and those which result from an inflammatory process. The noninflammatory opacities are usually temporary or transient in nature. Pressure opacities occur in cases with increased intraocular tension. These are transient and disappear when the pressure within the eye subsides. In a sense they are an edema of the cornea and give the center of the cornea a cloudy appearance which is rather uniform in its outline. The edema affects principally the epithelium of the cornea.

Striae or striate opacities of the cornea occur as the result of traumatism to the eye. In a few cases they are also seen with inflammatory lesions of the cornea, such as ulcus serpens. These striae are caused by a wrinkling of Descemet's membrane. There is no cellular infiltration, but the lymph spaces are dilated from a distention with fluid. A common example of this condition is found in so-called striped keratitis, following cataract operation. Here, fine vertical striations are found in the cornea resulting from the traumatism of operation, particularly the wound made in the section of the cornea. The striations can usually be observed on the following day and for several days following, after which they gradually disappear. They do not cause any inflammatory symptoms. A similar condition is sometimes observed after an eye has been covered with a pressure bandage.

Contusions of the cornea may result in opacities in the center of the cornea which are found to consist of fine interlacing striae. The opacities are usually

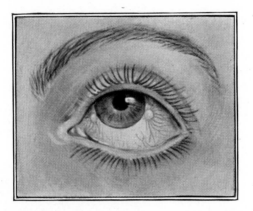

Fig. 47.—Phlyctenules at the limbus of the cornea.

in the middle and deeper layers of the cornea, and their presence has been designated under the name of keratitis profunda. These striae are very transient in the ordinary case, but in more severe injuries, they are round and larger, and are called annular opacities. Folds of Descemet's membrane and Bowman's membrane often occur following contusions of the cornea and are associated lesions.

Erosions may be found in the form of excoriations in the superficial epithelium of the cornea, as the result of injury from scratches, abrasions, and contact with rough materials. These are accompanied by pain and marked signs of irritation. The epithelium of the superficial cornea is removed with vesicular formation. The vesicles quickly rupture. This condition often leads to ulceration.

Drug opacities are occasionally produced in the cornea, as for example, by the use of cocaine. This drug in many cases causes a diffuse grey haze in the epithelium which is present for several hours after instillation of a weak solution. In stronger concentration it causes discrete spots throughout the cornea from destruction of the epithelium.

Opacities resulting from inflammation are of a more or less permanent nature and cause an impairment of vision corresponding to their location, size, and extent. Ulcer of the cornea is the most common cause. These opacities are more marked and usually denser when they are recent, and thin out, becoming more faint with age. Opacities result from interstitial keratitis, phlyctenular keratitis, and other forms of keratitis.

Maculae.—Sometimes called nebulae, these are faint, hazy spots in the cornea which have a bluish-white tint and result from former small ulcers. They are very often so faint that they are difficult to see and are often overlooked. They can be observed best with oblique illumination and are at times found to be rather diffuse. They can also be seen when the eye is examined with the ophthalmoscope by using one of the higher power lenses, and on examination with the slit lamp.

Leucoma is a dense opacity in the cornea which is usually white or greyish-white in color and of a permanent nature. It results from thickening of the epithelium on the surface of a scar. In some cases it follows perforation of a corneal ulcer. A corneal leucoma is usually fairly well outlined. The surface of the cornea at the site of the leucoma is slightly elevated. It can be rather plainly seen on ordinary inspection, or with oblique illumination, and on examination with the slit lamp.

Scars are another form of opacity in the cornea resulting usually from ulceration. They are well defined and may be faint or dense. They are usually white in color and are caused by the formation of cicatricial tissue. They occur on any part of the cornea, depending on the site of the primary lesion, but are very common on the margins. They can be seen on direct inspection with ordinary or oblique illumination, and on examination with the ophthalmoscope and slit lamp.

Ectasia.—Sometimes called keratasia, ectasia is a protrusion of the cornea or corneal tissue. Noninflammatory ectasia of the cornea occurs in keratoconus and keratoglobus. In this type of ectasia the cornea is uniformly clear, whereas in ectasia following inflammation, the cornea is opaque. In the latter variety the ectasia is produced by a thinning out of the superficial layers of the cornea following ulceration, so that the posterior layers can no longer hold back the pressure of the ocular contents. It may occur following interstitial keratitis, pannus, and various types of ulcers.

Staphyloma is an ectasia of the cornea caused by perforation which is characterized by a bulging scar. The scar contains the iris which was prolapsed into the wound when the perforation took place. Either a part of or the entire cornea may be involved by the staphyloma. They are white or bluish white in color and may be covered by several vessels coming from the conjunctiva. They are opaque and prevent any examination of the deeper structure of the eye. They are plainly visible on direct inspection.

Nodules may occur on the cornea principally in tuberculosis and in leprosy. In tuberculosis the nodule may be present near the limbus as an infiltrative lesion, and tends to spread into the cornea as a grayish opacity. It may also occur as a secondary tubercle which springs from the conjunctiva primarily.

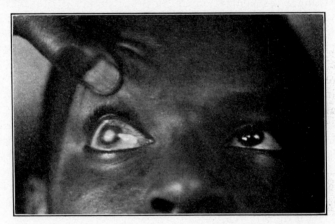

Fig. 48.—Maculated cornea. (I. S. Tassman, Wills Hospital.)

Nodules occur in leprosy at the limbus of the cornea and may be associated here with nodules of the conjunctiva and sclera. They are firm, yellow spots described as miliary lepromas and contain lepra cells and bacilli.

Blood Stain may occur near the periphery of the cornea after a subconjunctival hemorrhage. Hemorrhage into the anterior chamber might cause blood staining of the posterior cornea. All, or nearly all, of the cornea may be involved. When fresh, the stain has a dark red color which fades out into a dark brown as it becomes older. The staining is caused by the products of the broken up blood corpuscles which are absorbed through Descemet's membrane. It may be mistaken for a dislocated lens, which it resembles very much in appearance. It usually requires a long time to clear up.

Pigmentation.—Pigmentation of the cornea is perhaps best illustrated by the presence of a Kayser-Fleischer ring. Here, the pigmentation produces a ring around the periphery of the posterior cornea which is rather typical in appearance. It occurs close to the limbus and is about 1 to 3 mm. in width. It therefore presents the appearance of a rather bright band made up of a number of different colors usually including brown, green, blue, and sometimes yellow. The brown predominates while the entire spectrum gradually fades out at the inner border. The pigment consists of fine, closely clumped granules just under the epithelium. They reach Descemet's membrane but do not penetrate it. The Kayser-Fleischer ring has been said to occur in cases of disseminated sclerosis and pseudosclerosis, but it is considered to be a characteristic finding in Wilson's Disease. The condition can be observed on examination with oblique illumination, but should be studied with the slit lamp.

Pterygium is a degenerative process in which a triangular area pointing toward the limbus from the conjunctiva encroaches on the cornea. It may be present in one or both eyes and occurs more commonly on the nasal side of the cornea, although both sides may be affected simultaneously. The early sign of pterygium of the cornea is the appearance of small gray spots of infiltration which gradually fuse into a spot forming the head. This is continuous with the conjunctival portion. The pterygium is sharply outlined on its upper and lower borders and can be lifted up between the blades of a forceps. It can readily be examined on direct inspection (see Pterygium of the conjunctiva).

Dystrophy is the occurrence of opacities in the cornea which are supposedly produced by degeneration. There are several different kinds of dystrophies, but they are described in general by Fuchs as chronic disturbances of nutrition, in which an opacity gradually develops in the cornea, and steadily increases in extent in the course of time; although they are, as a rule, progressive in their course, they are not accompanied by external signs of inflammation. In most of the dystrophies there takes place either a fatty or hyaline degeneration, while in others, there are deposits of calcareous material.

Arcus Senilis is considered to be a physiologic change in the cornea which takes place with oncoming age. It is characterized by a lipoid infiltration of the stroma which produces a ringlike opacity around the periphery, just inside the limbus from which it is separated by a small, clear zone. It is grayish white in color and can be seen in many older people on direct inspection of the eyes. Early in the condition it may appear only as a peripheral haze in the upper and lower portions of the cornea. When it occurs in younger people, it is known as arcus presenilis, or arcus juvenilis. It nearly always affects both eyes, and is commonly seen in the colored race.

Band-Shaped Opacity is sometimes called zonular opacity and is a form of degeneration in the cornea characterized by the appearance of a horizontal band occurring just below the pupil and occupying the space of the palpebral fissure. There is a clear zone of cornea above and below. The band is gray in color and is very gradual in its onset and progress. It has been said to occur either primarily or in eyes which were formerly affected with some inflammatory condition, such as iridocyclitis and interstitial keratitis. The occurrence of rheumatism is sometimes a factor in some of the cases affected. Calcareous deposits are said to take place in the bandlike area.

Sclerosis of the Cornea develops after degenerative pannus. The cornea is white in color and resembles the appearance of the sclera.

Groenouw's Nodular Dystrophy.—The center of the cornea is occupied by a number of white spots which are under Bowman's membrane. They are grouped together in a round or irregularly shaped mass. They may be found in any number and progress slowly in the course of time, gradually appearing in the deeper portions of the cornea.

Another type of nodular dystrophy is known as Salzmann's corneal dystrophy. This is also a progressive condition affecting the superficial cornea where the nodules show degenerative changes. Signs of irritation are usually absent, but the vision becomes impaired. The small nodes give the appearance of prominences on the corneal surface. The condition is said to occur in eyes previously affected with phlyctenular keratitis. Nodular thickenings on Descemet's membrane, which are known as Hassall-Henle bodies, occur around the periphery of the cornea and project into the anterior chamber. They occur in younger people and appear as dark round holes in the epithelium, when examined with the slit lamp; but they were described by Vogt as drop-like protuberances.

Epithelial Dystrophy (Fuchs) is a rare condition occurring mostly in females over 50 years of age. It is characterized by the appearance of an early edema of the central epithelium, which gradually spreads to the periphery. The vacuoles later form groups and burst, leaving superficial gray opacities in the cornea. The sensation of the cornea decreases with progress of the condition and eventually the entire cornea may become involved. The vision in the affected eye is diminished. Severe pain may be a disturbing symptom because of recurring bullae. Both eyes often become affected and glaucoma is a common complication.

Endothelial Dystrophy is a condition characterized by very fine spots with a gold color or gleam on the posterior surface of the cornea. Large black circles or spheres appear in the arrangement of the endothelial cells. Because of the small size and location of the lesion, it can best be studied on examination with the slit lamp. The cells become fewer in number with vacuole formation on the posterior surface. Pigmentation of the posterior cornea increases, which later has the appearance of a brown film covering the cornea, with impairment of vision resulting. In the late stage the condition can be seen with oblique illumination and on examination with the ophthalmoscope.

Abnormalities of the Sclera and Episcleral Tissue

The sclera will be remembered as a fibrous protective coat of the posterior eye which becomes continuous with the cornea in the anterior portion at the limbus. Here it can be seen clearly to give the eye its white color. Compared to most of the other structures of the eye, it is not commonly affected, and the lesions occurring there are fewer in number. It is mostly avascular, but vessels pass through it, in entering and leaving the interior of the eye. The episcleral tissue which connects the conjunctiva with it is very vascular, however, and is more commonly affected by inflammation, often of endogenous origin, than the sclera itself. It is very often difficult to separate an inflammation of the episcleral tissue from that of the sclera once the one may develop into the other.

Congestion and Inflammation.—Congestion and prominence of the episcleral vessels may occur as an early sign of inflammation of the episcleral

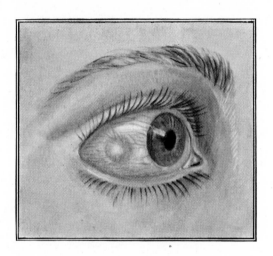

Fig. 49.—Nodule of the sclera, showing bluish colored swelling on the temporal side covered by conjunctival vessels.

or scleral tissue. The vessels of the episclera can be seen to stand out rather prominently across the white of the eye and under the conjunctiva, in a lateral direction. The congestion or inflammation may affect only a certain area, very often well back from the cornea, while in other instances, it will be found to be more diffuse. The conjunctival vessels may also show a congestion at the same time, but these are seen more superficially. When inflammation of the episcleral tissue occurs, it is known as episcleritis, while inflammation of the sclera itself is designated as scleritis.

Nodules occur in the episclera in a form of episcleritis and also in leprosy. In the latter condition lepra cells are plentiful in the episcleral tissue, and it is thought by some that this is their portal of entry. (See Leprosy.) The nodules found in the episcleral tissue are more common in episcleritis. In this condition they are the manifestation of a local inflammatory focus which is benign in nature. The nodules are usually round or nearly round, and may be large enough in size to be distinctly seen on direct inspection of the eye. They are firmly attached to the sclera below, but the conjunctiva is free and loose above. Distention of the episcleral vessels is an accompanying feature and gives the nodule a purple color. They are very sensitive and are accompanied by signs of inflammation. After a period of several weeks, the nodule may subside, leaving a pale, atrophic area in the sclera to which the conjunctiva may become attached. Recurrences are frequent, and the lesions may be multiple in rare instances, so that the process remains for a much longer time. This form of episcleritis and scleritis is considered to be associated with rheumatic conditions, articular rheumatism, and foci of infection, principally those occurring in the teeth and tonsils. Inflammation of the sclera may also be an accompanying factor in the presence of syphilitic or tuberculous involvement. Gumma of the sclera is a rare occurrence, but it might be present in the form of an injected nodule which is seen in the neighborhood of the corneal limbus. These are usually secondary manifestations of gumma of the ciliary body which have extended into the sclera. They may go on to ulceration and perforation of the eyeball if the patient does not receive antisyphilitic treatment.

Tubercle of the sclera occurs occasionally as a manifestation of a tuberculous focus which has been conveyed to the sclera through the circulation. The bacilli have probably reached the sclera from the anterior chamber through the network around the angle of the iris. These tuberculous nodules, like others, are attached firmly to the sclera with the conjunctiva freely movable above. They are hard and have a yellowish color, and their size may be almost that of a pea, which is raised, so that they can be clearly seen by direct examination. After a time, the tubercle may break down and ulcerate.

Ulcer is not a common finding on the sclera, but it may result subsequent to tubercle, or other nodular formation, traumatism, or infection. When ulcers do occur, they are characterized by a pitting at the site of the lesion, to which the conjunctiva will later become attached.

Cysts of the sclera are also rare, but when they occur, they are probably formed from the conjunctiva and are due to injury or operation. These are characterized by a vesicular swelling which is rather soft, fluctuating, and has a thin outer wall. The posterior wall may appear dark, due to the presence of uveal pigment. They gradually increase in size and may become as large as marbles.

Ectasia and Staphyloma.—This condition of the sclera is characterized by a bulging forward. When the entire sclera is involved, the ectasia is total, and when the bulging occurs only in a certain area, it is considered to be a partial ectasia. The ectasia is produced either because of a great increase of the intraocular pressure or a thinning out and lack of resistance of the sclera. An ectasia may result from the presence of a former pathologic process, such as a tubercle, scleritis, wound, etc. Wounds and injuries to the eyeball are a common cause of ectasia and staphyloma. A thinning or destruction of the sclera lowers the resistance of that portion of the anterior eyeball from the pressure of the intraocular tension behind, which results in the ectasia and staphyloma. When injuries occur in the neighborhood of the ciliary body, the latter may be found prolapsed into the staphylomatous area, giving it a darker color. Staphyloma of the sclera may be associated with enlargement or even staphyloma of the cornea, such as occurs with injuries at the corneoscleral margin. In staphyloma of the sclera, the surface appears irregular with ridges occurring on the inner surface. The color in nearly all cases is dark, due to pigment from the uveae which degenerated. Here and there may be found one or more bands of sclera which are still resistant and, with the atrophied tissue on either side, give it the appearance of a bluish lobulated saclike formation. When touched by the finger, this saclike formation pits easily, and on transillumination, it transmits the light more clearly in some portions than in others, because of the difference in density in the sacculated area. With gradual progression, the entire eyeball may become very much enlarged with accompanying pain, displacement, and degeneration of the contents, so that eventual enucleation of the eye is indicated. In a few cases, however, the condition may become more or less stationary, so that a fatal termination is avoided unless the eyeball is subjected to further injury.

Examination of the Anterior Chamber

The anterior chamber should be examined especially to determine its depth and to note the presence or absence of any foreign material in its contents. This is accomplished by direct illumination, oblique illumination, examination with the slit lamp, and ophthalmoscopic examination.

Bounded in front by the posterior surface of the cornea, and behind by the iris, lens, and ciliary body, the anterior chamber is often subjected to alterations in its depth because of changes and diseases affecting these structures. Keratoconus, posterior dislocations of the lens, retraction of the iris, and posterior synechiae will result in an increase in depth of the chamber.

Examination of the Angle of the Anterior Chamber (Gonioscopy).—This is the term applied to the examination of the angle of the anterior chamber by means of focal illumination. It has been attempted in the past without much success by placing a contact glass with flat sides over the cornea and raising the illumination of the slit lamp.

More recently, a gonioscope has been devised by Troncoso for this purpose. This is based on the principle of a periscope. A contact glass is placed over the cornea and with the illumination of the gonioscope, the angle of the anterior chamber can be examined in detail. This will reveal the inner line of the sclera at this point as a white band, the concave inner part of the cornea, Schlemm's canal, the narrow brown band of the ciliary body with the root of the iris attached, the iris itself, and the pupillary border of the iris. Any abnormalities in this region can be detected and an examination can be made of any injuries, inflammatory processes, gummata, tubercles, and tumors. Most important, however, is the detection of posterior synechiae in this location, and the study of the condition of the angle of the anterior chamber with reference to glaucoma.

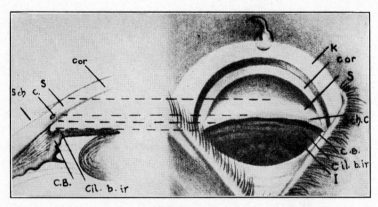

Fig. 50.—The normal angle of the anterior chamber as seen by the gonioscope. *K,* Dome of the contact glass. *Cor,* Cornea. *S,* Sclera. *Sch.C,* Schlemm's canal. *C.B.,* Ciliary body. *Cil.b.ir,* Ciliary root of iris. *I,* Iris. (After Troncoso, from Duke-Elder: Text-Book of Ophthalmology.)

Transillumination

Examination by transillumination or diaphanoscopy is employed principally for the detection of intraocular tumors. It has been used for a great many years, and many different instruments have eben devised for this purpose. The most recent and the one in common use at the present time is known as Würdemann's transilluminator.

The examination is made in a dark room. The eye to be examined is anesthetized, and the pupil is dilated. As a general rule, the patient is directed to look in a designated direction, and with the eyelids separated, the tip of the instrument is placed against the opposite side of the eyeball. This is repeated several times, while the patient is instructed to look in different directions. At the same time, the examiner determines whether the light of the instrument is transmitted through the eyeball without obstruction.

The anterior portion of the eyeball can be transilluminated by passage of a strong beam of light into the pupil. The light of the slit lamp may be employed, and in this way, the ciliary region and angle of the anterior chamber can be fairly well examined, especially for the presence of pigmented tumors.

Transillumination through conjunctiva and sclera consists in placing the tip of the instrument against the eyeball behind the cornea. In a normal eye the pupil reveals the red light reflex. If a growth is present inside the spot on the sclera through which the light is projected, the pupil will appear black. Very small growths may not cause sufficient obstruction to the passage of the light, while on the other hand, extensive hemorrhages or exudates, if present, will obstruct the passage of the light. In some patients such as negroes, with deep pigmentation, the passage of light may also be interfered with. Cataract of the lens does not interfere with transillumination, and foreign bodies can be detected in the lens in this way, even in the presence of cataract.

The eye can also be examined directly during transillumination by using the ophthalmoscope with a lens of high power. In this way the region anterior to the equator may be examined for tears, wounds, foreign bodies, and solid growths.

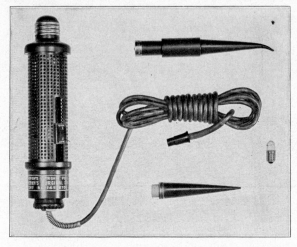

Fig. 51.—Ocular transilluminator. (From Block: Arch. Ophth., March, 1940.)

Abnormalities in the Anterior Chamber

The aqueous content of the anterior chamber may reveal the presence of foreign material when examined with the methods described.

Hemorrhage in the anterior chamber (hyphemia) may occur as the result of trauma and inflammation. It is a common occurrence following a blow to the eye and following operative procedures, such as iridectomy. In these conditions the hemorrhage occurs almost immediately and can be observed on direct inspection with the aid only of direct illumination. The free fresh blood can be observed in the lower portion of the chamber between the iris and the cornea. Before clotting takes place, the blood can be seen to change its position with tilting of the patient's head from side to side. Such hemorrhage in the anterior chamber is ordinarily rapidly absorbed, so that its presence is no longer noted after twenty-four to forty-eight hours. In other instances, however, especially in diseased eyes and where the hemorrhage is more profuse, a longer period of time is required for absorption to occur. When the hemorrhage is of longer standing, it takes on a dark brown color, and in older cases, the only signs may be a dark brown pigment staining on the posterior cornea or on the iris.

Pus in the Anterior Chamber (Hypopyon).—The presence of free pus in the bottom of the anterior chamber between the iris and posterior surface of the cornea may occur in a large number of inflammatory conditions of the iris and cornea, as well as a metastatic involvement resulting from more remote foci of infection. The free pus is yellowish in color and can be observed on inspection with only ordinary direct illumination. When very recent, it can be seen to change its position with tilting or movement of the patient's head. The pus is absorbed and disappears in a short time in many instances, but it may become organized and remain for a long time.

Floating Particles in the Aqueous.—Examination with the illumination of the slit lamp may reveal the presence of foreign material in the anterior chamber. Floating particles of colloid material which give rise to the aqueous flare may be observed as evidences of early or low-grade inflammatory conditions. The aqueous may be found to be uniformly cloudy or even turbid because of the presence of fine dustlike particles which may be either cellular debris, cholesterin, pigment particles, or the products of inflammation. These may be found with inflammatory conditions of the uveal tract and as the result of trauma.

The Intraocular Tension or Pressure.—Since the depth of the anterior chamber is dependent on the position of the structures which mark its boundaries, and secondly, on the intraocular tension, it is necessary and important in nearly every examination of the eye to obtain a knowledge of the state of the pressure within the eye. The method of determination of the intraocular pressure is known as tonometry. This term, however, refers principally to the measurement by use of the tonometer. Although this affords the most exact determination available, the state of the intraocular tension can also be estimated by finger or digital palpation. The method and instrument employed in measuring the tension should always be specifically stated and recorded, as for example: "tension by finger palpation," or "tension by tonometer" (naming the particular type of instrument).

To estimate the degree of the intraocular tension by finger palpation, the patient can be either sitting or standing with the head erect. The examiner stands almost directly in front of the patient who is directed to look downward toward the floor. The tip of the index finger of each hand is then placed on the upper eyelid, back of the location of the ciliary body, and just under the superior rim of the orbit. The thumbs of each hand swing free, while the remaining fingers can rest easily on the forehead of the patient, just over the eyebrows. Gentle pressure is then made on the eyeball through the lid, with first one finger, and then the other, in fairly quick succession. The pressure made should be just sufficient to enable the examiner to sense the fluctuation of the eyeball from the tip of one index finger to the other, and thereby form some opinion as to the degree of the intraocular pressure. It is necessary, however, to have some conception of the "feel" of the normal eyeball, and this can be obtained only from practice and experience in the routine palpation of every eye which comes to the attention. The procedure is somewhat similar to palpation of an abdomen to determine the nature of distention and the degree of resistance to palpation encountered. It should be remembered, however, in testing the tension of the eye by palpation, especially in the presence of an inflammatory or irritable condition, to make gentle pressure and to avoid causing pain. Moreover, continued or repeated palpation of the eyeball will cause a reduction in the intraocular tension. The results obtained provide only a general idea of the condition, but to one with experience, it should not be difficult to determine the presence of an increased or high tension, and in other instances, the presence of low tension, and whether or not the eye is softer than usual. It is often advantageous to compare the finger tension of one eye with that of the other, so that the tension in an affected eye can be determined in comparison to that of its fellow, which is known to be normal. The results of finger tension are also designated roughly as +1 or –1, +2 or –2, and +3 or –3, according to the degree of hardness or softness encountered on palpation.

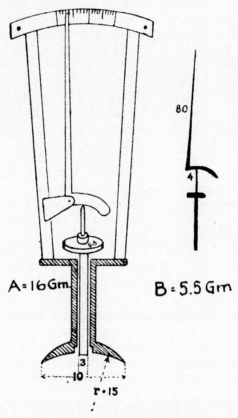

Fig. 52.—Diagram of Schiötz tonometer. (From Posner: Arch. Ophth., September, 1935.)

The Tonometric Measurement.—The instrument employed for more accurately measuring the intraocular pressure is known as the tonometer. Several different types of these are available, the most popular of which is the one devised by Schiötz in 1905, and which is known as the Schiötz tonometer. This consists of an upright or vertical arm at the upper extremity of which is a cross bar with a series of about twenty graduations. The lower portion of the tonometer consists of a rod which passes through a sleeve, so that it can move freely upward and downward. At the bottom of this sleeve is a concave foot plate with a radius of curvature which corresponds to the curvature of the average cornea. The upper extremity of the rod is threaded to receive the weights which are of four different grades, and which can be easily slipped over the tip of the rod. Attached to the lower end of the vertical arm is an indicator which swings freely in a lateral direction, at its upper extremity, and when at rest is checked by a small stud on either side of the upper crossbar. When assembled for use, therefore, the tonometer has the shape of a large letter T with a wide handle with which it is held, at the junction of its lower and middle third. The weights employed are 5.5, 7.5, 10, and 15 Gm. The smallest weight necessary to obtain a satisfactory reading in any case is fitted over the lower rod of the tonometer. To obtain a satisfactory result, the weight which will give a reading of at least 2 on the upper crossbar, should be employed. If the weight employed gives a reading of less than 2, the next heavier weight should be used. Before using the tonometer, it is to be tested on a small curved metal test plate which accompanies the instrument. The indicator should correspond to zero on the scale.

One or two drops of a local anesthetic, such as holocaine, 1 per cent, or butyn, 2 per cent, are placed in each eye. Cocaine should be avoided since it might affect the intraocular tension and is also damaging to the corneal epithelium. The patient is placed in a recumbent position, with the eyes open and looking directly upward. An attempt should be made to fix the gaze. The lids of the eye to be tested are gently separated by the thumb and index finger of one hand, while the tonometer held by its handle in the other hand, is brought to rest very gently on the center of the cornea. While the patient maintains a fixed gaze on a spot directly above and with the instrument in a perfectly vertical position, when it comes to rest, the indicator will be seen to swing over to a certain point on the scale of the upper crossbar. The reading at this point is noted, and the instrument is gently lifted from the cornea. After a moment or two at rest, the procedure is repeated with the same care, and the reading at the upper scale again noted. This should correspond closely to the former, and any great difference indicates an error in technique. A greater number of tests should be avoided, however, since this tends to lower the pressure with a lower reading on succeeding tests. A graph accompanies every Schiötz tonometer which transposes the reading obtained on the scale of the instrument to a result which is supposed to correspond to a mm. Hg in the final result. It is therefore necessary now to refer to this graph on which is plotted a series of curves, one for each weight belonging to the instrument. These curves indicate the intraocular tension for the various readings obtained on the scale of the tonometer. For example: If the reading obtained on the scale of the tonometer is 7 with a 10 mg. weight, the curve for this weight is then followed on the graph to 7, which will indicate the intraocular tension as 36. This is then recorded as the result in the eye tested. In patients with an abnormal cornea, as in keratoconus or staphyloma, the tonometer cannot be employed with any degree of accuracy. Other types of tonometers, such as the McLean tonometer, give slightly higher results for the normal than those obtained with the Schiötz instrument.

There is no fixed tonometric measurement for the normal eye, but the intraocular pressure may range normally between a measurement of 15 mm. to 28 mm. with the Schiötz tonometer. Above 28 should be considered as an indication of increased intraocular tension. The test is employed otherwise to follow the course and progress of the state of intraocular pressure over a period of time in any diseased eye.

Glaucoma

Glaucoma is a disease which is characterized by increase of the intraocular tension, supposedly due to a disturbance of the circulation of the fluids of the eye. The latter include the aqueous, vitreous, the blood, and lymph. An important factor in the production of glaucoma is the filtration of the fluid which takes place through the canal of Schlemm, and it is considered that some interference occurs with the outflow from the anterior chamber of the eye. The important local cause of glaucoma is an obstruction at the angle of the anterior chamber. This pathologic change is a constant finding in the disease and is the etiologic factor in all secondary glaucomas. Another characteristic change in the disease occurs in the optic nerve. In the latter there is first a deep cupping of the disc which is produced because the lamina cribrosa is forced back by the intraocular tension, the nerve fibers being also drawn back. An atrophy of the nerve fibers is produced where they pass over the edge of the scleral canal. Atrophy of the optic nerve is the ultimate result of the increased intraocular tension in glaucoma.

The angle of the anterior chamber is affected by peripheral anterior synechiae which are either annular or partial. The base of the iris becomes adherent to the posterior surface of the cornea.

In the cornea an edema and a vesiculation take place in the anterior layers. A thinning of the corneal lamellae occurs and newly formed fibrous tissue develops between Bowman's membrane and the new epithelium. A zonular hyaline and calcareous opacity of the cornea develops late in the disease.

In the iris areas of necrosis occur early in the process, and later, pronounced atrophy takes place with shrinking of the iris so that in advanced cases, it can scarcely be seen clinically. The ciliary body exhibits a swelling and edema of the epithelial cells, and the ciliary processes are swollen. In cases of long duration a pronounced atrophy of the ciliary body and processes takes place.

The choroid and retina show vascular changes with hyaline degeneration of the vessels, and later, an atrophy of the retina and choroid.

Clinical Causes.—The causes of glaucoma may be designated as predisposing and exciting causes. The specific cause is unknown. The disease usually occurs in older people, the ages ranging from 50 to 70. The possibility of the occurrence increases with the increase in age. This is probably due to such factors as sclerosing of the tissue at the angle of the anterior chamber, gradual increase in the size of the lens, increasing vasomotor instability, and other changes coming on with senility. It occurs equally in the two sexes, with perhaps a greater prevalence among women. With the latter, the emotions and menstrual changes occurring with age may be factors.

Glaucoma may occur as a hereditary condition, although this is not necessarily an important factor. Certain structural defects which are inherited may act as a cause, especially in true congenital glaucoma. The condition is quite common in the Jewish race, and among some foreign groups. It is quite common also in the Negro race.

The refractive state of the eye, especially when hyperopia is present, has been considered to be a predisposing cause of chronic simple glaucoma particularly. When the hyperopia remains uncorrected, the chronic congestion of the ciliary body which is produced by the action of the accommodation is said to be an important factor in causing the disease. It has often been pointed out that a patient with a small cornea is predisposed to glaucoma.

Shock has also been considered as a predisposing cause, especially in those who are affected with a vasomotor instability. The latter may produce an increase in intraocular tension in an eye after the fellow eye has been operated upon. In these instances a large pupil with retraction of the iris into the angle of the anterior chamber has been considered the causative factor, and as a general rule, such pupils are usually contracted by miotics as a preventive measure before operation is performed to the other eye.

Glaucoma may supervene or occur secondary to some acute infectious diseases and other inflammatory conditions, such as herpes zoster ophthalmicus. Such instances are comparatively rare, however.

Clinical Signs.—The increased intraocular tension may affect the various structures of the eye in different ways. This depends usually on whether the increase is sudden or gradual. With a sudden increase in the tension, for example, the eyelids will be found to be swollen and edematous to a moderate degree, while this is absent in the chronic form.

The conjunctiva reveals a marked chemosis and venous congestion with occasional hemorrhages when the rise in tension is very sudden or abrupt, while it is thin and shows a loss of elasticity, and tears very easily in the chronic form.

The sclera in the acute form shows a change in color becoming violaceous in appearance as a result of the venous congestion which takes place. In the chronic form there is continued pressure with thinning of the sclera which causes a bluish color produced by the uvea just beneath it. In cases of long-standing absolute glaucoma, ectasia of the sclera around the ciliary body may occur.

The cornea is very hazy and steamy in acute glaucoma. This is caused by the edema which is present in the epithelium and the anterior layers. It, therefore, loses its transparency and luster. There is accompanying loss of sensitivity. Later on in the condition, vesicles and bullae may occur. In chronic glaucoma, the cornea may show slight change and only a slight reduction in sensitivity. Vesicles and bullae also occur in the later stages, and in cases of long duration.

The aqueous will show a slight turbidity in the acute form, but the clouding may also be caused by the swelling of the cornea and discoloration of the iris. The anterior chamber is very shallow and, in some cases, almost completely eliminated. Narrowing in the depth of the anterior chamber also occurs in chronic simple glaucoma, but in secondary glaucoma, the depth may be increased.

The iris is found to be retracted and the pupil irregularly dilated in the acute form of the disease. This is caused by pressure on the ciliary nerves and changes in the iris vessels. The pupil may be also enlarged in chronic glaucoma, but this may not be much greater than normal. In late stages of the disease and in complicated glaucoma, the iris becomes atrophic, brittle, and paperlike, so that it tears easily when handled in any operative procedure.

The lens may be displaced forward early in glaucoma with resultant changes in the refraction. Cataract of the lens is a very common occurrence especially in chronic glaucoma. The ciliary body is markedly edematous in the acute form of the disease, and because of the change of direction of the ciliary processes, the latter may press against the lens which produces a narrowing of the anterior chamber. In the late stages of the disease, the ciliary body becomes atrophic.

The vitreous may show little change with perhaps only some opacities being found in the chronic form of the disease.

The choroid may show an increased thickening, due to the congestion in the acute form of the disease. This may result in an atrophy of the retina. In the chronic form the vessels undergo hyaline changes in their walls, and late in the disease, an atrophy is produced by pressure. The retina is affected in the acute form by the decreased amount of blood in the vessels resulting from pressure. This is accompanied by decrease in the vision. In the chronic form, various alterations occur in the visual fields from the effect produced on the nerve fiber layers, and on the blood vessels. In the latter a smaller amount of blood circulates to the retina, and a pressure is exerted on the circulation at the margin of the scleral canal. The nerve fiber layer of the retina is affected by a stretching of the fibers at the lamina and also a pressure at the edge of the excavation.

In the optic nerve the glial tissue in the nerve head and also in the nerve trunk is destroyed. The pushing of the lamina backward is the principal factor in causing the cupping of the optic nerve head. The nerve fibers are also pulled over the edge of the scleral canal with resultant stretching and compression.

Classification.—Glaucoma can be divided into a primary and a secondary variety. Primary glaucoma includes acute congestive (inflammatory type), chronic congestive (inflammatory type), and chronic simple glaucoma. The secondary variety includes those which result from obstruction to the outflow of fluids, changes in composition of fluid, congenital malformations of the eye, elevation of pressure in the vitreous, and congenital glaucoma (buphthalmos). These types may at times be difficult to differentiate. An acute attack may occur during the course of chronic or subacute glaucoma.

Acute Congestive Glaucoma.—Although this type of glaucoma may occur rather suddenly, certain prodromal symptoms may be noted as a result of the congestion which occurs. The patient may complain of very transitory dimness of vision and will state that halos are occasionally observed around lights. The eye will appear congested, and the pupil somewhat large. With the onset of the attack, the cornea is found to be steamy, the eye may show intense congestion, the pupil is considerably larger than normal, and the tension is increased to a moderate degree. The pain in the eye is very severe and radiates to the face, and also to the top of the head, being confined principally to the area of the fifth nerve. A marked reduction in the vision occurs early, and reflex symptoms such as nausea and vomiting may be present. The eyelids and conjunctiva of the eyeball show a moderate chemosis. The anterior chamber is either very shallow or entirely obliterated. On palpation, the eyeball will feel hard, and with a tonometer may be found to range from 60 to 80 mm.

This acute attack may last for a period of several weeks to several months, but the painful symptoms reach a maximum before the end of the first week. The acute congestion may gradually subside, especially if operation is performed at this stage (see Treatment). If no operation is performed, subsequent attacks may occur and will affect the excavation of the optic nerve and the vision to a greater extent.

Treatment.—The acute congestive form of glaucoma requires almost immediate surgical treatment. The operation usually performed in these cases is iridectomy. This is followed by almost immediate relief from pain and the intense congestion. Prior to the operation, hot compresses may be applied and local anesthetics instilled for the pain. Following operation, the patient will recover from the effects of the acute attack in about one week. Usually, there will be little or no impairment of vision, and the optic nerve head remains practically unaffected. The patient should remain under observation for an indefinite period and the intraocular tension should be tested regularly during this time.

Chronic Congestive Glaucoma.—In this type of the disease the eye is nearly always affected with a moderate amount of congestion which is accompanied by a moderate amount of impaired vision, increased tension, narrow anterior chamber, and enlarged pupil. An acute attack may supervene at almost any time. The visual fields on examination will show an enlargement of the blind spot and pronounced changes in the periphery. On examination with the ophthalmoscope the cornea is found to be slightly hazy, which will somewhat impair a view of the fundus. However, the retinal vessels are congested, and the optic nerve head will show glaucomatous excavation. The condition runs a more or less chronic course, and the patient is disturbed by intervals of pain, and a gradual increase in visual disturbances.

Treatment.—The treatment of these cases is either operative or nonoperative. In many instances it is necessary to employ both. The nonoperative treatment consists in the use of miotics in order to control the tension, and the occasional use of hot compresses for pain. The results obtained from nonoperative treatment are usually unsatisfactory, and some form of operative procedure must sooner or later be resorted to. The results from operative procedures are also uncertain, and in many cases unsatisfactory. As a result most of these cases run an unfavorable course.

Chronic Simple Glaucoma.—This type of glaucoma may take place at any age, but its occurrence is somewhat rare before the age of 50. It occurs more frequently with increasing age. Both sexes are equally affected, and heredity is apparently a factor in some instances. The Jewish race seems to be very susceptible. While the disease may begin simultaneously in both eyes, there is usually a noticeable difference in the progress of the condition when it comes under observation.

Signs and Symptoms.—Certain prodromal signs and symptoms usually appear first. A recession of the near point may frequently occur and necessitate a change in reading glasses. There is fatigue of the eyes in near work, while the eyeball feels full. Because the dark adaptation has slowed down, the patients cannot adjust quickly going from light to dark. The patient may notice a dimness of vision which may be only transient at first and later more prolonged. This may be accompanied by the appearance of halos around lights. These symptoms may be aggravated by emotional stress, worry, and fatigue.

The objective signs include an early narrowing of the chamber, with the pupil dilated in subdued light to an abnormal extent. At this time, no fundus changes may be observed.

During the progress of the case, the subjective symptoms show only slight change, while the objective signs become more numerous and pronounced. The anterior chamber becomes more shallow and anesthesia of the cornea occurs. The pupil is unusually large even in ordinary light and reacts poorly to light stimulation. The central retinal vessels become dilated and more tortuous. The tension by palpation may still appear to be normal but the tonometer should be employed at intervals to determine any periods of increased tension. The glaucomatous condition becomes certain when the tension is found to be elevated and the excavation of the nerve head becomes pronounced. Subsequent to this stage, the progress of the disease is more rapid, with oncoming changes in the visual field, continued increase in the intraocular tension, and further cupping of the optic nerve. The sensitivity of the cornea may be slightly diminished, the pupil is always larger than normal, but the visual acuity may not be necessarily affected. However, there may be a concentric contraction of the form field when tested with a 5 or 10 mm. test object at 330 mm. In other instances there may be found a relative contraction in the nasal field. The central fields are taken on a tangent screen with a 2 to 6 mm. test object at 1000 or 2000 mm., and may reveal a number of characteristic changes, such as enlargement of the blind spot, usually in its vertical diameter; a Seidel scotoma may be found as an early defect characterized by a finger-like scotoma which extends from one or both vertical borders of the blind spot toward fixation. With its concavity toward fixation, this additional scotomatous area is crescentic in shape. A "Bjerrum" scotoma, which is wider than the former and also extends toward the fixation point, may also be present at the upper or lower border of the blind spot, or it may extend from both borders and become a ring scotoma.

In the nasal area the changes observed are as follows: The field on the nasal side extends farther out above the horizontal meridian than it does below, or it may extend farther out below than above. This is called the "Rönne" nasal step. In advanced cases paracentral and central scotomas may appear; these may be independent of the scotoma forming the Rönne step, or the Rönne step may include fixation. In some cases the Bjerrum scotoma also extends around to include the fixation point.

Accompanying these field changes and with the progress of the disease, the depth of the excavation in the nerve head is found to increase, and there is a constant daily change in the intraocular tension. The condition continues in this way over a period of years, and eventually terminates in blindness.

Ophthalmoscopy.—The excavation in the optic nerve head can be seen to extend to the edge of the disc. For a brief period in the early stage of the disease, the nerve head may not reveal involvement in its entirety, but the blood vessels will soon be found to bend over the edge of the disc abruptly. Somewhat later, they disappear entirely after crossing over the edge and are only observed again in the floor of the excavation. They appear on the inner side of the nerve head and cannot be focused clearly with the retinal vessels. The latter may show the arteries to be smaller in size while the veins appear normal or slightly larger.

The depth of the glaucomatous excavation can be estimated by noting the difference in refraction between the edge of the excavation and that of the floor. With continued progress of the condition and the persistent elevation of the intraocular tension, with intervals of slight remission during the day, the nerve head gradually becomes more pale and atrophic, so that when it has reached the absolute stage, its appearance is almost unmistakable.

The final stage of the glaucoma is considered to be absolute. The vision is lost, while the cornea is thin and the sclera bluish in color and also thin. The iris has become atrophic, frequently to such an extent that only a narrow rim can be seen in the angle of the chamber with a band of pigment at the pupillary margin. The pupil assumes a greenish color, and the lens may become cataractous. The eyeball is now very hard. Secondary changes in the cornea are present in the final stage of absolute glaucoma. These are characterized by the formation of vesicles and bullae on the surface. Pannus may also occur. Finally, a zonular opacity which contains calcareous deposits and hyaline masses may develop in the central area of the cornea.

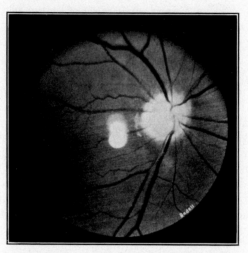

Fig. 53.—Glaucoma of right eye in a 47-year-old male. Complete glaucomatous excavation. (Courtesy of Dr. Arthur J. Bedell.)

Treatment.—The treatment of chronic simple glaucoma includes operative and nonoperative procedures. In most cases the former will sooner or later be found necessary. The patient should, however, receive medical treatment both locally and generally before or until operation is decided on. Careful attention should be given to the general condition of these patients, with special reference to the cardiovascular system, the blood pressure, renal function, and gastrointestinal system. The patient should receive plenty of rest. Reading should be almost entirely restricted and should be done only with good illumination. The patient should receive proper management with regard to the refraction of the eye, the diet, metabolism, and also the state of the nervous system. Many of these patients show a nervous temperament, are easily disturbed, may suffer with arteriosclerosis, and also high blood pressure. In short, the general health of the patient should receive necessary consideration.

The local treatment consists in the regular instillation of miotics into the affected eye. In the early stages of the disease weak solutions of pilocarpine may be employed in the strength of about 1 gr. to 1 ounce with satisfactory results. The state of the tension should be regularly observed. The miotics should be instilled at least three times a day, since the effect is only transient. If it is found that the intraocular tension of the eye is not controlled by the initial strength employed, this should be increased, and if this fails, a drug which is known to be stronger should be employed. For this purpose, eserin salicylate is commonly used in the strength of ⅛ to ¼ per cent. These drugs, especially in increased strength, may also cause a spasm of the vessels with a temporary impairment of vision. When this is noticed, they should be temporarily discontinued, and hot compresses applied locally, or vasodilators prescribed by mouth. Headache, irritation of the eyeball, and twitchings of the eyelids may also be complained of. For the relief of the latter, the strength of the miotic employed may be temporarily reduced. The use of these drugs is intended principally to reduce the size of the pupil and control the intraocular tension. For the same purpose, adrenalin has also been employed either alone or with a little cocaine dropped on a very small piece of cotton which can be inserted under the upper eyelid to remain there for a few minutes.

During this period, the visual acuity and the visual fields should be tested regularly, and the results accurately recorded. If the central vision holds, and the visual fields show no signs of undue impairment, while the intraocular tension is reduced to within normal or close to the normal limits (25 to 30 as high normal), the use of the miotics might be considered to be effective. Each case, however, must be studied according to its individual characteristics. If the vision shows signs of impairment and a decrease in the visual fields is noticed after several examinations, and the intraocular tension remains above normal limits, operative procedure should be indicated. In younger patients especially, surgery should be decided on after the diagnosis is established, since it would be otherwise necessary to continue the use of miotics for too long a period of time. In other cases where, for some reason, surgery is not performed, the use of miotics must be carried out regularly and continuously in order to obtain a satisfactory result.

The Operative Treatment.—The operative procedures for the control of glaucoma include basal iridectomy, and those which produce a filtering bleb, such as the Lagrange operation, and a sclerocorneal trephine (Elliot's operation) for the same purpose. The latter is most commonly employed and probably affords the best results in the experience of most surgeons. In some instances, however, complications may occur following operations. These include opacities in the lens and changes in the refraction and, occasionally, marked reduction in the vision which results from the sudden reduction in tension. No improvement in the vision can be expected as a result of operation, since the latter is indicated only for the reduction of intraocular tension. The loss of vision in glaucoma is evidently due to pressure and atrophy of the nerve fibers, and since the latter cannot be regenerated, the vision which has been lost cannot be regained. However, with reduction and control of the intraocular tension, further loss of vision may be prevented. Other operations which are occasionally performed are iridotasis and cyclodialysis. The last-named is occasionally performed with satisfactory results in secondary glaucoma, and in long-standing cases of simple glaucoma.

Secondary Glaucoma.—Secondary glaucoma occurs as the result of an interference or obstruction to the drainage of the intraocular fluids, at the angle of the anterior chamber. One of the most common causes is iridocyclitis, which is accompanied by annular synechiae in the formation of "iris bombé." Congenital anomalies, especially those in the neighborhood of the angle of the anterior chamber, intraocular growths, swelling, and forward dislocation of the lens may all result in secondary glaucoma. The forward dislocation of the lens may occur as a congenital condition or as the result of injury. This type of glaucoma may also occur occasionally as a complication of other long-standing inflammatory conditions of the eye.

References

1. Leucutia, T., and Price, A. E.: Mikulicz's Disease and Mikulicz's Syndrome. Treatment by Irradiation, Am. J. Roentgenol. 24: 491, November, 1930.

Conjunctivitis

2. Thygeson, Phillips: Treatment of Conjunctivitis, Arch. Ophth. 19: 586-608, April, 1938.

Trachoma

3. Thygeson, Phillips: "Viruses and Virus Diseases of the Eye" Viruses of Ocular Importance, Arch. Ophth. V. 29 No. 4: 635, April, 1943.
4. Lindner, Karl: "Trachoma," In Beren's, The Eye and Its Diseases, Saunders, Philadelphia, 1936.
5. Loe, Fred: J. A. M. A. 111: 1371-1372, Oct. 8, 1938.

CHAPTER V

STRUCTURAL ABNORMALITIES AND MANIFESTATIONS
—Cont'd

Examination of the Iris

The iris can be examined by all of the methods described and should be studied by all of the means at hand in the order named, i.e., by inspection with direct illumination using a loupe, oblique illumination, ophthalmoscopy, and slit lamp examination. Examination by direct illumination with the aid of a loupe, which is supplemented by examination with the slit lamp, provides the best means for studying the normal or pathologic condition of the iris in all its details.

The principal features to be observed in the course of the examination are: (1), the color of the iris; (2), the condition of its markings; (3), the character of its outline and the presence or absence of adhesions; (4), the size and character of the pupil, and a comparison with that of the other eye; (5), the presence or absence of foreign materials or abnormal growths.

The color of the iris changes as the result of inflammatory processes, especially those of long standing. Moreover, differences in the color of various portions of the iris, known as heterochromia may be present as a congenital condition. The iris may assume a muddy color in cases of plastic iritis. In some of the inflammatory diseases, especially those of long standing, the markings of the iris may become altered or obscured. With atrophy of the iris, its structure shrinks and becomes friable. This occurs commonly in cases of chronic glaucoma, complicated by iritis or iridocyclitis.

The pupillary margin of the normal iris should be regular in outline and round. In some cases the pupillary margin may appear to be serrated in its outline. In other instances the outline is such as to alter the shape of the pupil. As a result, the pupil instead of being round, is found to be oval in shape with one diameter greater than the other. Inflammatory adhesions may result from the presence of iritis and iridocyclitis. The iris is, therefore, found to be attached in certain places to the cornea in front, the condition being known as anterior synechia. In other instances portions of the iris may be seen to be attached to the anterior capsule of the lens behind, in which case the alteration is described as posterior synechia. In some cases in which the pupil is small, it might be necessary to instill a mydriatic before the presence of adhesions can be determined.

The pupils should be compared in the two eyes to determine whether they are equal in size and to study the reaction to illumination and to convergence.

The Pupillary Reactions.—The reaction to direct illumination can be studied best in a darkened room by using a small electric bulb or the illumination of the slit lamp. When the iris has relaxed by looking off in the distance, the light flashed into the eye will cause the iris to contract immediately with an accompanying reduction in the size of the pupil. Each eye is tested separately and both should react in a similar manner to direct light stimulation.

When one eye is exposed to direct light in this manner, the fellow eye if observed, will also be found under normal conditions to show a contraction of the iris. This is known as the consensual light reflex.

The reaction of the pupil to the act of convergence can be observed after controlling the exposure to illumination to eliminate the effect of the latter. While the eyes are fixed on a distant point, a small object is held up in front of the eyes. When the patient fixes on this, the pupils will be seen to contract in the act of convergence. Absence of the reaction to light with preservation of the reaction to convergence is described as the Argyll-Robertson pupil.

All cases should be examined for evidences of foreign materials, pigment stains, exudates, or growths on the iris. The latter may occur on either the ciliary or pupillary border and should be studied in detail with the slit lamp. The position of the iris, to note whether it is displaced from its normal position, should also be observed. In dislocation of the lens the iris frequently loses its posterior boundary; as a result, iridodenesis can be observed, characterized by a quivering of the iris when the eyeball is quickly rotated.

Abnormalities of the Iris and Ciliary Body

The iris is scarcely ever affected by disease without simultaneous involvement of the ciliary body. Since they are similar, especially in structure, nerve supply, blood supply, and in other respects, it is to be expected that they are nearly always affected earlier or later by the same disease. It is, therefore, logical to consider the abnormalities affecting each of these structures under the same heading.

Abnormalities Due to Trauma.—The iris may present alterations in shape or position as the result of trauma and injury. A hole in the iris might result. Coloboma of the iris is found following iridectomy, an operative procedure preliminary to cataract extraction. This is usually at the upper pole. Stretching of the iris may occur as the result of injury with a perforating wound of the cornea or perforation of the cornea from ulceration. A portion of the iris is caught in the wound and, if not released, the pupil becomes eccentric and altered in its shape.

Prolapse of the Iris.—The iris may protrude through a wound in the cornea. This occurs frequently after operations for cataract. Failure to replace properly the cut edges of the iris into the anterior chamber results in a prolapse, through the wound, while healing takes place. The amount of iris tissue protruding through the wound may continue to increase and may even prevent complete closure of the wound. The prolapsed portion can easily be seen at the limbus of the cornea and has the appearance of a small, black bead. In marked cases it is necessary to excise the portion of the iris which is presenting and to cover the area with a flap of conjunctiva. After a short period of time the conjunctival flap retracts to its normal position and seals the opening at the site of the prolapse. The same condition might result from an incised or perforating wound of the cornea over the limbus and can be treated in the same manner.

Prolapse of the Ciliary Body.—This may occur as the result of serious injury to the eyeball with perforation near the limbus of the cornea. It may be difficult to determine definitely that the ciliary body is prolapsed, and it must be determined from the location of the injury and the appearance of the wound. Any perforation of the eyeball just behind the limbus of the cornea is likely to result in injury to, or prolapse of, the ciliary body. In such cases there may be considerable hemorrhage into the anterior chamber and a great deal of pain; the prolapsed tissue in the wound is dark blue in color. In these cases there is great danger of the occurrence of sympathetic ophthalmia, and it is advisable to enucleate the eye.

Displacement of the Iris.—The iris can be displaced forward or backward. The former is much more common and results in a decrease in the depth of the anterior chamber. It occurs most frequently after a loss of aqueous such as results in cataract operations or other injuries. With closure of the wound and a reformation of aqueous, the anterior chamber regains its normal depth with return of the iris to its normal position.

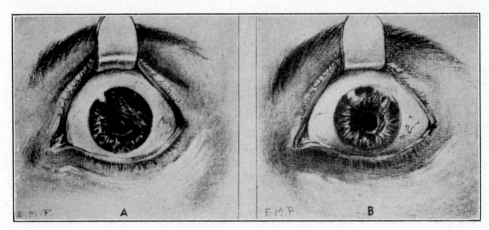

Fig. 54.—Iridodialysis. *A*, Before operation; *B*, one year after operation. (From Key: Arch. Ophth. May, 1932.)

Swelling of the lens with cataract results in a pressing forward of the iris. Tumors of the ciliary body may also cause a forward displacement of the iris. Increased intraocular tension and glaucoma nearly always cause the iris to be pressed forward, resulting in a shallow anterior chamber. In some instances the iris may approach the posterior surface of the cornea, almost obliterating the anterior chamber.

The iris may be found displaced backward in a retrodisplacement of the lens. In otherwise normal eyes, it also sometimes appears to be located farther back than usual. This is occasionally seen in myopic eyes of high degree.

Iridodialysis is a tearing or loosening of the insertion of the iris and usually follows an injury to the eye, such as perforation of the cornea and iris by a foreign body or sharp-pointed instrument. The condition might result from operative procedures, especially in the removal of a foreign body enmeshed in the stroma of the iris near its base.

Synechiae.—Synechiae are adhesions of the iris which frequently occur as the result of inflammation. They occur as anterior and posterior synechiae. With anterior synechiae, a portion of the pupillary margin of the iris becomes attached to the posterior surface of the cornea. With posterior synechiae, the attachment takes place on the anterior capsule of the lens. With an undilated pupil, it may be difficult to see the synechiae, and it is necessary to instill a mydriatic into the eye. The pupil is then usually seen to dilate in all portions except at the point of adhesion. Such synechiae or adhesions occur commonly in inflammatory conditions involving the iris and are very characteristic of iritis and iridocyclitis. In these cases the pupil is ordinarily contracted, and if not dilated early in the disease, the adhesions are caused by exudates and products of inflammation. As a result, when the pupil is dilated by use of a mydriatic, it is irregular in its shape and outline. With the early use of strong solutions of atropine or other mydriatics, it is sometimes possible to tear the iris away from the point of attachment, but in many instances, this is not possible. The pupil, therefore, remains permanently irregular in its outline.

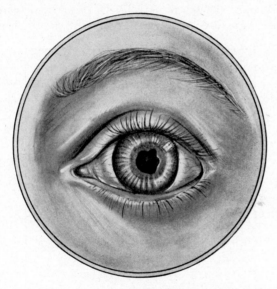

Fig. 55.—"Iris bombé" in iritis, showing irregular pupil and synechia.

The entire circumference of the pupillary border of the iris may become adherent to the anterior capsule of the lens, resulting in the condition known as iris bombé. The entire pupil is occluded as a result, and the iris is gradually pushed forward with increased narrowing of the anterior chamber. This condition also occurs frequently with recurrent attacks of iritis and iridocyclitis. Secondary glaucoma is a frequent complication, and these cases require the instillation of strong solutions of atropine, epinephrine, or other drugs, which have the effect of opening the pupil. When these fail, it might be necessary to resort to some operative procedure to release the iris and reduce the intraocular tension.

Iridodonesis.—Subluxation or dislocation of the lens results in a quivering of the iris which can be observed on direct inspection when the affected eyeball is quickly rotated. The quivering greatly resembles the shaking of jelly and is usually caused by injury or by a blow to the eye. With occurrence of the dislocation, the iris no longer rests on the anterior capsule of the lens at this point, as is indicated by the tremulous movement observed.

Foreign Bodies.—Almost any variety of foreign body might be found in the iris or ciliary body as the result of injury. These include fine splinters of wood, steel, iron, glass, and copper. More rarely an eyelash may be found to have entered the anterior chamber and is located here or in the iris.

The diagnosis of metallic foreign bodies in the iris can often be confirmed by means of x-ray examination. Particles of glass, however, in the anterior chamber or iris may be difficult to diagnose. Particles of copper which have entered the eyeball usually prove serious if not removed. They usually become surrounded by a fibrinous material and cause a purulent exudation. The reaction is very severe and may result in the loss of the eye.

Iron particles in the anterior chamber or in the iris result after a time in a partial solution of the iron with a deposition of iron pigment granules on the iris, known as siderosis. These are dark brown in color and can be observed on examination either with direct illumination or with the slit lamp.

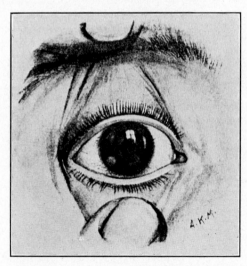

Fig. 56.—Nodule on iris (tubercle). (From Ramsay: Clinical Ophthalmology for the General Practitioner, Oxford Medical Publications.)

The treatment of foreign bodies consists principally of their removal and attention to the local reaction. Small splinters of wood or other foreign bodies located on the surface of the iris may be removed by entering the anterior chamber with a keratome and grasping the foreign body directly between the blades of a fine pair of iris forceps. Should the foreign body be enmeshed in the stroma of the iris, it is necessary to remove that portion of the iris holding the foreign body, by means of an iridectomy. When the foreign body is metallic, it might be removed by magnet extraction.

Papules.—In syphilitic uveitis papules may be found on the iris in the secondary stage of the disease. The occurrence of these papules may be only one of the manifestations of the inflammatory iritis. They are usually located on the ciliary or pupillary border and may be single or multiple in number. They are about the size of a pinhead, slightly elevated, and are brownish-yellow in color. They can often be seen on examination by direct inspection with ordinary illumination and on examination with the slit lamp. Treatment of the iritis and the syphilitic condition usually results in a resorption of the papules. (See Syphilis.)

Nodules (Tubercles).—Tubercles may occur on the iris in the form of small nodules in the course of tuberculous iritis and uveitis. When present, they are important in confirming the diagnosis of the condition. They may be single or multiple and have a dark gray color. They may be very small and difficult to observe by ordinary examination and must be studied with the slit lamp. The smaller tubercles are usually accompanied by the other evidences of uveitis and iritis, such as synechiae, deposits on the cornea, infiltration of the vitreous, and other external signs of inflammation.

Treatment of the tuberculous nodules consists in local treatment of the inflammation and treatment of the general condition. (See Tuberculosis.)

Hyperemia.—Hyperemia of the iris is a symptom and is present early, as a manifestation of an irritation or inflammation such as that which occurs in iritis. To the beginner hyperemia might be difficult to recognize, since it generally produces a greenish appearance of the iris. It is difficult to observe the distended blood vessels with the unaided eye, but these can be examined with the slit lamp and are found to produce a fullness of the iris. The pupil is at the same time contracted because of the distention and spasm of the sphincter. The reaction to light is decreased. Increased lacrimation, photophobia, and pericorneal injection are usually accompanying symptoms.

Exudation.—This is another sign of inflammation of the iris and can be seen either with or immediately following hyperemia. In the presence of exudation the iris appears muddy and discolored, swollen, and rigid. The pupil is small and constricted, and reacts poorly to light. The swelling of the iris is due to the outpouring of cells which also causes the hazy appearance of the iris markings. The exudation of cells may go forward into the aqueous, causing the latter to become turbid in appearance, and it may extend backward into the posterior chamber and capsule of the lens. Organization of the exudate may take place in the center of the pupil which can lead to the condition known as occlusio pupillae (occlusion of the pupil) and subsequent interference with the vision.

Coagulation of fibrin in the exudate may occur which is gray in color and has the appearance of a gelatinous mass. In other instances the fibrin shrinks with expression of all liquid content which causes it to resemble a spongy mass. The exudative material may disappear almost completely in about a week, and leave just one or two strands connected with the iris at its pupillary border. In cases of long standing the exudation may extend to the cornea and manifest itself on the posterior surface in the form of small dots or deposits smaller than a pinhead in size, dark brown in color, and known as precipitates.

In many cases exudation on the iris and the deposition anterior to the cornea and posterior to the anterior capsule of the lens can be distinguished on examination by oblique illumination with the aid of a loupe, but in more detail and to better advantage with the slit lamp. Deposits on the iris may be difficult to see because of the color of the iris, but they become darker when old and leave pigment granules as the cellular material breaks down and becomes absorbed.

With the outpouring of the exudative material, the pupillary border of the iris may become attached to the posterior cornea in front or to the anterior capsule of the lens behind. These attachments (see Synechiae) form at the height of the inflammatory process, and when the iris is constricted. On dilating the pupil, the retinal pigment of the posterior iris remains adherent.

The ciliary body may become infiltrated with exudate and may produce exudation itself into the anterior chamber, posterior chamber, and into the vitreous.

Iritis and Iridocyclitis.—An inflammatory condition of the iris and ciliary body characterized by some of the alterations in these structures already described, i.e., principally early hyperemia of the iris, exudation on the iris and into the anterior and posterior chamber, a turbidity of the aqueous, deposits on the posterior surface of the cornea and anterior capsule of the lens, a small pupil, pericorneal injection, and the presence of anterior or posterior synechiae, when the pupil is dilated, especially after instillation of homotropine or atropine. The intraocular tension should not be altered.

All of the objective signs can be observed on examination with oblique illumination and the loupe, and by slit lamp examination.

In nearly all cases the inflammation of the iris is associated with that of the ciliary body. This is indicated principally by the outstanding subjective symptoms which include (1) pain in the eye; (2) reduced vision; and (3) ciliary tenderness. The pain complained of is nearly always severe, and the patient will state that it is usually worse at night, to the extent that sleep is impossible. This is characteristic. The ciliary tenderness is complained of when the closed upper eyelid is gently touched by a finger just behind the limbus of the cornea. In addition, the patient complains of photophobia to the extent that he tries to avoid direct light. Lacrimation is also a disturbing symptom.

In the acute cases these inflammatory symptoms may become marked, but they run a rather short course. The inflammation begins to subside after a period of a few weeks. The pain and injection are gradually relieved, especially if treatment is started promptly. With the use of atropine, the pupil is dilated, and the condition improves. In chronic cases, however, the duration is longer and drawn out. Although the irritative symptoms are now very slight, with only moderate injection and photophobia, the deposits and results of the exudative process are usually clearly visible. The deposits are found on the posterior cornea and lens, while synechiae are always present. The vitreous may be found to contain opacities, and the choroid may show some exudation indicating an involvement of the entire uveal tract or uveitis. The manifestations in the posterior segment, i.e., the vitreous and choroid, should be observed with the ophthalmoscope. In acute cases the condition may be confined to only one eye. In long-standing cases of chronic iridocyclitis or uveitis, both eyes are likely to be affected. A number of synechiae, either anterior or posterior, may be found, or the pupil may be completely occluded. The iris later may become atrophic, opacities may occur in the lens, the vision of the patient will be impaired, and even blindness may result. The deposits may be present in the various structures affected for a long time, after which they might disappear to a great extent by resorption.

The principal complication of iritis, iridocyclitis, or uveitis is secondary glaucoma. This is more likely to occur in the chronic form, especially with occlusion of the pupil. The intraocular tension should be constantly observed and every effort should be made to maintain a dilated pupil.

Recurrence of the condition is quite common, but a subsequent flare-up is usually less severe than the initial attack. These recurrences may be due in many instances to a prolonged activity of the primary cause in the form of the systemic disease. Each recurrence, naturally, leaves added pathologic changes in the structures affected.

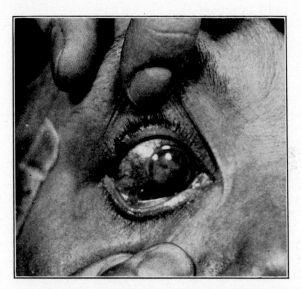

Fig. 57.—Plastic iritis. (Wills Hospital.)

Etiology.—Iritis and iridocyclitis occur very frequently following or in association with inflammation of an adjacent ocular structure. Almost any form of conjunctivitis, keratitis, or scleritis might lead to the occurrence of iritis and iridocyclitis. In these cases the immediate cause might be considered a local one, and the inflammation of iris and ciliary body is a secondary involvement.

The condition might result primarily from some external source, such as traumatism, in which case it is designated as traumatic iritis or iridocyclitis. Almost any direct traumatism to the eyeball will produce it. These also include foreign bodies on the eyeball, as well as those which penetrate the eyeball, lacerations, infections from external sources, and chemical burns. Traumatic iridocyclitis usually runs a protracted course and may be accompanied by other pathology, such as hyphemia (blood in the anterior chamber), dislocation of the lens, and detachment of the retina.

In extensive lacerations of the eyeball, especially those which involve the ciliary body, the iridocyclitis is very severe and is likely to result in a sympathetic involvement of the fellow eye. This is known as sympathetic iridocyclitis, or sympathetic ophthalmia. The latter may also occur as the result of other forms of iridocyclitis. Sympathetic ophthalmia usually occurs at the height of the inflammation in the injured eye. This is about six weeks to two months after the injury. If the eye originally injured recovers fully and remains quiet with no signs of irritation or inflammation present at any time, the danger of sympathetic involvement of the second eye is very slight. If the injured eye remains irritable and is the seat of a chronic inflammation, it should always be regarded as a possible source of infection of the second eye, especially when acute attacks of iridocyclitis suddenly recur at later periods.

The exact mode of transmission of the disease to the second eye is not definitely known. It has from time to time been variously suggested that this might be brought about by means of the ciliary nerves, although these do not communicate directly in the two eyes. The transmission of bacteria or toxins has been said to take place through the circulation and by way of the uveal tract, or by way of the optic nerve. It has also been attributed to the occurrence of anaphylaxis. With the latter, the second eye becomes sensitive to infection by the transmission of infected uveal tissue from the first eye. None of the theories has been proved, and as yet no one cause is generally accepted. Theobald[1] found that the greatest frequency of sympathetic cases occurs in the first decade, and that the diagnosis can be made only histologically, each eye being sectioned serially and at least every tenth section carefully examined.

The clinical diagnosis is extremely difficult. The appearance of precipitates on the back of the cornea of the second eye is given as proof that sympathetic ophthalmia occurs.

A third group of causes of iritis and iridocyclitis includes infections and infectious diseases and internal diseases localized in other structures and organs of the body. The systemic diseases which are known to cause iritis and iridocyclitis are: (1) Syphilis, in which the condition is described as syphilitic iritis; (2) Tuberculosis, in which the uveal inflammation is designated as tuberculous iritis, iridocyclitis, or uveitis; (3) Other infectious diseases and foci of infection. Among these may be included influenza, erysipelas, small pox, typhoid fever, herpes zoster, relapsing fever, gonorrhea, including gonorrheal arthritis and prostatitis, rheumatoid arthritis and infections from the teeth, tonsils, and sinuses. Metabolic glandular diseases, such as hyperthyroidism, gout, gastro-intestinal disturbances, and occasionally diabetes may also be primary causes.

Iritis or iridocyclitis occurring with, or as the result of, any of these conditions is of endogenous origin, and in most of them, it can be considered as a metastatic involvement.

Syphilitic iritis or iridocyclitis is probably the most common form and will be described in a later chapter as a manifestation of that disease. Suffice here to state that it might occur infrequently as a manifestation of hereditary syphilis and of infection before birth, but more commonly as the result of acquired syphilis. In the latter, it usually occurs in the secondary stage and may be accompanied by the formation of papules or small nodules on the iris. Nodules may also occur on the ciliary body. Gumma may be associated with iritis in the later stage of syphilis. (See Syphilis.) Tuberculous iridocyclitis and uveitis are usually present at the same time. In addition to inflammation by involvement of the iris and ciliary body, other manifestations might also be present in other portions of the uveal tract. The detailed description of tuberculous uveitis will be found under "Tuberculosis." Briefly, however, tubercles may be found on the iris in the form of nodules. Deposits and exudation are present, fine dustlike opacities may be present in the vitreous, and tubercles and exudate may be found in the choroid. Another frequent cause is probably localized foci of infection, such as those found in the teeth, nasal accessory sinuses, and tonsils.

Treatment.—The treatment of iritis and iridocyclitis includes both local and general treatment. The latter must be determined by the causative factor and nature of the primary disease or infection.

In the local treatment the prompt use of atropine is the first indication. It can be instilled into the eyes, employing one drop of atropine sulphate, 1 per cent, three times daily. This will produce a dilatation of the pupil, placing the iris at rest, and prevent the formation of synechiae. The dilatation of the pupil should be maintained as long as possible during the presence of the inflammation.

Local anesthetics, such as butyn, 2 per cent, or holocaine, 1 per cent, may be instilled into the affected eye as required for the relief of pain. Hot wet compresses can also be applied to the eye for a period of fifteen minutes, three or four times daily, for the relief of pain and to promote healing. This is frequently followed by almost immediate relief. The use of sodium salicylate (gr. x—4 times daily) is also beneficial in these cases. Diaphoresis, in the form of hot packs, electric light baths, hot drinks, or even the use of pilocarpine, is of value, when not otherwise contraindicated.

The use of mercury by inunction and administration of potassium iodide by mouth are of value in helping to absorb the exudate and products of inflammation.

The use of leeches or application of an artificial leech to the temple on the affected side may assist in reducing the degree of inflammation.

The eye affected with iritis or iridocyclitis should not be bandaged. The patient should wear a pair of black glasses, and use of the eyes should be restricted. The diet and elimination should receive attention.

While the local treatment is being carried out, every effort should be made to determine the primary cause. A careful examination should be made of the teeth, tonsils, nasal accessory sinuses, and other possible foci of infection. When such a focus is found to be present, the proper treatment for its removal should be instituted.

When syphilis is known to be the cause, the inflammation usually responds favorably to prompt and active antisyphilitic treatment. Here, mercury by inunction, giving one dram daily, is very beneficial. At the same time, other forms of antisyphilitic treatment ordinarily employed in different cases may be carried out.

When it is determined that the condition is tuberculous in origin, the use of tuberculin may be employed as well as any other measures indicated in the treatment of the systemic disease. (See Tuberculosis.)

Gumma.—The occurrence of gumma on the iris or ciliary body is rare. When present, however, it appears late in the disease in the form of a nodule. When present on the ciliary body, it may increase in size and may be seen behind the pupil. It might also extend into the sclera. It must be differentiated from such other growths as sarcoma and tuberculous nodule. With active antisyphilitic treatment the growth will disappear if it is a gumma.

Atrophy.—Degenerative changes and atrophy may follow severe inflammatory conditions of iris and ciliary body of a chronic nature. The iris changes in color, becomes thin, the vessels are obliterated, and it becomes crisp and paper-like in texture. This causes it to crumble on being handled, especially if any operative procedure is attempted when it has reached this stage. Following iritis and glaucoma of long standing, the ciliary muscle also becomes atrophied, and the ciliary process becomes flattened. The stroma becomes thick, and later shows hyaline degeneration. In the late stages, necrosis might take place.

Small sections of iris may show defects in the pigment layer, especially after acute iridocyclitis, and glaucoma. Dark spots about the size of a pinhead may be found in the stroma which result from the former presence of nodules occurring in tuberculosis. Other alterations, such as vitiligo, have been found in the irides, following inflammatory conditions and tuberculosis. Atrophic changes in the pigment layer of the iris are also found sometimes in diabetes. A swelling takes place with an accumulation of fluid and the liberation of pigment.

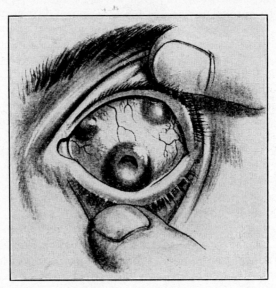

Fig. 58.—Staphylomas of the ciliary body. (From Ramsay: Clinical Ophthalmology for the General Practitioner, Oxford Medical Publications.)

Cysts of the Iris and Ciliary Body.—Cysts of the iris are rare, but may develop within the stroma of the iris and appear as small transparent vesicles containing a clear serous fluid, and some few fibers with pigment. They gradually increase in size, approaching the posterior surface of the cornea, causing a clouding of the latter as a result of contact. Again, a cyst may grow into the pupillary space, resulting in the alteration of the size and shape of the pupil with a corresponding reduction in the amount of vision. With continued growth, the cyst might include the anterior chamber and result in the increase in intraocular tension. Such a cyst might result from trauma, or penetrating wounds of the eyeball with implantation of epithelium on the iris.

The treatment consists in surgical removal. This can be done by making an incision at the limbus of the cornea introducing a pair of forceps and withdrawing the cyst to be excised.

Tumors of the Iris and Ciliary Body.—These consist principally of melanoma and sarcoma. Melanoma occurs in two forms. First, a tumor which is black in color, growing from the stroma of the iris, extends into the anterior chamber. It arises from a proliferation of chromatophores of the iris. The second variety originates at the pupillary margin, and develops from the cells of the retinal pigment layer at the point where it is reflected onto the anterior surface of the iris at the margin of the pupil. Small brown or black outgrowths occur which project into the pupil. A melanoma grows to a certain size and is benign in nature. In some instances, however, it has been known to develop into sarcoma.

Sarcomas of the iris are pigmented tumors, dark brown in color. They gradually increase in size, extending into the anterior chamber, and might involve the entire eye. A sarcoma of the ciliary body is usually concealed at first by the iris and after reaching a sufficient size might be seen to project as a small brown body behind the iris. Sarcoma of the ciliary body itself is rare, and when it does occur, it also may push the iris well forward until it reaches the cornea.

These tumors must be differentiated from other nodular tumors of different origin. Included among these are syphilitic nodules, gumma of the iris, tubercles, and granulation tumors. Syphilitic papules are usually found at the pupillary and ciliary borders, while the other tumors originate at any point on the surface of the iris. Iritis accompanying a tumor occurs later than the iritis in syphilis and tuberculosis. In addition, the general physical condition of the patient and the presence or absence of generalized syphilis or tuberculosis will aid in the differentiation. Nodules of syphilitic origin clear up with anti-syphilitic treatment, and tuberculous nodules may also clear up after a certain time.

The treatment of tumors of the iris consists in early removal wherever possible. Small tumors of the iris can be removed by iridectomy and excision of that part of the iris involved. Large tumors of the iris and ciliary body necessitate early enucleation of the eye involved.

Examination of the Lens

The crystalline lens is, perhaps, the most important structure in the refractive media of the eye. It can be examined by using the ophthalmoscope with a plus 10 D. to 20 D. lens, and in more detail by the use of the slit lamp. Any alteration which is present on ophthalmoscopic examination of the lens should be studied by slit lamp examination before a thorough knowledge of the condition can be obtained. It should be examined for its transparency, its general appearance, and the position. In spite of the fact that the lens has no direct blood supply, it very frequently is indirectly affected by diseases present in other organs, as well as by inflammation and other pathologic conditions affecting the adjacent structures of the eye. If the eye under examination is known to have a normal refractive state, a plus 10 D. lens on the ophthalmoscope will, in all probability, provide a satisfactory examination. In the course of this examination, the details of the posterior of the eye, including the retina and optic nerve, will not be visible. If the lens has a normal transparency, the illumination of the ophthalmoscope will be transmitted without obstruction.

Any opacities that are present will stand out as dark spots of varying degree in contrast to the rest of the illuminated field. In observing an opacity, an attempt should be made to determine principally the size, location, and, if possible, the nature of the opacity. An idea of the location can be obtained by asking the patient to rotate the eye up and down, and right and left, while continuing to observe the opacity with the ophthalmoscope. If it is located in the anterior portion of the lens, it will appear to move in the same direction as the eyeball. If it is in the posterior portion, it will appear to move in the opposite direction from the rotation of the eyeball. The apparent size can be determined from the amount of illumination obstructed and the extent to which the lens is involved. In some instances, the appearance on ophthalmoscopic examination might afford some idea as to whether or not the opacity indicates the presence of a foreign body.

Anything of a pathologic nature present in the lens should be examined with all forms of slit lamp illumination in order to determine the various features of the abnormality. The narrow beam of the slit lamp will be found to have different intensities of light when reflected through different layers. Since, in the course of its growth, the more recent fibers occur in the peripheral portion of the lens, it can be divided into various sections according to their age. In this way it is possible to designate the most recent portion or the newest fibers in the periphery; next, the adult nucleus; the next portion represents that which was developed between the time of birth and puberty; and, lastly, the fetal or embryonic nucleus.

The anterior capsule of the lens being less dense, affords the best reflection of any part of the lens. In younger patients, it is somewhat bluish, has a forward convexity, and with a wide beam appears as a glistening curved surface. It can be seen to be slightly roughened resembling grained leather. This is designated as "shagreen." It is probably caused by a reflex of the lens fibers. A fine, delicate line just back of the capsule is known as the subcapsular line, and has been variously designated by Graves as a reduplication line, by Vogt, as a cleavage line, and by Koeppe, as a line of disjunction.

The adult nucleus is separated from the cortex by an anterior band which can sometimes be seen, and which has a greater curvature than the capsular band. The anterior and posterior surfaces of the fetal nucleus can be determined by the location of the Y sutures. The vertical Y is found on the anterior embryonal nucleus. The area between the two is the first portion of the lens to develop.

The cortex is located between the adult nucleus and the subcapsular layer. It is a much softer portion of the lens and increases in thickness with age.

The reflex of the posterior capsule on examination shows a line which is somewhat less bright than that of the anterior capsule and is curved posteriorly. It also shows shagreen similar to the anterior capsule when examined with the wide beam, and has a golden-yellow color.

When the broad beam is reflected onto the posterior capsule, a small white ring may be seen which indicates the point at which the hyaloid artery was attached to the posterior capsule, just inside and below the center.

It can be understood from the above, therefore, that an opacity in the lens can be studied not alone with regard to its location, but with the recognition of the location, the length of time the opacity has been present may be determined.

Abnormalities of the Lens

Dislocations.—It should first be determined whether or not the lens occupies its normal position in the eye. Any change in position must be recognized as a displacement, and it is then considered to be either partially or completely dislocated. Dislocation may occur either as a congenital or acquired condition. The former is described in the chapter on congenital abnormalities.

An acquired dislocation can be caused by traumatism, or may be the result of a diseased process in an adjacent structure. The former are the most common and are usually produced by direct injuries to the eyeball which loosen the zonule of the lens. Such injuries may occur from foreign bodies striking the eye or from blows such as from a fist or other objects. Occasionally, a blow to the orbit may result in dislocation of the lens. Among the diseased conditions which might result in a dislocation are severe degenerations and inflammations resulting from very high myopia, iridocyclitis, and detachment of the retina. Tumors in any adjacent structures may also cause a change in the position of the lens as the result of pressure.

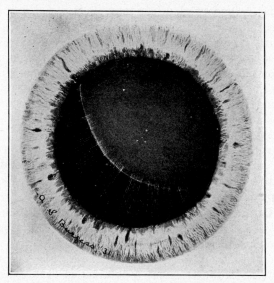

Fig. 59.—Ectopic lens. (From Clapp: Cataract Etiology and Treatment, Lea & Febiger.)

The symptoms of dislocation are usually characterized by an interference with the vision which depends principally on the direction in which the lens is displaced. Astigmatism nearly always results. If the lens is partially displaced, so that one-half of the pupil is clear, and the other half is occupied by a portion of the lens, a diplopia may be complained of by the patient.

If the lens occupies the central portion of the pupil, it will refract most of the light which enters the pupil, and the vision of the patient may not be seriously impaired. If only a small portion of the lens is found in the pupillary space, and most of the light entering the pupil passes outside of the edge of the lens, the eye is practically aphacic, and the vision is greatly reduced.

On objective examination, it can readily be determined as to whether the dislocation is partial or total. A partial dislocation is designated as a subluxation. A slight rotation of the lens resulting in a partial dislocation can be indicated by a variation in the depth of the anterior chamber. When one edge of a lens is displaced forward, the anterior chamber over this portion is seen to be more shallow. This can be observed on examination with the oblique illumination, with the ophthalmoscope, and with the slit lamp. Examination with oblique illumination will also reveal the presence of iridodenesis or tremulous iris, indicating a break in the attachment of the lens and the presence of a subluxation.

With total dislocation of the lens, the iris will be found to be loosened around the entire pupillary border, and the anterior chamber will be deeper. On examination with the ophthalmoscope, the eye appears to be aphacic, and the retina, retinal vessels, and optic nerve are seen immediately with the higher power lenses of the ophthalmoscope. In anterior total dislocation, the lens may be found in the anterior chamber. In total dislocation posterior, the lens may be found in the vitreous. It may come in contact with the ciliary body, or be well back at the retina. The latter is unusual, however. Dislocation into the anterior chamber may result in iritis or iridocyclitis, and, because of crowding the angle, secondary glaucoma may occur.

The treatment of dislocation of the lens depends principally upon its type and extent. With subluxation, refraction and correction by lenses should be attempted, especially in those cases where the greater portion of the lens is still in normal position. If most of the lens is dislocated, however, it may not be possible to improve the vision satisfactorily on refraction, and removal of the lens by surgical procedure would be indicated. This should be preceded, however, by an attempt to force the lens into the anterior chamber, which facilitates its removal. This is sometimes accomplished by having the patient maintain a position in bed with face downward for a period of time. The lens can then be extracted in its capsule, after performing a wide iridectomy, in a location satisfactory for this purpose. The occurrence of secondary glaucoma should indicate the prompt removal of the lens wherever possible.

Opacities (Cataract).—The occurrence of an opacity in the lens is ordinarily considered as cataract. Clinically, however, and from the standpoint of a patient affected with minute opacities, some consideration might be given to the use of the term cataract, especially with those which are known to be nonprogressive in type. However, since a cataract is defined as any opacity occurring in the crystalline lens, these may be classified in a number of different ways. With regard to their time of occurrence, cataracts may be classified as congenital, which includes those that were present at the time of birth; juvenile, those which develop in childhood; presenile, those which occur in early adult life; and senile, those which occur after middle life.

Cataracts may also be classified according to their location. First, subcapsular, usually a circular opacity in the region of the equator. These may be seen with senile cataract, but more often in the complicated variety. Second, cortical cataracts, which occur between the subcapsular line and the adult nucleus. These are first seen in the periphery and extend centrally. Third, nuclear cataracts, in which the opacities are found in the embryonic nucleus in the incipient stage. The entire lens may later become cloudy with the gradual loss of vision following sclerosis of the nucleus. This occurs usually after middle life.

According to their development, cataracts may be classified as stationary and progressive. The former obtain a certain size and increase no further, while the latter continue to increase in extent until most of the lens is involved. This is characteristic of ordinary senile cataract.

Cataract may also occur as a result of traumatism (traumatic cataract); as a result of chemical intoxication, illustrated by thallium cataract, ergot cataract, dinitrophenol cataract, and naphthalene cataract. Excessive exposure to ultraviolet light, radium, and x-ray may also result in cataract. Dietary deficiencies, glandular dysfunctions, and metabolic diseases have been accompanied by the formation of cataract. Diabetic cataract may be an illustration of the latter.

Workers engaged in certain occupations may develop cataract, as illustrated by the electric cataract, glassblower's cataract, and furnace worker's cataract. These might also be included under the heading of traumatic cataract. Any contusion, concussion, or penetrating wound of the eye may result in the formation of a traumatic cataract.

Complicated cataracts result from the presence usually of an inflammation, or alterations in other structures of the eye. They can be illustrated by the cataract occurring as a complication of iritis and iridocyclitis; also, those which sometimes are found to follow operations, especially trephining for glaucoma. Complicated cataracts may occur with certain other anomalies of the lens, such as lenticonus, or coloboma. Complicated cataracts are also considered as secondary cataracts. When the latter are old and of long standing, they may be found to shrink and contain calcareous deposits.

Senile Cataract.—Senile cataract is ordinarily intended to include those opacities in the lens which occur about the time of middle life or later. It might be found in a patient who would not necessarily be considered senile, since the age for the occurrence of the ordinary type of senile cataract might range from about 50 years upward. The earliest opacities are usually in the lower nasal portion of the lens. Senile cataract may also be designated according to its location, i.e., subcapsular, peripheral, cortical, and nuclear cataract. These have already been described. According to the extent of lens involvement or stage of development, they are also classed as incipient, immature, mature, and hypermature. These may at times vary in color as the opacity develops, and may range anywhere from a white to an amber or even black color.

In the incipient stage the cataract may show nothing more than early vacuoles beneath the capsule of the lens. There will be an irregular refraction of the suture lines which are separated by the fluid present. A short time later, these are characterized on the ophthalmoscopic examination by the appearance of short, dark spicules which are found in the extreme periphery of the lens and resemble short spokes which radiate toward the center. The spicular opacities in this stage do not cause any noticeable visual impairment.

The immature stage of cataract is characterized by the appearance of opacities which have progressed and increased in size and extent. They may now interfere with the vision to some degree. On examination with the ophthalmoscope they will be seen around the entire periphery of the lens which appears more or less opaque, while the center of the lens appears more clear. A swelling of the lens may take place to a slight extent as fluid is taken up and the volume increased. In a later stage of immature cataract, almost the whole lens may be clouded, and it is reduced in volume by the loss of fluid.

In the mature stage the lens is found to be completely opaque, and again back to normal size. Light reflected into the eye should cause no shadow of the iris on the lens, and the pupillary space is completely filled with the gray or grayish-white opacity behind the iris. Extraction of the lens by operation is usually performed when the cataract has reached this stage.

The hypermature stage of cataract is characterized by a completely opaque lens which has begun to undergo degeneration. The remainder of the fluid present is absorbed, the cortex becomes liquefied, and deposits may take place in the lens mass. The anterior chamber is found to be deeper, the capsule of the lens becomes wrinkled, and the nucleus is shrunken. If this change continues to progress, it develops into a morgagnian cataract. The nucleus sinks to the lower part of the capsule, the latter becomes hard, further swelling takes place, and the cataract appears milky. The lens is loose in consistency and is difficult to extract when it has reached this stage.

Symptoms.—The principal subjective symptoms complained of by the patient are decreased vision, in proportion to the extent and location of the opacity. Peripheral opacities ordinarily cause little interference with the vision. Small opacities, especially those at the posterior pole, also cause little impairment of vision. Opacities in the center of the lens and in the nucleus cause a greater decrease in the vision. The vision may also be found to vary with changes in the size of the pupil. When the pupil is dilated, especially with a moderate light or in the dark, these patients have better vision, whereas in direct light or in ordinary daylight, the vision is reduced. Diplopia and metamorphopsia are frequent complaints in the course of development. In older patients a myopia may develop with progress of cataract because of the refractive change in the lens. This may result in improved vision for reading. There is no pain associated with the development of cataract, but difficulty from exposure to light is often troublesome. Occasionally, the patient might complain of his color vision; "watering" of the eye may also be a regular complaint.

When a senile cataract has reached the stage of maturity, consideration must be given to the ability of the eye to project light, to the condition of the intraocular tension, and to the reaction of the pupil. When a patient has been under examination during the course of development of the cataract, it is possible for the examiner to have a thorough knowledge of the condition of the posterior portion of the eye. Occasionally, however, a patient comes under observation when the cataract has reached a stage of maturity, and examination of the fundus of the eye is no longer possible with the ophthalmoscope. In such instances the light projection of the eyes should be tested with the patient seated in a dark room. The opposite eye is carefully covered, and with the patient looking directly ahead, a small beam of light is directed into the eye from various directions. The patient is requested to state from which direction the light appears to come. If the light projection is found to be good in all directions, it would indicate that the posterior portion of the eye is, in all probability, normal. If the projection should be faulty in one or more directions, it would indicate the possibility of pathology behind the lens and a poor prognosis from the standpoint of visual improvement after removal of the cataract.

The pupil should dilate regularly and should react promptly to direct light. Increased intraocular tension might indicate the presence of glaucoma and would complicate the condition.

Treatment.—The treatment of senile cataract in the stage of maturity is surgical. Having reached this stage of development, the vision of the eye is reduced to light perception or hand movements at best, and the patient should be admitted to a hospital for extraction of the cataractous lens. The type of operation employed will depend on the practice and judgment of the surgeon in charge of the case.

In cases where the patient is under care and observation during the course and development of senile cataract, the treatment should be concerned principally with the management and care of the patient. Since there is as yet no known medical treatment for the prevention or arrest of cataract, the management of the case may be regarded as a preparation for the time of operation, or what might be termed preoperative management.

During this period, the patient should be seen for examination at regular intervals, which may increase in frequency as the cataract approaches a mature state. In addition to the care of the eyes themselves, the management should be directed principally toward improving the general physical condition of the patient. This would, therefore, include attention to the cardiovascular system, the gastrointestinal tract, the mental condition, and the presence of any low-grade foci of infection.

With regard to the cardiovascular system, the blood pressure should be controlled. The cardiac action should receive attention. Plenty of rest should be prescribed. The elimination of hard work is important, but, at the same time, the patient should be permitted to follow his regular activities if not too exacting. In the latter respect the use of the eyes for excessive close work should be restricted. A mild eyewash should be prescribed in order to reduce the possibility of local infection. A number of different drugs have been advocated from time to time for use in the eyes, in order to check the further development of the cataract. These include the use of solutions of dionin and mercury cyanide which are intended to increase the local blood supply and nutrition, lens antigens which are injected for the purpose of establishing an immunity to the further development of cataract. The use of combinations of glandular extracts has also been advocated because of the possibility that senile cataract is caused by alterations in glandular function accompanying senescence. Thus far, no satisfactory clinical evidence has been provided to warrant the use of these or other drugs in order to check the progress or cure senile cataract without surgical means.

Attention to the diet and elimination of the patient is of considerable importance. These may be affected by the mental state, for a patient knowing that he has a cataract often becomes depressed and is apt to look forward with some apprehension to the time of operation. As a result, the appetite may suffer. A general tonic may be prescribed in addition to fresh air and exercise in the form of walking. The diet of the patient should consist principally of green, leafy vegetables and should include the daily use of carrots, orange juice, and lemon juice, because of the high vitamin A and C content. If the patient is very old, and generally debilitated, ample quantities of vitamin B complex should be supplied. The elimination of the patient should be regular and thorough. Since senile cataract occurs in later life, these patients frequently are affected with constipation of a more or less chronic nature. The abdominal muscles are usually relaxed and efforts for proper elimination are difficult and often unsatisfactory. In these instances it is well to prescribe an enema at regular intervals, and in some cases, even a high colonic irrigation in order to prevent and overcome intestinal stasis.

As much as possible, the patient should be relieved of mental stress and worry, particularly with regard to his own physical condition and the outcome of the contemplated operative procedure. This is of especial importance as the time for operation approaches, for a patient who is confident and mentally prepared is a better subject for operation than one who is highly nervous, and under great mental stress at the time of the operation.

Lastly, the condition of the mouth, nose, throat, and respiratory tract should all receive attention, and any focus of infection should be removed. Any defective teeth, infected roots, apical abscesses, should be removed. A chronic cough should be relieved especially at the time of operation. Anything which might prove to complicate the condition of the patient immediately after operation, especially the presence of any low-grade infection in any remote part should be cleared up before the time of operation.

Examination of the Vitreous

The vitreous is examined with the ophthalmoscope to determine principally the presence or absence of foreign particles. Under normal conditions the vitreous is clear and should present no obstruction to the passage of reflected light back to the retina. A plus 8 or 10 D. lens on the ophthalmoscope to examine the media of the eye usually affords the clearest focus on the vitreous. The patient is then directed to rotate the eyeball in different directions, and then to fix directly ahead. In this way, any opacities or particles which are present in the vitreous will be seen to float about. Such opacities are commonly found in a large variety of conditions. In some instances their origin can be determined, while in others, it will remain more or less obscure.

Abnormalities of the Vitreous

Opacities.—Opacities occur in the vitreous in several different varieties. They are probably the commonest abnormalities observed here, and they range from numerous, fine, floating, dustlike opacities, such as those sometimes seen in tuberculous uveitis, to large, membranous, sheetlike opacities, sometimes seen with degenerative conditions, very high myopia, and detachment of the retina.

The opacities seen in uveitis are ordinarily very small, closely packed, and can be seen to move slowly and as a group, on rotation of the eyeball. Close observation on the part of the examiner is often required to determine their presence.

A single opacity is frequently complained of as a subjective symptom by patients who state that they can see the opacity moving about at times with rotation of the eyeball. These are sometimes seen on examination with the ophthalmoscope, but it is frequently difficult or even impossible to determine their etiology. They are often discovered, or rather suddenly noticed by the patient, who is otherwise apparently well. Opacities of this kind, however, are usually considered to be of systemic origin and are frequently seen in those who suffer with gastrointestinal disturbances.

The opacities occurring with high myopia are often large and usually not difficult to observe. They move about freely with rotation of the eyeball and occur in this condition as a result of the degenerative changes which have taken place.

Opacities are frequently found on the vitreous resulting from inflammatory and degenerative changes in the choroid and retina. Hemorrhages are usually followed by the presence of opacities which are dark in color and can be observed in the vitreous for some time. They occur in choroiditis, diabetes, and in diseases with alterations in the blood and blood vessels. Detachment of the retina is usually followed by the appearance of foreign particles in the vitreous which usually occur with the incidence of the detachment.

Recurrent vitreous hemorrhages with periphlebitis of the retinal veins may occur in tuberculosis. This may lead to extensive formation of connective tissue followed by detachment of the retina and loss of vision.

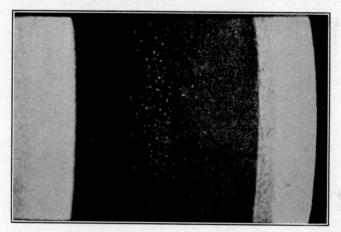

Fig. 60.—Floating particles in anterior vitreous. (From Kirby: Arch. Ophth., February, 1932.)

There is no direct treatment which can be recommended for opacities of the vitreous, but in many instances, they will absorb after a period of time. This is especially true of those occurring as a result of inflammatory conditions which have subsided with treatment. Those found with a degenerative condition, and with the changes accompanying high myopia, usually persist for a long time and do not lend themselves well to treatment. Those which occur as a result of hemorrhage are usually absorbed. Opacities in the vitreous which are found to be associated with some internal diseases may clear up with the treatment and improvement of the primary condition. The iodides, mercury, sweats, and purgation can be employed.

A condition in which the vitreous presents numerous small shiny particles on examination with the ophthalmoscope is known as *synchysis scintillans*. The opacities in this condition are observed when the patient rotates the eye. Large numbers of small, shimmering goldlike particles can be seen to move about like a shower in the vitreous and gradually come to rest in the bottom of the chamber. These particles have a smooth surface, reflect light well, and are said to consist of cholesterin. They occur mostly in older patients and do not cause interference with the vision.

Samuels[2] classified opacities in the vitreous microscopically as: 1, physiologic opacities, and 2, pathologic opacities, according to shape and size.

The physiologic opacities included (a) embryonal, (b) senescent. The embryonal variety was mostly the remains of Cloquet's canal or of the hyaloid artery. These are often difficult to differentiate from products of inflammation or degeneration. The senescent variety is characterized by the type of opacity which usually occurs in the older patients who complain of suddenly seeing a "fly" floating in the visual field. The opacity represents a thread or tangle of threads which have become detached either whole or in part and can be seen with the ophthalmoscope. They occur because of a breaking-down and disappearance of the delicate central meshwork of the vitreous.

The pathologic opacities were described as (a) cells from exudation, such as lymphocytes and leucocytes; (b) red blood cells, from extravasations of blood either on the surface or in the stroma; (c) pigmented cells, either as intact cells from the iris or ciliary body occurring in the vitreous as the result of injury, or cells which are broken up and the granules released into the vitreous; (d) blood vessels in the vitreous arising from the vessels of the ciliary body, retina, or optic nerve; (e) connective tissue, resulting from hemorrhage and interference with the circulation leading to a chronic reaction with organization of the entire vitreous. Massive exudates or hemorrhages undergoing organization may be difficult to distinguish from growths; (f) single strands or cords may be seen as a result of proliferation from a primary focus; (g) cell spheres, occurring as globular masses; (h) tissue spheres without pigment, described as round bodies which have a different origin from that of the cell sphere. They consist of hemogeneous masses thrown into folds between which are flattened cells. They are free in the vitreous and arise from remnants of broken-down coagulated stroma which become globular with cells becoming adherent to them; (i) tissue spheres with pigment. These contain pigment granules and are probably products of pigment epithelium which have passed through the entire thickness of the retina.

Examination of the Choroid

It should be remembered that the choroid, the iris, and the ciliary body constitute the major portion of the uveal tract. The choroid, therefore, is also necessarily affected in the course of many of the inflammations involving the iris and the ciliary body. Moreover, because of its close proximity to the retina, it is nearly always involved whenever the retina is affected by inflammation and degeneration. The choroid is examined together with the retina by means of the ophthalmoscope. Since the retina is the innermost coat of the eye, lesions in this structure usually lead to an affection of the choroid, and the condition of both is, therefore, ordinarily studied at the same time. The choroid is examined principally for the presence of hemorrhages, exudative lesions, inflammation, nodules, growths, detachments, and changes resulting from injury.

Abnormalities of the Choroid

Rupture.—This usually occurs as a result of direct trauma to the eyeball and is evidenced by the presence of a tear or separation concentric with the disc and located usually between the disc and macula. It sometimes occurs in another portion of the choroid, and can be recognized as a narrow area, crescent-shaped, and white or yellowish white in color. It may be covered with a slight hemorrhage, especially when recent. The upper and lower pole of the rupture are pointed. The overlying retina is usually damaged at the same time. Rupture of the choroid may be of almost any size, but usually it is about as large as the disc, or slightly larger. It may be single or more than one may be found in association with dislocation of the lens, retinal hemorrhages, and detachment. When the macula is involved, it will result in the loss of central vision. Small ruptures occurring in the periphery, however, may not seriously impair the vision.

Hemorrhage.—Hemorrhage occurs from the choroidal vessels and takes place either between the sclera and choroid or into the choroid itself. The area of choroid involved is usually yellowish in color. Late in the stage of hemorrhage, it is accompanied by the deposit of pigment. In profuse hemorrhage from the choroidal vessels, the retina may be involved and extravasation may also take place into the vitreous.

Sclerosis of the Choroidal Vessels.—The arteries, especially, undergo a thickening of their walls, and later degeneration occurs in arteriosclerosis, with occlusion of the lumen of the vessels. The nutrition of the retina is affected as a result of interference with the choroidal circulation, and degenerative changes followed by atrophy of the retina as well as that of the optic nerve may result. Pigment may be found in the retina, and a corresponding impairment of vision takes place.

Degeneration.—Degeneration of the choroid occurs as a result of nearly all inflammatory conditions affecting the retina and choroid. Any interference with the retinal or choroidal circulation usually terminates in a degenerative condition. Degeneration also is observed in the choroid with oncoming senility. This is usually found near the macula and often close to the disc. The retinal pigment layer and the choroid become atrophied. The large choroidal vessels are visible on examination with the ophthalmoscope, but are found to be smaller than normal. The smaller vessels cannot be seen.

Small yellowish-white hyaline areas often located centrally are sometimes found, especially in older people, indicating the presence of a form of choroidal degeneration known as Tay's choroiditis. The condition is bilateral. Another variety of this form of choroiditis is similar in appearance but occurs in younger people and is considered to be congenital.

The choroid undergoes degenerative changes in very high myopia. This is ordinarily more marked at the margin of the optic disc where a large white crescentic area is often found, especially among older patients. The retina also is affected in the pigment epithelial layer with an accompanying loss of pigment, the vessels of the choroid being prominent on examination with the ophthalmoscope. Nearly all cases of degeneration of the choroid ultimately result in atrophy.

Tumors.—The choroid may be affected by occasional sarcoma which might occur primarily or secondarily, and carcinoma. The latter is also rare and occurs most often as a metastatic involvement. One or both eyes may be affected. Tumors of the choroid usually result in increased intraocular tension and secondary glaucoma, detachment of the choroid and retina, and loss of vision of the eye.

Inflammation.—When the choroid alone is the seat of an inflammation, there may be no external evidences, and the only subjective symptom will be interference with the vision. However, if the anterior portion of the uveal tract is also involved, it will be observed externally by the presence of iritis and iridocyclitis. Inflammation of the choroid is usually designated as choroiditis. It may occur either as an acute or chronic condition. Acute choroiditis may be either of exogenous or endogenous origin. The former is more rare and is usually due to perforating wounds of the eyeball. Endogenous choroiditis, which is acute, is usually caused by infection being transmitted through the blood stream in the course of infections localized elsewhere in the body, acute infectious diseases, septicemia, puerperal fever, endocarditis, and other septic conditions. In these instances the local manifestations are accompanied by symptoms caused by the primary infection.

Choroiditis in the chronic form usually occurs as an ocular manifestation of some internal disease, such as syphilis, or tuberculosis. It may also be distinguished as a suppurative or nonsuppurative condition, depending upon whether or not the exudates present disappear by absorption or result in the formation of pus. The nonsuppurative variety is known as exudative choroiditis and is more common than the suppurative. In the presence of the latter, the other structures of the eye are usually involved, and in extreme cases, panophthalmitis may result.

In ordinary exudative choroiditis, scattered, isolated foci of inflammation are found over the choroid. On examination with the ophthalmoscope these appear grayish yellow in color and lie beneath the retinal vessels with their margins poorly outlined. The edges of the spots usually appear fuzzy. The choroidal vessels are not visible in the affected area. These reappear and the choroid can again be seen when the exudate disappears. It is now changed in appearance, however, being lighter in color and atrophic. With oncoming atrophy, the area appears white and the underlying sclera is now visible. A proliferation of pigment may also take place in the affected area. In the later stages also, these spots are more sharply outlined than they appear when recent. The retinal vessels are usually seen crossing the area above. In old cases the choroidal pigment may migrate into the retina, where it is seen to cover the retinal vessels.

A chronic variety characterized by the occurrence of a number of round or regular spots seen over the fundus is designated as disseminated choroiditis. As these spots occasionally clear up, they are replaced by other more recent ones. In older cases of long standing the choroid is found to be covered with many discreet areas which in some places become confluent. The retina and optic nerve are usually also involved, and the condition results in atrophy, with some impairment in vision. This might not be marked, however, unless the macula is involved.

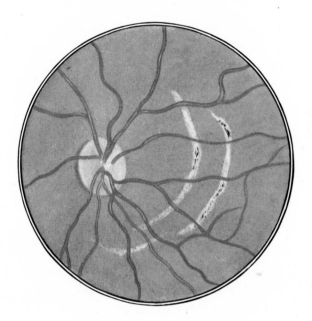

Fig. 61.—Ruptures of the choroid.

Syphilitic affections of the choroid may be characterized by changes in the vessels and the occurrence of choroiditis with large round spots throughout the fundus. They vary in size up to half the diameter of the disc. The condition is designated as an anterior choroiditis, and the spots are usually poorly defined, pale brown in color, with their edges rather hazy. The retina may also be affected and pigment spots may fringe the involved area over which the retinal vessels can be seen to pass. (See Syphilis.)

The choroid reveals characteristic inflammatory lesions in tuberculosis. These lesions may be either single or multiple and are characterized by the presence of patches which can very often be seen on examination with the ophthalmoscope. Discreet patches are found which are usually yellowish in color with poorly defined edges. Their size varies to about one-third that of the size of the disc. New patches may occur from time to time in the fundus. They are usually known as tubercles in the choroid and are conveyed here through the blood stream. Usually only one or two are present, although sometimes a larger number can be seen. Pigment spots are usually absent. These tubercles, when found, indicate a miliary tuberculosis of the choroid and are significant of a general miliary tuberculosis.

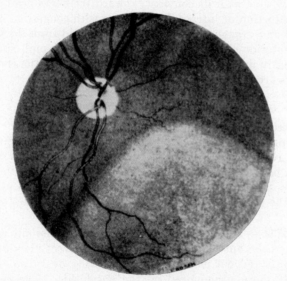

Fig. 62.—Flat detachment of choroid. (From O'Brien: Arch. Ophth., October, 1935.)

A large single focus of choroidal inflammation may be seen in the neighborhood of the disc or macular region in chronic tuberculosis. This is considered as a single nodule elevated in appearance, and which may be as large as the disc. In the later stages they become absorbed, leaving an area of atrophy with some pigment in the choroid. These are also indicative of the presence of general tuberculosis, although the latter may not be definitely diagnosed. Very large solitary tubercles indicative of tuberculosis are occasionally found on ophthalmoscopic examination. These sometimes break down and rupture through the sclera. They occur mostly in young people and are rather rare. When they occur, however, the condition usually results in loss of the eye.

Atrophy.—As has already been indicated, inflammation and degeneration of the choroid ultimately result in atrophy. This occurs around the disc in myopia and glaucoma, as well as in some ordinary senile conditions. It is very often associated with retinal degeneration and atrophy; a circumscribed white patch is usually found where the area of atrophy occurs. These are usually covered by the choroidal vessels.

Detachment.—The choroid may become detached as a result of a long-continued inflammatory process with proliferation which exerts a traction or pulling in different directions. Hemorrhages beneath the choroid may also result in detachment. This usually occurs after a sudden expulsive hemorrhage. Sarcoma and extensive exudation under the choroid may also be the cause. A choroid which is detached appears as a dark elevation projecting into the vitreous when examined with the ophthalmoscope. The opportunity for examination of these cases, however, is not often afforded.

According to O'Brien,[3] detachment of the choroid may occur at the time of, or shortly after, cataract extraction. He found it in forty-one cases following intracapsular extraction and in nine after extracapsular operation. It appears in the periphery of the fundus as a translucent elevation, the border of which is a dark shadowy line with its convexity toward the nerve head. The cause was said to be the reduction of intraocular pressure with congestion of the uveal vessels and a rapid and exaggerated transudation of fluid from the veins of the ciliary body and anterior choroid into the perichoroidal lymph space. The visual acuity is apparently unaffected, and the prognosis is good, the choroid invariably returning to its normal position.

Examination of the Fundus

Ophthalmoscopic examination of the fundus ordinarily includes an examination of the optic nerve head, fundus vessels, retina, and macula, in the order named. If the refractive state of the eye is normal and that of the examiner emmetropic, the best focus of the fundus details would be obtained with the lens of the ophthalmoscope marked zero. The refraction of the eye examined, as well as that of the examiner, will determine which lens to use to obtain the best detail.

The Optic Disc.—The patient is directed to look just slightly to the nasal side. This brings the optic disc or nerve head in direct view of the examiner. It can be seen to stand out as a round or vertically oval disc of a pinkish hue which is slightly more pronounced on the nasal side. The color of the disc varies somewhat also with age, appearing more of a yellowish-red in older people. It stands out in contrast to the darker color of the remainder of the fundus.

The actual size of the diameter of the disc is about 1.5 mm. Its margins are normally clearly seen and should present a sharp outline. A white ring is often seen surrounding the border which consists of connective tissue and is called the scleral ring. Another type of ring is also very often seen surrounding the margins of the disc either wholly or in part. This is black in color and is usually more pronounced around the outer border. It consists of pigment in the margin of the choroidal opening through which the optic nerve passes. The second ring is designated as a choroidal or pigment ring. Alterations in the shape of the sclerochoroidal canal through which the optic nerve passes, sometimes produces a crescent or conus which is seen with the ophthalmoscope, usually on the temporal margin of the disc. This is called a scleral crescent or conus and is more common in myopic eyes.

Normally the disc lies in the same plane with the retina and is not elevated. In the central portion is an excavation or depression, which is usually small in size and is produced by the early separation of the optic nerve fibers. In some instances this excavation may appear large and deep, occupying the entire temporal portion of the disc. It is whiter in color than the rest of the disc and is known as the physiologic excavation or cup. The depth and appearance should always be noted since these are altered in many diseased processes. The dark gray dots seen in the bottom of the excavation indicate the lamina cribrosa. A physiologic excavation never takes in the entire disc but leaves a portion of the disc usually on the nasal side, unaffected.

The Fundus Vessels.—The central vessels of the disc can be seen to emerge from the nasal or inner side of the excavation, where they divide into branches which pass over the edge onto the retina. Here the arterioles continue to branch off and subdivide into small twigs which finally connect with the veins. They therefore comprise a terminal system which has no communication with any other vascular system. This is of importance in the production of retinal lesions in many diseased conditions. The central artery and vein each divide into a superior and inferior branch. With the ophthalmoscope these can be seen to bifurcate into a superior nasal and superior temporal artery and vein as well as an inferior nasal and inferior temporal artery and vein. These supply the respective portions of the retina. The temporal vessels arch around the macula above and below with their smaller branches terminating outside of the macula itself.

The retinal arteries and veins can be differentiated by their size and color. The veins are darker in color than the arteries, larger in caliber, and somewhat more wavy in their course. The arteries are usually seen to pass above the veins where they cross. Pulsations of the central vein are sometimes seen in the center of the disc as a normal occurrence. An arterial pulsation, however, is indicative of a pathologic condition. Occasionally, a venous pulsation may be transmitted in such a way as to create the impression of an arterial pulsation being present and may require closer observation to eliminate the latter.

The Fundus.—On examination with the ophthalmoscope the normal retina, being transparent, is not seen. It is the retinal vessels which are exposed to view on a background of reddish fundus reflex. The normal color of the fundus might be described as a light or pinkish red and depends principally on the amount of pigment present in the retina and the color of the choroidal vessels. With little pigment present in the retina, the color of the fundus is much lighter than normal. In albinotic eyes which contain practically no pigment, the color is very light because of reflection of the white sclera behind. This is designated as an albinotic fundus. The color may vary, therefore, from one extreme of pigmentation to the opposite. In older people and in some dark-skinned races, the pigmentation is more pronounced, and the color of the fundus is a darker red. When the dark pigment epithelial layer is seen, it gives the retina a dotted or stippled appearance, sometimes called "stippled fundus." With marked decrease of the pigment epithelium, the choroidal vessels are exposed to view and can be observed together with the retinal vessels. They lie deeper than the latter, however, and are larger and lighter in color. Areas of choroidal pigment are exposed and can be seen lying between the choroidal vessels, giving the fundus a tessellated appearance. This is called a "tessellated fundus."

Light reflexes are often seen in the fundus, especially in young patients. These may shift about and present a shimmering appearance, especially on movement of the ophthalmoscope. These are less noticeable in the darker fundi and in older patients. They may prove annoying to the examiner and might, in some instances, simulate the appearance of pathologic bands or stripes, especially when seen about the vessels.

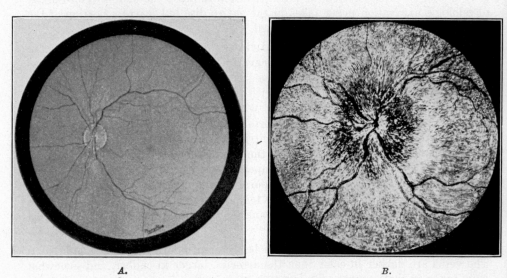

A.   B.

Fig. 63.—A, The normal fundus. (From Duke-Elder: Text-Book of Ophthalmology.) B, Papilledema.

Any structure or lesion observed in the fundus should be studied with especial reference to its size, location, and appearance. The size and location are determined by comparison and with relation to the size and location of the disc. For example, the object observed may be said to be about one-half the size of the disc and about one disc-diameter above and to the temporal side of the disc. Knowing the actual measurement of the disc to be 1.5 mm., a knowledge of the size and location of the structure under observation can be obtained.

Differences in level in the fundus can be determined on examination with the ophthalmoscope. An area in the fundus which is depressed or elevated can be determined by the difference in power of the lenses of the ophthalmoscope which focus the normal and abnormal level. Three diopters are considered to be equal to 1 mm. difference in level.

The Macula.—The macula and its fovea centralis are observed with the ophthalmoscope about 1½ to 2 disc-diameters to the temporal side of the disc. Its color is slightly darker than the rest of the fundus, and it is devoid of vessels. Normally, the fovea can be seen in the center of the dark red macula, to stand out as a small, glistening, yellow spot. The nerve fibers to the center of the macula run nearly straight, while the more peripheral fibers are curved and form an arch meeting beyond the macula. The fibers themselves cannot be distinguished, but the area occupied in their course between the disc and macula and that around the macula are the most sensitive parts of the retina. This area should, therefore, receive close attention on ophthalmoscopic examination, since it is frequently affected by traumatism, inflammations, and other pathologic processes.

Abnormalities of the Optic Disc

Hyperemia.—Ordinary hyperemia of the optic nerve is characterized by an increased redness in the color and by a haziness of the margins. As a result, there is a tendency for the nerve head to blend more in color with the surrounding fundus. There is also some dilatation and increased tortuosity of the vessels. Hyperemia of the disc is frequently observed and is an accompanying manifestation of inflammation of the nerve, retina, and choroid. It may be present in one or both eyes and may be found in many inflammatory conditions of the anterior segment of the eye.

Inflammation.—The optic nerve may be affected by inflammation almost anywhere in its course. When the nerve head is involved, it is visible on ophthalmoscopic examination and is designated as *optic neuritis* (papillitis). With inflammation of the nerve behind the eyeball there are no signs visible on examination with the ophthalmoscope, and this form is designated as *retrobulbar neuritis*. When inflammation of the optic nerve head is accompanied by inflammation of a fair-sized area of surrounding retina, it is known as a *neuroretinitis*.

Optic Neuritis (Papillitis).—Optic neuritis is an inflammatory condition of the optic nerve which is usually unilateral, although it may occasionally be bilateral. Functionally, it is characterized by early and marked visual loss, visual field changes as concentric contraction, central and paracentral scotoma, enlargement of the blind spot, impairment of dark adaptation.

It may result from many different causes. These include: (1) Traumatic infections of the interior of the eye. (2) Purulent infections in the teeth, sinuses, or orbit. (3) Acute infectious diseases and exanthemas, such as measles, mumps, scarlet fever, diphtheria, small pox, erysipelas, and typhoid fever. (4) Syphilis and tuberculosis. It occurs more commonly in the former and may become very marked. It is more rare in tuberculosis but may be found accompanying tuberculous involvement of the choroid. (5) Demyelinating diseases of the central nervous system, although these are more often accompanied by retrobulbar neuritis. (6) Intoxications (a) exogenous, e.g., lead, alcohol and tobacco, arsenic; (b) endogenous, such as that occurring in diabetes, nephritis, menstruation, lactation, and pregnancy. (7) Inflammations of the brain, such as meningitis with extension of the inflammation to the orbit and optic nerve producing a descending neuritis. (8) Severe anemia, especially occurring with certain diseases of the blood, and also severe secondary anemias. Clay and Baird[4] reported seven cases which they concluded were an acute infectious optic neuritis, the cause being an unknown virus with predilection for the optic nerve.

Symptoms.—The symptoms of optic neuritis are usually sudden in onset, with marked loss of vision and amaurosis. Pain is not so marked with optic neuritis as with retrobulbar neuritis. The pain may be present in the eyeball or in the back of the eye; it may be described as a headache; it may occur on ocular movement, or on the application of pressure to the eyeball. As the inflammatory process subsides, visual acuity improves with partial or complete restoration of vision; in some instances, the disc may regain a normal appearance. If the inflammatory process is severe, optic atrophy with permanent changes in the disc and defects in the visual field result.

On objective examination, the pupils may be found dilated and immobile. With the ophthalmoscope, the disc appears swollen up to 2 or 3 diopters, but rarely more; the swelling is cloudy; the disc margin is blurred and cannot be outlined. The disc is larger and much redder than normal. The arteries are slightly contracted and obscured by the swelling, while the veins are dilated, tortuous, darker, and kinked at the disc margin. Small hemorrhages, either round or linear, are found on, or near, the disc. Small grayish-white exudates may also be present. As the inflammatory swelling extends to the surrounding retina, a neuroretinitis develops. As the disease process abates, the swelling of the disc gradually decreases with the disappearance of hemorrhages. As the disc outline becomes visible, it shows a grayish pallor with blurred edges. The excavation is shallow, being filled in with organized inflammatory debris.

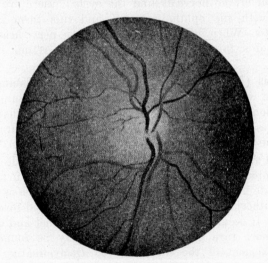

Fig. 64.—Mild optic neuritis. (From Wilmer: Atlas Fundus Oculi, The Macmillan Co.)

The diagnosis is made by the early loss of visual acuity, the visual field defects, the ophthalmoscopic appearance, and investigation of the cause. The latter includes a careful examination for any involvement of the teeth, tonsils, sinuses, ears, orbit, and examination for the presence of any systemic infections or intoxication.

The prognosis for vision depends on the severity of the disease process and elimination of the cause. When optic atrophy develops (postneuritic atrophy), the central vision especially may be permanently impaired.

Treatment.—The treatment is directed at removing the underlying cause, such as any focus of infection in the structures already mentioned. In the presence of systemic disease the specific treatment, if any, should be instituted. Various drugs are employed, such as sodium salicylate, potassium iodide, and mercury, especially when the etiology of the condition is not revealed. Good results are obtained from the use of some form of foreign protein or fever therapy. Boiled milk is given intramuscularly, beginning with about 3 c.c. and increasing until reaction is produced. Typhoid vaccine may be employed intravenously, beginning with 10 million and increasing to 20 or 30 million. Locally, the patient should wear dark glasses, the eyes should be given absolute rest, and one drop atropine sulfate (1 per cent) instilled, three times a day. The applications of leeches to the temples may also prove beneficial.

Papilledema (Choked Disc).—Papilledema is a noninflammatory swelling of the optic disc, usually, but not always, resulting from increased intracranial pressure. The outstanding, single cause of papilledema is intracranial tumor, being found in about 80 per cent of these cases (Paton). In the early stages disturbance of function is slight; hence, vision is unimpaired and patients have relatively few ocular complaints. If the intracranial pressure is unrelieved and the papilledema persists, optic atrophy invariably ensues with appreciable visual loss. The swelling is usually bilateral and there may be little difference in the amount of swelling in the two eyes. According to W. R. Parker, the eye with the lower intraocular pressure will manifest a greater amount of swelling.

Subjectively, blurred vision and transient, momentary attacks of blindness occur. Visual acuity and visual fields remain intact for a long period. The only exception may be an enlargement of the blind spots; with onset of optic atrophy, the peripheral field is the first to be affected, then the central field, and finally, total amaurosis.

In addition to brain tumors, there are numerous other causes of choked disc as brain abscess, cerebral syphilis, tuberculosis, hydrocephalus, meningitis, nephritis, blood dyscrasias, anemia, cysticercus of brain, sinus thrombosis, deformations of the skull (tower skull), and wounds of the skull with subdural hemorrhage. According to Benedict[5] the most common ocular sign of brain abscess is choked disc, which is present in about a third of the cases.

The pathogenesis is based on the increased intracranial pressure with a consequent increase in the pressure of the central retinal vein. With the venous engorgement an increased sheath pressure leads to lymph stasis and obstruction. These two factors, therefore, appear to be responsible for the resulting edema, although the exact point at which the obstruction takes place has not been determined.

Watkins, Wagener and Brown[6] reported three cases of thrombocytopenic purpura with bilateral choked optic discs in the absence of any demonstrable extraneous intracranial process or lesion. No intrameningeal or intracranial bleeding could be proved in any of the cases. (See Purpura hemorrhagica.) They felt that the mechanism of production of the papilledema was a local reaction of the tissues of the optic nerves to anoxemia that resulted from loss of blood and they concluded that edema of the brain arising from the same cause might be a factor in the development of papilledema.

Leinfelder and Paul[7] also suggested that edema of the brain is responsible for the increased intracranial pressure occurring with papilledema in the course of some of the general diseases.

Ophthalmoscopic Findings.—The disc appears redder than normal due to the increased capillarity. Earliest changes in the form of a swelling appear at the upper and lower borders of the disc and nasally, while the temporal margin may remain clear. The center of the disc is indistinct due to separation of the internal limiting membrane. According to Schieck, this is the earliest sign of papilledema. The arteries are reduced in size, while the veins are fuller, darker, and tortuous. The edema is usually transparent, and the elevation varies anywhere from 2 or 3 to 8 diopters of choking. The occurrence of hemorrhages is variable; usually, there is little or no hemorrhage, but when present, it is located peripherally.

In advanced stages the amount of swelling is greater, the disc margins are obliterated except for radial streaks, and the size of the disc is markedly increased as the swelling infiltrates into the surrounding retina. Also, the transparency of the retina diminishes, the arteries are obscured by the swelling while the veins are dilated, tortuous, and darker due to the venous stasis. Occasionally, a macular star is seen due to rupture of the fibers of Müller (Paton) and small, white fluffy exudates are found near the disc as a result of the swelling and degeneration of the cement substance of the nerve fibers.

As the stage of swelling subsides, the disc becomes atrophic. The veins become smaller and the margins of the disc become more normal and can now be outlined, although they will always appear blurred on examination with the ophthalmoscope. This may require a long period of time during which connective tissue forms to replace the nerve fibers which have been destroyed.

The diagnosis of papilledema is ordinarily not difficult, except possibly in the early stage when it must be differentiated from optic neuritis. As already stated in the description of the latter, the vision is diminished early in this condition, whereas in papilledema, the vision may remain unaffected until very late in the condition. The light adaption of the patient is affected in optic neuritis, whereas in papilledema it is normal. The physiologic excavation remains deeper and the lamina cribrosa visible in papilledema, whereas in optic neuritis, the excavation is either shallow or filled in, and the lamina cribrosa is not seen. In optic neuritis the perivascular sheaths are clearly observed outside the vessel walls, while these are not visible in papilledema. Examination of the visual fields reveals usually a central scotoma and an enlarged blind spot, while in papilledema, there is only an enlargement of the blind spot and perhaps a slight contraction of the peripheral fields.

The extent of the papilledema occurring with brain tumors depends more on the location of the tumor than on the size of the tumor. Bilateral choked disc is most common in tumors located in the posterior cerebral fossa and cerebellum, because of compression here of the aqueduct of Sylvius and the production of intracranial tension from the obstruction to circulation of the cerebrospinal fluid in the ventricles. Tumors occurring in the cerebellopontine angle may produce papilledema associated with involvement of the facial and auditory nerves.

Treatment.—The treatment of papilledema depends mainly on the cause. An attempt should be made to localize the tumor or other primary cause, and this must be determined and the treatment decided on, after thorough study by a competent neurologist and neurosurgeon. In tumors other than a posterior fossa tumor, where lumbar puncture is contraindicated, this procedure might reduce the papilledema. This is only a temporary or palliative measure, however, and not a cure. When the tumor is localized, a decompression operation is usually performed by the neurosurgeon. Papilledema resulting from other causes requires treatment of the primary cause when the nature of this is determined.

Retrobulbar Neuritis.—When an inflammation is localized in the orbital portion of the optic nerve behind the globe, it is designated as retrobulbar neuritis. This form of inflammation in the optic nerve is not transmitted to the optic disc and is sometimes known as an axial neuritis. On examination with the ophthalmoscope, therefore, the disc may show no abnormal changes which would indicate the presence of the inflammatory condition. In the late stages, however, when atrophy occurs, this may be recognized on examination of the disc. The condition must, therefore, be diagnosed by other means, such as the nature of the symptoms and their location.

The papillomacular bundle of the optic nerve and the myelin sheaths around the cylinder axes behind the lamina may be affected either alone or together in retrobulbar neuritis. Inflammation of the papillomacular bundle in axial neuritis may be either acute or chronic. This form usually results from infection which starts either in the nerve itself or in the surrounding tissue. It may become involved as a result of the infection being conveyed through the circulation, or by the extension of the inflammation from the neighboring structures in the orbit.

Retrobulbar neuritis has been divided into two groups from an etiologic standpoint (Troncoso). The first is that which occurs as a form of axial neuritis and is caused by infections or inflammations which are transmitted from neighboring structures as well as those which are caused by acute infectious diseases, such as influenza, pneumonia, erysipelas, scarlet fever, etc. Among the infections the most frequent causes are those which arise in the nose, throat, and sinuses, and by direct spread to the optic nerve or by convection through the blood stream, produce a retrobulbar neuritis. (See Infections of the Nose, Throat, and Sinuses.) Such involvement can occur because of the close anatomic relationship between the optic nerve and the sphenoid and ethmoid sinuses, the latter being separated from the orbit by a very thin wall. In the examination of 100 skulls, Francis and Gibson found this to be only $\frac{1}{4}$ mm. in thickness in 38 per cent. Onodi found that the optic nerve is often separated from the posterior ethmoidal cells by a thickness of $\frac{1}{2}$ mm. The second group are those cases of retrobulbar neuritis which occur with the demyelinating diseases, such as disseminated sclerosis, neuromyelitis optica (Devic's disease), acute disseminated encephalomyelitis, and encephalitis periaxialis diffusa (Schilder's disease). These will be described under diseases of the nervous system.

In the past, nearly all cases of retrobulbar neuritis were considered to be due to the presence of sinus infection, but in recent years, the condition has been attributed more frequently to the presence of disseminated sclerosis.

In the study of 100 patients with retrobulbar neuritis, Carroll[8] found this condition to be associated with the following diseases:

Multiple sclerosis	37
Leber's disease	9
Encephalomyelitis	8
Arachnoiditis	3
Vascular disease	3
Sinus disease	2
Syphilis	2
Postspinal anesthesia	1
Neuromyelitis optica	1
Unknown etiology	34

The number of cases of sinus disease is here very small. Some of those listed otherwise also suffered with sinus disease.

He pointed out that a unilateral central scotoma may be the first sign of a neoplasm either primarily intraorbital or intracranial or metastatic to the optic nerve. Careful studies of the visual field characteristics are of importance in establishing the causative factor. Carroll also differentiated tobacco-alcohol amblyopia from retrobulbar neuritis. The former condition is always bilateral, tends to occur in older persons, especially males, and is always associated with bilateral centrocecal scotoma. It is also gradual in onset and recovery and is not accompanied by pain on movement of the eyeball or by tenderness of the eyeball. Moreover, it is associated with a history of excessive use of tobacco and alcohol and lack of vitamin B in the diet.

The possibility of infection in the teeth and tonsils, periosteitis, and other orbital infections about the optic canal, must be kept in mind in searching for the cause of a retrobulbar neuritis. Syphilis and, less frequently, tuberculosis are also fairly common causes. It may occur as the result of alterations in the female generative organs, such as menstruation, pregnancy, and also during lactation. Leber's disease, which is described as an hereditary optic neuritis or hereditary optic atrophy, is also characterized by a loss of central vision and the presence of a central scotoma.

According to Benedict,[9] who reviewed the records of more than 400 cases of retrobulbar neuritis seen at the Mayo clinic from 1920 to 1940, "it would seem reasonable, in the absence of signs or symptoms of other causes of retrobulbar neuritis, to presume that the condition is due to multiple sclerosis, even though the etiologic basis of the disease cannot be established on any other grounds." (See Disseminated sclerosis.)

Symptoms.—The subjective symptoms consist principally of pain, especially on movement of the eye, and tenderness when slight pressure is applied to the eyeball. Severe headache is usually a prominent complaint. The onset is accompanied by a marked impairment of the vision which may go on to almost total blindness. In most cases the condition is found only in one eye, although both may be occasionally affected.

On examination with the ophthalmoscope, the objective symptoms may be very few in number, or entirely absent. This depends on how close to the disc the inflammatory condition occurs. The fundus may be entirely normal, but the retinal veins may appear somewhat enlarged and the arteries constricted. Late in the disease, especially in severe cases, an atrophy of the papillomacular bundle occurs which results in pallor, especially noted on the temporal side of the disc. In this stage the vision of the patient may also improve to some extent.

Examination of the visual fields reveals the characteristic finding of a central scotoma in the affected eye. The size of the scotoma depends on the severity of the condition and may extend from fixation out as far as 40 or 50°. The peripheral field beyond the area of the scotoma may be unaffected. In many cases the scotoma is smaller, although the entire central area and the blind spot are usually involved.

The disease may run a variable course which depends principally upon the causative factor. After a period of time the central scotoma becomes smaller and may gradually disappear, especially in mild cases. This is accompanied by a return of vision, but in the more severe cases it may be present for an indefinitely longer period. With degeneration of the nerve fibers either in whole or in part, optic atrophy occurs. This is accompanied by a loss of vision in proportion to the extent of the atrophy.

Treatment.—The treatment of retrobulbar neuritis depends principally upon the underlying cause. An attempt should be made to reveal the presence of any infection, such as in the nose, throat, sinuses, teeth, or other parts. When such a focus is found to be present, the treatment should be directed toward its removal. When any other disease which is known to be an etiologic factor is found, this must also be treated, according to the nature of the condition. The treatment may otherwise include the administration of salicylates, mercury, iodides, and diaphoretics. Locally, one drop of atropine sulfate, 1 per cent solution, should be instilled into the eye about twice daily to keep the eye at rest. The patient should refrain from any use of the eyes, especially for close work. Black glasses should be worn, and the diet and elimination of the patient should receive careful attention.

Optic Atrophy.—There are two principal forms of atrophy of the optic nerve: (1) primary or simple atrophy, and (2) secondary optic atrophy. The pathology in the former occurs primarily in the nerve itself, while in the secondary form, the atrophy results from inflammatory diseases of the eye. Destruction of the nerve tissue is common in both, but with the difference that there is no replacement of the tissue destroyed in the primary form, whereas, the defect may be replaced with organized inflammatory exudates in the secondary form.

Optic atrophy may occur as the result of inflammatory, degenerative, and vascular conditions which impair the nutrition of the nerve.

The inflammatory atrophy is further to be divided into (a) postneuritic atrophy, which is the end result of optic neuritis or retrobulbar neuritis, and (b) ascending atrophy, occurring as the result of diseases which primarily affect the retina and choroid.

In the degenerative atrophies, cerebrospinal diseases are the most common cause, for example, tabes dorsalis, multiple sclerosis, and general paralysis. Optic atrophy occurs in 10 to 15 per cent of tabetics as an early sign and often precedes other signs of the disease by a period of years. It is nearly always bilateral, although the amount of the destruction on the two sides may differ in extent. It is slowly progressive over a period of years and generally leads to total blindness. Primary atrophy also occurs after injuries to the optic nerve, such as laceration or compression of the nerve by bone fragments resulting from fractures. It may also follow hemorrhage in the optic canal, orbital tumors, tumors producing chiasmal syndrome, and sclerosis of the carotid artery.

Vascular disease produces a degenerative atrophy, such as that which follows thrombosis or embolus of the central retinal artery and arteriosclerosis of the retinal vessels. Extreme posthemorrhagic anemia is also a cause of true atrophy.

In glaucoma a degenerative atrophy is produced as a result of the increased intraocular pressure. This is indicated on ophthalmoscopic examination by the deep pathologic excavation of the nerve head.

Optic atrophy may occur also from mechanical pressure which is exerted on the nerve fibers along the course of the optic nerve or tract, and also secondary to alterations in the circulation and innervation which might result from pressure. These are known as pressure atrophies and may appear very similar to the form described as primary degenerative atrophy. This type of atrophy is found occurring as a result of tumors which, because of their location, produce pressure on the optic nerve. In other instances, by bony changes in the skull or bones of the orbit, the pressure results on some part of the optic nerve or tract.

Symptoms.—A gradual loss of vision is the outstanding symptom of optic atrophy. In addition, foggy vision, difficulty in recognizing colors, and early loss of dark adaptation occur. In tabes, fleeting diplopia may be complained of. The visual field test will show an early contraction for red and green, with retention of the field for blue and yellow. Later there is a complete loss of the color field, with concentric contraction of the peripheral form field. The fields, however, may be extremely variable, even to the occurrence of sector-like defects. The picture is not necessarily characteristic, except for the presence of a concentric contraction of the peripheral fields, and the positive presence of an enlarged blind spot.

Ophthalmoscopic Examination.—

1. Primary or tabetic type.—Here the disc displays a prominent white pallor, or even a pure white color. The capillaries of the disc are obliterated, and no longer evident. The disc margin is sharp and clearly outlined; there is no obliteration of the physiologic excavation, which on the contrary, may be exceedingly deep, with the blue dots of the lamina cribrosa standing out prominently. Changes in the retinal vessels are characterized by a gradual constriction and narrowing, especially affecting the arteries. This is found to be rather marked, especially late in the disease.

In glaucomatous atrophy there is extreme cupping of the optic disc which is known as a pathologic or glaucomatous excavation. It is characterized by a sharp bending of the retinal vessels as they cross over the disc margin. The color of the disc is grayish white, and the lamina cribrosa is also visible in the excavation.

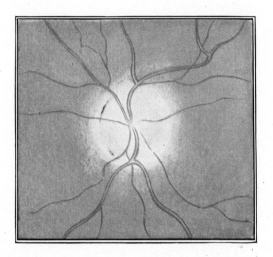

Fig. 65.—Postneuritic optic atrophy, showing a pale disc with blurred margins and a shallow excavation in the center.

In obstruction of the central artery by thrombosis or embolus, the disc shows primary atrophy of the tabetic type with marked changes in the vessels which are characteristic of the vascular condition, and which suggest the diagnosis.

2. Secondary atrophy (postneuritic).—The disc here shows a grayish-white color, which may later assume a more profound white color. The excavation is central but obscured because of the organized exudate which fills it in. The margins of the disc are indistinct and nearly always show blurring to some extent. These ophthalmoscopic findings serve as important factors in differentiating this condition from the primary optic atrophy. The vessels show evidences of inflammatory change. The veins are tortuous and congested, while the arteries are narrowed in caliber and their perivascular sheaths bordering the vessel walls are prominent. Some discoloration and slight pigment changes may be observed around the area of the disc.

Abnormalities of the Retinal Vessels

Angiospasm.—This is a form of occlusion of the retinal arterioles which occurs in sclerosis and hypertension, affecting either a part of or the entire vessel as a result of constriction. It may occur in the central artery of the retina, or any one of the branches, and produces an interference with the blood supply and interference with the vision. In the central artery its occurrence would cause a pallor of the disc and blurring of the margins, together with some edema, and a cherry-red spot in the macula. Such a spasm may be of a temporary or a permanent nature. If the occlusion is released, the optic nerve or part affected resumes its normal condition. With the permanent obstruction, however, the affected portion becomes atrophic.

Aneurysm.—An aneurysm may occur in the central artery resulting in a dilatation of the vessels which can be seen to pulsate synchronous with the systolic heart beat. This occurs rarely, but in other instances, smaller aneurysms may be found in the arteriolar branches which are accompanied by an edema in the surrounding retina.

Sclerosis.—Sclerosis of the arteries of the retina frequently occurs in association with generalized arteriosclerosis, but it may also occur as a localized condition in the retina. A generalized sclerosis may be found in senility, hypertension, nephritis, and as a result of syphilis. The changes in the smaller arteries of the retina are similar to those occurring in the small vessels elsewhere. This is considered usually to begin in the media with the formation of connective tissue which is followed by hyaline degeneration and results in thickening. Later, the intima becomes involved, the endothelium proliferates, and occlusion may take place. A pressure results from sclerosis of the artery, and thrombosis of the veins may occur. The blood supply is diminished in the parts supplied as a result of the vascular changes which take place, and the nutrition of the retina is impaired. This is followed by degeneration and atrophy of the part involved. Later, the formation of new connective tissue may result in a further sclerosis.

On examination with the ophthalmoscope, the retinal vessels in sclerosis will first show a change in the walls of the arteries which become visible as a yellow stripe. The color gradually changes to pale red. Later, the vessel walls become opaque, and white lines are seen on either side of the column of blood. This stage is known as perivasculitis. The lumen of the blood vessel becomes gradually constricted with a narrowing of the blood column itself.

In the late stage this continued thickening of the vessel walls terminates in an obliteration of the vessel which, on examination, has the appearance of a white cord.

In early stages spasm of the artery is localized to certain portions of the vessel. In other instances the angiospasm is noted along a greater length of the vessel and appears more uniform. In still other instances constriction in the vessel may take place at short intervals which gives the appearance of beadlike formations.

Tortuosity in the retinal vessels can be noted early, with the ophthalmoscope, and may become so marked as to have a corkscrew shape, especially in the smaller vessels around the macula.

Increase in the appearance of the light streak in the artery is also observed. This results from the reflection caused by the contrast between the lumen of the vessel and the vessel wall. In advanced cases it resembles a copper wire in appearance and is sometimes called a "copper-wire" artery. In some instances the vessel wall becomes white, and on examination in advanced sclerosis it resembles a silver wire, giving rise to the name, "silver-wire" artery.

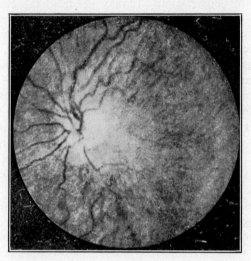

Fig. 66.—Tortuosity of the retinal vessels in arteriosclerosis.

In the course of progressive sclerosis, at the point where a retinal artery crosses a vein, an indentation or compression sometimes is visible, especially in those cases further advanced. The walls of the veins which are somewhat more elastic, are compressed by the artery, so that the former appear to be indented and not visible at the point of crossing, when examined with the ophthalmoscope. Continuous sclerosis of the artery impedes the venous circulation which results in a gradual dilation and distention, especially between points of crossing. In marked cases this will give the vein the appearance of having varicosities.

In the course of sclerosis the vessel walls become more brittle, and small ruptures may occur which result in hemorrhages. These hemorrhages may be as small as a pin point in size when they are caused by rupture of the smaller capillaries. When they come from the larger vessels, they can be seen to occur much larger and take on various shapes in the nerve fiber layer of the retina.

Sclerosis of the retinal vessels may result in an edema around the disc with an increase in the redness of the color of the disc, and later optic atrophy as a result of the interference with the nutrition of the structure.

Obstruction (Embolism; Thrombosis).—The central artery of the retina or any one of its branches may be the seat of an embolus. This results in a mechanical obstruction to the circulation in the affected vessel and a sudden stopping of the blood supply to that portion of the retina involved. Some nutrition may still be supplied by the adjacent vessels of the choroid, but the retina becomes atrophic. The patient becomes suddenly blind in the affected eye.

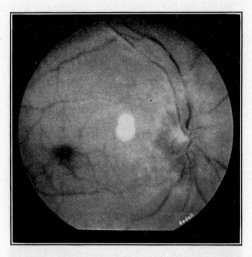

Fig. 67.—Embolism of the central retinal artery in the right eye of a man aged 51 a few hours after sudden and complete blindness; white edema, pink nerve head, and red macula. (From Bedell; J. A. M. A., March 18, 1939.)

On ophthalmoscopic examination the evidences to be seen are characteristic of the condition. When the central artery is affected, the retina presents an appearance of general anemia. The arteries are all extremely narrow, and the smaller arterioles are not visible. The veins are not much changed, and the optic disc is pale with its margins blurred. A bright red spot in the fovea is seen, which is surrounded by a large white area. The white area is that portion of the inner layers of the retina which has become opaque. Since there are no inner layers at the fovea, the red choroid shows through at the spot surrounded by the large white opacity. This produces the characteristic picture known as a "cherry-red" spot in the macula and is observed immediately after the embolus occludes the artery. It does not remain long, however, for after a time, the retinal vessels again become filled, and as this takes place, columns of blood can be seen to move spasmodically through the veins especially. The white opaque area around the macula gradually disappears and the optic disc becomes white in color. Its margins can be clearly outlined, and the vessels are very narrow and thin, while the smaller branches cannot be seen. In cases where a cilioretinal vessel is present, the blood supply of the retina might not be completely cut off, since these vessels are supplied with blood from the posterior ciliary arteries.

In cases where only a branch of the central retinal artery is occluded by an embolus, the resulting changes are confined to that part of the retina supplied by the affected artery. Total blindness does not occur as in embolus of the central artery, but only the affected portion of the retina is blind. This can be definitely demonstrated and outlined as a defect or blind area in the visual field.

Embolism of the central retinal artery occurs in valvular heart disease, especially endocarditis. It affects one eye only and is accompanied by the sudden loss of vision and practically no other subjective symptoms.

In certain purulent conditions an infectious embolus may be conveyed to a retinal vessel and result in a suppurative retinitis. This extends to the surrounding parts of the eyeball and causes a metastatic panophthalmitis.

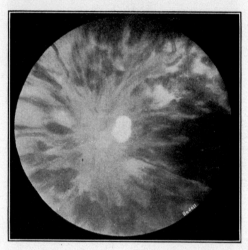

Fig. 68.—Thrombosis of central retinal vein in a 49-year-old male. Complete destruction of the vein; widespread hemorrhages. (Courtesy of Dr. Arthur J. Bedell.)

In many cases it is difficult to determine whether the obstruction is caused by an embolus or a thrombus. This necessitates a consideration of the primary internal disease. For example, rare cases of bilateral occlusion might occur as the result of the thrombosis, such as might be found with arteriosclerosis. With endocarditis in young children the condition is embolic. In older patients with proliferating endarteritis, obstruction is probably caused by thrombosis. In the latter the condition is usually produced by local causes. A sudden fall in blood pressure in any case may result in obstruction of the central retinal artery.

The treatment of occlusion of the central artery consists in an attempt to dislodge the obstruction. This might be possible by dilatation of the vessels if the case is seen early. For this purpose amyl nitrate inhalation should be employed immediately. The effect, however, does not last long, and nitroglycerin, $\frac{1}{100}$ gr., should also be administered. Acetylcholine has also been injected in order to produce vasodilatation.

Obstruction of the Central Vein (Thrombosis).—When the central vein of the retina becomes obstructed the venous circulation becomes impeded and a distention in the veins of the retina results. With increase in the distention the veins also become tortuous and hemorrhages which may be large and extensive cover the retina. The arteries are found to be smaller and very narrow. The vision of the patient is reduced in the eye affected and may even be entirely lost. When total loss of vision results, however, it is usually not as sudden and abrupt as in embolism of the central artery. The hemorrhages usually recur and new ones may be found from time to time. They may be present in all shapes and sizes, and together with the venous distention, they may obscure the entire disc. An edema of the retina may be found around the disc in which portions of the congested veins are lost to view.

An obstruction may occur in one of the branches of the central vein, in which case the hemorrhages and other changes described are confined to the area supplied by the affected vessel. In some cases a collateral circulation may be established which may compensate to some extent with the interference in the affected vessel.

The obstruction is said to be caused by an endophlebitis and usually occurs in older patients with syphilis and arteriosclerosis and diabetes. It may also occur in those suffering with inflammation of the orbit and orbital cellulitis following erysipelas. The vein becomes involved by extension of the inflammation or by an infected thrombus.

The prognosis of thrombosis of the central vein is not good, although somewhat better than with embolus of the artery. Recurrence of hemorrhages may cause loss of a great part or nearly all of the vision.

As a result of venous thrombosis and distention, the intraocular tension is frequently increased and secondary glaucoma results. This does not respond well to treatment in these cases and makes the prognosis more unfavorable.

The treatment of the condition depends principally on the nature of the primary disease. Therefore, general rather than local treatment is indicated. In addition to treatment of the general disease, some form of calcium and the iodides may also be prescribed.

Abnormalities of the Retina

The retina is examined in detail with the ophthalmoscope with particular reference to the color, the presence or absence of hemorrhages, pigmentation, exudates, edema, elevation, and as to the condition of the retinal vessels. It is often affected following pathologic involvement of neighboring structures, such as the choroid, the sclera, iris and ciliary body. Exudative choroiditis, for example, may cause secondary retinal involvement. Abnormalities in the retina may occur at some time in the course of almost any of the internal diseases. They may result from transmission of infection by direct extension and from toxins, or products of degeneration and inflammation which are conveyed through the circulation. Changes in the general vascular system result in alterations in the retinal vessels which also in turn may cause abnormalities to be found in the retinal tissue. Generalized arteriosclerosis, vascular hypertension, diabetes, nephritis, syphilis, and tuberculosis, are only a few of the diseases which may lead to disease of the retinal vessels and the retina itself.

Hyperemia.—Hyperemia, which is arterial, will accompany nearly all inflammatory conditions of the retina, and the adjacent structures. This is evidenced by marked tortuosity and swelling of the retinal arteries. Dilatation and tortuosity of the retinal veins characterizes a venous hyperemia. In the latter, the arteries are often smaller than normal. This occurs mostly in glaucoma with increased intraocular tension. The veins are compressed in the excavation of the nerve head. In optic neuritis also, the veins are compressed with swelling of the nerve head. In cardiac disease and in arteriosclerosis a hyperemia may be present as the result of general congestion in the veins. Dilatation of the retinal veins may be accompanied by a haziness of the retina around the optic disc, and a few hemorrhages might be present. Usually this change occurs in only one eye and sometimes in a definite area of the retina, depending on the primary cause. Normal eyes sometimes show a marked tortuosity of the vessels, but in these instances, they are both affected similarly, and it is unaccompanied by other lesions. With hyperemia, the normal pinkish color of the retina changes to a more pronounced red color.

Hemorrhage.—Retinal hemorrhages occur in various sizes and shapes and appear usually as small extravasations of blood which can be seen with the ophthalmoscope as dark red spots or streaks surrounded by the brighter red of the adjacent retina. They are described as having a flame shape when they occur in the fiber layer of the retina, because of the fact that the extravasated blood spreads in the direction of the fibers. Hemorrhages which are irregular in shape or round are usually found in the deeper layers of the retina, and sometimes between the retina and the choroid. Large round hemorrhages may occur in the macular region and are anterior to the retina protruding into the vitreous. These are known as preretinal hemorrhages, and sometimes as subhyaloid hemorrhages. They are eventually absorbed without impairment of vision. Extensive preretinal hemorrhages, however, may be present for a very long time and finally result in the formation of connective tissue and a proliferating retinitis. They cause a corresponding loss of vision. Hemorrhages occurring in the retina take on a darker brown appearance when they become older and are very slowly absorbed. Pigmentation might be present at the former site of the hemorrhage.

Their presence is usually due often to local alterations in the retinal vessels, and they are found in many of the internal diseases, as e.g., arteriosclerosis, renal disease, diabetes, syphilis, and tuberculosis. The vascular changes which take place with generalized hypertension are a common cause. They also occur after occlusion of either the central retinal artery or central retinal vein or any of their branches. Diseases which are characterized by alteration in the composition of the blood, such as the primary anemia, secondary anemia, and leucemia, are characterized by the presence of numerous hemorrhages. In newborn infants, retinal hemorrhages are sometimes found as a result of trauma sustained during instrumental delivery.

Edema usually occurs in the retina near the disc as a result of inflammation in the optic nerve, and in other instances, as an early manifestation of inflammation of the retina itself. It may be present about the disc as an early sign of toxemia of pregnancy. In inflammation of the retina it may be localized in one particular area, or it may be more diffuse. When observed with the ophthalmoscope, it has the appearance of a more or less pronounced haze, and the retina appears somewhat elevated. Signs of edema due to the presence of serum may be seen around the region of the macula after injuries to the eyeball, while circumscribed areas might be found in the neighborhood of inflammatory lesions of the choroid.

Exudates usually occur as more or less circumscribed patches in the retina in association with various inflammatory and degenerative conditions. They can be found as retinal manifestations of renal disease, syphilis, and certain forms of exudative retinitis or chorioretinitis. The exudates seen in true inflammatory conditions usually appear white or grayish-white in color and may vary in size. In some instances they are slightly larger than a pinhead, while in others, they may be as large as the disc, with their edges blurred and fuzzy. These are usually found in the more superficial layers and lie between the retinal vessels. The latter are also seen in the retina affected by renal disease and are described as "cotton-wool patches." Exudative areas show a tendency to gravitate toward the macula, and in many instances, they form a star-shaped figure around the macula. This is due to their infiltration into the separation between Müller's fibers. In other conditions, such as diabetes and circinate retinitis, a large number of small areas are seen. These are more or less round, well demarcated, and glistening-yellow in color. These coalesce and arrange themselves in a circular or U-shaped pattern around the macular area, where they may be present for a long time. Exudates occurring in inflammatory conditions sometimes clear up after a period of time. The accompanying visual disturbance will depend on their location and extent. If the macula should be involved, a central scotoma is present, whereas the vision may not be seriously impaired when other portions of the retina are involved.

Anemia.—In a few diseases which are characterized principally by a loss of blood or profound general anemia, the retina may also be found to show an anemia. This occurs principally in some of the primary anemias as pernicious anemia, chlorosis, and leucemia. It may also occur following some of the more severe secondary anemias, such as those following intestinal hemorrhages in typhoid, occasional severe uterine hemorrhages, and those occurring with carcinomatous conditions of the gastrointestinal tract. In some of the chronic diseases of long standing, an impairment of nutrition may occur which will result in an anemia of the retina.

Such an anemia can be observed on ophthalmoscopic examination, as a general pallor of the retina and retinal vessels. In acute cases whitish patches of edema may be noted around the disc. The optic disc can be seen to appear pale. The retinal vessels themselves are lighter in color than normal and are smaller in size. The vision in anemia of the retina is decreased and will continue to decrease as long as the anemia progresses. With improvement of the circulatory disturbance, however, the vision might improve.

Retinitis (Retinosis).—The term retinitis has always been employed to describe the abnormal and pathologic condition of the retina which follows an impairment of the circulation and nutrition. In recent years, however, the term retinosis has been proposed by Troncoso, to be more properly applied to this condition, since the pathology found is one which should be considered as the result of a degenerative rather than an inflammatory process. The abnormal appearance of the retina which is characterized by the presence of those alterations already described as hemorrhages, exudates, edema, hyperemia, and anemia, are usually a part of a degenerative process and ultimately lead to a degenerative condition of the retina itself. Such retinal changes occur in the diseases which affect the vascular system and the circulation, those which alter the constituents of the blood, many of the metabolic and glandular diseases, as diabetes, nephritis, senile degenerations, and some of the hereditary and familial conditions already described.

A true inflammation of the retina may occur, however, in the form of a more diffuse retinitis in association with choroiditis. This is found especially in syphilis and tuberculosis, septicemias, and purulent infections which lead to a septic retinitis, and after certain external influences, such as excessive direct sunlight, electricity, acetylene torches, radium, and x-rays. The retinitis caused by the external influences is accompanied by pigmentation, small white and yellow spots, and occasional hemorrhages. A central scotoma may be present for a variable period of time, and the visual acuity is impaired, depending on the length of exposure.

In the septic conditions white spots and hemorrhages may be found in the retina, especially around the disc and neighborhood of the macula. The retinitis occurring as the result of infection conveyed by the circulation from distant parts is part of a metastatic endophthalmitis and is characterized by the presence of suppuration usually involving the entire eyeball. In other cases, the inflammation may lead to an abscess formation extending into the vitreous which becomes encapsulated and limited in its progress.

In syphilis and tuberculosis the retinitis is associated with inflammation of the choroid. In the former disease the condition was described by Foerster as syphilitic retinochoroiditis, which is characterized by the presence of edema and exudates occurring over the fundus, more especially around the nerve head and macula. The nerve head is somewhat discolored and grayish, while the entire fundus may appear clouded because of vitreous infiltration. Small areas of exudate are present around the macula in many cases. Late in the disease, the fundus details may become more visible following clearing of the vitreous. Localized pigment deposits with oncoming atrophy may now be observed in the areas occupied by the exudates. The walls of the retinal vessels now reveal signs of the inflammatory process, with narrowing in their caliber and prominence of the perivascular sheaths. The vision of the patient is decreased during the progress of the condition and may become reduced to only light perception. (See Syphilis.) The retinitis occurring in tuberculosis (see Tuberculosis) is usually characterized first by the changes in the retinal vessels, since the tubercle bacillus is conveyed here by the circulation, lodging in the choroidal and less commonly, in the retinal vessels. The inflammation, therefore, usually originates in the choroid and then involves the retina.

A form of retinitis was described by Jensen as *chorioretinitis juxta-papillaris* which was formerly thought to occur with syphilis, but now is considered as being due to tuberculosis. It is characterized chiefly by the presence of a large area of exudation which is grayish white in color and indistinct in outline. It is seen with the ophthalmoscope to lie close to the disc and overlying the retinal vessels. It may also be accompanied by some deposits on Descemet's membrane. The visual field of the affected eye reveals a typical sector-like defect which includes the blind spot and extends out into the periphery.

Pseudoglioma.—When a suppurative process in the eyeball is confined to the posterior segment alone, it may result in the formation of an abscess which becomes encapsulated in the vitreous. When such an eye is examined some

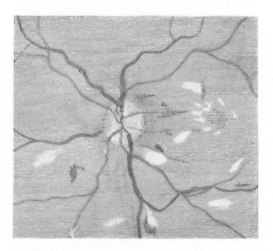

Fig. 69.—Drawing showing edema, hemorrhages, and exudates (cotton-wool patches) in the retina. (From Tassman: Medical World, October, 1936.)

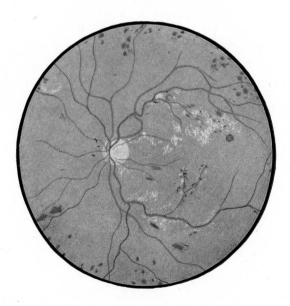

Fig. 70.—Retinosis in diabetes (Hirschberg), showing typical hemorrhages and exudates in the retina. (From Troncoso: Internal Diseases of the Eye and Atlas of Ophthalmoscopy, F. A. Davis Co.)

time after the acute process has subsided, the anterior segment of the eye may appear normal and reveal no evidences of the condition except possibly a few posterior synechiae and retraction of the iris. The abscess formation is replaced by cicatricial tissue which by combined contraction results in detachment of the retina and atrophy of the inner eyeball. The vision of the affected eye is almost or even entirely lost. On examination with the ophthalmoscope, in this late stage, the appearance resembles very much that which is present with glioma (retinoblastoma). This is especially true in cases occurring in children, and they are, therefore, designated as *pseudoglioma*. The eye can be seen to reveal a large gray area in the posterior segment which is very bright and stands out prominently, giving off a reflex, especially in the dark, which resembles the appearance of a cat's eye. For this reason, it is sometimes called an "amourotic cat's eye." To differentiate this condition from true glioma of the retina, the age of the patient and the history of a previous inflammatory or suppurative condition present in the eye are of great importance. Glioma usually occurs in very young children and is not of an inflammatory nature. Pseudoglioma implies the presence of a former inflammation or suppuration. The latter may follow some of the acute infectious diseases, as measles and scarlet fever, or septic and purulent conditions occurring for other reasons. The intraocular tension in pseudoglioma may be unchanged or lower than normal, while in glioma it might be increased above normal. In glioma, deposits of calcium take place in the tumor which are revealed by x-ray examination and are considered pathognomonic of the growth, when they are present. These are absent in pseudoglioma. The latter condition also remains stationary, whereas glioma is liable to progress to a fatal termination.

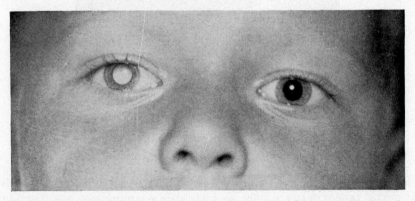

Fig. 71.—The white pupillary reflex in the right eye caused by a retinoblastoma in a boy aged 4 years. In one year this patient showed a metastasis in the bones of the skull and later throughout the entire body. (From Reese: South. Surgeon, June, 1938.)

For this reason, therefore, enucleation of the affected eyeball is usually indicated, and it is necessary often to differentiate between the two in order to avoid euncleation unnecessarily. In very doubtful cases, however, especially with a sightless eye, it might be necessary to enucleate, even though the diagnosis of glioma has not been definitely established.

Pigmentation.—When the structural elements of the retina are diseased and later destroyed, including the pigment epithelial layer and the rods and cones, melanin granules are conveyed through the aperture in the limiting membrane. This is considered by some to be brought about by the lymphatic system, and by others, the pigment granules are said to be conveyed into the retina by phagocytes. Such pigmentation may be seen on examination with the ophthalmo- scope to be present in any part of the retina, either localized or generalized, lying in some conditions alongside the retinal vessels, while in others, between the retinal vessels. It may occur as round concentric spots of definite size; in other instances, in irregular accumulations varying in shape and size.

Tumors and Cysts.—Tumors of the retina may be congenital in origin and occur in such diseases as tuberous sclerosis (Bourneville's disease), angio- matosis retina (von Hippel's disease) and in neurofibromatosis (von Reckling- hausen's disease). They are usually accompanied by congenital spots and nevi in the skin and other structures. They occur also in association with tumors in the brain and other organs. The disease in which these tumors are found have been grouped by van der Hoeve under the name of phakomatoses. (See Congenital and hereditary eye manifestations of the retina.)

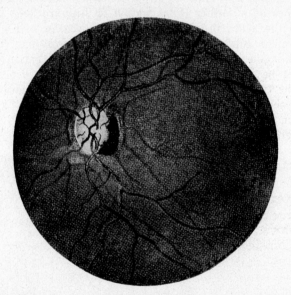

Fig. 72.—Angioid streaks of the retina. (From Clay: Tr. Sect. Ophth., A. M. A., May, 1932.)

In the eyes of some older people who have been suffering with disease, small cystic spaces occur which, on histologic examination, may be found in the entire nuclear layers of the retina. When such a cyst becomes large, it might be observed on ophthalmoscopic examination either in the periphery of the retina or in the neighborhood of the macula. In the latter location, it might occasionally result in the formation of a hole in the macula.

Angioid Streaks are radiating dark red or brownish striations in the retina, in the neighborhood of the disc and encircling the latter. They have the appearance of retinal vessels and resemble the latter, but they lie deeper in the structure of the retina. They are usually present in both eyes and although no definite cause is known, they have been described many times in the literature and have been found in association with a large variety of conditions affecting other parts, as diabetes, Paget's disease, tuberculosis, and inflammatory conditions of the choroid. Pigmentation as an end result of inflammation has often been given as the cause of their occurrence.

Detachment of the Retina.—The retina may become detached in the course of, or as an end result of, almost any of the severe inflammatory, exudative, or degenerative processes affecting the eye. It occurs in cases of intraocular tumor, following traumatism, extensive inflammation, and exudative conditions of the choroid. In some instances it is produced by a loosening and pushing forward of the retina from behind either by fluid or a solid growth. In others it occurs as the result of a pulling from in front, such as may be caused by the contraction of cicatricial tissue or bands, following severe inflammations and also by contraction of the vitreous. In addition to this form of detachment of the retina occurring as a secondary condition, it may also be found as a primary or idiopathic condition, the cause of which cannot be definitely determined. Many cases occur with high myopia and following traumatism. The former is very commonly found to result in late detachment, especially when the patient has a very high degree of myopia, and the eye shows evidences of degenerative changes. Nearly all cases of detachment have been shown to be associated with a tear in the retina. This has been explained in various ways, principally as the result of a pulling effect exerted by the vitreous in its forward retraction.

Traumatic detachment may follow injuries and blows to the head, especially in cases where the eyes are highly myopic or otherwise pathologic. A fall or sudden severe effort or exertion may serve as the cause. The detachment in some cases may not occur for some time after the injury or mishap.

Senile changes and degeneration predispose to detachment. Tumors, exudative conditions of the choroid and severe inflammatory conditions of the outer coats of the eye and of the orbit produce a detachment by continued pressure and force being exerted from behind the retina. A tear in the retina may not be present with detachment following severe inflammations and exudation in the neighboring structures.

A detachment of the retina is not always readily detected and requires a detailed examination with the ophthalmoscope. Very close and repeated observation is also required in many cases to determine the presence or absence of a tear. The pupil should, therefore, be well dilated in order to permit a careful search of the entire periphery of the fundus, where a tear is most likely to be found. A tear may occur in almost any size and in any shape, although they usually appear either irregular or crescentic in shape and outline. They are also occasionally round and their edges rather sharply outlined. Surrounding a tear, the retina appears gray in color in contrast to the adjacent red of the normal fundus. It is also elevated and sometimes appears to lie in folds. On rotation of the eyeball, the detached part of the retina can be observed with the ophthalmoscope to float or lift up and then recede again into its original position. Following detachment, the vitreous is usually infiltrated with numerous floating opacities which can be observed on examination with the ophthalmoscope. Many of these may later disappear leaving the vitreous more clear.

With detachment caused by the presence of an underlying tumor, the retina may be seen as a smooth elevation which can be rather well localized to the area of the growth and definitely separated from the surrounding normal retina. The detachment appears more solid or firm and does not appear to float on movement of the eyeball, as with a serous detachment. The elevation may appear irregular in its surface outline, however, especially when an underlying tumor is irregular or has nodules on its surface. With detachment due to intraocular tumor, the tension is likely to be elevated and on transillumination, the eyeball will fail to transmit light, whereas in serous detachment, the eye can be transilluminated without obstruction.

The earliest subjective symptoms of detachment of the retina are the appearance of streaks and flashes which are complained of by the patient. The light sense in the affected eye may also be complained of early and then floating specks are observed by the patient. If the visual fields are tested at this time, they may reveal the presence of indistinct color areas and spots that are cloudy. With occurrence of the detachment, a positive scotoma will be revealed corresponding to the affected area of the retina.

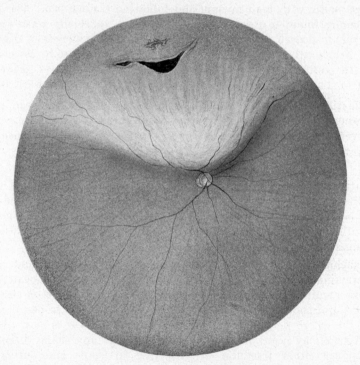

Fig. 73.—Detachment of the retina, showing large crescentic hole. (From de Rötth: Arch. Ophth., November, 1939.)

The prognosis of detachment of the retina depends primarily on the nature and cause of the condition. In any case it should be considered as serious, and the prognosis with regard to reattachment and recovery of vision should be very guarded. The extent of the detachment and length of duration will also influence the prognosis. Extensive and old detachments offer practically no chance for reattachment and recovery. Those which offer the best prognosis are comparatively recent detachments of traumatic origin.

The treatment consists in first confining the patient to bed and keeping him flat on his back. The movement of the eyes is restricted by the use of **goggles**

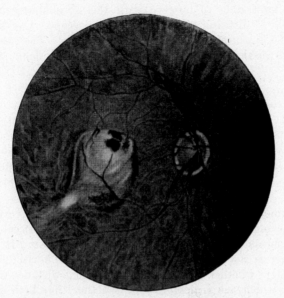

Fig. 75A.—Disciform degeneration of the macula in the right eye. (From Adler: Arch. Ophth., September, 1933.)

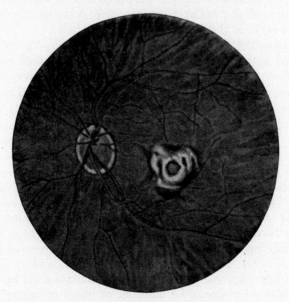

Fig. 75B.—Disciform degeneration of the left eye. (From Adler: Arch. Ophth., September, 1933.)

Cystoid degeneration occurs in the macula as the result of a previous edema. This is almost impossible to observe with the ophthalmoscope but may be examined with the Gullstrand binocular ophthalmoscope. Cystoid degeneration is followed by the appearance of a hole in the macula. The condition has been called retinitis atrophica centralis when it follows an inflammation.

Examination of the Orbit

The eyeballs occupy the orbits, and their positions relative to each other and to the rest of the face are in great part due to the configuration of the skull. Large deep orbits with well-developed superior margins and frontal sinuses are mostly responsible for deep-set eyes. Shallow orbits necessarily locate the eyeballs farther forward, making them prominent. Less frequently, with the same sized orbits, a difference in the size of the eyeballs can vary the degree of prominence.

Facial Symmetry.—Perfect symmetry of the face is rarely found, but only when the asymmetry is so marked as to be readily noticeable upon inspection, has it any special bearing on the ophthalmic diagnosis. It is important to determine whether or not the eyes are on the same line horizontally, and if not, which one is higher; whether or not they are the same distance from the median line, and if not, which one is nearer; also, whether they both project forward to the same extent or whether one is proptosed farther forward than the other. The presence of asymmetric position of the eyeballs should not be mistaken for squint, which is a deviation of the visual axes. When one side of the face is underdeveloped, it lacks the fullness or roundness of the opposite side. The frontal eminence and the malar bone, the two principal landmarks, are less prominent. The orbit is, therefore, smaller, the eyeball lower, nearer the median line, and in a plane posterior to that of the fellow eye. The better side of the face is considered normal, and if by alternate screening, each side of the face is inspected, the more fully developed will be seen to be the stronger.

Hyperostosis, periostosis, acromegaly, and tumor may all cause an enlargement of one side of the face, with great asymmetry.

Abnormalities of the Orbit

Fracture.—Almost any portion of the orbit may suffer a fracture as the result of direct injury. The outer wall is probably the strongest and best protected, so that it is the least affected by fracture. Deep fracture of the orbit is accompanied by hemorrhage and sudden appearance of exophthalmos. The vision might be suddenly impaired following injury in these cases, and the optic nerve may be injured with the occurrence of hemorrhage into the sheath. The condition may be similar to that produced by fracture of the base of the skull, but in the latter, exophthalmos will be absent, and involvement of the conjunctiva and lids may not occur until some time after the injury. An x-ray examination of the orbit should be made in all cases of injury in this region.

Inflammation.—When any of the bones of the orbit are affected by an inflammation, the condition is known as a periostitis. This occurs more frequently at the margins of the orbit and is characterized by a thickening or swelling of the bone, accompanied by edema and swelling of the lids and the conjunctiva. There may be some pain and tenderness to touch. When the inflammation occurs in the deeper parts of the orbit, its presence may not be recognized until later when abscess formation takes place.   A periosteal abscess may occur at the orbital margin with proptosis caused by swelling of the tissues behind the eyeball. The rotations of the eyeball are restricted, and paralysis of movement may occur.   With involvement of the optic nerve the vision is also impaired.   It is accompanied by pain, headache, and sometimes severe systemic and cerebral symptoms.   When abscess formation occurs, the lids may become involved, and rupture occurs through the skin of the lids.   This is followed by gradual healing. The infection may, however, spread to the cranial cavity and result in brain abscess or meningitis.   In other cases the condition may gradually subside with absorption of the inflammatory material and a return to normal.

Orbital cellulitis may result from injury, inflammation, or infection in adjacent structures, such as the nasal sinuses, from dental infections when the alveolar process of the superior maxilla is involved, and also from infections in the petrous bones, the pharynx, and parotid glands.   It may also occur in some of the infectious diseases, such as erysipelas, influenza, scarlet fever, meningitis, and smallpox.

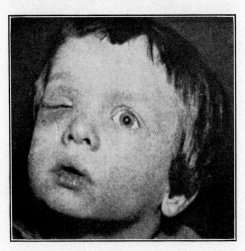

Fig. 76.—Periostitis of lower rim and wall of the orbit due to trauma. (From Gamble: Arch. Ophth., October, 1933.)

Edema.—Obstruction to the circulation in the orbit may result in an edema with accompanying proptosis and exophthalmos.   The skin of the lids may become edematous, and the bulbar and palpebral conjunctiva may be intensely chemotic and red from venous distention.

Emphysema.—Emphysema develops in the orbit and lids as the result of trauma and fracture.   Air enters the anterior part of the orbit and can be felt through the lids.

Exophthalmos.—Unusual protrusion of the eyeball from the orbit is recognized as exophthalmos.   A small degree of protrusion which is limited to one eye may be difficult to diagnose and should be studied with reference to the position of the other eye.   It might be present in any degree up to a complete prolapse of the eyeball in front of the lids.   In such marked cases, it may interfere with complete closure of the eyelids. The direction of the protrusion depends usually on the cause and may be straight forward or forward and to one side. The degree of exophthalmos can be measured by means of an exophthalmometer. This consists of a light metal frame which can be placed against the outer angle of each orbit. The frame has a miror on either side which reflects the image of each eyeball. Below the mirror is a scale which indicates the distance in millimeters. That point on the scale which corresponds to the position of the anterior cornea in the mirror, denotes the amount of proptosis of the eyeball from the anterior plane of the orbit. A comparison also is made in the reading obtained for both eyes.

Exophthalmos may occur in a variety of conditions which include principally: exophthalmic goiter, thickening of the bones of the orbit, tumors of the orbits, distention of the orbital blood vessels, and inflammation of the orbital structures already described.

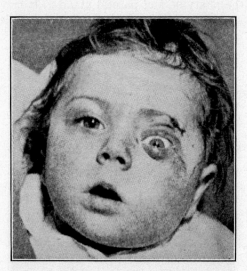

Fig. 77.—Discharging fistula in upper lid; loose piece of bone felt with probe. (From Gamble: Arch. Ophth., October, 1933.)

When present in marked degree, exophthalmos may result in serious complications. The eyelids are first widely separated and much of the eyeball is exposed. It becomes increasingly more difficult to close the eyelids completely, with the result that a portion of the cornea may be constantly exposed. This leads to a drying of the exposed portion and eventually to keratitis, which may progress to ulceration and loss of the eye. The position of the eyeball becomes fixed in marked cases, and movement is restricted. Diplopia may occur when one eye is displaced to the side.

The treatment of exophthalmos depends principally on the etiologic factor and its removal wherever possible. Locally, the treatment consists in protection of the cornea and the attempt to prevent ulceration. The palpebral fissure should be closed by holding the lids together with adhesive tape properly applied or by a bandage. This should always be done in marked cases when the patient prepares for sleep. In other instances, it is well to instill a few drops of albolene to protect the cornea or to keep the cornea moist by applying a watch glass or shield over the eye containing a small piece of wet cotton. When these measures fail, it might be necessary to resort to some form of surgery, such as tarsorrhaphy, in order to facilitate the narrowing of the fissure and more closely approximate the edges of the lids in closing.

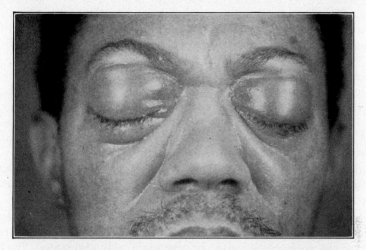

Fig. 78.—Bilateral exophthalmos. (Clinic of Dr. L. Lehrfeld, Wills Hospital.)

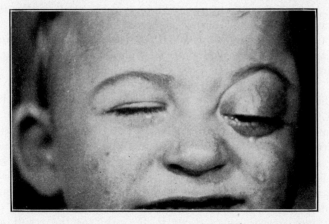

Fig. 79.—Exophthalmos and displacement of left eye in a child with orbital tumor. (From the clinic of Dr. Frank Parker, Wills Hospital.)

Tenonitis.—An inflammation of the eyeball which involves Tenon's capsule will result in a tenonitis. This is characterized by pain and tenderness, together with a fair amount of edema of Tenon's capsule which results in chemosis of the bulbar conjunctiva and a moderate protrusion of the affected eyeball. This may occur with traumatic iridocyclitis after injury and in such diseases as rheumatism, gout, influenza, and sometimes after brief exposure to severe cold.

The treatment of tenonitis includes the treatment of the causative agent or disease. Locally, the use of astringents such as zinc sulfate, adrenalin, and warm or cold compresses, as indicated in the individual case, can be employed. Active diaphoresis will also favor reduction in the amount of edema.

Enophthalmos.—When the eyeball is found to be recessed into the orbit, the condition is known as enophthalmos. This is the opposite to exophthalmos and is due to a decrease or loss of orbital tissue, such as fat and water. It may also occur after injury, such as fracture of the orbit, or as the result of paralysis of the sympathetic. Sometimes enophthalmos is only apparent rather than actual, the condition being simulated by the presence of other abnormalities, such as ptosis, and spasm of certain of the extraocular muscles occurring after operations.

Tumors.—Most of the tumors occurring in the orbit will produce exophthalmos, and the latter must be differentiated from that which is caused by inflammation. This is usually done without much difficulty, since exopthalmos resulting from tumor growths is very gradual in its onset and progression. Occasionally, however, a tumor growth in the orbit might be simulated in such diseases as syphilis and tuberculosis.

The direction of the displacement and the motility of the eye may often indicate the location of the tumor. Wherever possible, the tumor growth should be palpated in order to determine the size, motility, and form.

The tumors occurring in the orbit may be of various kinds. Dermoid cysts, in most instances, are congenital, although they may increase in size after birth. Vascular tumors, such as are caused by aneurysm, may also occur. The latter are often produced by rupture of the carotid artery into the cavernous sinus, occurring after injury, such as fracture of the base of the skull. Other tumors of the orbit are osteomas, which arise from the bones forming the wall of the orbit, the most common being the frontal bone. Others may arise from the sinuses adjoining the orbit, such as the antrum of frontal sinus. Osteomas are very hard and progress slowly in size. In time, they displace the eyeball and may compress the optic nerve. They are difficult to remove by operation, and it is often necessary to remove the eyeball, especially when the vision has been greatly impaired and considerable displacement has taken place.

Malignant tumors also occur primarily in the orbit. Orbital sarcomas may arise from the bone and periosteum, and also from the optic nerve. These are usually rather soft and well circumscribed, being enveloped in connective tissue. Sometimes sarcoma and glioma perforate into the posterior orbit. Carcinoma may arise from the lacrimal gland and enter the orbit, but the tumor rarely occurs as a primary growth in the orbit.

Other tumor growths may occur in the orbit as the result of metastasis and in the course of diseases characterized by changes in the blood, such as leucemia. Lymphosarcomas, leucemic growths, and chloromas may occur, especially in younger patients who suffer with alterations in the number of erythrocytes, leucocytes, and myelocytes (Fuchs).

The diagnosis of tumors of the orbit can often be aided by x-ray examination.

References

1. Theobald, Georgiana Dvorak: Frequency of Sympathetic Ophthalmia, Tr. Am. Acad. Ophth., October, 1929.
2. Samuels, Bernard: Opacities of the Vitreous, Arch. Ophth. 4: 838, December, 1930.
3. O'Brien, C. S.: Detachment of the Choroid After Cataract Extraction, Arch. Ophth. 14: 527, October, 1935.

4. Clay, Grady E., and Baird, J. Mason: An Unclassified Type of Optic Neuritis, Arch. Ophth. 18: 777, November, 1937.
5. Benedict, William L.: Brain Abscess, Tr. Am. Acad. Ophth., 1929.
6. Watkins, Charles H., Wagener, Henry P., and Brown, Robert W.: Cerebral Symptoms Accompanied by Choked Optic Discs in Types of Blood Dyscrasia, Am. J. Ophth. 24: 1374, 1941.
7. Leinfelder, P. J., and Paul, W. D.: Papilledema in General Diseases, Arch. Ophth. 28: 983, 1942.
8. Carroll, Frank D.: Retrobulbar Neuritis, Arch. Ophth., Verhoeff Number 24: 44, July, 1940.
9. Benedict, William L.: Multiple Sclerosis as an Etiologic Factor in Retrobulbar Neuritis, Arch. Ophth. 28: 988, 1942.

CHAPTER VI

CONGENITAL AND HEREDITARY EYE MANIFESTATIONS

CONGENITAL ANOMALIES AND MALFORMATIONS OF DEVELOPMENT

Hereditary and Heredofamilial Diseases

The congenital and hereditary conditions affecting the eyes include those which occur in the various ocular structures as anomalies and malformations in anatomic development, and those conditions which result from certain defects or imperfections in the individual (stigma) which are transmitted from either one of the parents or through the parents from members of former generations of the same family.

As examples of the first group we have such conditions as microphthalmos, anophthalmos, lenticonus, colobomas of the various structures, aniridia (absence of the iris), and others. In the second group are those conditions which manifest themselves principally as degenerations in the ocular tissues and are discovered immediately after birth or some time later. They can be exemplified by the abiotrophies or tapetoretinal degenerations such as retinitis pigmentosa, amaurotic familial idiocy (Tay-Sachs' disease), hereditary optic nerve disease, hereditary macular degeneration, congenital familial cataracts, albinism, and other similar conditions which usually occur in more than one member of a family and in successive generations of the same family.

The Lacrimal Apparatus

Congenital Absence of the Puncta and Canaliculi.—The puncta and canaliculi may be either entirely absent or imperforate at birth. This condition is accompanied by constant lacrimation of the eyes from the time of birth. It is the characteristic sign and should attract attention to the lacrimal apparatus in general and the puncta in particular.

When it is determined that the puncta are absent, an attempt should be made to learn whether or not the lacrimal sac is present. It is possible that the puncta are simply covered by a membrane, which when opened will lead into a canaliculus and sac. Other cases occur occasionally, however, in which the canaliculus as well as the punctum is absent. An attempt can be made by surgical means in such instances to provide a canaliculus which will communicate with the lacrimal canal in the nose.

The author had a case in a boy 6 years of age who suffered with epiphora and lacrimation in both eyes since birth. Examination revealed the papilla to be present but the puncta were all imperforate. These were successfully opened and found to lead into the canaliculus. The condition was subsequently improved.

Goar[1] described a case in a young woman 22 years of age in whom the papilla and puncta of the upper and lower lids of the left eye were entirely absent. This case was operated on with complete success. Goar, in his report, also reviewed the literature on this condition and found twenty-two cases reported of congenital absence of canaliculi.

Supernumerary Puncta and Canaliculi.—A congenital anomaly in which more than one punctum or canaliculus is present at the same site. Charamis[2] reported two such cases. In one, the patient had a second punctum in the lower lids which was situated about 1.5 mm. outside the first. This was explained on an embryologic basis. In the second case there were two openings into the cul-de-sac on each side.

Fistula of the Lacrimal Gland.—This condition is rarely encountered in ordinary practice, but such cases have been reported occasionally. It is characterized by the presence of a small opening in the eyelid somewhat removed from the punctum. On passing a probe, it will be found to communicate with the lacrimal gland. They conduct tears when the secretion is stimulated and they may become infected.

The treatment consists (Schornstein[3]) in an attempt at surgical excision of the fistulous tract.

Cyst of the Lacrimal Sac.—Congenital cysts of the lacrimal sac may occur either alone or in association with other abnormalities. The cysts can be readily recognized by their appearance and by palpation. They may vary in size from that of a pea to a marble and are located in proximity to the lacrimal sac.

Silverman[4] described a rare case occurring in a female twin who presented a microphthalmic right eye with a coloboma of the iris, and a cystic structure in the position of the lacrimal sac of the left eye.

Congenital Stenosis of the Lacrimal Sac.—The lacrimal sac and duct are often the seat of a congenital stenosis, in which case an infant or young child suffers with almost constant lacrimation of varying degrees on the affected side. The condition is usually noted by the mother of the child as early as the first week after birth. It is characterized by a "watering" of the eye due to a failure of the tears to drain through the lacrimal sac which is obstructed. The watery discharge may later become mucopurulent, and in cases of longer duration it becomes purulent. The condition can be readily diagnosed by the history, dating the condition back to a very short time after birth and by expression of the secretion or pus from the affected punctum, by gentle pressure or massage at the inner angle of the eye.

The treatment of this condition should be carried out early. This consists of careful dilation of the affected punctum with a very sharply pointed dilator. The point is introduced into the punctum and the dilator is then held parallel to the lid which is held taut and gently maneuvered through the canaliculus to the nose. It is then turned vertically and carried down into the sac relieving any obstruction present. This procedure should be carried out, however, only by an ophthalmologist who has a knowledge of the anatomy of the area and who has the ability to introduce the dilator properly. This will, in most cases, entirely correct the condition, and it can be performed as early as the age of one month. In these cases, there is a great tendency to delay in the hope that the condition will clear up spontaneously or with local medication. On the contrary, however, the lacrimal sac usually becomes infected and the child usually comes to attention at a later age (7 or 8 months) when the condition is more difficult to relieve, and it might be necessary to employ more radical dilatation in order to remove the obstruction and to clear up the infection now present.

The Eyelids

Several congenital anomalies of the eyelids of rather infrequent occurrence include: ablepharon, in which there is a partial or total absence of eyelids, either single or bilateral; ankyloblepharon, in which there is a union of the eyelids which, in most cases, is partial. There is usually an opening between the lids, especially at the inner canthus. Epiblepharon is another anomaly in which a fold of the lower lid covers the margins and cilia on looking downward. Cryptophthalmia is characterized by a continuity of skin with the eyeball and usually occurs with anophthalmos or microphthalmos. It is very rare.

Epicanthus.—This is a deformity in which broad folds of skin occur at the inner canthus and curve down over the bridge of the nose, giving the lid a slanting appearance. It may be associated with ptosis and is present in nearly all mongolians. They usually conceal the inner sclera, caruncle, and the puncta.

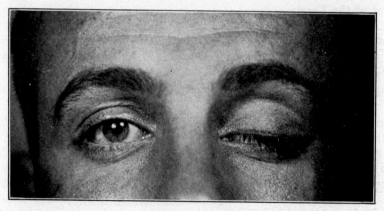

Fig. 80.—Congenital ptosis, later corrected by operation. (I. S. Tassman, Wills Hospital.)

Congenital Ptosis.—This condition occurs principally as the result of a poorly developed levator muscle. It may be either bilateral or unilateral and may occur either alone or in association with other anomalies of the eyes. It is not uncommon to find an associated paralysis of one or more of the extraocular muscles, frequently the superior rectus or one of the obliques.

Congenital bilateral ptosis may occur with complete ophthalmoplegia. A case was described by deSchweinitz[5] which was associated with complete bilateral congenital exterior ophthalmoplegia in a woman aged 44 years. In a review of the subject he cited a number of other similar cases in the literature and stated that nystagmus also is not uncommon in these cases.

The treatment of congenital ptosis consists of correction of the condition by surgical means. Good results can be obtained with operations for shortening and advancement of the levator muscle, or employing the superior rectus muscle if normal, by attaching the lid to its tendon. In other instances a procedure has been used to substitute the action of the occipitofrontalis muscle for that of the levator.

Jaw Winking.—This is a condition first described by Marcus Gunn in 1883, which is characterized by the presence of a unilateral ptosis, with ability of the patient to raise the affected eyelid only when the mouth is opened or when the lower jaw is moved in a lateral direction. It is described by Fuchs as an abnormal association of movements of the lids which have been ascribed to peculiarities in nerve communication. A number of cases have been reported occurring in infants and young children. According to Foster Moore, the lid is raised on opening the mouth, and when the jaw is moved to the side, the external pterygoid produces a further upward movement.

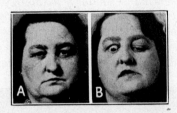

Fig. 81.—The jaw winking phenomenon (Marcus Gunn). *A*, The condition at rest. *B*, On movement of the jaw to the left. (From Cooper: Arch. Ophth., August, 1937.)

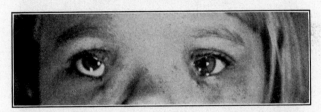

Fig. 82.—Coloboma of eyelid. (Courtesy of Dr. E. B. Spaeth.)

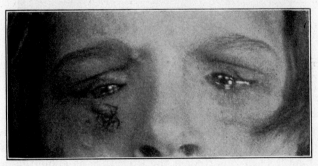

Fig. 83.—Coloboma of eyelid after surgical correction; sutures are still seen. (Courtesy of Dr. E. B. Spaeth.)

Congenital Coloboma.—Congenital coloboma of the eyelids is a rare condition. It may occur, however, either alone or in association with other conditions. Horner and Cordes[6] recorded a case of congenital coloboma of the upper eyelid associated with dermoid cysts of the cornea and an aberrant lacrimal gland, which was determined by laboratory diagnosis.

Congenital coloboma of the eyelid may also occur in association with other congenital anomalies, such as epicanthus, coloboma of the iris and other structures, and also with such defects as harelip and cleft palate.

The defect is plainly visible in the eyelid in which a portion of the structure is absent. It occurs as the result of aberrations associated with the closure of the fetal cleft and is characterized by the presence of a notch in that portion of the lid which is missing. The upper lid is nearly always affected. Coloboma of the eyelids sometimes occurs in more than one member of the family.

Congenital colobomas of the lower lid in three children of one family was reported by Spaeth.[7] Each of the three children had in addition, varying degrees of congenital defects of the lacrimal puncti, canaliculi, sacs and lacrimal-nasal ducts with complicating secondary pathology. They were otherwise normal. The parents of the children were normal and without any known congenital defects themselves. The unusual occurrence of this condition in three children of one family suggested an hereditary character. Surgery performed in all three resulted in an excellent correction of the condition.

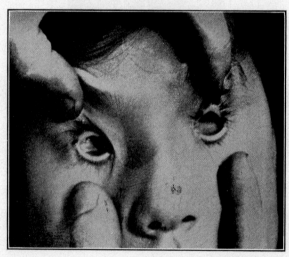

Fig. 84.—Patient with congenital anophthalmos. (From Rosenbaum: Arch. Ophth., June, 1931.)

The Eyeball

Anophthalmos and Microphthalmos.—These two congenital conditions are named together because it is generally agreed that most of them, on close pathologic examination, are found to be cases of microphthalmos, although a large number have been reported in the literature as anophthalmos. The latter condition constitutes a congenital absence of the entire eyeball, but nearly always some form of a rudimentary eye is found to be present, so that these cases are more properly designated as microphthalmos. The author has a case of microphthalmos under observation at the present time in a 5-year-old girl. The orbit on the left side is somewhat smaller than its fellow and the palpebral fissure is narrower and smaller than normal. A small rudimentary eye can be palpated in the posterior part of the orbit. In these cases the lids and palpebral fissure on the affected side are usually underdeveloped because of the absence of a normal-sized eye. This condition may also be associated with other congenital anomalies occurring in the orbit and the lacrimal apparatus. In cases of unilateral anophthalmos, the opposite eye may also show evidences of congenital anomalies, such as microphthalmos, nystagmus and coloboma of any of the ocular structures.

The treatment depends on the nature of the condition presents. In order to avoid an underdevelopment of the parts in later life, it is advisable where possible in cases of this kind, to employ some early means for promoting the normal development. In some cases this can be done when the child is young, by surgical enlargement and widening of the palpebral fissure after removal of a rudimentary eye. A gold ball of proper size can be inserted under the conjunctival lining of the orbit which would serve to replace the eyeball. The gold ball can be replaced with one of larger size from time to time as required by the growth of the child. As soon as the child is old enough, the socket should be fitted with a prosthesis.

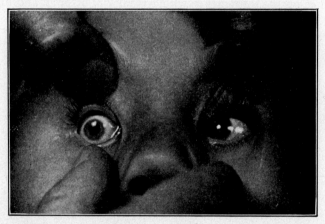

Fig. 85.—Microphthalmos. Right eye of a 4-year-old child. (From the clinic of Dr. J. M. Griscom, Wills Hospital.)

Buphthalmos (Hydrophthalmos).—A fairly common congenital condition, which is characterized by an abnormally large cornea in the eyes of infants or very young children. It usually occurs as part of a general increase of the size of the eyeball (hydrophthalmos). Because of the increased intraocular tension which is present in this condition, it is sometimes known as infantile glaucoma. The increase in intraocular tension leads to a general enlargement of the eye because it produces a stretching of the sclera. The characteristic sign in buphthalmos is the presence of fine, faint, crossed striae in the posterior cornea which are caused by spontaneous ruptures in Descemet's membrane. These striae can be observed with oblique illumination or on examination with the slit lamp. The edges of the rupture will appear as a very small pair of parallel lines. This form of infantile glaucoma is differentiated from megalocornea and megalophthalmos by the increased intraocular tension which is absent in the two latter conditions. In these, an overdevelopment takes place with an exceptionally large cornea and eyeball. The ruptures affecting Descemet's membrane in buphthalmos are absent in megalocornea and megalophthalmos.

Buphthalmos is usually unaccompanied by pain. The principal signs and symptoms are the decrease in vision, increased intraocular tension, enlargement of the cornea and enlargement of the eyeball. It affects either one or both eyes and may occur either alone or in association with other abnormalities of the eye, such as coloboma of the lids, lens, or iris, or an absence of the entire iris (aniridia). Cases have been reported as occurring in more than one member of the same family. The condition apparently has some hereditary origin and usually results in almost complete blindness. In some cases it has been spontaneously arrested, but usually the eyeball becomes very large in size.

The treatment consists principally in surgical procedures, such as trephining, intended to lower the intraocular tension and limit the progress of the condition. The prognosis for improvement of vision, however, is poor. In some cases the increase in the tension and the growth of the cornea and eyeball can be checked by the operation, but the high intraocular tension usually causes pressure on the optic nerve which results in atrophy and loss of vision.

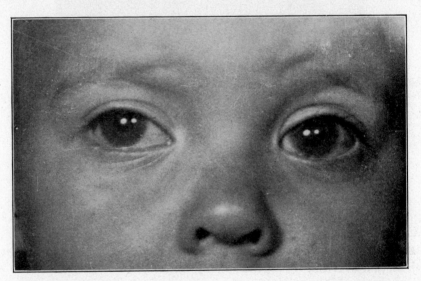

Fig. 86.—Hydrophthalmos (buphthalmos). (I. S. Tassman, Wills Hospital.)

Megalophthalmos.—Enlargement of the eyeball is called megalophthalmos. Because the enlargement is confined mostly to the anterior part of the eye, it is sometimes designated as "anterior megalophthalmos." It is characterized especially by an enlargement of the circumference of the cornea, deep anterior chamber, and atrophy of the iris. The condition is of hereditary origin and is restricted almost entirely to males. It is nearly always bilateral. Vail[8] found cataracts of various types to be commonly associated, but no evidences of glaucoma except as a complication arising later. The condition closely resembles buphthalmos, but the latter condition is often unilateral and occurs equally in both sexes.

Keratoconus (Conical Cornea).—This is a fairly common condition sometimes called conical cornea because it is characterized by an excessive anterior curvature or forward bulging of the cornea. It is congenital in nature and is recognized usually early in life when the patient complains of a marked impairment of vision. The condition is ordinarily bilateral and can be recognized with oblique illumination when the examiner stands to the side of the patient. The cornea will then be seen to taper forward almost into the shape of a cone instead of presenting the normal regular and uniform anterior curve. In marked cases, the apex of the cornea is drawn out almost to a point which

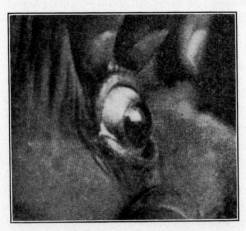

Fig. 87.—Megalophthalmos. (From Vail: Tr. Sect. Ophth., A. M. A., June, 1931.)

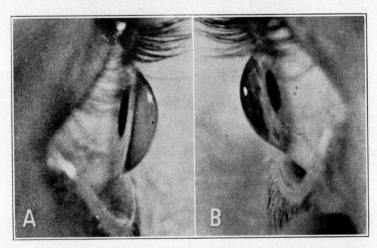

Fig. 88.—*A*, Sideview of right eye of patient showing thickened cornea two years after acute hydrops. *B*, Keratoconus in the left eye. (From Rychener and Kirby: Arch. Ophth., August, 1940.)

causes an opacity that can be observed on examination with the ophthalmoscope. A marked stretching and thinning out of the cornea itself takes place and leads to a rupture of Descemet's membrane similar to that which occurs in buphthalmos (Fuchs). The abnormal curvature of the cornea also causes a very high degree of astigmatism which is usually myopic, and as a result, the vision in such an eye is greatly reduced and limited. The cause of the condition is not known, but it has been found to occur more commonly in women than in men. Some basic impairment probably exists in the eyes of these individuals which leads to the abnormal curvature. It has been attributed at times to disturbances of the endocrine glands. Cases have been known to occur in different members of the same family. In one family reported by Abelsdorff[9] a mother and daughter had keratoconus of both eyes. In another instance, a patient with keratoconus had two cousins who were affected with the same condition. Another patient had an uncle with two daughters, all of whom had keratoconus. It is of interest to note that Abelsdorff's patients all lived in a city located at a very high altitude, where keratoconus was very common.

The treatment of keratoconus consists principally in attempting to improve the vision in the affected eye and also limiting the tendency toward further increase in the conicity of the cornea. The former can be accomplished in some mild cases by careful refraction and prescribing a lens, usually a cylinder of high power. This may improve the vision only to a limited degree, however, especially in the more severe cases.

The latter have been found to show a marked and satisfactory improvement in vision when fitted with a contact lens. As a matter of fact, the most satisfactory results from the use of contact lenses have been obtained in these cases. Moreover, the use of a contact lens properly fitted may have the additional benefit of checking the further bulging of the cornea. The principal effect of the contact lens is to provide a new corneal curvature or refracting surface and thereby eliminate all of the corneal astigmatism. The author has prescribed a large number of contact lenses in these cases with uniformly good results. In many instances the vision in the affected eye can be improved to nearly normal. These patients become tolerant to the use of the lens and learn to wear it for a number of hours without inconvenience.

Another method of treating cases of high degree with opacity at the apex of the cornea is by keratoplasty (Castroviehjo). This consists in surgical removal of the anterior conical portion of the affected cornea, and transplanting a section with normal curvature from a donor eye. It has been performed in some cases with a satisfactory degree of success.

Dermoids of the Cornea.—Dermoids may occur on the cornea as well as on other structures of the eye. They vary in size and may appear as a single mass or in association with other malformations of the eyeball. They can be excised and the diagnosis confirmed by laboratory examination.

Congenital Ichthyosis (Keratodermia).—Ichthyosis is a rare congenital disease of the skin, characterized by a rough, dry, scaly condition which is usually present at the time of birth or may appear early in life. The cause is unknown, but it is considered to result from a congenital impairment of nutrition of the epidermis and the fatty layers of the skin. The possibility of a glandular origin was also suggested when changes were found in the thyroid and adrenal glands.[10] The skin of the face, scalp, and extremities may be affected in generalized ichthyosis.

Eye manifestations in these cases are rare. Ichthyosis involving the skin of the face may, however, in some instances extend to the skin of the lids. The cilia are covered at their roots with whitish scales which adhere closely and prevent growth of the lashes. Severe cases of face and lid involvement may result in ectropion.

In ordinary cases the process involves the conjunctiva and cornea. The conjunctiva of the lids and the palpebral conjunctiva are red and swollen. The bulbar conjunctiva may be thick and infiltrated with granules.

Two types of corneal manifestation have been described. In the one, only the corneal cells are involved in association with generalized ichthyosis. In the second, the corneal nerves alone are involved without generalized ichthyosis. The latter is designated as familial corneal disease.

Cordes and Hogan[11] reported a case of bilateral involvement of the conjunctiva and also the right cornea, in association with generalized ichthyosis. The conjunctiva was red, thickened, and showed no papillary or follicular formation. The right cornea was infiltrated from the lower limbus to the center and showed pannus formation. These changes were considered to be secondary to the conjunctival lesions. They described several forms of ocular involvement in cases of ichthyosis of the skin as follows:

''(a) There may be asymptomatic involvement of the cornea in the nature of a dystrophy of the corneal cells and nerves. This form is seen only with the slit lamp or other means of magnification.

''(b) There may be an inflammatory form, showing smooth or papillary hyperplasia of the conjunctiva, with involvement of the cornea due to mechanical irritation, which causes secondary changes.

''(c) The cornea may be involved primarily by a keratosis in which the scales correspond to the scales present in the dermatologic lesions.''

A case of congenital ichthyosis which presented multiple corneal nodules, in a 9-year-old boy with marked photophobia, was reported by Vail.[12] Specimens from the cornea in this case, when examined microscopically, were found to resemble closely those seen in Salzmann's corneal dystrophy. The similarity between this condition and corneal dystrophy was also noted in other cases.

Treatment: Vail's case received chiefly large doses of vitamins A and D, which produced marked relief from the photophobia and improvement in the vision. No specific treatment of any kind is available. A mild eyewash should be employed locally, and any other symptomatic measures which might be found necessary.

Congenital Syphilis.—The important eye manifestation of congenital syphilis is interstitial keratitis. This condition may seriously involve the cornea with marked impairment of vision or even total loss of sight. It affects chiefly children and young people who exhibit no other manifestations of active syphilis. This condition will be described in more detail in the chapter on syphilis.

The Ocular Muscles

The ocular muscles may present a variety of congenital anomalies, especially in connection with their origin and insertion, structure and function. The latter would, as a matter of course, be altered by the two former, but the impairment of function of the extraocular muscles may also be of nuclear origin. Injuries at the time of birth may also be responsible for paralysis of the extraocular muscles occurring in infants. One of the most common forms of congenital paralysis is that affecting the superior rectus muscle which in some cases is accompanied by congenital ptosis. Congenital paresis of the inferior rectus muscle is also common, but the external rectus muscle seems to be affected just as frequently as the vertical muscles. Head tilting is not uncommon in children who are affected with a congenital paralysis of an extraocular muscle. When present, it may be so pronounced that it may resemble a torticollis.

Hereditary Ophthalmoplegia Externa.—This is a hereditary condition which usually occurs early in life and which is characterized by a slow but progressive paralysis of each of the external ocular muscles in turn (Treacher Collins). The levator palpebrae superioris may also be affected. A number of cases have been described by Wilbrand and Saenger. The origin of the condition is supposed to be nuclear, and it has also been classed as a slow degeneration or abiotrophy. The internal ocular muscles are never involved.

Complete bilateral congenital external ophthalmoplegia and double ptosis may occur, but the condition is rare (deSchweinitz). A number of cases with "minimal excursions" have been described with accompanying manifestations, such as rotary, horizontal, and irregular nystagmus. The pathology is said to be concerned with imperfect development or defects of the nuclei of nerve supply of the external ocular muscles. In a number of instances, the muscles, when examined, have been found to be atrophied and very few fibers were found.

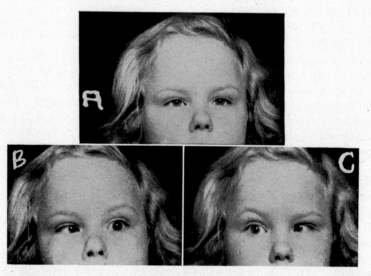

Fig. 89.—Bilateral congenital deficiency of abduction with retraction. *A*, Position of eyes in primary position looking straight ahead. *B*, Left eye fails to rotate externally in rotation to the left. Right eye is the fixing eye and shows retraction and narrowing of the palpebral fissure in adduction. *C*, Right eye limited in rotation to the right. Left eye is the fixing eye with retraction and narrowing of fissure in adduction. (From Mengel: Arch. Ophth., June, 1935.)

Congenital Paralysis of the External Rectus (Abducens or Sixth Nerve Palsy).—The external rotation of one or of both eyes may be either partly or completely restricted because of a palsy of the affected external rectus muscle. Although this is considered to be a rare congenital anomaly, a number of cases have been reported in the literature. The condition is, in most instances, bilateral when it is not due to an injury. It may also be associated with other anomalies. A case of congenital bilateral palsy of the abducens with internal strabismus was found to be associated with so-called "status thymicolymphaticus'' (Phillips, Dirion, and Graves[13]). At autopsy, there was a complete absence of both abducens nerves with diminutive sixth nerve nuclei and the presence of a marked thymic hyperplasia, the thymus weighing 36 Gm.

In this particular case an attempt was made without knowledge of the underlying condition to correct the convergent strabismus present by operative procedure and employing gas-ether anesthesia. The 5-year-old patient failed to recover from the anesthesia of the operation. The authors emphasized the possibility of thymus enlargement being present in these cases, and, as a result of their experience, pointed out the need for a careful investigation of the thymus.

Paralysis of the abducens nerve may also occur as a hereditary condition of the familial type. A case of this kind was described by Laughlin,[14] in which the mother revealed a typical Duane syndrome and five members in three generations of the same family were also afflicted. The condition was found to be present mostly in females, and the left eye was the one most commonly affected.

Congenital paralysis of the lateral rotator muscles of the eyes in association with paralysis of the muscles of the face may occur as a result of pathology, possibly congenital hypoplasia of the brain stem (Möbius' syndrome).

This would result in complete paralysis of abduction and adduction or paralysis of abduction with paresis of adduction when the two medial recti are only partially involved. Both facial muscles are also paralyzed or paretic to some degree. This condition may occur in association with other congenital anomalies and is due either to trauma at birth or to absence of innervation of the lateral recti muscles. Although the location and extent of the lesion are not definitely known, they probably vary somewhat in different cases. Theories to explain the nature of the disease stress principally congenital aplasia of the brain stem. Hicks,[15] in reporting four cases of Möbius' syndrome of different degrees, refers to Möbius' theory of intrauterine nuclear disease, Kann's theory of congenital aplasia of part of the brain stem and Hübner's theory of hypoplasia of the brain stem. He, himself, concludes after a study of these cases that the anomaly is due to an unknown pathologic process involving the brain stem. This condition is also considered by some to be hereditary and familial.

The Retraction Syndrome (Duane's Syndrome).—A congenital impairment of external rotation. It is due to paralysis, usually partial, of the external recti and paresis of the internal recti muscles. The condition was first described by Duane in 1905. Mengel,[16] who reported a case in a 5-year-old girl, described the following characteristics: (1) Deficiency of abduction. (2) Partial deficiency of adduction. (3) Retraction of the globe when the eye is adducted. (4) Oblique movement when adduction is attempted. (5) Narrowing of the palpebral fissure during adduction, and (6) deficiency of convergence. The clinical picture may vary in different cases, some features being more constant and more marked than others. Deficiency of abduction is said to be the most constant finding. This is accounted for by the replacement of the external rectus muscle by fibrous cords. These cordlike muscles contain more muscle fibers in some cases than in others, and sometimes the internal rectus muscle is abnormally inserted. Facial paralysis may be an accompanying feature which is due to involvement of the seventh nerve. This will indicate a lesion of the nuclei as the causative factor. The condition may be either unilateral or bilateral. Zentmayer[17] described three of these cases occurring in three generations of the same family, i.e., the child, the mother, and the maternal grandmother.

Operative treatment for these cases has been attempted, but in most instances, it has proved unsuccessful.

The Sclera

Blue Sclera.—This is a rare condition which occurs in infants and young children of either sex. In the eye it is characterized by the presence of a blue-colored sclera which is also very thin. It may affect several members of a family and different generations of the family. The blue color of the sclera is said to be caused by the color of the ciliary body which is visible through the thin sclera. The bones of the patient are very fragile and easily fractured. Multiple fractures of the long bones, which may occur without trauma, are common in these cases. Partial deafness is another important feature of the condition and is usually noted at the age of about 20 years. This symptom was first described as occurring in association with the other symptoms of the condition in 1918 by van der Hoeve, and since that time, it is sometimes called van der Hoeve's syndrome.

The syndrome is hereditary and familial. The patient usually presents a small body, a large head with little hair, scoliosis or kyphosis, and poor teeth. Sometimes exophthalmos is present. Roentgenogram of the skeleton usually reveals slender bones, generalized osteoporosis and deformities resulting from multiple fractures. The conjunctiva may be pale, and occasionally, other ocular defects in the choroid and lens may also be present. The condition may also occur in association with buphthalmos, syndactylism, and congenital heart disease.

Dessoff,[18] who published a comprehensive review of the subject of blue sclerotics, stated that 60 per cent of the adults with this condition suffer with deafness. This was said to be generally due to otosclerosis, sometimes complicated by labyrinthine disease and nerve deafness.

Fragility of the bones with multiple fractures is also said to occur in 60 per cent of the cases. These usually occur in early childhood and become less frequent after puberty. They usually heal rapidly and are not accompanied by much pain.

A number of theories has been advanced for the cause of the condition, but the exact etiology is unknown. A prominent cause has been described as a supposed disturbance of calcium and phosphorus metabolism due to defective function of the thyroid, parathyroids and adrenal glands. According to Rados and Rosenberg,[19] however, the variations in the values for calcium, phosphorus, and phosphates are not sufficient, in the ordinary case of blue sclera, to warrant a supposed endocrine disturbance. They pointed out that blue sclera was associated with proved parathyroid disorders in only a few rare instances, and they believed that the hyperparathyroidism had been superimposed on a pre-existing congenital anomaly.

No special form of treatment has any particular effect on the condition. Ultraviolet irradiation and raying of the parathyroids in combination with calcium therapy has been employed, but the results are uncertain. The use of hormones has been tried but found unsatisfactory.

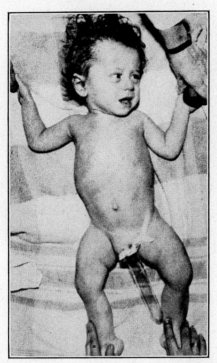

Fig. 90.—Clinical appearance of patient with blue sclera. (From Rados and Rosenberg: Arch. Ophth., July, 1936.)

The Iris

Most of the congenital anomalies of the iris are inherited and may occur in more than one member of the same family. Both eyes of an individual may be affected and the vision in such patients will be correspondingly decreased. The condition may be associated with congenital anomalies in other structures of the eye.

Aniridia or Irideremia.—This is a condition characterized by a complete congenital absence of the iris. In some cases, there may be a very small root portion present, but the iris is missing practically in its entirety. As a result, such a patient is found to have a full-sized pupil so that there is no check on the amount of light which enters such an eye. The patient may develop normally otherwise, but the affected eyes are always sensitive to light. This defect is often accompanied by other eye defects such as congenital opacities in the lens, coloboma of the lens, choroid, or both.

According to Neher,[20] the condition follows the mendelian law in that: "one-half of the offspring have aniridia while the other half have a normal iris. Moreover, when the offspring with aniridia marry normal individuals and have children, 50 per cent have aniridia and the remainder have a normal iris; the normal offspring who marry normal individuals never have borne children with aniridia."

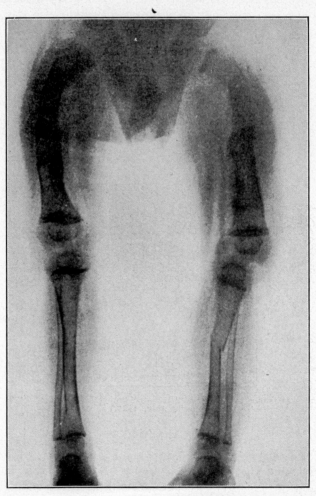

Fig. 91.—Roentgenogram of the lower extremities of the patient. In addition to general- ized osteoporosis, evidences of eight new and old fractures are visible. (From Rados and Rosenberg: Arch. Ophth., July, 1936.)

Congenital Coloboma.—This always occurs at the lower pole of the iris and is characterized by an absence of a small portion of the iris at this point, so that the pupil is elongated downward, presenting the shape of a pear with the narrow end at the lower border of the cornea. The form, however, may vary in different cases and may resemble a keyhole in appearance or may assume some different shape. Coloboma of the iris may be associated with coloboma of the lens, choroid, or ciliary body. In patients who have only a coloboma of the iris, the vision may not be seriously impaired, but they may be rather sensitive to the effect of light or glare. The impairment of vision may be greater in those in which the condition is associated with a similar defect in the lens and choroid, and the latter may, on refraction, show a rather high degree of astigmatism. There is no treatment to be instituted for the condition.

Persistent Pupillary Membrane.—Occasionally a fine strand or dark filament will be found which crosses the pupil to connect one margin of the iris with the opposite. There may be one or two such strands present in the same eye, and they can be readily seen on close examination with the ophthalmoscope, as well as with the slit lamp. In some instances, however, they may be so thin that they can be overlooked with the ophthalmoscope, especially in a hurried examination. These so-called membranes occur quite frequently and are sometimes attached to the anterior capsule of the lens. They ordinarily cause no interference with the vision of the eye or with the normal function of the iris. Furthermore, they require no treatment or attempt at removal and are only of interest in being recognized. Occasionally, when found to be present in infants, they may disappear in later life.

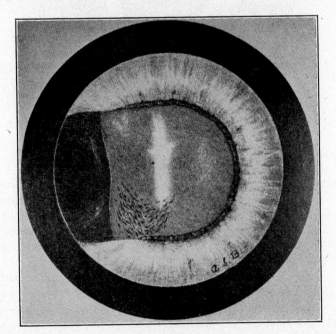

Fig. 92.—Coloboma of iris and lens. Defect in the zonular fibers can be seen in the center of coloboma. (From Rones: Arch. Ophth., August, 1930.)

Iritis.—A form of low-grade iritis may occasionally be found in a very young child as the result of hereditary syphilis. Or, as the result of syphilitic iritis which occurs during intrauterine life, the eyes at birth may be found to present an occlusion of the pupil. The pupil will be contracted, and the iris is either completely bound down and cannot be dilated, or synechiae are present by which the iris is adherent in places to the cornea or to the anterior lens capsule. The vision of the patient's eye is decreased to a corresponding degree and depending on the extent of the inflammation present in the eye.

As soon as the condition is recognized, treatment should be instituted which consists of attempts to dilate the affected pupil by the use of mydriatics in the eye, such as atropine. If syphilis is known to be the cause of the condition, the patient should receive the necessary general treatment. Since this condition should properly be considered as a manifestation of an infection, even though this occurs during intrauterine life, it will also be described later under the classification of syphilitic manifestations.

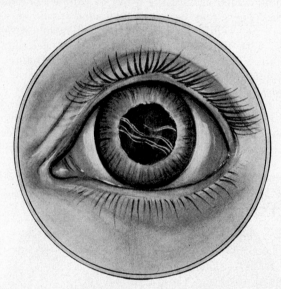

Fig. 93.—Retained pupillary membrane.

The Lens

Congenital Aphacia.—A congenital absence of the entire lens is a very rare condition, but such cases are occasionally encountered. It may occur in connection with other congenital defects affecting either the same or the opposite eye. In total absence of the lens the iris may be seen to move or shake on movement of the eyeball, the affected eye will be highly hyperopic, and the vision correspondingly reduced.

If the eye is otherwise unaffected, the condition might be aided and the vision improved by refraction and prescribing a lens found to be indicated. If the light or glare should be annoying to the patient, the lens can be prescribed in a tint sufficient to reduce the effect of the glare.

Lenticonus.—This is a congenital condition in which the lens shows a conical formation on its anterior or posterior surface. The latter is more frequently encountered than the former. The difference occasioned in the curvature of the affected surface causes a marked disparity in the refractive power of the various portions of the lens, the conical portion being much more highly myopic. Posterior lenticonus affects the posterior pole of the lens, which is marked by a small opacity at the apex of the cone, similar to that described as occurring in keratoconus. Sometimes other congenital anomalies may be present, and these include retained pupillary membrane, coloboma, and remnants of hyaloid artery. The condition has been said to be due to inflammation occurring in fetal life and to fetal rupture of the capsule of the lens. There is no treatment for lenticonus other than to secure the best vision obtainable by means of refraction.

Coloboma.—A notch or partial notching sometimes occurs on the lens or edge of the lens, either alone or often in association with coloboma of the lid, iris, or choroid. It is always congenital and is due to a defect in development. A coloboma may vary in size and shape in different cases, but it requires no treatment. In ordinary cases they cause no serious impairment of the vision.

Dislocation of the Lens.—Although it may occur as an acquired condition, dislocation of the lens is frequently congenital. Being displaced internally from its normal anatomic position behind the iris, it is sometimes referred to as subluxation of the lens or ectopia lentis. The displacement may occur in any direction. When completely displaced so that none of the lens occupies the pupillary space within the iris, it is referred to as a complete or total luxation. Both eyes are usually affected, and the condition in many instances has an hereditary origin. When partially dislocated, the vision is interfered with according to the degree of displacement of the lens. If it is such that most of the lens is in the pupillary space, it may function as part of the refractive system of the eye. If completely dislocated internally, so that most of the lens is beyond the pupil, it cannot take part in the refraction of the light through the eye. This would cause such an eye to be highly hyperopic.

Subluxation of the lens can readily be studied with the ophthalmoscope, the free border being clearly defined in the pupillary space. That portion of the fundus oculi observed through the lens may appear as it would if the lens were not dislocated, and the refraction will appear normal for the eye, whereas that portion seen outside of the lens will appear more highly hyperopic. The optic disc and other structures in the fundus appear much smaller than when viewed through the lens.

Since the lens is dislocated, the iris is free and has no resting place at the pupillary border. It can therefore be seen to shake or flutter when the eyeball is rotated quickly in any direction. This condition is known as iridodonesis and is indicative of dislocation of the lens.

If the dislocation is only of slight degree, it requires no treatment, but in more marked cases, operative removal of the lens may be indicated. Depending on the direction and extent of the dislocation, the operative procedure employed would be either discission followed later by the linear extraction of the lens or, in other cases, removal of the lens in toto. Great care must be exercised in either case, and such procedures are only undertaken by an experienced ophthalmic surgeon after careful study of the case.

A forward dislocation of the lens in the anterior chamber of the eye would predispose to increased intraocular tension and secondary glaucoma.

Arachnodactyly (Marfan's Syndrome).—Congenital bilateral dislocation of the lens is present at birth. Those cases in which the congenital dislocation of the lens is associated with later changes, such as abnormally long bones of the legs, arms, hands, and fingers, and a scoliosis, have been described by Marfan in 1896, and many cases have since been reported. The condition should not be difficult to recognize, since the patient complains first of an interference with the vision because of the malposition of the lens. In addition, the length of the fingers and abnormally long bones of the extremities should attract attention. The spinal column reveals a curvature, usually a scoliosis, and the trunk of the patient is long and narrow. A large number of these cases are also said to suffer with congenital heart disease. Lloyd,[21] who reported a number of cases of arachnodactyly, among them five in one family,

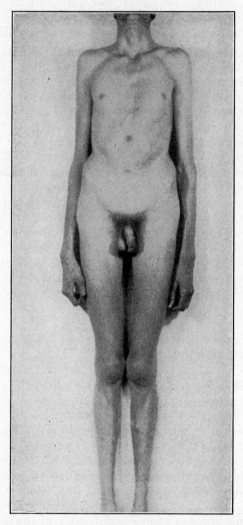

Fig. 94.—Clinical appearance of patient with arachnodactyly. (From the clinic of Dr. Warren Reese, Wills Hospital.)

described the following characteristics: The condition is familial and heredi-tary, occurring in males more often than in females. The thinness and length of the long bones are prominent features, as well as the weak musculature and frail spinal column, which accounts for the scoliosis. There is a congenital miosis present which cannot be overcome by the use of atropine. This is due to the rigidity of the iris framework and not to the lack of dilator fibers. There is some difference of opinion as to whether or not it should be considered as a mesodermal dystrophy because the zonule and the dilating fibers of the iris do not originate from the mesoderm. Laval[22] stated that he obtained dilatation of the pupils in his cases with either homatropine hydrobromide or cocaine hydrochloride. He also suggested that the condition might be a dystrophy of mesodermal or ectodermal origin.

Rados,[23] who reviewed most of the cases reported in the literature up to the time of his report, summarized the dislocations in arachnodactyly and showed that they may occur in almost any direction. They are usually incomplete but may develop into the complete form. Many of the cases have a lenticular myopia, although axial myopia of high degree may also occur.

The pathologic cardiac changes result from the presence of an open duct of Botalli or an open foramen ovale. There is said to be a probable congenital inferiority of the heart structure in many cases which may favor the development of rheumatic infection and other forms of cardiac involvement following infections.

The vision in the eyes affected is reduced according to the extent of the lens dislocation. When this is sufficient to handicap the patient and cannot be improved on refraction, an attempt can be made by an ophthalmic surgeon to remove the lens. The procedures are the same as those previously described for congenital dislocation of the lens. After successful removal, the eyes can be refracted and glasses affording the best vision obtainable are prescribed.

Congenital Cataract.—Congenital opacities in the lens may occur as the result of aberrations which take place in the development of the lens. Such opacities are known to occur principally as anterior polar cataract, posterior polar cataract, zonular cataract, fusiform cataract, punctate cataract, coralliform cataract, and others.

Anterior polar cataract consists of a small dotlike opacity at the anterior pole of the lens. It is usually bilateral and is sometimes associated with disc-shaped cataract in which there is an absence of the nucleus and the lens is flattened from before backward. When present alone, anterior polar cataract will cause no serious interference with the vision of the eye. The dotlike opacity can be observed with the ophthalmoscope and can be seen to move in the same direction as that in which the eye is rotated.

Posterior polar cataract occurs as a small dotlike opacity at the posterior pole of the lens. It also causes no serious interference with the vision, but should be differentiated from posterior lenticonus. In the latter condition, there is a gap in the posterior capsule which is very thin at the pole of the lens and which bulges outward into the vitreous. On examination with the ophthalmoscope a posterior polar cataract will appear to move opposite to that of the movement of the eyeball. It cannot be observed with oblique illumination. Most posterior polar cataracts are considered to be the point of attachment of the hyaloid artery in fetal life. They may occur in association with posterior lenticonus or with a persistent hyaloid artery. Since it causes no serious interference with the vision, it requires no treatment.

Zonular cataract, sometimes called lamellar cataract, is the most common form of congenital cataract. Observed with the ophthalmoscope through the dilated pupil, it appears as a disclike cataract in the center of the lens, of varying size and having a grayish color. A peripheral transparent zone

through which the fundus can be seen surrounds the opacity. The condition
is usually bilateral and hereditary in origin. It interferes with the vision
of the eye according to the density rather than to the size. Defects of other
structures, especially of the teeth, may be found in association.

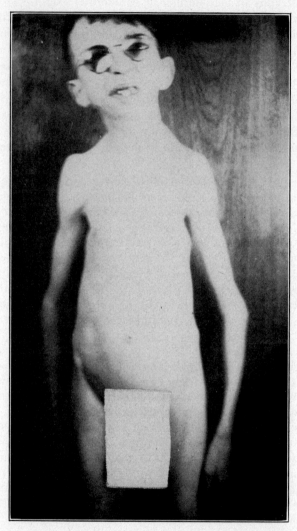

Fig. 95.—Patient aged 18 years with deformity of chest and upper extremities and bilateral
congenital cataracts successfully operated. (I. S. Tassman, Wills Hospital.)

The treatment of zonular cataract depends principally on the degree of
visual impairment which it produces. When the vision can be improved
satisfactorily by refraction, nothing further is required. When this is not
satisfactorily improved, it may be necessary to resort to an operation procedure. Such operations usually consist of discission and linear extraction.

Fusiform cataract is a type of congenital axial opacity which extends
through the center of the lens from the anterior to the posterior pole.

Punctate cataracts consist of small, white, dotlike opacities found uniformly throughout the entire lens. They are located principally, however, in the cortical layers of the peripheral lens. They may occur in fairly large numbers. They fail to develop to any extent, and being in the periphery, they do not cause any serious interference with the vision. They are usually bilateral and may occur in more than one member of the family. No treatment for punctate cataract is required.

Coralliform cataract is a form of congenital cataract in which the opacities radiate out from the center in a forward and lateral direction. They terminate in a sort of bulb-like formation just under the capsule. They are probably due to some disturbance which occurs in the line of sutures in the anteroposterior plane of the lens.

Hereditary Cataract (Presenile and Senile Types).—Many cases of congenital cataract of a hereditary nature have been reported as occurring in several members of the same family and different generations of the same family. In 1905, Nettleship[24] made a complete report on hereditary cataract from a review of the literature and his own records. From these he offered six rules concerning the occurrence of cataract in families, which rules seem to apply to most cases. 1. The descent is direct. No generations are skipped, but children of a family not having cataract can feel assured that none will develop. 2. If the children in one family have cataract, the liability of the next generation is increased. 3. Transmission from like sex to like sex is most common. 4. The cataracts tend to appear earlier in life in succeeding generations. 5. The age of onset is approximately the same in persons of the same generation. 6. The families with cataract are not affected as to fertility, health, or longevity.

The Vitreous

Persistent Hyaloid Artery.—This is probably the most common or most frequent congenital anomaly of the vitreous which we encounter. It is due to an aberration which arises in connection with the disappearance of the fetal vascular system of the vitreous. In a newborn infant, the hyaloid artery as a result remains as a slender fiberlike cord which normally disappears during the first year of life. In some instances, however, the remains of the hyaloid persist and can be observed in these patients with the ophthalmoscope as a filamentous band which extends out into the vitreous from the nerve head and can usually be traced forward to the posterior pole of the lens. Other projections which extend into the vitreous may simulate a persistent hyaloid artery, but these can be eliminated when the filamentous or fibrous band is present and is seen to connect with the central vessels at the nerve head. The condition may be associated with congenital opacities in the posterior lens, such as posterior polar cataract and posterior lenticonus.

Retained Hyaloid Canal.—When a wide tubular-like band projects forward from the optic nerve head into the vitreous, it represents the remains of the hyaloid or Cloquet's canal. When observed with the ophthalmoscope this is similar in appearance to that of a persistent hyaloid artery, and it may also be associated with posterior polar cataract.

Congenital Cysts of the Vitreous.—A rather rare condition which has been variously described. Congenital cysts appear as round or spherical bodies which occur in the vitreous and are usually transparent and vary in size from one-half to two disc diameters. They may be seen to float usually in the central or lower part of the vitreous. Most of the cases reported were described as pigmented, but the apparent pigmentation has been termed an illusion (Cassady[25]) since it was found that the tiny hyaline-like plaques on the surface appear to be streaks or spots of dark pigment on the light background of the fundus. These vitreous cysts float or move about with rotation of the eyeball and come to rest when the movement stops. They apparently give no serious interference to the vision. Their origin was formerly considered to be from degenerative adenomatous cysts of the vitreous processes, but from a consideration of the factors concerned, Cassady suggests the primary vitreous as the site of the cyst.

Congenital Vascular Veils in the Vitreous.—The condition is rather rare, but three cases were reported and described by Mann and Macrae[26] in which a thin transparent veil lies well forward in the vitreous and in front of the retina from which it is independent. Vessels could be seen in the veils which were both retinal and arising from the vitreous. Their origin was said to have been in the vitreous condensation which was supposed to take place.

The Retina

Medullated Nerve Fibers.—This is not really a congenital anomaly, but rather a developmental defect which begins very shortly after birth. The intraocular nerve fibers in the optic disc and adjoining retina remain with a medullated sheath. The retina around the disc, therefore, has the appearance of a bright white spot when observed with the ophthalmoscope. This spot may vary in size in different patients, and can be plainly seen to stand out in strong contrast to the color of the surrounding fundus. The edges of the white spot are usually irregular and the fibers are drawn out into a flame-shaped appearance. These are sometimes called "opaque nerve fibers." They usually occur at the upper or lower border of the optic disc, but in some cases they may surround it entirely. The fibers cover the retinal vessels in places, and although the vision of the patient is not usually interfered with, there may be a slight enlargement of the blind spot. They cause no other disturbance and require no treatment.

Ablatio Falciformio Congenita (Congenital Retinal Folds).—This condition is an abnormality of development in the retina which is familial and hereditary in type and in appearance may resemble an inflammatory process or a pseudoglioma. The folds occur commonly in the temporal and inferior part of the retina and may be associated with other noninflammatory abnormalities of development. Among these are congenital cataracts, persistent pupillary membrane, persistent hyaloid artery and nystagmus. The condition is bilateral in 50 per cent of the cases, and in these the folds are symmetric in both eyes. The cases studied revealed that the retina showed an imperfect differentiation which was due to a disturbance of growth of the whole of the inner layer of the optic cup. Weve,[27] who reported a number of these cases, stated that there was consanguinity of the parents in at least seven of his patients.

Congenital Retinal Hemorrhages.—This condition in most instances is assumed rather than diagnosed. However, it is usually indicated by the presence of nystagmus associated with amblyopia in very young children. The nystagmus is present at birth, and although it is determined that the visual acuity in the eye is very poor at a later age, no evidences of any pathology which would account for the poor vision can be found on ophthalmoscopic examination. It has been found in the newborn, especially among premature and immature infants, that as many as 41 per cent show evidences of retinal hemorrhage incurred either before or during birth (Edgerton[28]). These hemorrhages clear up after a time and leave no signs of their former presence, except that the vision is considerably reduced in these eyes. It has been suggested that the occurrence of such hemorrhages is the cause of the poor central vision in these instances. In Edgerton's series of 458 newborn infants, examination revealed the presence of nystagmus 89 times.

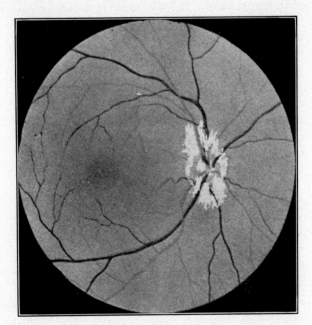

Fig. 96.—Medullated nerve fibers.

Grouped Pigmentation of the Retina.—This congenital condition is characterized by the presence of grouped pigmentation spots which are to be differentiated from solitary patches of pigment. They are usually located in some certain part of the fundus and have the appearance of black or dark brown spots. These may vary in size from that of a pinhead dot near the optic disc, to much larger ones farther off in the periphery. The condition is not uncommon, and a number of cases have been reported. These were reviewed by Perera[29] with the report of a case, and the following characteristics were pointed out: (1) The condition is usually unilateral and more commonly found in males than females. (2) It is not hereditary and consanguinity is not a factor. (3) No other congenital deformities or changes are necessarily present. (4) The condition is stationary. (5) The fundus is involved in sections and the macula is usually unaffected.   (6) The pigment spots lie deep to the retinal vessels.   (7) The vision in the affected eye is not decreased, and night blindness is absent.

Pigmentary Retinosis (Retinitis Pigmentosa).—One of a group of degenerations of the retina considered under the designation of "tapetoretinal degenerations." These are characterized by their progressive nature, hereditary tendency and occurrence primarily in the neuroepithelial layers of the retina. The degeneration usually leads to an atrophy of the retina and the optic nerve.

The initial and probably the most important lesion is a disappearance of the visual cells.   This is sometimes accompanied by other developmental anomalies, such as polydactylism and deafness.   The condition is more common in males than in females and appears rather early in life.   It is distinctly hereditary in nature and consanguinity in the parents or in earlier generations has been noted in many cases.   It may occur in several members of the same family.

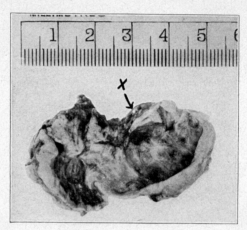

Fig. 97.—Gross specimen of a cerebellar hemangioendothelioma in Lindau's disease.   (From McDonald: Arch. Ophth., March, 1940.)

The symptoms are characterized first by an inability to see in poor light or in the dark.   This becomes more pronounced, with night blindness (hemeralopia) being the most troublesome symptom.   The vision later decreases in daylight with a gradual contraction of the field of vision in the periphery.   Early in the disease, ring-shaped or U-shaped scotoma may be found in the visual field, within about 30° fixation.   The central vision remains unaffected until very late in the disease, when this becomes very narrow and greatly contracted, so that ultimately, the patient may experience difficulty in going about even in daylight.   Both eyes of the patient are affected, and the condition is practically the same in each.   The course is chronic, and the disease may be complicated later by glaucoma and cataract of the lens.

On examination with the ophthalmoscope, the outstanding lesion is the almost characteristic pigmentation of the retina.   This can be seen early in the disease, usually to the nasal side of the optic disc and consists of an increasing number of individual pigment lesions or spots which are grouped

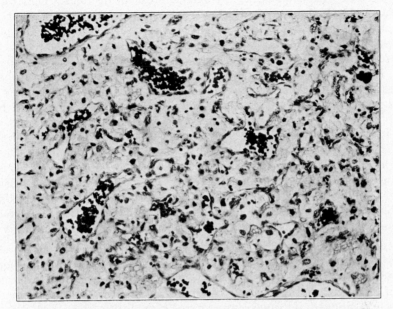

Fig. 98.—High-power photomicrograph (×85), showing the detail of the angioplastic cerebellar tumor shown in Fig. 97. (From McDonald: Arch. Ophth., March, 1940.)

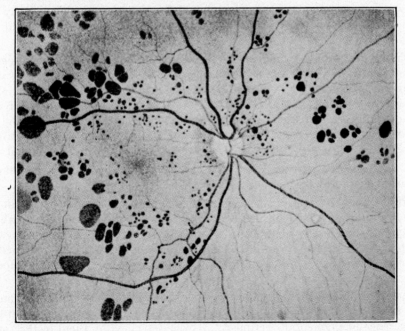

Fig. 99.—Congenital grouped pigmentation of the retina. (From Perera: Arch. Ophth., January, 1939.)

and connected with one another, by extensions or projections. They therefore resemble individual bone corpuscles in appearance, and together present a network throughout the fundus which is more or less striking. The pigment is black and penetrates the sheaths of the vessels which it encircles. It also increases as it approaches the optic disc and eventually reaches the disc margins. The retina later becomes atrophic and the pigment heaps up between the vessels of the choroidal circulation which is seen to be exposed. The retinal vessels themselves are very greatly constricted and later become thread-like. Early in the disease, the optic disc may appear to be of normal color, but this gradually changes to a grayish or waxy color resembling that of parchment. Later in the disease, it becomes more atrophic. The optic nerve head may also present a granular appearance, as the result of accompanying small colloid spots, resembling drusen. Other conditions occasionally observed in association are pigmentary degeneration of the macula and retinitis albescens. There are no signs of any inflammatory process found in the fundus. The prognosis is poor, but patients may not become totally blind.

Differential diagnosis of pigmentary retinosis is not necessarily difficult in most cases, but it should not be confused with retinal and chorioretinal degeneration which, in their terminal stages, principally, show an accumulation of pigment throughout the fundus. This might resemble the "bone corpuscle" pigment in appearance. Late in syphilitic chorioretinitis, an accumulation or migration of pigment might occur secondarily into the superficial layers and invade the perivascular sheaths. The early occurrence of the characteristic pigmentation in primary retinosis, together with its progressive increase, its hereditary origin, night blindness, and gradually concentric contraction of the visual fields, should all serve to diagnose the condition.

Treatment consists principally of regulation and general management with attempts to provide the best vision obtainable by refraction. Since it was considered that contraction of the retinal vessels was caused by action of the sympathetic system, which resulted in the degeneration, a number of cases were operated on with removal of the first sympathetic ganglion for the purpose of producing a vasodilatation. Satisfactory results were reported in enlarging the field of vision, but no permanent improvement was obtained.

Complications, such as cataract formation and the possible occurrence of glaucoma, should be treated accordingly.

Pigmentary Retinosis Sine Pigment.—Pigmentary retinosis without pigment is the same as the former condition but the pigment spots are absent. The symptoms are the same as in actual pigmentary retinosis, and it is believed by some that this condition is an earlier stage of the real pigmentary retinosis. However, it has been found to remain unchanged for a number of years.

Lawrence-Moon-Biedl Syndrome.—This condition may occur in one or more members of the same family, and the principal ocular manifestation is the presence of pigmentary retinosis. It was described by Biedl in 1922 and is characterized otherwise by a retarded mental development in the patient, hypogenitalism, polydactylism, and obesity of the Fröhlich type. The fat is increased in the trunk and lower extremities, and the obesity is present in varying degrees.

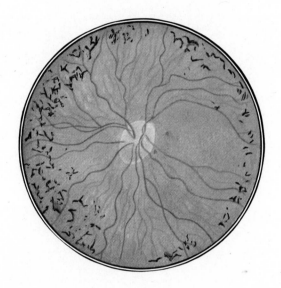

Fig. 100.—Pigmentary degeneration of the retina, showing typical "bone corpuscle" pigment spots.

The body contour in the male resembles that of the female, and in the latter the contour is exaggerated. Both sexes are equally affected. The vision of the patient is decreased, and in most cases, it continues to diminish. Sometimes the pigmentary retinosis is atypical. Skull roentgenograms in this condition showed the sella to be normal. No changes in the hypophysis have been found to be present.

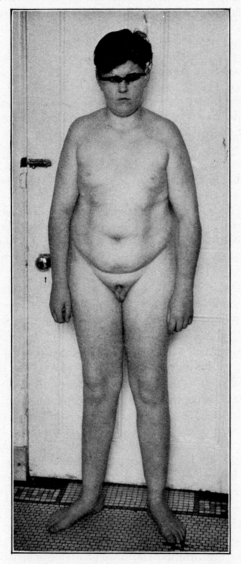

Fig. 101.—Patient with obesity of the Fröhlich type, commonly found in cases with Laurence-Moon-Biedl syndrome. (From Meakins: The Practice of Medicine, The C. V. Mosby Co.)

The condition is usually progressive, and the prognosis for improvement is poor. The treatment has consisted principally of the use of glandular extract since these cases have been attributed to glandular dysfunction. This treatment is by no means specific, however, but rather empiric. In one case treated by Biedl with thyroid and pituitary extract, the vision was improved, the menses re-established, and the weight reduced thirteen pounds.

Hereditary Macular Degeneration.—There are several degenerative conditions which affect the macular region and are considered to be closely related in nature to pigmentary retinosis, since they are of congenital origin, although they may not become evident until sometime after birth. These conditions have been grouped with the hereditary and familial degenerations and variously described as abiotrophies and tapetoretinal degenerations. There is some defect in all which affects the nerve cells of the macula as a result of an impairment in embryonic development. Defective central vision in particular is found in those patients so affected. Their etiology and classification are not clearly understood, but in some of these patients, the lesions may become evident shortly after birth, while in others, they may not appear until later in life. Both eyes are nearly always involved, and females are more commonly affected than males.

The infantile type of hereditary macular degeneration, which was described in detail by Stargardt, is characterized by a lesion around the macula in each eye which is nearly as large as the disc. It is composed of a number of small yellowish spots which are encircled by numerous fine pigment dots. Later, the yellowish discoloration of the macula may increase in size and contain a larger black pigment mass. The yellow area may vary in size, and when observed with the ophthalmoscope, it is seen to present a well-defined margin and a glistening appearance. No other evidences of pathology may be found in the fundus.

The vision gradually diminishes, and a central scotoma develops. Night blindness is also a common finding. When the disease occurs early in life, it may be associated with cerebral symptoms characterized by paralysis, idiocy, and dementia.

Although the condition has at times been attributed to glandular dysfunction and to syphilis, its association with these is rare. The etiology is unknown, and there is also no known form of treatment.

Retinitis Punctata Albescens.—This is another form of degeneration which may affect the peripheral retina as well as the macular region. While it is also related to pigmentary retinosis, there are no pigment spots present in this condition. The lesions consist of numerous, small white dots, with rather well-defined margins, and are scattered at short intervals over almost the entire fundus. They can be readily observed with the ophthalmoscope, and with the exception of a moderate contraction of the vessels, no other pathology is present.

The condition is bilateral, hereditary, and is accompanied by a very gradual impairment of the vision. There is no treatment known.

Amaurotic Familial Idiocy (Tay-Sachs Disease).—This is a hereditary, familial disease affecting infants who present a characteristic ocular manifestation of the systemic degeneration. The principal structure involved outside of the eyes is the central nervous system. It often affects children of Jewish birth, but it also occurs among foreign groups. The disease becomes evident at the age of 3 to 6 months, and the patients usually die in one or two years. The ocular changes consist mainly of a grayish-white area in the macula which is about the size of the disc or slightly larger, in the center of which is a cherry-

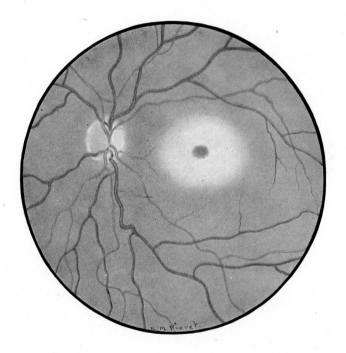

Fig. 102.—Typical ophthalmoscopic picture of amaurotic familial idiocy (Tay-Sachs disease). (After Reese, from Troncoso: Internal Diseases of the Eye and Atlas of Ophthalmoscopy, F. A. Davis Co.)

red spot, similar to that seen in cases with obstruction of the central artery of the retina. The optic nerve head becomes pale and goes on to a complete optic atrophy, so that the patient is usually blind before death. The retinal vessels themselves may show no changes. The condition is always bilateral. The pathologic lesions in the eye, as in the brain and spinal cord, are due to a degeneration of the ganglion cells, as the result of deposits in the cells of a lipoid substance of a peculiar nature. According to J. Friedenwald, there is a great amount of swelling of the cells with a loss of Nissl granules. The cells which are filled with a granular amorphous substance have their nuclei displaced. The degeneration of the ganglion cells around the macula leaves the area here white, so that the central red area within stands out in strong contrast. The condition was described in detail by Gouterman and Winkleman.[30]

The general symptoms of the patient consist of a general muscular weakness, the child being unable to sit up or to hold the head erect. They are usually apathetic, mentally dull, and may suffer with paralysis which increases until death. The ocular lesion is pathognomonic of the condition and, when seen, will determine the diagnosis in otherwise doubtful cases. The age of the patient and the mental and muscular symptoms, together with paralysis, will also aid in the diagnosis.

The disease should be differentiated from obstruction of the central artery, but although the eye changes are similar, the latter condition occurs usually in older people and is not accompanied by the other general symptoms. The ophthalmoscopic appearance of the eyes is usually so typical that other conditions, such as inflammation of the retina, pigmentary degeneration, central choroiditis, and other congenital macular defects, can be readily excluded.

A juvenile form of the disease has also been described in older children. These patients are apparently healthy at birth, and the condition is first observed at the age of 6 to 8 years. In this group the macular changes consist of a diffuse pigmentation which extends somewhat into the surrounding retina. The optic nerve head is grayish white in color and becomes atrophic. The retinal vessels are somewhat smaller than normal. This condition is also progressive, and death usually occurs at the age of about 12 years. It is also apparently race selective.

A third form also has been described as occurring in individuals at the ages of 14 to 16, or even 20 years. In this group, the condition does not appear to be race selective, but the macular changes are similar to the former type, and the visual disturbances are perhaps less marked. A central scotoma may be present; there may be loss of muscle power, and no dementia. This variety is not considered to be fatal.

Occasionally, an atypical form of the disease may present itself, particularly in children of 1 to 2 years of age. The fundus change might be modified to an extent so that it appears as a discoloration around a red macula, or a clouded mist around the macula which will gradually blend with the rest of the retina.

There is no known specific treatment for the condition.

Niemann-Pick Disease.—Another familial disease which occurs in infants and presents an ophthalmoscopic picture similar to that of Tay-Sachs disease. According to Goldstein and Wexler,[31] the cherry-red spot in the macula is similar to that seen in amaurotic familial idiocy, but the changes in the optic disc may differ. The color is yellowish, due to deposit of a lipoid substance in the nerve, while in Tay-Sachs, the disc becomes atrophic. In Niemann-Pick there is a disturbance of lipoid metabolism, and the pathology is that of a general histiocytosis. The cells contain lipoid and the excess of lipoid is taken up by the histiocytes which appear as "foam cells." The changes in the ganglion cells of the retina are similar to those occurring in Tay-Sachs disease, but are more severe. Some of the foam cells are found in the choroid and contain pigment.

In Niemann-Pick disease, other organs, such as the liver and spleen, are affected, whereas in Tay-Sachs disease, the changes are confined to the nervous system. The skin may become discolored and the abdomen of these patients distended, because of enlargement of the affected organs. The blood smear also has been said to reveal a large number of vacuolated lymphocytes. Goldstein and Wexler described the following features: Degeneration of ganglion cell layer of the retina, closely resembling that described in Tay-Sachs disease; vacuolation of the cells of the nuclear layers, causing a striking honeycombed appearance; pigmented vacuolated cells in the choroid; vacuolated histiocytes about the scleral vessels and in the episclera and an infiltration of these cells among the fibers of the sclera; a group of ganglion cells in the episclera, in intimate contact with the ciliary nerves, showing changes similar to those of the cells of the brain and ganglion cells elsewhere; granular degeneration of Nissl's substance, swelling of the cell and vacuolation of the cytoplasm.

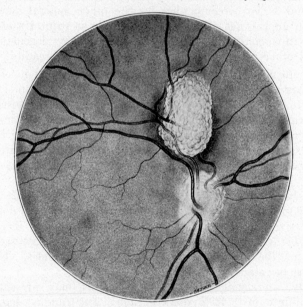

Fig. 103.—Tuberous sclerosis, showing typical mulberry-like tumor of the retina and optic nerve.
(From Reese: Arch. Ophth., July, 1940.)

Angiomatosis Retinae (Von Hippel's Disease).—An abnormality of the retinal vessels, which has a congenital anlage and which may not be recognized until sometime later in life, is characterized by an aneurysmal formation with one or two new vessel formations which connect with a tumorlike body in the retina. Von Hippel first described the condition as a distinct clinical entity, and a fair number of cases have been reported since. It occurs in one eye, is chronic and of long duration, usually being discovered in young people of adolescent age. Cases have been reported in patients as young as 2 years and as old as 30 years or more. Occasionally, the condition may be present as part of a systemic process, with angiomas occurring primarily in the cerebellum, and tumor growths also present in other organs, such as the suprarenal glands, pancreas, and spinal cord. Skin moles may also be found. When a generalized angiomatosis is present in a patient, the condition is known as Lindau's disease.

The retinal lesion has been described as a small, spherical body into which a pair of large tortuous vessels, springing from the disc, disappear (Troncoso). The tumor may vary in size and is considered to be primarily an angiomatosis, although such tumors have been variously considered as angioplastic tumors, nevi of the central nervous system, and glial tumors.

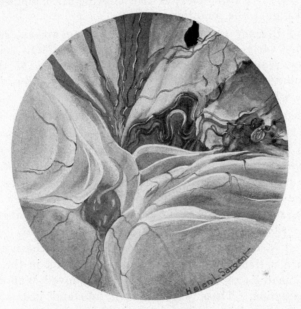

Fig. 104.—Angiomatosis retinae, showing cystlike dilatations in the periphery, dilated vessels, and detachment of retina. (From McDonald and Lippincott: Arch. Ophth., December, 1938.)

Pressure on the eyeball has been said to cause the spherical tumor to disappear and a pulsation to start in the artery. The disease has a familial tendency, and a number of cases have been reported occurring in more than one member of the same family. The condition may be followed by iridocyclitis, detachment of the retina, secondary glaucoma, and loss of vision with ultimate blindness. The prognosis for life in these patients is also poor, since it may be complicated by cerebral manifestations which terminate fatally. When the condition becomes generalized, as in Lindau's disease, the tumors occurring in other organs, such as the pancreas or kidneys, may also bring about a fatal termination.

Bedell[32] called attention to a fullness of the retinal veins as one of the earliest signs. Later, the dilation takes on a cystlike, or aneurysmal, formation, usually in the periphery. Sometimes these vascular tumors are multiple.

Surrounded by a rather large area of whitish exudate extending out over the retina, the condition might easily be mistaken for Coats' disease or other forms of exudative retinitis. Hemorrhages may be present in the retina or vitreous; proliferation of glial tissue occurs around the mass, and finally, the entire retina may become detached. McDonald and Lippincott[33] reported a case in a boy, 5 years of age, with both eyes affected, although the right eye had suffered an additional traumatism and was blind. On discovering the angiomatosis in the left eye, the right eye was enucleated and the diagnosis confirmed on microscopic examination.

Treatment of the condition has consisted principally of electrolysis diathermy, radium applications and x-ray therapy, in the absence of any known specific treatment. McDonald and Lippincott's case received 1405 mg. hours of radium over the left orbit, four treatments being given one week apart, with no apparent change in the condition.

Cordes and Hogan[34] reported a case in a young woman, 20 years of age, who was treated early in the disease with a course of high voltage roentgen therapy. They reported a definite decrease in the size of the tumor and amount of exudate after a period of seven months. No alteration in the condition of the vessels was noted, however.

In a subsequent report by Cordes and Dickson[35] the eye of this patient showed a marked improvement after three and one-half years of irradiation. These authors also reported definite improvement in another eye with early involvement after two years of irradiation. An eye with a more advanced lesion became progressively worse with ultimate loss of vision, complete detachment of the retina and gliosis. From their experience they concluded that in early cases, x-ray therapy offers a safe, convenient means of treatment. The advanced lesions do not respond to any type of treatment.

Guyton and McGovern[36] reported good results by the use of diathermy coagulation in a patient with early angiomatosis retina in the right eye and advanced angiomatosis of the left eye. They employed Walker pins as in a detachment operation. These were inserted into and just surrounding the tumor mass, their position being determined by frequent ophthalmoscopic examinations. A current of approximately 15 milliamperes was applied for three seconds through each pin. The angiomatous masses were obliterated and the sites of the masses became scars. The dilated retinal vessels were reduced in size and vision was completely preserved in the right eye. Although no vision was regained in the left eye, the ophthalmoscopic appearance of the eye was improved.

Lindau's Disease.—When angiomatosis retinae occurs with multiple hemangiomas of the central nervous system, principally in the cerebellum or other organs, the condition is known as Lindau's disease. Like von Hippel's disease, it is also of hereditary and familial incidence. In this disease the kidneys, pancreas, liver, bones, and many other structures may also be involved. The condition usually occurs in the second or third decade of life and may be present in several members of a family, as well as in members of other generations of the family. A. E. MacDonald[37] reported finding the

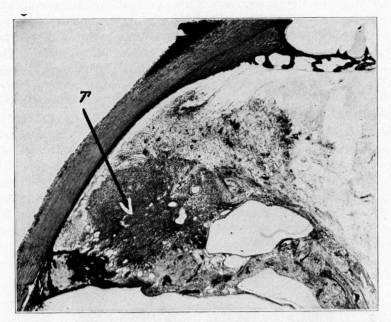

Fig. 105.—Low-power photomicrograph of a hemangioendothelioma in the anterior retina behind the ciliary body in Lindau's disease. (From McDonald: Arch. Ophth., March, 1940.)

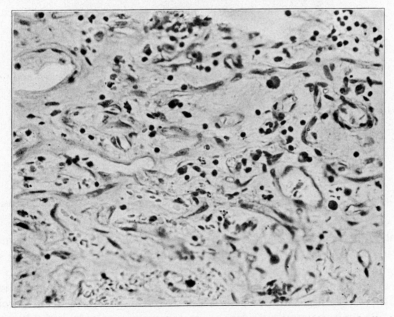

Fig. 106.—High-power photomicrograph (×165), showing the detail of angioplastic tumor in Fig. 105. (From McDonald: Arch. Ophth., March, 1940.)

condition in six of eleven members in two generations of a family in which the diagnosis was confirmed by pathologic examination in two of the cases in which the patients are living. In one of his cases, the patient was blind from an obscure cause until after a sister's operation for cerebellar tumor. When the affected eye was enucleated, the diagnosis of retinal hemangioendothelioma was made. This patient was also suffering with a cerebellar tumor which, on removal, was found to be a typical hemangioendothelioma. Another sister of these two patients had a conjunctival nevus.

The treatment of the condition consists principally in the application of radon seeds which thus far seem to have given favorable results. MacDonald employed 4 radon seeds, 0.7 millicurie each, which were attached to a silk suture. These were applied to the sclera opposite the tumor about 4 mm. apart and for a period of seven days. The prognosis of the condition is guarded. The vision in the affected eye may be saved by irradiation, but complications such as cataract and glaucoma may occur. When the disease has progressed very far and is discovered late, the termination is usually fatal.

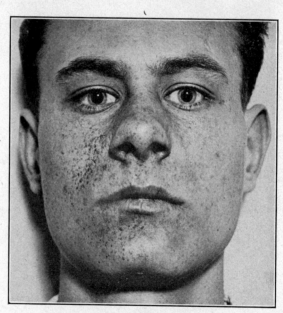

Fig. 107.—Patient with typical adenoma sebaceum in tuberous sclerosis. (From Messinger and Clarke: Arch. Ophth., July, 1937.)

Tuberous Sclerosis (Bourneville's Disease).—A rare congenital condition which is characterized by a tumor formation in the fiber layer of the retina which consists of neural fibers, neurocytes, or both (van der Hoeve). They nearly always contain cysts, and these cells may readily become malignant. In addition to the lesion in the retina, the condition also affects the cerebrum. It may also be associated with tumors in other organs, such as the heart, kidneys, thyroid, bony structures, and the central nervous system. The patients affected may be mentally defective and epileptic. Adenoma sebaceum may appear on the face, particularly around the nose and lips, early in life.

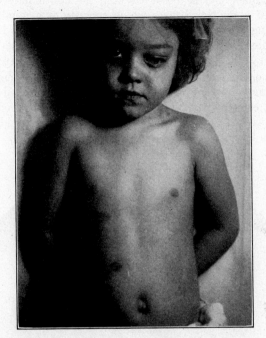

Fig. 108.—Neurofibromatosis of the left orbit. (Spaeth.) Note the "café-au-lait" spots on the body.

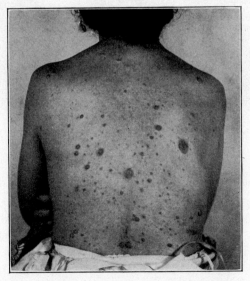

Fig. 109.—Mother of patient shown in Fig. 108 with neurofibromatosis. The mother shows multiple nodules over the entire back.

The retinal tumor can be observed with the ophthalmoscope and presents the appearance of a mulberry mass which consists of a number of very small nodules protruding forward into the vitreous. It is usually found near or adjacent to the optic disc.

In addition to adenoma sebaceum, other skin lesions may be present, such as fibromas, pigmented nevi, and some resembling neurofibromatoses. Although rare, an increasing number of these cases have been reported in the literature since 1927. The condition is said to be closely related to angiomatosis retinae (von Hippel's disease) and neurofibromatosis (von Recklinghausen's disease) with which it has been grouped as an allied disease.

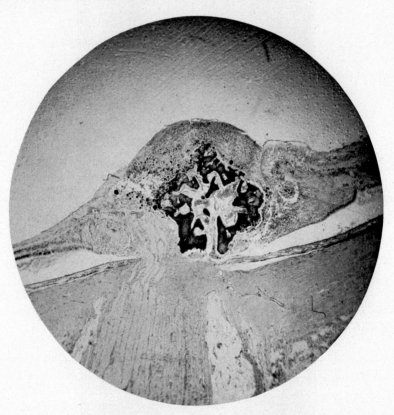

Fig. 110.—Low-power photomicrograph of a section through the nerve head, showing location and extent of tumor in tuberous sclerosis. (From Messinger and Clarke: Arch. Ophth., July, 1937.)

Since they are all congenital in origin and hereditary in tendency and are accompanied by lesions on the skin such as adenoma sebaceum and nevi, they have been grouped under the name of Phakomatoses (from phakoma, "birthmark"). In addition to their presence on the skin of the eyelids, conjunctiva, and retina, these phakoma may also occur on the iris and optic nerve. Most authors today also include Sturge-Weber's syndrome with this group. In this condition malignant blastomas develop. In some cases of tuberous sclerosis, the retinal tumors may undergo malignant changes. Lowenstein and Steel[28] reported a case of Bourneville's disease in a 3½-year-old boy with no history of hereditary defect and he presented no sebaceous adenomas. They feel that all these diseases form one entity with no sharp borderline against malignant blastomas. They stressed the opinion also that Bourneville's disease is a primary ectodermal growth and that the angiomatous reaction of the mesoderm is secondary, whereas angiomatosis retinae is a primary mesodermal growth with the glial reaction of the ectoderm secondary. In all of these conditions, moreover, the normal balance of the germinal layer is disturbed at some point of development by the growth of certain undifferentiated cell groups. The drive of growth is assumed to be a chemical one like the carcinogenic substances, which in excess produces a growing tumor. A defect produces various regressive metamorphoses which are known as familial degenerations of the tissues.

Neurofibromatosis (von Recklinghausen's Disease).—A disease characterized by a type of multiple tumor syndrome, congenital in origin. A tumor of the optic nerve or retina is accompanied by cutaneous pigmentation with multiple tumors of the cranial and peripheral nerves as well as of the sympathetic system. The involvement of the trunks, meninges, and central nervous system was described as a hyperplasia of the cells due to an irritant or stimulus which is followed by a true neoplastic growth of the cells. Since they are not true neuromas, the growths were called a neurofibromatosis by von Recklinghausen because they originate from the connective tissue sheath of the nerves.

A patient may at birth reveal pigmentation of the skin. The tumor which sometimes affects the optic nerve may progress and produce an optic atrophy from pressure. Pressure may also cause a displacement of the eyeball. A great variety of manifestations may accompany neurofibromatosis, but they are never all found in the same individual. These include multiple neurofibromas, flat pigment moles, fibrous mollusca, neuroma plexiform, tumors of the auditory nerve and other nerves, fibroendothelioma of the lids and orbit. Buphthalmos may also be an ocular manifestation of multiple neurofibromatosis. Cysts and other tumors in the retina also occur.

The Choroid

Coloboma of the Choroid.—A coloboma of the choroid is a defect in the lining membrane which exposes to view the underlying sclera. Since coloboma of the choroid is often found with coloboma of the retina, they will be considered together. In complete coloboma of the retina, the vessels are discontinued at the edge of the colobomatous area. In coloboma of the retina and choroid, there is present a defective patch through which the white sclera can be seen when viewed with the ophthalmoscope. Coloboma of the choroid is sometimes associated also with a coloboma of the iris or of the optic nerve. The visual acuity and visual fields in these cases may be found to be affected according to the location and extent of the coloboma. They are usually oval in shape or may be pearshaped. Their size may vary. The smaller ones might be about twice the size of the optic disc while the others may occupy a very much larger section of the choroid. They may extend forward to the ciliary border or backward to the optic disc. Their edges may be surrounded by pigment. The vessels at the edges of the coloboma are usually retinal vessels and appear more superficial than the body of the coloboma. Within the coloboma may be seen a few choroidal vessels interspersed with connective tissue. The exact etiology is not definitely known but it has been attributed to a nonclosure of the fetal cleft probably from the presence of mesoblastic tissue which prevented complete closure.

When a choroidal coloboma is located in the macula, it is known as a central coloboma. In this location it will prevent central vision. The area may be very deep and appear to be about the size of the optic disc. Pigment is also seen around the edges.

More rarely, a coloboma of the choroid may be found outside the macula and outside of the location of the fetal cleft. These may resemble lesions resulting from an inflammation, but no other signs of the latter are present. They can also be differentiated from connective tissue by their depth. There is no treatment for the condition.

Melanosis.—This is a condition in which an excessive amount of retinal and choroidal pigment has been developed with the result that the appearance of the fundus with the ophthalmoscope is darker and more brownish than normal. The conjunctiva at the corneal margin and the sclera are darkly pigmented, while the iris also has a dark brown color. The condition is not pathologic and causes no real interference with vision.

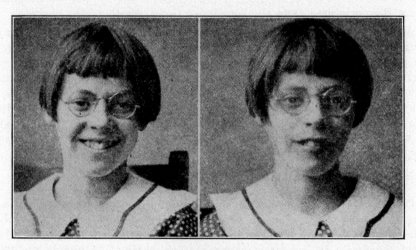

Fig. 111.—Monozygotic twins with bilateral macular coloboma. (From Gesell and Blake: Arch. Ophth., June, 1936.)

Albinism.—A congenital and hereditary condition in which there is an absence of normal pigment in the eye with perhaps a slight amount in the choroid around the fovea. Pigment cells themselves are present but contain no pigment. As a result, these patients are much more sensitive to light than the normal. The lack of pigment in the eye is associated with a lack of pigment in other structures, so that the skin and hair are unusually light. The iris itself transmits light, and the pupil in marked cases has a light or pinkish reflex. Often the lashes and even eyebrows are light in color, giving an almost characteristic appearance to the patient. More than one member of a family may be affected.

The visual acuity in these cases is nearly always poor, and the eyes have a rather high refractive error which is usually found to be myopia and astigmatism. Nystagmus is often present. Various degrees of albinism may be encountered in different patients, and in some, only patches of absent pigment may be found in the periphery.

The treatment of the condition consists principally in proper refraction and the prescribing of lenses which are tinted sufficiently to overcome the photophobia present in the individual case. In marked cases it is difficult to improve the vision beyond a limited point.

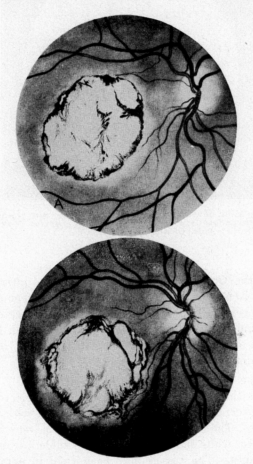

Fig. 112.—The coloboma in the right fundus of each of the twins shown in Fig. 111. (From Gesell and Blake: Arch. Ophth., June, 1936.)

Posterior Vortex Veins.—This is a rare condition in which short, projecting veins branch off from around the optic disc or from the conus which is present in myopic eyes. They terminate suddenly in a looped end entering the sheath of the optic nerve.

Choroideremia.—A rare form of congenital degeneration characterized by an absence of the entire choroid with the exception of a small area around the macula. As a result, the entire fundus appears white, with the exception of the small red area in the macula. According to Fuchs, in some cases there may be a peripheral white lobulated ring which surrounds a more or less intact central red area. The condition may affect more than one member of a family, and the field of vision in such cases is reduced to almost central vision.

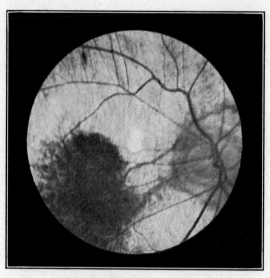

Fig. 113.—Fundus in an advanced stage of choroideremia, with retention of the choroid in the macular region, a circumpapillary dark ring and a white sclera. Vision 3/200. Field small and tubular. (From Bedell: Arch. Ophth., March, 1937.)

The Optic Nerve

Coloboma of the Optic Nerve.—Coloboma of the optic nerve rarely occurs alone, but it is nearly always associated with coloboma of the choroid which has been previously described. A number of cases have been recorded, however, and Shipman, in reporting a case which he believed to be a coloboma of the optic nerve not involving the choroid, but with posterior lenticonus, gave a detailed review of the condition.[39]

Coloboma of the optic nerve may be round or vertically oval, and the size may be many times that of the normal disc. The optic nerve head will, therefore, appear to be correspondingly larger than normal with the lower margin irregular in outline. The excavation will appear to be very deep, and the surface white or grayish white in color. It may resemble a marked glaucomatous cup in its appearance. The vessels may be normal in arrangement, or they may emerge from the lower portion or from the very edge of the circumference. In Shipman's case, the pseudo-optic disc appeared to be about twice the normal size and revealed an excavation of from about 5 to 10 D. The color was grayish white with the margins sharply outlined and a thin ring of pigment temporally.

The condition is also attributed to an interference with normal closure of the fetal cleft. The vision may vary in these cases from normal to very defective vision. Coloboma of the optic nerve is usually confined to one eye, although it may rarely be bilateral. In addition to its association with coloboma of the choroid, lens, or iris, it may also occur with any of the other congenital anomalies.

Hole or Pit of the Optic Nerve Head.—A rare congenital anomaly of the optic nerve head which is characterized by a marked depression, usually at the lower border of the disc. The hole may be very deep (9 to 15 D), and a few vessels may be seen to emerge from its margin. The color is usually grayish white or grayish blue, and in some cases, pigment spots have been found to be present. These holes have been considered to be allied to coloboma of the nerve.

Crescents of the Margins of the Optic Disc.—A congenital anomaly in which a crescent is seen at the margin of the optic disc, usually at the inferior temporal or nasal border. This is sometimes described as a conus, and sometimes a few vessels may be seen to emerge from the border. The color is usually a dark gray; being thin, the sclera may be seen at a different focus from that of the rest of the fundus. A certain amount of astigmatism is usually present, and there may be some amblyopia also.

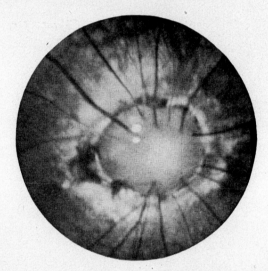

Fig. 114.—Coloboma of the optic nerve. (From Shipman: Arch. Ophth., March, 1934.)

Pseudoneuritis.—This may be considered as a congenital condition in which the margins of the optic disc are blurred as in optic neuritis, but here it is due to irregularities in the shape of the disc, or to the presence of high hyperopia and astigmatism. The retinal vessels may also appear to be more tortuous than normal. It may be impossible to obtain a clear focus of the disc margins by direct ophthalmoscopy. This may be accomplished, however, by the indirect method, and the condition thus differentiated from a true optic nerve neuritis. The remainder of the fundus may appear normal, and the visual fields are normal. When there is an associated hyperopia or astigmatism of high degree, the refractive error should be accurately corrected.

Hereditary Optic Neuritis (Hereditary Optic Atrophy) (Leber's Disease).—Leber's disease is a hereditary and familial disease of the optic nerve which has been described as a subacute retrobulbar neuritis and optic neuritis. It is usually seen in young adults up to the age of 30 or 40 years and affects males much more frequently than females. Cases have been traced through a number of generations.

The ocular symptoms are characterized by a rather sudden and rapid loss of vision. Both eyes are usually affected, although not necessarily simultaneously at the onset. Usually the central vision decreases to a certain point after which the condition might become stationary. The peripheral vision is usually good, and the patients can go about alone fairly well. They scarcely ever become totally blind.

Examination of the fundus usually reveals a grayish-red color of the optic nerve head. When the patient first comes to the attention of the physician, the optic nerve head is already in the atrophic stage. It seems that the optic neuritis which was present earlier is probably one of low grade, and is scarcely ever observed. There may be no other pathology seen.

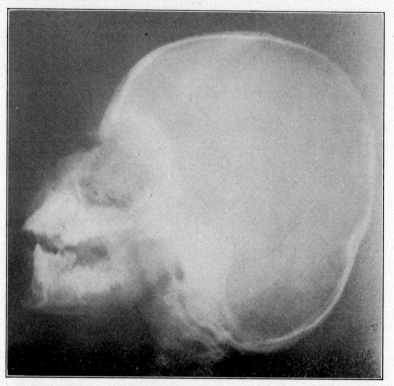

Fig. 115.—Microcephalic skull of a child with congenital optic atrophy. (Clinic of Dr. W. H. Harrison, Wills Hospital.)

Examination of the visual fields reveals a central scotoma which is usually rather large, round, and sometimes irregular. According to Traquair, the defect is approximately pericentral in position. It is usually dense and absolute. The peripheral vision for color and white is impaired, but a fair-sized white test object may show a normal field.

The specific cause of Leber's disease is not known, but it has been attributed to a transitory disturbance of the pituitary gland which makes itself manifest at the particular age period (Fisher). The condition has also been considered to be an abiotrophy. It might be mistaken for a form of toxic amblyopia and must be differentiated from the latter. However, a history of intoxication will probably be lacking, and the visual field changes present characteristics which will differentiate it from tobacco amblyopia and chiasmal changes in particular.

Although it has been reported that some cases recovered, there is no known treatment for the condition.

The Orbit

Anophthalmos, microphthalmos, and similar conditions which might be considered as congenital anomalies of the orbit have been previously described as congenital anomalies of the eyeball.

Cysts of the Orbit.—Dermoids are the commonest form of cyst of the orbit and are congenital, although they may increase in size some time after birth. They are usually superficial and found mostly on the upper border at either angle. They can be palpated under the skin and are found to be freely movable. They may vary in size from a small nodule to the size of a walnut.

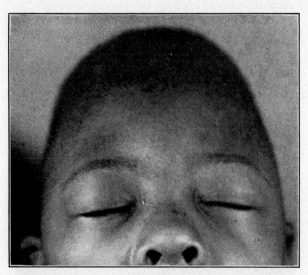

Fig. 116.—Tower skull (oxycephaly). (Wills Hospital.)

A dermoid cyst does not displace the eyeball, but may be prominent and unsightly in appearance. Treatment consists in complete extirpation of the entire cyst, being careful not to collapse the sac which would render complete removal more difficult.

Congenital Vascular Tumors of the Orbit.—Telangiectasis is a congenital form of hemangioma which is located primarily in the eyelids from which it gradually extends into the orbit (Fuchs).

Lymphangiomas of the orbit have been reported by Radnot[40] in two patients, one a boy aged 3 years, and another in a woman aged 34. In the former, a moderate ptosis was present. A bluish-red subconjunctival tumor about the size of a pea was seen under the eyelid. It consisted of endothelium-lined cavities separated by vascular connective tissue septa and contained principally small hemorrhages, transudates, and occasional lymph cells. Considerable pathologic change was found in the blood vessels.

In the case of the woman there was a marked exophthalmos and advanced optic atrophy of long standing. The eyeball and the two large tumor masses were removed, and found to be similar histologically to that in the first case. Pigment cells, fibroblasts, and accumulations of lymphocytes were found. The entire tissue resembled lymphoid tissue because of the large number of lymphocytes. Radnot considered these as congenital tumors having the appearance of lymphoid tumors rather than true lymphangiomas.

Oxycephaly (Tower Skull).—A malformation of the skull due to a premature synostosis of the sutures, principally the coronary or sagittal. This results in a decrease in the anteroposterior diameter of the skull and an increase in the vertical, so that the head of the patient becomes elongated or tower-shaped. With growth and increase in the size of the brain, pressure is exerted by the diminished cranial cavity; as a consequence, there takes place an increase in the intracranial pressure. Pressure is also exerted on the orbit which results in a reduction in the size of the latter with displacement of the eyeball. A reduction in the size and shape of the optic canal has also been found.

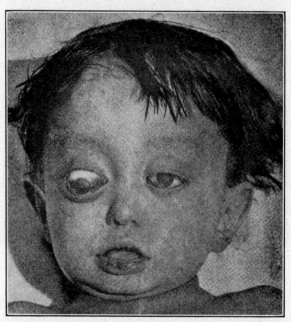

Fig. 117.—Exophthalmos in case of xanthomatosis. (From Heath: Arch. Ophth., January, 1931.)

The eye changes in oxycephaly may, therefore, include exophthalmos of varying degrees. In some cases this may be very marked and accompanied by lagophthalmos with corneal ulceration. A case of complete forward dislocation of the eyeball was reported (Sherne[41]) in a girl aged 8 months. It was explained that spasm of the orbicularis during a fit of crying was so great as to dislocate the globe from the orbit, the resistance from the fascia and muscles being overcome. Divergence of the eyes may occur because of a change in the axis of the orbit, resulting from the malformation. Pressure on the optic nerve because of the narrowing of the orbit and the canal may lead to a pressure atrophy. Atrophy of the optic nerve and blindness may also result from the choked disc sometimes present in this condition. Oxycephaly may be occasionally associated with other anomalies such as syndactyly, highly arched palate, and coloboma of the iris.

Treatment of the condition includes attempts at reduction of intracranial pressure by decompression operations and skull trephine in severe cases. In others, lumbar puncture may be employed. No improvement in vision can be obtained, however, especially when optic atrophy is already present.

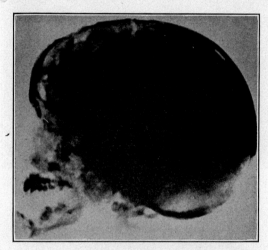

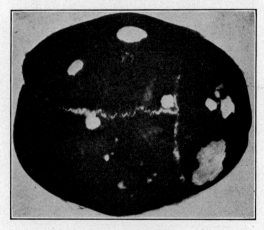

Fig. 118.—Multiple defects in the bones of the skull in xanthomatosis. (From Heath: Arch. Ophth., January, 1931.)

Schüller-Christian-Hand Disease or Syndrome (Xanthomatosis).—A diffuse liporeticular disease of young children which has been designated by various names and which is characterized by degeneration and lipoid deposits in the bones, especially those of the skull, exophthalmos, and diabetes insipidus. The pathologic changes involve the so-called reticulo-endothelial system, and the signs and symptoms follow as a result of the location of deposits and erosion (Heath[42]). Diabetes insipidus is a common symptom, and

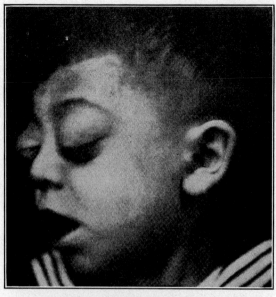

Fig. 119.—Exophthalmos in diabetes insipidus. (From Wheeler: Arch. Ophth., February, 1931.)

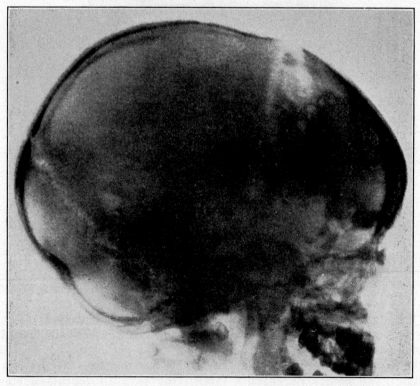

Fig. 120.—Roentgenogram showing defects in skull and destruction of bone in orbital region of case shown in Fig. 119. (From Wheeler: Arch. Ophth., February, 1931.)

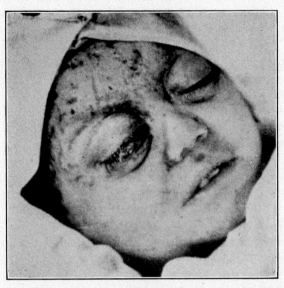

Fig. 121.—Schüller-Christian disease, showing lesions of the skin and bilateral exophthalmos with destruction of right cornea. (From Wheeler: Arch. Ophth., January, 1934.)

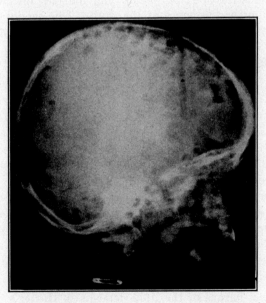
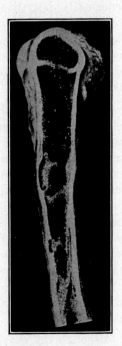

Fig. 122.—Showing changes in bones of skull and xanthomatous invasions of the femur in Schüller-Christian disease. (From Wheeler: Arch. Ophth., January, 1934.)

according to Heath, it results from pressure at the base of the brain and on the hypophysis or from proliferation, storage, or both, within the hypophysis. It has also been accounted for by a lesion of the posterior lobe of the pituitary body.

The exophthalmos is usually bilateral, although it may occur on one side. It might become quite marked and may be accompanied by changes in the optic nerve and retina with loss of sight. Exposure of the cornea due to the marked exophthalmos may lead to ulceration and keratitis. The exophthalmos has been explained as being due to pressure and loss of bony support at the apex of the orbit. Heath considered the ocular signs chiefly as a reaction from a metabolic disease, the pathology affecting the reticuloendothelial system.

The defects in the bones of the skull may be numerous and have been found at autopsy to contain a soft gummy substance which could be removed or pushed out, leaving an irregular hole in the bone.

Wheeler[43] described a case in which the diabetes was very marked, and the defects in the bones of the skull were present as well as marked exophthalmos. He felt that the hyperplastic process which takes place in the disease invades the orbit and causes the exophthalmos. In a case of a 3-year-old white boy, later reported by Wheeler,[44] the necropsy revealed: generalized xanthomatosis of the bones, dura mater, hypophysis, infundibulum, periosteum, orbits, skin, thymus, pleura, lungs, heart, peritoneum, liver, pancreas, lymph glands, splenomegaly, fatty liver ascites, subcutaneous edema.

The diagnosis of this syndrome can, therefore, be readily made in a young child presenting a condition of marked exophthalmos and diabetes insipidus associated with areas of softening in the bones of the skull. This should immediately lead to further study and the diagnosis of the condition as xanthomatosis.

Dysostosis Multiplex (Hurler's Disease)

This is a rare congenital disease also called gargoylism because of the grotesque appearance of the patient. It was first described by Gertrude Hurler in 1919, and since that time about fifty cases have been reported in the literature. The syndrome is also familial in nature and is classed with the diseases in which there is a disturbance of lipoid metabolism with a deposit of the lipidlike material in the tissues. These include Tay-Sachs disease, Niemann-Pick disease, Schüller-Christian-Hand and Gaucher's disease. In Tay-Sachs disease and Niemann-Pick disease, the pathology is found principally in the central nervous system, muscles and glial cells and the deposits are in the form of a phosphotide. In Schüller-Christian-Hand disease the bones are principally involved and there is diabetes insipidus, while the deposits are said to be cholesterol and its esters. Gaucher's disease affects the abdominal organs, principally the liver and spleen and the lipid is kerasin.

Although the exact chemical nature of the lipid deposits in Hurler's disease is not definitely known, it is said to appear in the form of fine, curved, rod-shaped granules and is believed to be a complex compound of lipid and protein. The infiltration occurs principally in the liver, spleen and central nervous system.

The appearance of the patient with dysostosis multiplex is typical and striking, presenting a dwarfed body with a large head and prominent frontal bones. The orbits are widely separated, the nose bridge is flat with wide nares, the neck is short and the tongue thick, flabby and protruding. The bones of the extremities are short and thick and the hands short and stubby. There is a kyphosis and a prominent distended abdomen with an umbilical hernia often present. The bony changes are not due to the lipid disturbance. The liver and spleen are enlarged. At the time of birth the abnormalities other than a possible enlargement of the head may not be evident. During the first

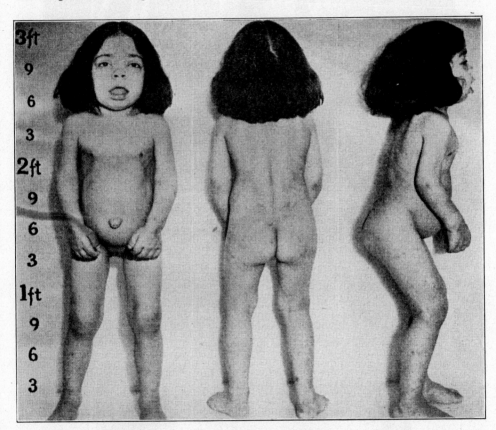

Fig. 123.—Clinical appearance in dysostosis multiplex (Hurler's disease). (From Cordes and Hogan: Arch. Ophth., April, 1942.)

year, however, the patient fails to develop normally and later is unable to walk, talk or eat properly. At the age of about 3 years the dwarfed appearance becomes more evident with failure of development in the long bones and vertebrae. The musculature also develops poorly and there is limitation of motion of the extremities. The sex organs remain infantile. Later there is mental retardation and imbecility. This is due to the infiltration of the nervous system.

The prognosis is poor since in most of the patients death occurs before the age of 20. This usually results from some infection or cardiac failure.

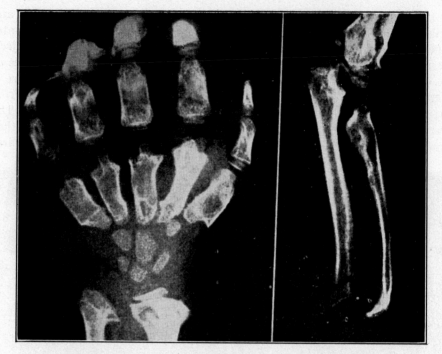

A.

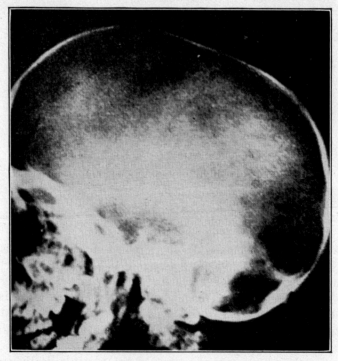

B.

Fig. 124.—*A*, Bony changes in dysostosis multiplex. *B*, Bony changes in skull in dysostosis multiplex. (From Cordes and Hogan: Arch. Ophth., April, 1942.)

Eye Manifestations.—The cornea is the structure of the eye which is involved in this disease. It shows an early diffuse cloudiness with infiltration of the lipid. Berliner[45] reported three such cases which he described as a lipin keratitis after slit-lamp and histologic examination of an eye. The slit lamp in optical section showed the opacification to be composed of a fine yellow-white granular deposit in the deeper corneal layers. Histologically, the lipid deposits were found in the spindle-shaped interlamellar spaces. The remaining structures of the eye are usually not involved. The eyeballs may be prominent, however, and the eyelids may be heavy with the eyes themselves set wide apart.

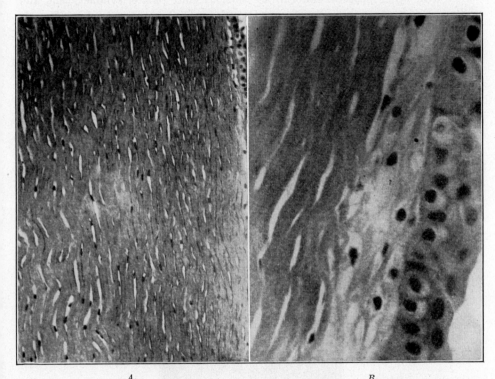

A.   *B.*

Fig. 125.—*A*, Paraffin section, showing thinning of Bowman's membrane and cellular infiltration in lipochondrodystrophy (dysostosis multiplex). Low power lens. *B*, High power. Complete replacement of Bowman's membrane by the large cells. Lipochondrodystrophy (dysostosis multiplex). (From Hogan and Cordes: Arch. Ophth., October, 1944.)

Cordes and Hogan[46] reported five cases in 1942, in all of which both corneas were involved. In four of the patients the findings were identical with those typical of the disease. Two of these patients from different families were twins and in each instance the other twin was unaffected by the disease. Two of the patients reported by Cordes and Hogan later died and the eyes of these patients together with those of a third were examined pathologically. The report stated,[47] "The corneal changes were confined to the region of Bowman's membrane and to the corneal corpuscles. The corneal opacities seen clinically were caused by (a) infiltration of numerous large phagocytic cells into the region of Bowman's membrane, and (b) swelling of the corneal corpuscles."

The phagocytic cells near Bowman's membrane and the corneal corpuscles showed numerous fine granules in their cytoplasm. They were present in frozen sections but were removed by fat solvents which indicated the possibility of their lipid nature. They did not, however, take the usual stains for fat.

Hypertelorism.—Hypertelorism is a congenital anomaly of the face and skull which produces an extreme separation of the orbits and thereby causes the eyes to be far apart. In most cases there is also a divergent squint which exaggerates the large interpupillary distance. The patient may be either normal or defective in mental and physical development. The condition may be associated with other physical deformities, such as cleft palate, syndactylism, and undescended testes, and may show a heredofamilial tendency. According to Weeks,[48] hypertelorism is a developmental defect of the lesser wings of the sphenoid bone which ossify early in intrauterine life and grow excessively, thereby resulting in the typical wide separation of the eyes. A case which occurred in a young woman, aged 31, was described by Berliner and Gartner.[49] The patient had an interpupillary distance of 84 mm. and a marked divergent squint; there was narrowing and malformation of the optic canals and the right eye showed a pallor of the disc, concentric contraction of the visual field, and a relative central scotoma.

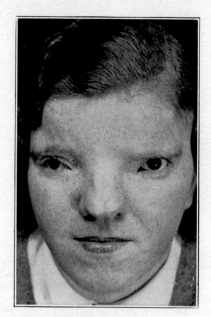

Fig. 126.—Hypertelorism. (From Berliner and Gartner: Arch. Ophth., October, 1940.)

Osteopetrosis (Marble Bones or Albers-Schönberg Disease)

A diffuse osteosclerosis in patients was first demonstrated by roentgenographic studies in 1904 by Albers-Schönberg. It had previously been mentioned in association with leucemia and pseudoleucemia, but after that time it was spoken of as "Albers-Schönberg's disease" and also "marble bones." Later, however, the condition was described as "osteopetrosis." A few of the patients with this disease have optic atrophy. In 1938, Clifton, Frank, and Freeman[50] reported a case in a 5-year-old boy who had bilateral optic atrophy. Later, Vigdoff and Bracher[51] reported a case in a white woman aged 30 years who had optic atrophy with blindness in both eyes. They were able to demonstrate roentgenologically the encroachment of the bony changes on the optic foramina. About 118 cases have been recorded. More recently Riser[52] made a later report on the case of Clifton and associates, especially from the ophthalmologic standpoint. He also differentiated the condition of osteopetrosis in children with optic atrophy from that of adult osteosclerosis in which optic atrophy is not a feature. In the latter condition, the marble bones were considered to be associated with a form of leucemia, showing the blood picture of leucemia and splenic enlargement.

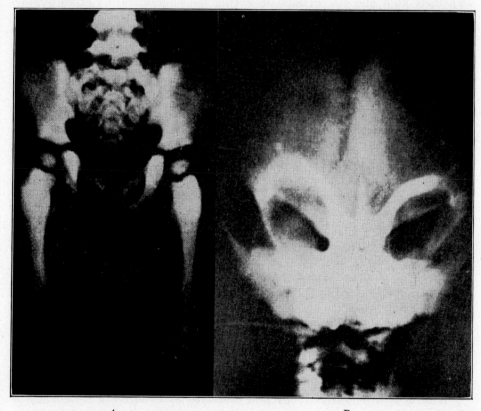

A.　　　　　　　　　　　　　　B.

Fig. 127.—A, Showing increased density, clubbing of long bones, and alternating lines of increased density and decreased density parallel to the epiphysis—marble bones. B, Showing the heaviness of the bones of the face in marble bones. (From Riser: Am. J. Ophth., August, 1941.)

Osteopetrosis is considered to be a disease of early childhood with a decided familial tendency. Parental consanguinity has been recorded in some cases. The patient is usually a child with a square forehead, stocky build, pigeon breast, bowed legs, arrested dentition and optic atrophy since early infancy. Hydrocephalus may be present. The diagnosis is made chiefly by roentgen studies which reveal a generalized increased density of the bones of the entire body with a loss of their normal structure. The shadow of the marrow cavity is reduced and sometimes obliterated. The greatest density is seen in the base of the skull, ends of the long bones, central part of the pelvis and the vertebral bodies. In addition to being more dense, the bones are also more brittle than normal. They are heavy, hard and thick, but their fragility predisposes to multiple fractures which are transverse and painless. In the patient of Clifton and associates roentgenologic evidence of marble bones was found on the tenth day of life and transverse lines of greater and lesser density in the bones were noted as early as the tenth week. They concluded that the process begins in utero.

Metabolic studies showed that a positive calcium balance was maintained with diets high and low in calcium during the administration of ammonium chloride and thyroid and parathyroid extract. The blood picture usually shows an anemia with variations, as well as extramedullary myelopoiesis or hemopoiesis.

There is no specific treatment known for the disease. Therapeutic measures are directed toward the relief of symptoms and the secondary conditions. The prognosis for life is poor in the cases occurring in infants and those who survive are greatly handicapped in their movements.

Eye Manifestations.—The ocular condition of prime importance in this disease is bilateral optic atrophy which, in most cases, occurs early and is an almost constant finding. It is caused by pressure on the optic nerves, probably most pronounced at the optic foramina. Blindness results or, at least, greatly impaired vision and sometimes lowered mentality. Hydrocephalus may be present in some instances.

The optic foramina have been shown in a few cases at autopsy to be narrowed. This has been difficult to demonstrate during life, but was shown roentgenologically in the case reported by Riser and also in the one by Vigdoff and Bracher. Clublike thickening may also involve the posterior clinoid processes with a narrowing of the sella turcica.

In addition to optic atrophy, other eye manifestations reported include ptosis, nystagmus, stabismus, hypertelorism, anisocoria, tortuosity of the retinal vessels and papilledema with hydrocephalus and increased intracranial pressure.

Hereditary Craniofacial Dysostosis (Crouzon's Disease)

A form of osseous dystrophy first described by Crouzon in 1912, which is hereditary in nature and characterized by cranial and facial deformities. Atkinson,[53] who published a review of the subject, described the distinctive characteristics as (1) cranial deformities; (2) facial malformations; (3) eye changes; (4) heredity.

The condition is not common and is first observed in the young infant. As the child develops, the appearance is rather typical of the craniofacial deformity. The frontal region is prominent and the anteroposterior ridge overhangs the frontal prominence and sometimes passes to the root of the nose. The head is brachycephalic with a large transverse diameter. There is an early synostosis of the frontal sutures and a basilar kyphosis. The upper jaw is underdeveloped, while the lower jaw is protruding. No satisfactory explanation has been given for the condition.

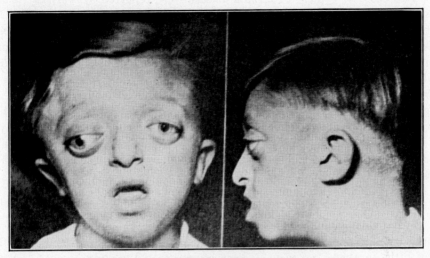

Fig. 128.—Patient with hereditary craniofacial dysostosis. (From Vorisek: Am. J. Ophth., September, 1941.)

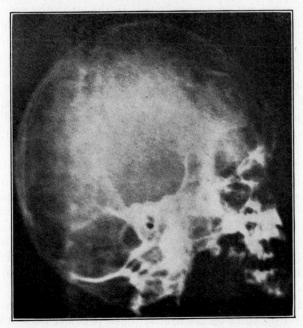

Fig. 129.—Skull roentgenograph in hereditary craniofacial dysostosis, showing decompression defect and digitations. (From Vorisek: Am. J. Ophth., September, 1941.)

Eye Manifestations.—There is usually a hypertelorism with divergence of the eyes and limitation of rotation outward. The eyes are proptosed and exophthalmos nearly always exists. The palpebral fissures are wide. Strabismus is nearly always present. Nystagmus is also common.

The optic nerve head may show an optic neuritis or choked disc, and blindness may result in one or both eyes.

Two cases of typical Crouzon's disease were reported by Vorisek,[54] in one of which a decompression of both cranium and orbit was performed. This patient, a 2-year-old boy, had excessive proptosis, marked hypertelorism, divergent strabismus and choked discs. At the age of 2½ years a decompression of the right orbit and the right subtemporal region was performed. This child, at the age of 7, showed considerable improvement in the degree of proptosis and in the ocular rotations. The condition of the optic discs was also improved. The second patient presented a moderate exophthalmos with both optic discs moderately elevated and both margins blurred and dirty gray in color. The vision seemed to be fair and the mentality normal. Decompressions were contemplated for this patient also. No other form of treatment has been recommended for the condition.

Congenital and Hereditary Conditions of the Nervous System

Nystagmus.—Congenital nystagmus should probably be regarded as the result, or manifestation, of some other congenital or hereditary condition. Very little or almost no visual power is present. A certain amount is necessary, however, in true nystagmus and the aimless movements which occur in totally blind eyes are not true nystagmus. In the latter the eyes can be seen to swing back and forth while in the primary position, making short, rapid and regular movements. These may take place in a lateral, horizontal, or rotary direction. The condition is always bilateral.

Congenital nystagmus is sometimes called visual nystagmus and results from conditions causing great loss of vision in both eyes, before or at the time of birth. Any of the ocular conditions, such as congenital cataracts, abnormalities in the retina or choroid, congenital opacities on the cornea, and other diseases causing almost total loss of vision at birth, might produce so-called congenital nystagmus.

Diseases of the brain and nervous system are also frequently responsible for the presence of nystagmus. In such diseases as hereditary ataxia, Little's disease (cerebral diplegia), and in some forms of idiocy, nystagmus is commonly found. In this form of nystagmus, head nodding is also sometimes found to be present. Spasmus nutans is a condition in which head nodding has been observed in infants in combination with nystagmus, during the first two years of life. Most observers have considered this, however, to be an acquired condition as the result of rickets and after being kept in darkened rooms.

Congenital Hydrocephalus.—Characterized by an enlargement of the head which produces a pressure on the orbits. Such pressure may cause downward rotation of the eyeballs with diminished vision. Optic atrophy is a common finding in this condition. The occurrence of papilloedema and optic neuritis in congenital hydrocephalus is considered as rare.

Mongolian Idiocy.—A very rare condition occasionally seen in very young children, principally of foreign birth, which is characterized by abnormalities of the eyelids and the orbits. The palpebral fissures are narrow and slant downward slightly toward the nose. The facial appearance as a result is peculiar, being accentuated by the fact that the mouth is nearly always open. The patients are mentally deficient or imbecilic and may present other anatomic abnormalities.

Congenital Myotonia.—Sometimes called myotonia congenita, a hereditary disease found in young children who present a spasm of the voluntary muscles which also affects the eyelids. Jerky movements are noted which are followed by a slow relaxation of the orbicularis, in opening and closing the eyelids.

Myotonia Atrophica (Dystrophia Myotonica).—A familial and hereditary disease sometimes called dystrophia myotonica. There occurs a wasting of the muscles of the face which produces a peculiar facial appearance. An atrophy of the muscles of the upper extremities and thighs also takes place. Cataract is a common ocular finding in this condition and may be found at a comparatively early age, usually 20 to 30 years. These cataracts may in some instances be the only sign of the disease and can be successfully removed by operation.

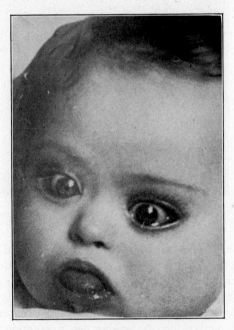

Fig. 130.—Mongolian idiocy.

Allen and Barer[55] who reported on twenty-two patients with dystrophia myotonica observed the lenticular changes in each case in which a biomicroscopic examination was made. Some of the patients offered no complaint of visual acuity. The early changes in the lens were found to occur in the anterior and posterior cortical layers close to the capsule. Many tiny, grayishwhite opacities are scattered between iridescent crystals, either in the superficial cortex or along the suture lines. Star-shaped figures may be found at the anterior and posterior poles. The posterior opacities usually occur earlier and are further advanced than the anterior. This was found to occur in all but one case.

In some cases the changes progress more rapidly than in others. The deeper layers of the cortex are involved with fine dustlike opacities and iridescent crystals which are followed after a while by water slits, lamellar separation and vacuolation, and development of a soft cataract with a small nucleus.

Both eyes are usually affected, with the rate of development nearly the same in each, although one may be more advanced than the other.

Other manifestations of the disease in the eyes were found to be ptosis which is nearly always present. Ectropion was an occasional finding and enophthalmos was manifest because of the loss of orbital fat.

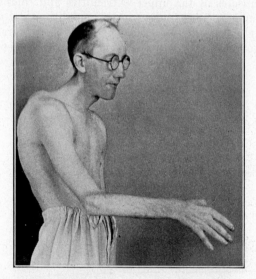

Fig. 131.—Patient with dystrophia myotonica, showing atrophy of muscles of forearms and hand. (From Allen and Barer: Arch. Ophth., November, 1940.)

Little's Disease (Cerebral Diplegia).—A congenital disease sometimes called congenital spastic paralysis was described by Little as a condition resulting from hemorrhages occurring during difficult labor. There is a mental impairment in these patients, with a rigidity or spasticity of the extremities which occurs shortly after birth. Usually, the lower extremities are affected first. The common ocular manifestations are nystagmus, ocular deviations, and optic atrophy. The condition has also been attributed to a defect in development which affects the cortical cells.

Friedreich's Ataxia.—A hereditary ataxia which is familial in type and which affects the cells of the postero-lateral column and cerebellar tracts. It is characterized by an ataxia of the upper and lower extremities and other deformities, such as scoliosis, speech defects, and absent or very weak knee and ankle reflexes.

The most common eye symptom in this condition is nystagmus which usually occurs in a lateral direction. Other ocular manifestations occasionally found are optic atrophy, paralysis of the external ocular muscles, and abnormal pupillary reactions.

Sanger-Brown's Ataxia.—A hereditary ataxia which affects the cells of the posterior column, spinocerebellar tracts, and Clark's column. The ocular findings are usually optic atrophy, ocular deviations with diplopia, ptosis, and ophthalmoplegia. Retinitis pigmentosa has also been occasionally observed.

Hereditary Cerebellar Ataxia (Marie's Ataxia).—A hereditary form of ataxia in which the eye signs are absence of the pupillary reflex, similar to the Argyll Robertson pupil, and decreased central vision with the accompanying field changes.

Congenital Word Blindness.—This condition is usually discovered when a child reaches school age, or later, and is characterized by an inability to read. It may vary from a total inability to read anything, to the recognition of certain letters of the alphabet. Numbers are usually recognized by such patients more readily. When the disability is first revealed, the patient is apt to be considered below the average in intelligence. On the contrary, however, they may excel in certain other subjects and might show ability along mechanical lines. The etiology has been described as a congenital impairment or developmental defect in the visual memory center in the left angular and supramarginal gyrus.

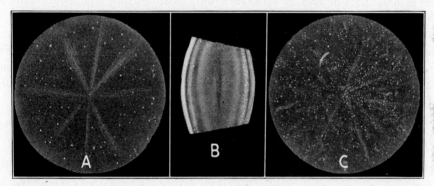

Fig. 132.—Early lens changes in dystrophia myotonica. *A*, Anterior subcapsular opacities. *B*, Schematic optic section of lens. *C*, Posterior subcapsular opacities. (From Allen and Barer: Arch. Ophth., November, 1940.)

Congenital word blindness is probably more common than might be assumed. A number of these cases might be overlooked in routine examinations, and the attention of the examiner can easily be misdirected.

The eyes reveal nothing of a pathologic nature, and the refraction is also found to be normal. It has been found to occur much more commonly in male than in female children.

The treatment includes efforts to overcome the defect by teaching the patient to read. This has been accomplished to a satisfactory degree in some cases, but requires a great amount of effort, individual training, and continued persistence on the part of special teachers.

Mirror-Writing.—A few children in early school years have exhibited a desire to reverse their writing or script. In other words, their tendency is to write "backward." They do this involuntarily at first, but in most cases these patients can be taught to write normally. They may come to the attention of the ophthalmologist for examination, but the eyes, on examination, will be found normal. The cause of the condition is not definitely known.

Congenital Color Blindness.—Color blindness may occur either alone or in association with other congenital or hereditary changes in the eye. It may occur as the result of degenerations and anomalies which were present in the eyes in members of former generations. In other words, it is a recessive symptom in these instances. The condition is familial and has been traced through a number of generations of the same family. Consanguinity is said to play an important part, and the condition is also sex linked. The color blindness may be present in some in association with such other lesions as congenital macular degeneration, pigmentary retinosis, and nystagmus. In a great many cases the eyes will be found normal in every other respect. The latter have been considered to be of central origin.

Red-green blindness is perhaps the most common form encountered, and quite often a patient himself is not aware of his own defect. These cases have a way of their own of interpreting standard or common objects which are colored. They might designate the color correctly after having learned how to interpret the color in which they are defective. Sometimes the color blindness is only partial and is concerned only with certain shades of standard colors. The basic color itself might be recognized or designated correctly.

In certain occupations a normal color sense is of utmost importance, and this is true especially among railroad workers and drivers of trucks and automobiles. Those with partial color blindness, especially, may be trained to recognize and designate the color properly, even though they see the color differently from those who are normal in this respect.

References

Lacrimal Apparatus

1. Goar, Everett, L.: Congenital Absence of the Lacrimal Puncta and of the Canaliculi, Arch. Ophth. **6:** 724, November, 1931.
2. Charamis, J.: Two Cases of Anomalies of the Lacrymal Passages, Arch. d'opht. **48:** 216, March, 1931.
3. Schornstein, T.: Congenital Fistula of the Lacrimal Gland, Arch. f. Augenh. **109:** 86, 1935.
4. Silverman, S.: Microphthalmos With Congenital Defect of the Lacrimal Apparatus, Brit. J. Ophth. **17:** 351, June, 1933.

Eyelids

5. deSchweinitz, G. E.: Complete Bilateral Congenital Exterior Ophthalmoplegia and Double Ptosis, Arch. Ophth. **5:** 15, January, 1931.
6. Horner, W. D., and Cordes, F. C.: Congenital Coloboma of the Upper Eyelid With Dermoids of the Cornea, Am. J. Ophth. **12:** 959, December, 1929.
7. Spaeth, Edmund B.: Congenital Colobomata of the Lower Lid, Am. J. Ophth. **24:** 186, February, 1941.

Eyeball

8. Vail, D. T., Jr.: Adult Hereditary Anterior Megalophthalmos, Tr. Sect. on Ophth. A. M. A., June, 1931.
9. Abelsdorff, G.: Heredity in Keratoconus, Arch. f. Augenh. **103:** 293, June, 1930.
10. Kingery, L. B.: Ichthyosis Congenita With Unusual Complications, Arch. Dermat. and Syph. **13:** 90, January, 1926.
11. Cordes, F. C., and Hogan, M. J.: Ocular Ichthyosis, Arch. Ophth. **22:** 590, October, 1939.
12. Vail, Derrick: Corneal Involvement in Congenital Ichthyosis (Keratoderma), Arch. Ophth. **24:** 215, July, 1940.

Ocular Muscles

13. Phillips, William H., Dirion, Josephine K., and Graves, Grant O.:   Congenital Bilateral Palsy of the Abducens, Arch. Ophth. **8**: 355, September, 1932.
14. Laughlin, R. C.:   Hereditary Paralysis of Abducens Nerve, Am. J. Ophth. **20**: 396, April, 1937.
15. Hicks, Avery M.:   Congenital Paralysis of Lateral Rotators of Eyes With Paralysis of Muscles of Face, Arch. Ophth. **30**: 38, 1943.
16. Mengel, Willard G.:   Bilateral   Congenital Deficiency of Abduction With Retraction (Duane Syndrome), Arch. Ophth. **13**: 981, June, 1935.
17. Zentmayer, William: Ann. Ophth. **24**: 30, January, 1915, and in discussion of Mengel's case.

Sclera

18. Dessoff, J.:   Blue Sclerotics, Fragile Bones and Deafness, Arch. Ophth. **12**: 60, July, 1934.
19. Rados, A., and Rosenberg, L. C.:   Relation Between Blue Sclera and Hyperparathyroidism, Arch. Ophth. **16**: 8, July, 1936.

Iris

20. Neher, E. M.:   Aniridia Congenita, Irideremia, Am. J. Ophth. **21**: 293, March, 1938.

Lens

21. Lloyd, Ralph I.:   Arachnodactyly (Marfan's Syndrome), Arch. Ophth. **13**: 744, May, 1935.
22. Laval, Joseph: Bilateral Congenital Ectopia Lentis With Arachnodactyly (Marfan's Syndrome), Arch. Ophth. **20**: 371, September, 1938.
23. Rados, Andrew: Marfan's Syndrome (Arachnodactyly Coupled With Dislocation of the Lens), Arch. Ophth. **27**: 477, 1942.
24. Nettleship, E.:   London Ophth. Hosp. Rep. **17**: 389, October, 1905.

Vitreous

25. Cassady, J. V.:   Congenital Cyst of the Vitreous, Arch. Ophth. **21**: 45, January, 1939.
26. Mann, I., and Macrae, A.:   Congenital Vascular Veils in the Vitreous, Brit. J. Ophth. **22**: 1, January, 1938.

Retina

27. Weve, H.:   Brit. J. Ophth. **22**: 456, August, 1938.
28. Edgerton, Ambrose E.:   Ocular Observations of New-Born, Arch. Ophth. **11**: 938, May, 1934.
29. Perera, Charles A.:   Congenital Grouped Pigmentation of the Retina, Arch. Ophth. **21**: 108, January, 1939.
30. Gouterman, Joseph I., and Winkelman, N. W.:   Tay-Sachs Disease, Tr. Am. Acad. Ophth., 1930.
31. Goldstein, Isadore, and Wexler, David: Nieman-Pick's Disease With Cherry-Red Spot in the Macula, Arch. Ophth. **5**: 704, May, 1931.
32. Bedell, A.:   Am. J. Ophth. **14**: 389, 1931.
33. McDonald, Robb, and Lippincott, Stuart, W.:   Angiomatosis Retinae, Arch. Ophth. **20**: 958, December, 1938.
34. Cordes, Frederick C., and Hogan, Michael J.:   Angiomatosis Retinae, Arch. Ophth. **23**: 253, February, 1940.
35. Cordes, F. C., and Dickson, O. C.:   Angiomatosis Retinae (von Hippel's Disease). Results Following Irradiation of Three Eyes, Am. J. Ophth. **26**: 454, 1943.
36. Guyton, Jack S., and McGovern, Francis H.:   Diathermy Coagulation in the Treatment of Angiomatosis Retinae, Am. J. Ophth. **26**: 675, 1943.
37. MacDonald, Alexander E.:   Lindau's Disease, Arch. Ophth. **23**: 564, March, 1940.
38. Lowenstein, A., and Steel, J.:   Retinal Tuberous Sclerosis, Am. J. Ophth. **24**: 731, 1941.

Optic Nerve

39. Shipman, James S.:   Coloboma of the Optic Nerve Associated With Posterior Lenticonus, Arch. Ophth. **11**: 503, March, 1934.

Orbit

40. Radnot, M.:   Arch. f. Ophth. **140**: 328, April, 1939.
41. Sherne, J.:   Brit. M. J. **1**: 565, March, 1938.
42. Heath, Parker: Xanthomatosis or Lipoid Histocytosis, Arch. Ophth **5**: 29, January, 1931.

43. Wheeler, John M.: Exophthalmos Associated With Diabetes Insipidus and Large Defects in the Bones of the Skull, Arch. Ophth. 5: 161, February, 1931.
44. Wheeler, John M.: Schüller-Christian-Hand Disease (Xanthomatosis), Arch. Ophth. 11: 214, January, 1934.
45. Berliner, M. L.: Lipin Keratitis of Hurler's Syndrome (Gargoylism or Dysostosis Multiplex), Arch. Ophth. 22: 97, 1939.
46. Hogan, M. J., and Cordes, F. C.: Dysostosis Multiplex (Hurler's Disease), Arch. Ophth. 27: 637, 1942.
47. Cordes, F. C., and Hogan, M. J.: Lipochondrodystrophy, Arch. Ophth. 32: 287, 1944.
48. Weeks, Webb W.: Ocular Hypertelorism: Report of a Case, Arch. Ophth. 20: 683, October, 1938.
49. Berliner, Milton L., and Gartner, Samuel: Hypertelorism, Arch. Ophth. 24: 691, October, 1940.
50. Clifton, W. M., Frank, A. A., and Freeman, S.: Osteopetrosis (Marble Bones), Am. J. Dis. Child. 56: 1020, 1938.
51. Vigdoff, B., and Bracher, G. L.: Osteopetrosis, Am. J. Roentgenol. and Rad. Therapy 44: 197, 1940.
52. Riser, R. O.: Marble Bones and Optic Atrophy, Am. J. Ophth. 24: 874, 1941.
53. Atkinson, F. R. B.: Hereditary Craniofacial Dysostosis or Crouzon's Disease, The Medical Press 195: 118, 1937.
54. Vorisek, E. A.: Hereditary Craniofacial Dysostosis, Am. J. Ophth. 24: 1014, 1941.

Nervous System

55. Allen, J. H., and Barer, C. G.: Cataract of Dystrophia Myotonica, Arch. Ophth. 24: 867, November, 1940.

CHAPTER VII

INFECTIONS AND INFECTIOUS DISEASES

The close relationship existing between internal diseases affecting the various organs and systems of the body is generally recognized. Thus, the diseases of the cardiovascular system are closely identified with those of the kidney and brain, and diseases of the endocrine glands are intimately associated with disorders of the autonomic nervous system and the diseases of metabolism. Then again, the disorders of the female generative organs and of pregnancy often occur with dysfunction of the endocrine glands, while a number of the diseases of the skin are apparently associated with nutritional disorders and digestive disturbances.

The infections and infectious diseases may occur in a number of different ways and result from various causative agents. They also present manifestations either simultaneously or at various periods throughout their course, in a number of different organs and systems of the body. Their classification is, therefore, sometimes difficult. Here, they will be described, as nearly as possible, according to the nature and type of the infection. Other diseases, which in many instances are degenerative in nature and effect, are described according to the organ or systems involved by the disease process. In a few instances, however, the disease is designated according to the causative nature, as illustrated by pellagra which is grouped with the diseases of nutrition and avitaminosis, although its manifestations are chiefly dermatologic.

ACUTE INFECTIOUS DISEASES

Scarlet Fever (Scarlatina)

An acute infectious disease which is considered to be caused by a hemolytic streptococcus and which is characterized by rapid onset of chills, headaches, fever, a cutaneous eruption over the face and body, and signs of general infection in some cases. The disease commonly affects children although it does occur, but more rarely, among adults. It occurs principally in the winter months in epidemics, although in certain localities it may be endemic. The portal of entry is undoubtedly through the nasopharynx. In children the disease may assume a mild form, while in adults it may cause severe prostration. It should be differentiated from measles, rubella, small pox, chicken pox, diphtheria, and drug rashes.

Eye Manifestations.—Eye manifestations are similar to those occurring in the eyes in measles. The most common form of ocular involvement is hyperemia of the conjunctiva and conjunctivitis. These are more common in children and occur early in the disease. The bulbar and palpebral conjunctiva especially is found to be uniformly reddened and congested. The eyes are "watery" and some photophobia may also be present. The patient may have conjunctivitis during the entire period of convalescence and even later. In some cases, the conjunctivitis may be more severe and has been at times described as a "streptococcic" or "diphtheritic" type.

The cornea may become involved with the occurrence of ulcus serpens. This may progress and involve a considerable portion of the cornea with resulting impairment of vision to a corresponding degree.

Involvement of the ocular muscles is rare, and ocular palsies are infrequent. Optic neuritis also occurs rarely.

The orbit may become involved with the occurrence of orbital cellulitis and orbital abscess. As a result the lids are found to be swollen and edematous with noticeable redness and edema of the conjunctiva. In marked cases the eyeball may be displaced. These complications usually occur, however, when the nasal sinuses have become involved as a result of the infection.

The retina is usually free of any pathology in an uncomplicated case of scarlet fever, but in the presence of nephritic complications, it is quite possible to find secondary lesions in the retina characterized by nephritic retinitis and blindness from uremia, should this occur.

Treatment consists principally in protection for the eyes and avoiding exposure to strong light. Conjunctivitis may require active treatment according to the severity of the case. In the state of ordinary congestion or hyperemia of the conjunctiva, a mild wash, such as boric acid or normal saline, may be employed about three times daily and can be followed by the instillation of one drop of zinc sulfate, 0.5 per cent to 1 per cent. More than this may not be required unless the condition is prolonged or the result of a smear reveals the presence of streptococcus. A stronger solution, such as mercurophen 1:10,000 or metaphen, may be employed as a wash or by instillation. In severe cases a solution of 2 per cent silver nitrate can be applied to the everted lids after the instillation of one drop of a local anesthetic. This may be repeated once every other day or so, but should not be continued for any length of time.

Corneal involvement, especially the presence of ulcus serpens, requires active treatment by the instillation of atropine, 1 per cent solution, one drop two or three times a day. Hot applications or hot packs should also be used about three times daily for about ten minutes each time. For corneal infections, Gifford recommends early touching of the involved area with trichloracetic acid with a wisp of cotton on the pointed tip of an applicator. Tincture of iodine may also be applied to the ulcer once a day. The local treatment may be supplemented by nonspecific protein therapy if necessary. If the infection progresses in the cornea, it might be necessary to employ more radical procedures, such as paracentesis of the anterior chamber or delimiting keratotomy.

Whooping Cough (Pertussis)

An acute, infectious and contagious disease characterized by severe paroxysms of coughing which terminate in a "whoop." The disease is common among children, but it may also affect adults. It is considered to be caused by a bacillus pertussis. The portal of entry is through the nasopharynx to the larynx. The patient may not be generally affected to any great extent, except during the paroxysms of coughing. The condition may last for many weeks and will subside very gradually.

Eye Manifestations.—These are few in number and severity. They include, principally, hemorrhages which occur in the conjunctiva and eyelids. These may be fairly common here and are more rarely found in the orbit, anterior chamber, and retina.

The hemorrhages are in all probability due to rupture of small vessels from the extreme pressure exerted during the violent paroxysm of coughing. The veins of the neck and head are usually greatly distended by the great effort made in coughing with an overdistention in the smallest terminal vessels, so that it is not uncommon for a rupture to occur. These hemorrhages may be small or rather extensive and may cover a large portion of the lids or conjunctiva. They may remain for a considerable length of time, gradually changing color and eventually fading out. When a hemorrhage occurs in the anterior chamber, it can be seen by direct and oblique illumination. It will cause a marked interference with vision but will gradually be absorbed.

Typhoid Fever

An acute, specific, infectious disease caused by the *Bacillus typhosus*. It has an insidious onset and is characterized principally by fever, leucopenia, bradycardia, enlarged spleen, and a characteristic skin eruption. Headache, malaise, lethargy, and anorexia are common symptoms. The eruption is characterized by rose spots usually found over the abdomen. These are small pink papules which fade out on pressure. The portal of entry is usually the gastrointestinal system via food and drink which is contaminated. The disease may manifest gastrointestinal symptoms, respiratory symptoms, hemorrhages, and symptoms of an affected central nervous system. A bacteriemia occurs early, and as a result, secondary lesions may occur in many organs.

Eye Manifestations.—These are not frequent in occurrence, but ulcers of the cornea may be found as well as iritis, metastatic choroiditis, and optic neuritis. Of 253 cases, Uhtoff found seventeen cases or 6.5 per cent of optic neuritis. Both eyes may be involved about the second or third week, or even later in the disease. With the ophthalmoscope the optic disc can be seen in this stage to be blurred around the margins. There may be a slight amount of edema around the disc or the surrounding retina (neuroretinitis). This may be due to the toxemia, or it may be secondary to cerebral involvement. The visual fields may vary with enlargement of the blind spot or the presence of a central scotoma.

In rare instances metastatic ophthalmia with loss of an eye or embolus of the central artery of the retina may occur. Sudden loss of vision in the affected eye may result from dislodgment of a septic embolus in endocarditis following typhoid fever.

Ocular palsies, hemorrhages in the conjunctiva, lids, and orbit may also occur. The ocular palsy will be indicated by inability on the part of the patient to rotate the eye in the direction of the affected muscle. Inflammation and abscess of Tenon's capsule may occur and will be indicated by pain on rotation of the eye, tenderness on palpation, and redness and swelling of the affected area.

Treatment.—This will depend, of course, on the nature of the particular form of eye involvement presented. Corneal ulcer and iritis can be treated locally along the same lines. Atropine sulfate, 1 per cent solution, should be instilled into the affected eye two or three times a day. Hot packs or hot compresses should be employed for about ten or fifteen minutes three times daily. This tends to ease pain which might be present and at the same time has a healing effect on the cornea. Meanwhile, the atropine instillations keep the pupil open and prevent adhesions of the iris which would otherwise occur because of the inflammatory process. The tension in the affected eye should be watched during the period of treatment.

Optic neuritis, ocular palsies, and metastatic choroiditis are difficult to treat locally since their extent and improvement depend on the course of the systemic involvement. With improvement in the general condition of the patient, they will also improve and gradually subside.

Apply hot compresses locally for hemorrhages in the skin and conjunctiva in order to promote absorption. Hot compresses may also be employed to quiet the pain resulting from the inflammation and abscess of Tenon's capsule. This should be done guardedly, however, in the presence of septic infection in the eye, since it is possible to spread the infection by the increased congestion and chemosis. Cleansing and antiseptic eyewashes, such as boric acid solution or mercurophen solution (1:10,000), can be used.

Influenza (La Grippe)

An acute infectious disease, endemic in origin and characterized by a nasopharyngeal catarrh and severe general reaction. It is readily complicated by pneumonia. The name is often applied to any severe infection of the nasopharynx with moderate or severe general symptoms which cannot be otherwise diagnosed. It is said to be caused by the *Bacillus influenzae* or *Hemophilus influenzae* and recently a filtrable virus has also been considered to play an important role in the etiology of the disease. The mucous membrane of the nasopharynx and respiratory tract is the portal of entry.

The primary pathologic lesion is a diffuse catarrhal inflammation of the whole respiratory tract. The paranasal sinuses, middle ear, and mastoid may also become involved.

At the onset the symptoms are chilly sensations, or rigor, fever, and prostration. Headache, pains in the limbs, signs of catarrhal nasopharyngitis, laryngitis, and tracheitis are present. Unproductive cough, flushed face, and an injected conjunctiva are likewise symptoms. The temperature usually ranges from 100° to 103°. Bronchitis is frequent, and bronchopneumonia is a common complication.

Eye Manifestations.—Almost any of the ocular structures may become involved during or following an attack of influenza. About 7 per cent of the cases show manifestations in the eye.

The *eyelids* may be affected by abscesses. These are rather frequent in occurrence. They may be single or multiple and vary in size and extent. They are rather superficial and can be readily seen and diagnosed on external examination.

These abscesses may fluctuate and become tense, causing pain and pressure. In this stage the treatment would consist of incision and drainage of the pus contained in them. They can be dressed with gauze eye pads soaked in boric acid solution or normal saline. They can then be treated as a superficial abscess in any other location.

The *lacrimal sac* may become infected in influenza with a resultant dacryocystitis. It is characterized by an accumulation of pus or mucopus between the lids of the affected eye, and on closer examination, the pus can be seen to come from the punctum at the inner third of the lid margin when gentle but firm pressure is made over the area of the lacrimal sac.

The treatment of this condition will depend greatly on the degree of infection of the sac and the time of occurrence of the complication. If it is present before the patient has entirely recovered from the attack of influenza, it is necessary to treat the condition by palliative measures, attempting to keep the eye clear of pus coming from the infected sac. This can be done by flushing the eye regularly throughout the day with solutions of boric acid, normal saline, or mercurophen. When the general condition of the patient permits, the lacrimal sac itself, if the discharge is purulent, can be flushed by using a special irrigator containing normal saline solution or mercurophen solution. To do this the punctum must first be sufficiently dilated, after which the tip or needle of the irrigator is inserted well into the canaliculus and the solution gently forced into the sac from the syringe, thereby slowly washing out the pus. This should be repeated as often as is necessary. If the condition of the patient does not permit this procedure's being carried out, an effort can be made to express the pus by gentle but firm upward massage with the finger over the region of the sac. This can be done several times a day. In the case of a severely infected lacrimal sac, it is necessary to remove the latter in its entirety by operative procedure. This cannot be done until the general condition of the patient warrants an operation, and the type of operative procedure employed would be determined by the ophthalmologist in charge of the case.

The *conjunctiva and cornea* are probably the most frequently involved in influenza. The conjunctivitis often found here is caused by the influenza bacillus which can be detected in the smear from the conjunctiva. The bulbar conjunctiva may be reddened and congested, or a mild mucopurulent accumulation may be present. The lids are often pasted and difficult to separate, especially after awakening from sleep. Both eyes are usually affected, but the condition may start in one eye and spread to the other. It may last for one or two weeks and then disappear, or it may occasionally become chronic and be troublesome to the patient for a much longer time. A serious complication is involvement of the cornea by ulceration.

The treatment of the conjunctivitis should supplement the treatment of the infectious disease. The eyes should be protected from light and dust by wearing dark glasses. In mild cases flushing the eyes with a solution of boric acid several times a day is sufficient treatment. Puffed or swollen lids may be reduced by the use of cold, wet compresses over the eye. These may be made of gauze or absorbent cotton squeezed in the solution and may be employed as often as is necessary. A mucoid or mucopurulent discharge may be treated with silver nitrate, two to four grains to the ounce, applied to the inner surface of the lids by means of an applicator. More serious cases may require the use of a stronger solution, up to ten grains to the ounce, the application of which should be followed by flushing with normal saline solution. In some cases other drugs, such as metaphen, zinc sulfate, grain two to one ounce, and acriflavine may also be employed.

The cornea is often affected in influenza by herpes, and less frequently, by a parenchymatous keratitis. These may affect only one eye and might, in rare instances, be associated with iritis or iridocyclitis. A parenchymatous keratitis is slow in onset and might not occur until after the attack of influenza has subsided. It is accompanied in the beginning by a rather pronounced pain which may last for several days. Small erosions and even ulcerations may take place on the surface. The episcleral vessels may be injected, and the stroma of the cornea itself will become hazy showing fine precipitates.

Treatment of the corneal involvement is the same in this case as in other corneal infections, namely, rest, the application of hot compresses soaked in boric acid solution, instillation of 1 per cent atropine sulfate solution, two or three times a day, and flushing the eye with a mild antiseptic solution. Strong solutions of iodine are applied to the affected portion of the cornea in herpetic keratitis. A corneal complication may require several weeks before healing, and an opacity might result in the portion of the cornea which was involved.

Iritis, Iridocyclitis, Uveitis.—These complications are more rare but may be seen in isolated cases. The onset of iritis is characterized by severe pain in the affected eye which grows worse at night. The pupil is small, and the conjunctiva is injected around the limbus of the cornea which is tender to the pressure of a finger on the upper lid directly over the limbus. Usually the ciliary body shows signs of inflammation at the same time or shortly after the involvement of the iris. In fact, the entire uveal tract may become involved at the same time. When this occurs, examination with the ophthalmoscope and slit lamp will show the posterior surface of the cornea to be covered with varying degrees of inflammatory deposits, and the vitreous will be found to be infiltrated. Metastatic ophthalmia may also occur.

The treatment of iritis and iridocyclitis consists of instillations of atropine sulfate, 1 per cent solution, one drop three times a day. Hot compresses made of gauze or absorbent cotton and soaked in boric acid solution should also be employed here. By keeping the pupils dilated with atropine solution, adhesions of the iris (synechiae) are prevented, and gradually the condition will subside with recovery from the source of infection. A local anesthetic, such as pontocain, 1 per cent solution, may also be instilled as required for the pain. When uveitis occurs, the condition usually runs a prolonged course.

The *retina* and *vitreous* might be the seat of hemorrhages which can be seen on examination with the ophthalmoscope. These are comparatively rare in this disease.

The Optic Nerve.—*Optic neuritis* usually occurs during the period of convalescence from the disease. This can be observed with the ophthalmoscope when the margins of the optic disc are found to be blurred in outline. The course of the optic neuritis is slow, and it is probably caused by the effect of the toxins. Examination of the visual fields in these cases will show an enlarged blind spot.

Retrobulbar neuritis has also been found to follow influenza. In this case, the visual acuity is reduced, and the visual fields show central and paracentral scotomas. On examination with the ophthalmoscope the fundi in these cases may appear to be normal shortly after the patient has recovered from influenza.

Ocular palsies are rather frequent in occurrence. Paralytic squint as well as acute ophthalmoplegia may be found. These are probably due to the effect of the toxins and usually offer a good prognosis, recovery taking place gradually with recovery from the disease.

Pneumonia

Lobar pneumonia, also known as fibrinous pneumonia or croupous pneumonia, is an acute infectious disease caused by the pneumococcus which produces a massive exudative lesion in one, and occasionally more than one, lobe.

It is characterized by a very acute onset, pain, chill, and dyspnea. The incubation period is probably a short one, and the disease very often follows or occurs as a complication of acute "colds," influenza, and other infectious diseases, especially those occurring in the upper respiratory tract. It frequently occurs also after chronic diseases, such as nephritis, diabetes, and alcoholism. It is not restricted to any age, occupation, or sex, but frequently occurs during the winter months and after exposure to cold and dampness.

The pneumococci enter the bronchial mucous membrane and invade the lobe of the lung by way of the lymphatics to appear in the alveolar spaces. This causes an interstitial inflammation in the perivascular and peribronchial tissues. Edema and polymorphonuclear infiltration occur with marked engorgement of the smaller vessels and capillaries. This also occurs in the lymphatics. The intense congestion of the vessels and the appearance of the polymorphonuclear exudate, with serum and fibrin, characterize the stage of so-called red hepatization. This active congestion recedes as the condition progresses. With progression of the cellular exudate, the alveoli become distended and blocked by leucocytes which gradually disintegrate. This characterizes the stage of gray hepatization. The two stages may blend into each other in the same lobe. Resolution follows with recovery of the lesion, beginning in the hilus and spreading to the more distant parts. Small areas of organization may occur in the interstitial tissues and also the alveoli.

Clinically, the patient suffers an elevation of temperature to about 103 to 105° F. which is continuous for several days. The disease terminates by crisis. There is an accompanying leucocytosis which averages about 15,000. The respirations are markedly increased in rate, and cyanosis, due to impaired aeration of the alveoli, is common. The venous blood which passes through the pneumonic areas is poorly aerated and, therefore, reduces the oxygen saturation of the mixed arterial blood. With progression of the lesion the flow of blood through the capillaries becomes more and more constricted. The early florid or purple type of cyanosis later becomes more pale in color and may be accompanied by sweating and other signs of vasomotor collapse.

The cough in most cases is short and irritating in character, and depends mostly on the nature of the exudate in the bronchi. The sputum may be mucopurulent and depends in its character on whether or not the disease was preceded by an infection in the upper respiratory tract. Occasionally, it may present a fresh tinge of blood, but ordinarily it is scanty, tenacious, and rusty brown in color.

Secondary lesions in pneumonia may occur as the result of direct extension to the surrounding structures or by way of the blood stream to more remote organs. These include pleurisy, pericarditis, purulent mediastinitis, peritonitis, upper respiratory lesions, otitis media, and involvement of the eyes. The metastatic lesions do not occur frequently, but they may occur as the result of a bacteriemia when suppuration takes place. The pus is usually thick, green in color, and contains much fibrin.

The central and autonomic nervous systems may be affected as the result of toxemia. Disturbances of the gastrointestinal tract and the circulatory system may result. The cardiac insufficiency which is an important factor is also said to be caused by the toxin of the organism. These secondary lesions are probably of greatest importance in a consideration of the eye manifestations.

Eye Manifestations.—Although the appearance of ocular lesions or manifestations in the course of a clear-cut case of lobar pneumonia is not common or frequent, it is necessary to remember that such involvement may occur principally as a secondary manifestation and in association with or resulting from other secondary lesions as previously mentioned. These may be grouped as those occurring during the acute stage of the disease, and which appear during the stages of hepatization and cyanosis; those which might occur as the result of suppuration; and those which occur during the course of the secondary affections and sequelae, such as pleurisy, cardiac insufficiency, empyema, and bronchiectasis.

The stage of intense congestion and cyanosis may be manifested in a similar manner in the vascular system of the eyes. The conjunctiva is usually pale, especially during the stage of marked impairment of circulation in the smaller vessels and capillaries. During the first stages of the disease the retinal veins can be found to be congested and the arteries narrowed. A mild and transient optic neuritis may be observed. Other than this, the eyes may reveal no further changes.

With the presence of suppuration, however, more serious manifestations may develop, although they are also comparatively rare. Principal among these is the occurrence of iritis and also a metastatic ophthalmia which can involve the entire eyeball. Such an infection could occur also as the result of one of the secondary lesions or complications of pneumonia. In pleurisy or empyema, or even in the course of a later bronchiectasis, the purulent material may be conveyed to the eye by way of the blood stream and produce a metastatic infection. This might be characterized rarely by the presence of an acute inflammation, but more commonly by fibrinous exudation in the iris and anterior segment of the eye with gradual occlusion of the pupil and accompanying infection of the vitreous. With the lodgment of infected material in the form of an embolus in the retinal vessels, hemorrhages will be found in the retina, optic neuritis, and an area of exudation and necrosis may occur. The latter may at first be localized and close to the vessels and later spread to the periphery and surrounding structures, eventually involving the entire eyeball. Panophthalmitis and loss of the eye are very infrequent but may result during the course of any of the suppurative sequelae.

With involvement of the central or autonomic nervous system, paralyses of the extraocular muscles may be found. These may occur in association with other manifestations of toxemia, such as gastrointestinal paresis, tympanites, and delirium. The pupils may become dilated, and the accommodation of the eyes and convergence may be impaired for some time after recovery from the disease.

During the period of convalescence and also as sequelae of the disease, the eyes may be affected in several ways. Conjunctivitis is often present during convalescence, especially as the result of extension along the lacrimal or Steno's duct.

The cornea may become involved during the course of the disease and in convalescence by herpetic lesions (herpes febrilis cornea). These are characterized by an eruption of small, transparent vesicles on the cornea which are accompanied by severe symptoms of irritation. They occur in small groups and are scarcely as large as a pinhead in size. They rupture and usually heal without leaving any signs of opacity or impairment of vision. These lesions are probably analogous to, and occur in association with, similar herpes of the skin, especially about the alae of the nose, lips, and eyelids.

During convalescence and especially in the presence of complications resulting in more or less prolonged infection of the upper respiratory tract, the cornea may be involved by dendritic ulcer. This is characterized by a linear, branching opacity in the superficial layers of the cornea. The edges of the ulcer are slightly raised, and the small knotlike thickening is seen at the end of the branches. On staining with fluorescein these ulcers can be plainly observed with the unaided eye. (See Fig. 46.)

Treatment.—The treatment of eye manifestations occurring in pneumonia or any of its forms and complications is principally local and symptomatic, depending on the nature of the involvement.

When conjunctivitis is present, it requires only local treatment which consists of the regular daily use of a mild eyewash such as boric acid, metaphen, or mercurophen solutions. If a smear can be obtained and the pneumococcus is found to be present, the use of optochin (ethyl hydrocupreine), 1 or 2 per cent, is considered to be specific.

The presence of corneal involvement and iritis requires the use of atropine in the affected eye and the application of hot, moist compresses for about ten minutes at a time, three times daily. The atropine, 1 per cent solution, should also be employed in the usual manner, by the instillation of one drop, two or three times daily, until the involvement subsides. The eyes should also be protected from light by the use of dark glasses.

The presence of metastatic ophthalmia involving the anterior segment of the eye is a serious manifestation which requires the use of atropine in the eye and the local application of hot, moist heat. The particular form of general treatment which is being administered to the patient, whether it be specific therapy, vaccine, or serum therapy, may also prove of benefit in this condition. For the presence of retinal or choroidal manifestations and metastatic ophthalmia involving the posterior part of the eyeball, local treatment is of little or no avail. The process will either run its course and terminate by resolution and organization with limited involvement and permanent impairment, or the entire eyeball may become involved with loss of the eye.

If paralyses of the extraocular muscles occur, they usually clear up with recovery from the disease.

Diphtheria (Membranous Croup)

An infectious disease due to the *Bacillus diphtheriae,* which is also known as the Klebs-Loeffler bacillus. The mucous membranes are mostly involved, and a fibrinous membrane is found on the surface of the area affected. The portal of entry is usually through the nose, throat, or other mucous membrane. The infection also occurs through the inoculation of an open wound. The disease affects the mucous membranes of the pharynx, larynx, and nose. The ocular conjunctiva and other parts may also be affected. The pathologic lesion is an exudative ulceration of the mucous membrane which produces a pseudo-membrane composed of coagulated exudate and bacteria. This is caused by the local effect of the toxins. The membrane adheres rather firmly to the underlying structure, and it leaves a bleeding surface when removed. Involvement of the deeper structures may occur which may lead to necrosis, gangrene, and loss of tissue. There is a definite relationship between the extent of the local lesion and the severity of the systemic symptoms. The toxins are absorbed from a local lesion and cause secondary lesions elsewhere. Extensive paralyses may occur as the result of involvement of the central nervous system, which is especially susceptible. The adjacent glands may become involved, causing an accompanying adenitis.

The disease is usually ushered in with headache, malaise, fatigue, and sometimes vomiting and diarrhea in children. When the pharynx is involved, there is accompanying sore throat and difficulty in swallowing. The general toxemia may vary in its severity. A child may show very mild symptoms, but in other instances there may be very high temperature and severe prostration and intoxication. It is one of the most severe contagious diseases. Convalescence usually begins after about seven days, but complications may develop as late as several months afterward. The disease is diagnosed definitely by the examination of cultures taken from the inflammatory lesions. It should be differentiated especially from acute follicular tonsillitis and Vincent's angina. The results of examination of the culture, however, should confirm the diagnosis. The prognosis depends principally on the age of the patient, location and extent of the lesions, the degree of toxemia, and the time at which specific treatment is begun.

Eye Manifestations.—The conjunctiva is the ocular structure most commonly affected and is characterized by the presence of a diphtheritic conjunctivitis. This is commonly observed in children and may affect both eyes. It is particularly common during epidemics of pharyngeal diphtheria. A culture should always be taken from the affected eye and examined microscopically. The diphtheria bacillus may be simulated closely by many other organisms found in the conjunctival sac, so that laboratory reports cannot always give a positive diagnosis. The virulence of the organism found should then be tested by subcutaneous injection of a pure culture into guinea pigs, and the result ascertained both with and without the use of diphtheria antitoxin. The animal which was injected with a virulent diphtheria bacillus and which had not received antitoxin previously will fail to survive the infection after a few days.

The eyelids in diphtheritic conjunctivitis are often reddened and swollen and are hot and painful to the touch. In severe cases they become hard and are difficult to evert. The lymphatic glands in front of the ear and in the neck may be swollen. The tarsal and palpebral conjunctiva is the seat of a purulent infection which spreads by contagion, and which has an infectious secretion. The exudation is profuse and has a tendency to coagulate either on the surface of the conjunctiva, to form a membrane, or within the structure of the conjunctiva. As a result, therefore, there are two forms of diphtheritic conjunctivitis to be distinguished—a superficial or croupous form and a deep form. (A nondiphtheritic membranous conjunctivitis may also occur.)

The superficial form is characterized by a grayish-white membrane which adheres closely to the surface of the tarsal conjunctiva but can be removed with a pair of forceps. Below the membrane the conjunctiva is found to be bleeding, reddened, and very much swollen. There is, however, no great loss of tissue. The detached membrane consists of a minute meshwork of clotted fibrin with embedded pus cells and epithelial cells. The croupous membrane covers the tarsal conjunctiva, but rarely the retrotarsal fold. In one or two weeks the membrane may disappear, showing an intense catarrhal inflammation which recovers without any permanent change in the conjunctiva.

In the deep form the condition runs a more serious course. Here the exudate coagulates within the tissue of the conjunctiva; as a result the vessels are compressed, and the mucous membrane may become necrotic. On everting the lids, therefore, one finds marked swelling and redness of the conjunctiva and spots in which the conjunctiva is depressed. This is usually accompanied by a swelling of the adjacent lymph glands and comprises the first stage of the condition which lasts five to ten days. After this, resorption of the exudate takes place, but the necrotic spots may remain and slough away. In this stage the secretion becomes more profuse, and suppuration occurs, characterized by blennorrhea. The third is the stage of cicatrization, in which the sloughs in the conjunctiva become smaller and are covered over with a new epithelial lining. A contracted conjunctiva and symblepharon may result.

The cornea may also be more seriously affected here than in the croupous form. The former is more serious in all respects and usually occurs in those cases in which the general disease is more severe.

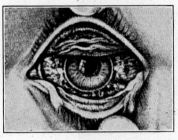
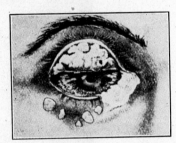

A.   B.

Fig. 133.—*A*, Pseudomembranous conjunctivitis. *B*, Diphtheritic, membranous conjunctivitis.
(From Duke-Elder: Text-Book of Ophthalmology.)

The prognosis of diphtheritic conjunctivitis is favorable in most cases, especially in the croupous variety. The iris is not as a rule involved. Optic neuritis is a rare complication, but paralysis of the accommodation is a rather common occurrence and can be seen in about 12 per cent of the cases. The severity of the infection does not seem to have a bearing on its incidence. It usually occurs about three or four weeks after the onset of the disease and is, as a rule, bilateral and complete, affecting those patients who are under 14 years of age. The average duration is about three weeks.

Extraocular muscle palsies usually occur after severe infections, the external rectus muscle being the one most frequently involved.

Treatment.—In diphtheritic involvement of the eyes the treatment should be both prophylactic and specific. The prophylactic treatment includes the isolation of the patient, the suspicious patient, and the contact. If the eye condition is unilateral, the unaffected eye should be protected. The specific treatment should be both general and local. Diphtheria antitoxin should be administered systemically in large doses and as early as possible. In doubtful cases, and also in the absence of positive bacteriologic diagnosis, the specific treatment should be employed without delay. The dosage may range from 2,000 units to 10,000 units of the serum, according to the severity of the condition. The serum can also be instilled into the conjunctival sac. Other local treatment should include the regular flushing of the eye with a mild lotion, such as boric acid solution. Stronger irritative antiseptic solutions should be avoided. Redness and swelling of the lids may require the application of cold compresses. In cases where the cornea becomes involved, use hot compresses. Atropine sulfate, 1 per cent solution, should also be instilled in the affected eye in such instances. In true diphtheritic conjunctivitis the condition will usually show improvement very soon after the injection of the serum is begun.

Erysipelas (St. Anthony's Fire)

A specific disease of the skin manifested by a spreading erythematous edema with a clear-cut margin. It is due to the hemolytic streptococcus and is found more commonly in women, especially during the middle decades of life. Debilitating and toxic conditions, such as acute illness, operation, chronic disease, and alcoholism, predispose one to its onset. It has a short incubation period of about three days, and a skin wound is the usual portal of entry.

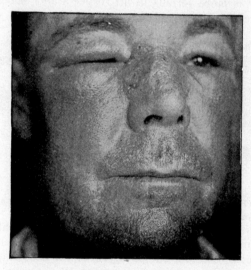

Fig. 134.—Erysipelas of the face. (From Sutton and Sutton: Diseases of the Skin, The C. V. Mosby Co.)

Symptoms appear suddenly with chills and rigors, then malaise, headache, anorexia, and fever. The face and nose are the sites of election, but other skin areas may be involved. It spreads over the cheeks in a butterfly-like distribution. The lesion appears as a bright red, moderately raised area which slowly spreads into the surrounding tissues. It is rather clearly defined and well demarcated, creeping forward by projections while the older areas show a recrudescence. Mucous membranes may also be involved. Bullae and vesicles may develop over the skin lesion, and local suppuration may occur, resulting from secondary infection. Constitutional symptoms are severe with extreme prostration and delirium. Pathologically, streptococci are found in the lymphatics of the skin but are absent in other parts of the lesion.

The diagnosis is made by inspection, but it must be differentiated from a simple erythema. The latter does not have a raised margin. An acute eczema or dermatitis can be excluded by the absence of fever and systemic symptoms.

Cutaneous phlegmon presents a much deeper inflammation with induration and does not have the clear-cut edematous margin found in erysipelas. The course is marked by relapses and recurrences, and usually it lasts for several weeks. The treatment is principally symptomatic and includes appropriate local applications to the site of the lesion.

Eye Manifestations.—Erysipelas of the face can be considered to be in great part a disease of the eyelids. In 130 cases of facial erysipelas observed by Bellows[1] over a period of six months, 103 cases, or about 80 per cent, showed involvement of the eyelids and adnexa. In seven of these he found the lids to be affected with superficial abscesses. Corneal ulcers were found in three cases. Orbital cellulitis, unilateral and bilateral, occurred six times. Three of the cases became blind, and two of these were bilateral. Thirteen of the 130 cases died and were listed variously as orbital cellulitis, pneumonia, cardiac disease, sepsis and uremia.

In many cases the inner canthi are the most frequent locations for the onset of the inflammation. With extreme swelling of the lids, the palpebral fissure is closed. Vesicles may form on the surface which may go on to suppuration and the formation of necrotic abscesses. Gangrene of the lids with loss of tissue may occur and result later in ectropion.

The conjunctiva may readily become involved, causing a conjunctivitis as a result of extension of the inflammation.

The cornea may become involved, with the formation of blebs and vesicles and the occurrence of keratitis. Involvement of the fifth nerve causing keratitis neuroparalytica has occurred. Paralysis of the first and second branches of the trigeminus nerve, palsy of the facial nerve, and optic atrophy on the affected side have all been reported.

Iridocyclitis, abscess of the vitreous, and suppurative chorioretinitis, as the result of metastatic involvement, are rare.

Orbital cellulitis and involvement of the optic nerve (retrobulbar neuritis) are rather common in erysipelas, and orbital phlegmon was reported in a number of cases. Thrombophlebitis is the chief anatomic finding described in most cases of orbital cellulitis. The scattered areas of infiltration around the veins may become confluent with the formation of an abscess.

The third, fourth, and sixth cranial nerves may become involved, with an accompanying involvement of the extraocular muscles supplied by them.

As a result of extension of the inflammatory process, principally along the veins, intracranial complications may occur. These may also occur as the result of extension from the orbit along the nerve sheaths. With involvement of the orbit in deep cellulitis behind the eyeball, the eye may be proptosed, fixed, and the tissues chemotic. The cavernous sinus may also become involved and lead to a fatal termination. The vision in about 50 per cent of these cases is usually impaired in one or both eyes.

Treatment.—Abscesses of the eyelids should be treated by incision and drainage. This may prevent extension to the deeper structures. Orbital cellulitis should be looked for early, and if an orbital abscess is present, it should be incised and drained.

In the absence of cellulitis or abscess, the skin of the eyelids should be kept clean and the eyes irrigated with mild antiseptic solutions. Hot or cold applications may be applied to the skin, according to which affords the most comfort. There is no specific treatment for the lesion, but magnesium sulfate, boric acid, and sulfanilamide have all been employed. Use of the latter has given satisfactory results in some cases.

Gonorrhea

An acute and chronic infectious disease caused by the gonococcus. It is most commonly observed as a venereal disease, although not necessarily so. The disease is usually contracted through sexual intercourse when one is infected. In young female children it may be contracted without sexual contact but by transmission through contamination and infection from towels, clothing, linen, and handkerchiefs. The gonococcus is a biscuit-shaped, gram-negative intra- and extracellular diplococcus. The incubation period of the disease is about four to five days. The portal of entry in the male is the urethra and in the female the vagina. The disease is characterized by a profuse urethral or vaginal purulent discharge. There may be a great number of accompanying symptoms which are present in the male patient as the result of involvement or disturbance of the urinary passages, and invasion of the neighboring structures. A systemic reaction may occur when the adjacent tissues or posterior urethra are involved. The disease may be prolonged and take on a chronic form. A focus in a neighboring structure may not drain properly and remain infected. This will act to prolong the local condition and also serve as a source for hematogenous and metastatic spread of the infection. The symptoms in the female are not so pronounced as in the male. There may be a burning sensation or pain on urination and such local signs as redness of the meatus and the presence of pus. The condition here may also become chronic and of prolonged duration. The vagina may contain some pus, but the cervical canal is more commonly affected by the discharge. Abscesses and cysts may occur, and the adjacent organs, such as the bladder, ovaries, endometrium, and pelvic tissues, may become involved. There may be low back pain, pelvic pain, and debility.

Systemic infection is not very common but may prove to be serious when it occurs. The inguinal glands may be enlarged and suppurate. Metastatic lesions may occur, however, when there is little or no evidence of persisting local disease. The gonococcus seems to show a particular selectivity for the synovial membranes of the joints and tendon sheaths, the endocardium, the skin, and the eye.

The most common manifestation of systemic involvement is gonorrheal arthritis, usually affecting the larger joints.

The endocardium may be the site of an ulcerative endocarditis. The skin lesions have been described as erythemas which are not especially characteristic. Certain hemorrhagic and bullous pustular eruptions may be quite suggestive. The lesions with hyperkeratosis are almost specific and are sometimes overlooked. They may be associated with or follow an arthritis and are due to a bacteriemia.

Eye Manifestations.—The ophthalmia which is seen in gonorrhea usually occurs in one of three ways. The first is that which results from introducing the pus directly into the eye by a patient's hands, handkerchiefs, towels, or other contaminated articles. This usually occurs among young children and adults and is known as gonorrheal ophthalmia or gonorrheal conjunctivitis.

The second is that form of purulent inflammation of the conjunctiva which occurs in newborn infants as the result of contact with the discharge during passage through an infected birth canal. This is known as ophthalmia neonatorum. The third form includes the eye conditions which occur as the result of metastatic involvement in a patient suffering with either a clinically infected focus elsewhere, or a systemic gonorrheal infection. These cases are known as metastatic gonorrheal ophthalmia.

Gonorrheal Ophthalmia is a specific purulent inflammation which affects the conjunctiva of the eye and is known as gonorrheal conjunctivitis. It results from the pus or discharge from a patient being brought into direct contact with the eye. This may happen to the patient already suffering from the disease or to some other individual who is infected innocently. It is not uncommon in children and it may occur in young girls who frequently suffer with gonorrheal vulvovaginitis. Among adults, the condition may be found with almost equal frequency in men and women.

In addition to the purulent infection and discharge of pus from the conjunctiva, the lids may be greatly swollen and reddened. The conjunctiva will become chemotic, and after a few days, gonococci may be found in the pus cells. Frequently, however, no organisms will be found on laboratory examination, and it is necessary to remove the large epithelial covering of the cells from the conjunctiva in taking the smear. The gonococci may then be found to have penetrated through the epithelial covering of the cells. They burrow deeply into the tissues, and later the epithelial cells become detached. An outpouring of exudate takes place with increase in the number of bacteria and repeated separation of epithelial cells. The production of toxins with edema and further separation of cells occurs. This is followed by a proliferation of new cells with an exfoliation of others. The proliferation occurring far in excess of the exfoliation leads to a marked thickening of the conjunctiva of the affected eyelid. An examination of the smear containing the new epithelial cells will show large numbers of gonococci in their cytoplasm. These cells have a phagocytic action on the bacteria.

In the early stages of the infection the eye may be very painful, and constitutional symptoms may be present. It reaches its height in about four or five days after which the discharge of pus begins to decrease. The redness and swelling of the lids decreases together with that of the conjunctiva. The acute inflammatory condition subsides nearly altogether in several weeks, and it then may take on a more chronic form which subsides very gradually.

The common complication in gonorrheal conjunctivitis is involvement of the cornea. This may become infected by direct extension of the inflammation from the conjunctiva. The cornea, moreover, is apparently very vulnerable to invasion by the gonococci. The earliest sign of corneal involvement is an oncoming haze or cloudiness which soon becomes grayish in appearance as infiltration proceeds. This infiltration becomes more dense and is followed by ulceration. The occurrence of corneal involvement seems to depend somewhat on the severity of the conjunctivitis and usually occurs during the height of the inflammation and discharge, or shortly after. When ulceration takes place, it may occur near the limbus or in the center of the cornea. Perforation of the cornea may follow ulceration. This is not ordinarily an unfavorable condition, however, since healing takes place rapidly, and it seems to limit the duration of the infection. Of course, a scar or opacity results in the cornea at the site of the ulceration and perforation. This will cause a future visual impairment of corresponding degree.

Iritis may prove to be a further complication especially in the presence of deep ulceration of the cornea. This will be accompanied by increased pain in the eye and increased lacrimation and photophobia. Other structures of the eye may also become involved with further extension of the inflammation, which, if not checked, may ultimately lead to a panophthalmitis.

Treatment.—The most important indication in a case of gonorrheal conjunctivitis is to keep the eye free from pus as much as possible. To do this, it is necessary to flush the affected eye almost constantly or at intervals of one-half to one hour. This can be done by using an ordinary solution of boric acid since it is the mechanical washing which is of importance. The patient should be kept in bed for this purpose, and a nurse should be constantly in charge. When only one eye is involved, the other eye should be protected from the infection by the use of a Buller shield. This can be made by placing an ordinary watch glass over the affected eye and holding it in place by strips of adhesive plaster. Absolute care and cleanliness should be enforced in the use of all materials by nurses and attendants. In the course of examination and treatment of the affected eye care should be used in separating the eyelids to prevent the pus from reaching any other part or person. The continuous flushing and irrigation of the affected eye should be carried out until the eye is free from discharge. This is the best way to prevent involvement of the cornea.

For the swelling and edema of the lids and conjunctiva, cold compresses should be employed whenever the eye is not being flushed or otherwise treated. If desired, the injection of foreign proteins, such as milk or typhoid vaccine, may be employed in order to produce a systemic reaction.

Other medication may include the application of silver nitrate (gr. 15 to oz. 1) to the conjunctiva of the lids. This should be followed by flushing with normal saline solution. It is necessary to continue to observe the condition of the cornea regularly. Should any signs of involvement be noted, the treatment should be modified. Instillations of atropine sulfate (1 per cent solution) will then be indicated, using about one drop two or three times daily, since the latter is more stimulating and healing in its effect on the cornea. If perforation of the cornea should occur, the condition will slowly heal as the inflammation subsides.

In addition to the above, metaphen and mercurophen solutions may also be employed.

Perhaps the greatest benefit in the treatment of gonorrheal ophthalmia has been obtained in recent years from the use of the sulfonamide preparations. This drug is administered orally on the approximate basis of one grain (0.065 Gm.) per pound of body weight daily. Many methods of administration and dosage have been recommended for sulfanilamide in gonorrhea, most of which are intended to produce a prompt high concentration of blood, and later maintain a reduced dose. It has been shown, however, that the blood concentration is not the most important factor, since some cases in which the blood concentration was low obtained good results, while others in which this was high showed poor results.

The usual method of administration in ambulant patients is to administer 60 gr. daily for the first two days. Thereafter, this may be reduced to about 40 gr. a day, maintaining this dose in the absence of toxic symptoms. Sodium bicarbonate in half or equal quantity may also be prescribed. In patients confined to bed the daily dosage may be slightly higher, but the patient should be seen daily and the drug discontinued with the onset of toxic symptoms, dizziness, or gastric distress. Sulfanilamide can also be employed locally in gonorrheal conjunctivitis by instilling about two drops of 0.8 per cent solution into the conjunctival sac about three or four times a day. It is commonly considered, however, that the principal effect is obtained from the oral administration of the drug although the local instillations may afford some additional benefit. The results obtained are in general most satisfactory. The duration of the disease in many cases has been reduced one-half, and the purulent discharge begins to subside soon after the use of the drug is begun. Corneal involvement has also been found to occur much less frequently following its use.

More recently, the use of sulfathiazole has been found to be even more effective in this condition. It is administered by mouth in doses of about 10 grains, four times daily, while it is also instilled in 5 per cent solution into the infected eye, three times daily.

Ophthalmia Neonatorum.—A purulent discharge from the conjunctiva caused by the gonococcus and occurring in newborn infants. The condition results from infection of the patient's eyes during its passage through the infected birth canal of the mother. Since involvement of the cornea with accompanying loss of vision is a serious complication, more blindness has resulted in the past from this condition than from any other infection.

The disease is characterized by a rather free discharge of pus from the conjunctival sac which may begin from the first to the third day after birth. In cases with profuse discharge it can be seen between the edges of the closed eyelids which, on being separated, reveal collections of the pus in the corners and over the conjunctival surface of the lids. This is usually accompanied by a swelling and puffiness of the lids to a fair degree. In some cases a chemosis of the bulbar conjunctiva may be noted. In severe cases the cornea is invaded and may lead to ulceration and perforation, with resulting impairment of vision. In less severe cases the disease may run a milder course without involvement of the cornea. Laboratory examinations should be made daily of smears taken from the infected eyes, and the condition should be considered active and serious until at least two successive negative reports have been received. In nearly all cases both eyes of the infant are affected.

Treatment.—This should include both prophylactic and active treatment. The purpose of the former is to prevent infections before and after the birth of the child. Before birth, the proper measures should be employed for cleansing of the birth canal by thorough irrigation and the use of vaginal antiseptics. Immediately after birth and washing of the child, the Credé method should always be employed. This requires the instillation of one drop of a 2 per cent solution of silver nitrate into each eye. This should be done with proper attention to all the details. The child can be laid on its back with the face turned upward, while the hands and legs are held by a nurse. The physician gently separates the eyelids until they are completely everted. The drop of silver nitrate solution can then be instilled without difficulty. When a physician is not in attendance, the midwife or nurse should see that this procedure is carried out. In many states it is compulsory that the Credé method be employed, and as a result, the incidence of ophthalmia neonatorum has been greatly reduced.

Other prophylactic measures to be employed, especially in the presence of a vaginal discharge in the mother, are thorough scrubbing and disinfection of hands of nurses, physicians, and other attendants, and the disinfection of towels, basins, sponges, and other utensils to be used.

The active treatment of ophthalmia neonatorum is practically the same as that already described for gonorrheal ophthalmia occurring in adults. If the eyelids are swollen, cold compresses can also be employed here. The conjunctival sac should be irrigated or flushed almost constantly, aiming to keep the eyes free from discharge. Boric acid solution can be employed and can be used in a large eye dropper or an irrigator. The lids should be carefully everted by the nurse and the entire cul-de-sac flushed with the solution. The inner surface of the eyelids can also be painted once daily with a 2 per cent solution of silver nitrate. The condition of the cornea should be studied constantly for the presence of any clouding. When this is observed, hot compresses should be employed to the eye, and one drop of 0.5 per cent atropine instilled about twice daily. The development of corneal ulceration and perforation may lead to serious impairment of vision. Too great stress in the treatment of this condition cannot be placed on keeping the eyes clear of pus by constant flushing.

Sulfathiazole can also be employed in the treatment of these cases just as in the case of adults. The drug is administered in smaller doses, according to the weight of the child and can be placed in the baby's bottle to be administered with the feedings.

Sorsby and Hoffa[2] treated sixty cases of gonorrheal ophthalmia in children with sulfonamides internally (sulfapyridine, sulfathiazole, sulfamethazine and sulfadiazine). Their results reported clinical cures in 51.7 per cent of the cases in three days and in 90 per cent of the cases in eight days.

The reports to date of the use of penicillin in the treatment of gonorrheal ophthalmia have also been very favorable. According to Keyes,[3] it is now the drug of choice in these conditions. He referred to the report of Florey and Florey who treated a case of ophthalmia neonatorum which failed to respond to sulfapyridine and other treatment after three weeks but which disappeared in two days after the instillation of 1,200 units per cubic centimeter of penicillin every hour. Sorsby also treated gonorrheal ophthalmia neonatorum successfully with penicillin therapy in thirty-six hours. In another case of a 24-year-old man suffering with gonorrheal ophthalmia and gonorrheal urethritis which resisted sulfonamide treatment for forty-six days, Griffey reported a cure after the intramuscular injection of 25,000 units of penicillin sodium every three hours for ten injections.

Metastatic Gonorrheal Ophthalmia (Metastatic Gonorrheal Conjunctivitis). —This form of eye involvement manifests itself usually as a conjunctivitis which results from the infection being carried to the eyes through the system in a case of chronic gonorrhea. The eye involvement is endogenous in nature and usually occurs in male patients and those who also suffer from gonorrheal arthritis. It may begin almost any time after the initial gonorrheal infection, but it usually starts several months later, or when the condition has become chronic.

The clinical appearance of the eye infection differs somewhat from the other forms of gonorrheal involvement in that the discharge is not so profuse and is mucopurulent rather than purulent in character. There may, however, be rather severe signs of inflammation present, and the conjunctiva may present a considerable amount of chemosis. In this form the presence of the gonococcus cannot be demonstrated in most cases, although the condition may be due to a metastasis of the organisms themselves, as well as to a metastasis of their toxins. A metastatic iritis may accompany the conjunctivitis or occur independently.

The treatment of this form of gonorrheal conjunctivitis differs very little from that already described for the others. The conjunctival sac should be flushed or irrigated regularly and carefully with a mild solution, such as boric acid. This should follow the application of cold compresses. In addition, a solution of metaphen or mercurophen (1:10,000) may be instilled about three times a day. Stronger antiseptics are not ordinarily required, and silver preparations should be avoided in the average case. An astringent, such as zinc sulfate, can be employed in $\frac{1}{4}$ per cent solution, instilling one drop two or three times a day. The conjunctivitis may run a rather long course while the discharge becomes more thin and watery, until it gradually subsides. The patient should receive adequate treatment for the systemic or other localized manifestations of the disease. Treatment with sulfathiazole should also be carried out in these cases in the same manner as has already been described.

In the presence of metastatic iritis, hot wet compresses should be applied, and atropine sulfate should be instilled three times daily.

Leprosy (Lepra Arabrum)

A bacterial disease caused by an acid-fast, curved or straight rod, discovered by Hansen in 1872. The disease occurs more commonly among certain dark-skinned peoples, such as Mexicans, Hawaiians, Puerto Ricans, Portuguese, Hindus, and Filipinos. It is rarely seen in the United States. Clinically the disease is classified as cutaneous, neural, or mixed. The cutaneous type is characterized by the thinning of the epidermis which is pushed into a nodular protrusion and separated from the leproma. The leprous bacilli become engulfed by the large monocytic cells of the leproma and form the foam cells. The neural lesions consist of an infiltration of the perineurium with lymphocytes, monocytes, and fibroblasts which eventually destroy the nerve fibers by pressure. The third or mixed type is a mixture of the cutaneous and the neural.

The incubation period may last several years. There are feverish attacks, changes in skin color and skin sensibility. The skin thickens, forming nodules which eventually ulcerate. The nerves thicken, causing loss of sensation. The disease is most prevalent in hot damp climates, and children and young adults are the most susceptible.

The bacillus is transmitted to others through long and close contact. It is less infectious than tuberculosis, and many advanced crippled nerve cases lose their infectivity.

Treatment consists of intramuscular injections of ethyl esters, intravenous injection of sodium salts, and sodium hydrocarpate injections.

Eye Manifestations.—Prendergast[4] reports that 29 per cent of the 350 lepers he examined were blind or nearly blind in one or both eyes, and 91 per cent had ocular involvement brought on by the disease. Eye involvement apparently occurs in an average of about 50 per cent of the cases. Middle-aged people and those who had a long history of leprosy had the most severe ocular disturbances.

There are several schools of thought as to the portal of entry into the eye. Some believe the bacillus enters externally from the conjunctiva or episcleral tissues, whereas others favor the theory of endogenous infection, since bacilli can be found in many internal organs at autopsy. The angle of the anterior chamber and the anterior point of ciliary body around the major circle of the iris are the commonest sites of primary ocular involvement, and it is felt that the bacilli are carried by the blood stream to the anastomosis of small vessels in this region. Some believe that the infection of the eye is secondary to a primary focus in the nose.

The adnexa of the eye are the site of many cutaneous lesions occurring in conjunction with lesions of the face. An absence of hair either in part or complete is common in nearly all cases. It may occur either with or without nodular formation on the lids and brows. The eyelids are the common site of nodular formation and hypertrophy. Xanthelasma also has been found quite often, especially over the leprous nodules on the eyelids. Dacryocystitis and other forms of tear sac involvement occur in a fair number of cases and are usually caused by infection from the nose.

The Extraocular Muscles.—Although strabismus has been found to occur in a small percentage of cases, the ocular muscles are rarely affected by the disease. This is attributed to the fact that being deeper ocular structures, they are fairly well protected from invasion. Paralysis of the facial nerve has been found to occur with resultant ectropion.

The fact that there are immune areas in the adnexa in the region of the folds in the upper and lower lids, an area well protected by bony structures, leads to the impression that protection is important as a prophylactic measure.

The Conjunctiva.—Conjunctivitis and involvement of the conjunctiva are evident in more than half of the lepers examined. Few of these, however, are of true leprous origin. The conjunctiva may become involved from the skin and nasal secretions, and internally from the episcleral tissues and the blood stream. The bulbar conjunctiva is probably most commonly affected, and this occurs in only a small number of cases. Most of the cases of conjunctivitis are evidently independent and of an irritative nature, not directly caused by the bacillus of leprosy.

Cornea.—The cornea seems to be the ocular structure most susceptible to the *Bacillus leprae.* Involvement is usually characterized by an infiltration in the deep layers of the stroma, of an amorphous, dull gray character. It resembles a syphilitic interstitial infiltration and usually starts at the upper and outer sides. A vascular net develops in its advanced stages.

Another common lesion is the occurrence of a superficial keratitis of leprosy which, microscopically, looks like cutaneous leprosy. Prendergast observed this following the infiltration, but others described it as primary leprosy. The infiltration usually starts from above and covers the deep haze with a network of pin-point dots described as "flour dust." (See Fig. 39.) Prendergast described these minute superficial areas surrounded by a grayish infiltration, and the corneal tissue between them is dull and lusterless. The entire area is sharply demarcated and when well advanced becomes vascularized and takes on the appearance of pannus formation. The epithelium is intact but irregular, and Bowman's membrane is either absent or pushed forward. The lamellae are separated, and corneal cells group themselves under Bowman's membrane and house numerous lepra bacilli. Sometimes beaded corneal nerves can be seen with the high-power slit lamp. These were considered by Prendergast to be analogous to generalized neural involvement. Corneal anesthesia is present only in cases of advanced superficial keratitis. Superficial ulcers are rare. Microscopic corneal lesions of leprosy are found at the limbus, and marked cellular infiltration may occur around the corneal limbus which causes a roll of the conjunctiva at the corneoscleral margin.

The most disfiguring type of gross corneal lesion is the immense leproma which covers the whole cornea. It appears to be extracorneal and dissects easily, but the microscope shows a hypertrophied epithelium separated from Bowman's membrane by lepra bacilli and fiber.

Lepra cells are plentiful in the episcleral tissue, and the inflammatory reaction may be localized or pericorneal but not deep. Yellowish nodules which are vascularized occur in the sclera near the limbus under the conjunctiva.

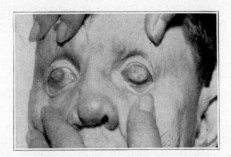

Fig. 135.—Immense corneal leproma. (From Prendergast: Arch. Ophth., January, 1940.)

The iris may be either seriously or mildly involved. The outstanding lesion seems to be the leproma or nodule which is white and globular in appearance. On examination with the corneal microscope they can be seen to protrude from the surface or to be enmeshed in its structure. Posterior synechia and pigment deposits on the anterior capsules are common. The pupils are usually miotic.

Acute inflammation and dense cellular infiltration of the choroid and ciliary bodies are rare. Choroiditis, vitreous opacities, optic neuritis, and optic atrophy occur in a small percentage of cases, and their frequency is in the order named.

Treatment.—For corneal infiltrates and opacities, ethylmorphine hydrochloride can be employed in gradually increasing strength up to 10 per cent solution three times a week. Prendergast reported that six out of eleven patients showed improvement in vision, but the slit lamp showed no change in the opacities. An ointment of quinine bisulfate (2 per cent) has also been recommended. Chaulmoogra oil in a 50 per cent solution with castor oil preceded by a 5 per cent solution of pontocain hydrochloride for irritation has also been given through the veins and by mouth. This, too, improves the vision but leaves the opacities unchanged, as seen on examination with the slit lamp. Thyroxin (2 mg. per c.c.), one drop instilled twice a day in each eye, gives the best results, according to Prendergast, since the vision is improved and the slit lamp reveals the interstitial infiltration to be clearer.

For uveitis and corneal scarifications one drachm (3.7 c.c.) calcium gluconate, given orally three times a day, produced improved vision in eight out of thirteen patients.

Acute ocular leprosy is best treated symptomatically with applications of heat and salicylates, and instillations of atropine. At the same time foreign protein therapy can be employed. Typhoid is said to have produced good results. Intravenous injections of gold sodium thiosulfate have also given satisfactory results in some cases. Ten milligrams are injected four times, increasing the dose to 25 mg. twice a week for a period of several months. The results of treatment with arsenical preparations have, according to reports, proved unsatisfactory.

In addition to medication, early segregation, early hygienic treatment, and careful attention to diet and rest have been found to be important in the treatment of leprosy.

Since leprous lesions of the eye are not primary but a response to a general pathologic condition, they are treated symptomatically. Many cases occur with an accompanying nasal involvement, and treatment of the nose indirectly benefits the eye.

Anthrax

Anthrax, which is also known as malignant pustule or malignant anthrax edema, is an acute specific infectious disease which occurs in man by infection through the skin and mucous membrane. It is caused by the *Bacillus anthracis* which occurs principally in cattle and sheep. These are infected when their food is contaminated by the spores of the bacilli which are found in pastures. It may occur in man principally among wool sorters by inhalation of the dust when sheep's wool is infected, or by contamination through cuts or abrasions in the skin while handling the hides.

The organism itself is a rather large, gram-positive nonmotile bacillus which grows quickly in bunched-up groups of filaments on a solid media. The spores of the organism resist heat and ordinary disinfectants.

The incubation period of the disease is about twelve to thirty-six hours. In the malignant pustule form the primary lesion is usually on the hands or face. This begins as a small red area which forms a vesicle which is surrounded by induration and edema. A black area of gangrene develops in the center with a spread of edema and adjacent clumps of vesicles. These coalesce and form a large, round, indurated necrotic area, which sloughs off. It is not accompanied by suppuration, but the adjacent lymph glands may become enlarged.

The other type of the disease, known as malignant anthrax edema, is a cutaneous infection without the presence of a pustule but with malignant edema. This form is more rare.

The patient with anthrax infection may not be very sick and may suffer no real pain. There is a moderate elevation of temperature accompanied by headache and nausea. The disease may occur in the gastrointestinal tract with the occurrence of a bloody diarrhea. When the respiratory tract is involved, it may lead to a systemic infection, with cerebral involvement, and terminate fatally. Ordinarily, the patient does not realize the seriousness of the condition, and if the avenue of infection is by way of the face or eyelids, death may occur very early.

The diagnosis of the condition depends on early recognition of the primary lesion and a knowledge of the patient's occupation requiring the handling of hides, skin, or wool from animals possibly infected. This is confirmed by finding the anthrax bacilli in the scrapings from the primary lesion.

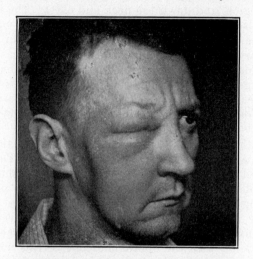

Fig. 136*A*.—Malignant anthrax edema. Early edema of lids and face. (From Ross and Shipman: Am. J. Ophth., July, 1935.)

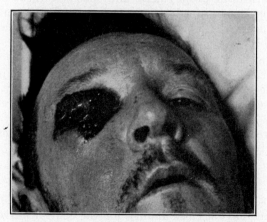

Fig. 136*B*.—Malignant anthrax edema; later stage. (From Ross and Shipman: Am. J. Ophth., July, 1935.)

The disease must be differentiated when it occurs on the face, principally from erysipelas and orbital cellulitis. With malignant pustule this should not be difficult because of the character of the lesion. In anthrax edema without the pustule, there is an absence of pain, no sharp line of demarcation of the area involved, no suppuration, and probably a typical history of exposure to this infection.

Eye Manifestations.—Since the infection is one which usually occurs in the face and begins around the eyelids, the edema and other lesions constitute the ocular involvement.

In reporting a case of malignant anthrax edema in a patient working with Brazilian goatskins, Ross and Shipman[5] described the clinical appearance as follows:

"The most common site of infection is the eyelids, usually starting in the upper lid and spreading rapidly, due to the loose tissues, to the lower lid, cheek, temporal region, and down the neck and chest. The buccal membranes and tongue may also be involved, but the arms are not usually affected. The chief characteristic of this edema is the absence of pain and suppuration. There is no primary pustule, although after the edema has been present for a few days, the lids usually show some vesicular formations, due to tension, and these form large dark crusts, underneath which there is a serosanguineous fluid. Positive smears and cultures for *Bacillus anthracis* are usually obtained from this fluid. The crusts finally slough off and disfiguring scars may be left, which sometimes give rise to ectropion."

The edema of the eyelid becomes so marked as to close the eye. Beginning in the lids of one eye, it may spread to the other eye. The extension takes place gradually, but not slowly, so that there is really no sharp line of separation of the affected area. There may be no tenderness or pressure, but there may be some pitting. The skin over the affected lids may be slightly reddened, with the skin over the edematous face waxlike in appearance. The eyeball itself remains uninvolved, but there might be some congestion of the conjunctiva. Examination with the ophthalmoscope reveals no pathology in the fundus.

Treatment consists of prophylactic and specific measures. The former is important and consists in sterilization of skins and hides which may be infected, and the vaccination of cattle, sheep, and men who are exposed to the infection through contact.

Specific treatment consists in the early administration of massive doses of antianthrax serum. This early and prompt treatment is emphasized. It can be given subcutaneously, intramuscularly, and intravenously. The doses are from 30 to 100 c.c. and may be repeated as often as required. In Ross and Shipman's case, a total of 440 c.c. of the serum was given. At first 300 c.c. were given intravenously and the remainder was given in doses of 20 and 40 c.c. intramuscularly. The patient recovered.

Tetanus (Lockjaw)

Tetanus or lockjaw is a specific infectious disease caused by the *Bacillus tetani*, whose toxins have a close affinity for the central nervous system. The disease is accompanied by local tonic and clonic spasms.

The *B. tetani* has a drumstick shape and a spore at one end. It is gram-positive and anaerobic, being found in the soil. It enters the body through penetrating or puncture wounds, such as those produced by nails, gunshot, shrapnel. The incubation period is from one to three weeks and may depend on the locality of the wound. The incubation is of shorter duration with wounds of the face and neck. The earliest symptoms are frequent yawning, restlessness, apprehension, and difficulty in opening and closing the mouth.

Tonic spasms of the masseter muscles later cause marked pain in opening or closing the mouth. The muscles of the face and neck nearly all become spastic, and opisthotonus may occur. Clonic spasms occur locally and generally. They are stimulated by light, air, and even contact with bed clothes. The symptoms increase in severity, with hyperpyrexia, exhaustion, and finally death. The mental state of the patient is usually clear to the end.

Eye Manifestations.—The ocular muscles are sometimes affected in cephalic tetanus. A spasm of the orbicularis may be the first symptom. Other muscles supplied by the oculomotor nerve may also be involved. This may occur in one or both eyes but is usually first in the eye on the same side as the wound. Wounds of the eyeball, especially those in or around the ciliary body, may lead to tetanus. Pentrating and puncture wounds of the cornea even with enucleation of the eye have resulted in tetanus. Sattler[6] reported a case of penetrating wound of the cornea with enucleation of the eye within twenty-four hours, which was followed by death from tetanus in eight days. Another case treated by Zentmayer[7] resulted in death from tetanus after a perforating wound of the eyeball with prolapse of the iris which was replaced. Extreme miosis may occur and the pupil will fail to react to direct light stimulation. The internal ocular muscles may not be otherwise affected.

Treatment.—The treatment of tetanus includes prophylactic and specific treatment principally. Every suspicious wound or burn from explosives should be cleansed, and a prophylactic injection of 1,500 units of antitoxic serum should be administered. This should be done in the case of eye injuries as well as with others. In fact, no case of penetrating wound of the eye should be permitted to pass without receiving a prophylactic dose of tetanus anti-toxin. The earlier that the antitoxin is administered, the better are the chances for preventing and overcoming the infection. If no prophylactic protection has been given, 50,000 units of the antitoxic serum should be injected into the subarachnoid space with the same amount injected intramuscularly as soon as the signs or symptoms appear. This is then repeated daily.

The local treatment of the eye depends on the nature of the ocular injury.

Polyarthritis

There are several conditions which involve the joints and are designated by the term "arthritis." These are produced by a number of different factors and are difficult to classify. They include acute rheumatic fever (subacute articular rheumatism or polyarthritis rheumatica), other forms of septic or infective arthritis, and chronic nonsuppurative arthritis, including rheumatoid arthritis and osteoarthritis. Gout, which is ordinarily considered to be a metabolic disturbance, will be discussed under that heading.

Rheumatic Fever.—Rheumatic fever is an acute infectious disease which is characterized principally by polyarthritis, pharyngitis, and cardiac infection. While the exact cause of the infection is not known, many associate a strepto-coccus or diplococcus with the primary lesions. These have at times been isolated from the blood stream. A filtrable virus has also been considered to be the cause and the streptococcus a secondary or associated factor.

The polyarthritis consists of a swelling of the joints and a congestion of the synovial membrane with serofibrinous exudate which contains a few leuco-cytes. The typical pathologic characteristic of the disease is the so-called "Aschoff body" which is microscopic in size and occurs as a small area of

necrosis around the smaller blood vessels. It is surrounded by polymorphonuclear leucocytes and large basophilic cells which are probably derived from
the endothelium of the small blood vessels and perivascular spaces. It occurs
in all the acute lesions and, with the subsequent microscopic scarring, is always
evidence of a former infection.

This disease has a tendency to recur, and there is always a danger of re-
activation of the infection which may occur after years of quiescence. The avenue
of infection appears to be by way of the throat, and pharyngitis or tonsillitis
ushers in the onset in more than one-half of the cases. This manifestation of the
disease, especially among children and young people, is at least as important as
the arthritic involvement. It is accompanied by malaise, temperature of 102°
to 104° F., sweating, rapid pulse, and prostration. Anemia is characterized by
a decrease in the erythrocytes and hemoglobin. There is a leucocytosis of from
15,000 to 25,000, principally of the polymorphonuclear cells. The spleen may
become enlarged, and skin eruptions, such as erythema multiforme and erythema
nodosum, are common.

The arthritis may involve one or more of the joints and is accompanied by
severe pain, redness, and swelling. The duration of this phase varies in different cases and may subside after several weeks, although it can recur after a
period of quiescence. In children especially, recovery takes place without
impairment of function.

The heart is also seriously involved by the same pathologic factor which is
found with the other manifestations of the disease. Myocarditis occurs with
serious impairment of function due to the presence here of many of the Aschoff
bodies. This is characterized by cardiac enlargement and disturbances of
rhythm. The valves may be affected by the same process, resulting in valvulitis
or endocarditis. This is characterized by murmurs and changes in the character
of the heart sounds. Mitral insufficiency, mitral stenosis, and aortic insufficiency are the principal manifestations. The Aschoff bodies are here also considered to be responsible. Pericarditis, subcutaneous nodules, kidney disease,
and pneumonia may all occur during the course of rheumatic fever.

Chorea occurs in association with valvular disease at times and is considered a visceral manifestation of rheumatic fever. With the possible exception of the onset after scarlet fever, chorea should otherwise be considered as
a manifestation of rheumatic fever. Even after scarlet fever it is also likely
to be a part of this disease.

Sydenham's chorea usually occurs between the ages of 5 and 15 years, but
occasionally it affects adults. It may begin suddenly or slowly. Acute tonsillitis or pharyngitis may shortly precede the onset. Fever, malaise, anorexia,
and sometimes vomiting occur. A polyarthritis may precede or even follow
the chorea. The disease is characterized by uncontrolled, jerky movements of
the skeletal muscles with weakness and ataxia. These movements may occur on
one side or both and almost at any time, with or without provocation. This condition may persist for a long time after signs of the rheumatic infection have
subsided. Simultaneous visceral rheumatic heart lesions occur in many of these
cases. As the infection subsides and the temperature becomes normal, the chorea
becomes less pronounced and the movements eventually disappear.

Chronic Arthritis (Rheumatoid Arthritis).—Under the heading of chronic
arthritis may be included several nonsuppurative varieties, namely, rheumatoid
arthritis, arthritis deformans, atrophic arthritis, osteoarthritis, and a number of

others. Principal among these, however, especially from the standpoint of ocular involvement, is rheumatoid arthritis. Eye manifestations in arthritic conditions are commonly designated as "rheumatic" ocular conditions, as for example, "rheumatic iritis," with no particular reference to the special type of rheumatic or arthritic condition which is the primary disease. The conditions described here do not include the gonorrheal arthritis and the associated eye manifestations which are discussed elsewhere. (See Gonorrhea.)

Rheumatoid arthritis is ordinarily considered as an infectious disease, although this is not definitely determined. Neither is the etiology definitely known. It is considered to occur following trauma, exposure to dampness and cold, constitutional factors, and heredity. Climate is also an important predisposing factor in the cause of the disease since it is more prevalent in temperate zones than in the warmer climates. The disease usually occurs in middle and later life. Focal infections in the teeth, tonsils, nasal sinuses, prostate gland, gall bladder, and intestinal tract are considered to be frequent contributory causes. It has also been considered to be caused by a streptococcus infection. A form of chronic arthritis occurring in children is known as juvenile arthritis deformans, or Still's disease.

The onset of arthritis may be either slow or rapid. Low-grade fever, malaise, headache, and lymphadenopathy may occur. The finger and knee joints are usually the first to be involved. These are followed usually by manifestations in the wrists, elbows, shoulders, ankles, and later almost all the joints. One or two joints alone may be affected for a long time, the affection gradually spreading to the others. Local swelling occurs in the joints which is accompanied by some pain, although this may not be present in the same degree. The fingers gradually assume a stiff and arched appearance. Contraction takes place, leading to deformities in the fingers and other joints. Hyperextension, flexion, swelling, redness, and effusion may be found. The patient's general condition usually exhibits an emaciation and anemia. A vasoconstriction of the capillaries and reduction in their number leads to an impaired nutrition of all parts causing a lowered surface tension, cold clammy skin, muscle atrophy, and susceptibility to involvement of other organs. The bones, especially around the joints, lose their contour and fusion eventually takes place, especially in the wrists and fingers. In the joints themselves the inflammatory condition eventually causes a complete destruction of the articular surfaces. Fibroid nodules resembling those that occur in acute rheumatic fever may also occur here.

Rheumatoid arthritis may resemble gout, acute rheumatic fever, or osteoarthritis. The last named is often difficult to differentiate, and may, in fact, be present at the same time, especially late in the disease.

Eye Manifestations.—Very few eye manifestations can be definitely established as being rheumatic in origin. A possible exception is the occurrence of the ocular manifestation associated with gonorrheal arthritis in which case the specific cause and primary disease can be established with a degree of certainty. In most of the other arthritic conditions, there are no typical manifestations in the eye which will indicate the presence of the specific primary disease. In those eye conditions which are considered to occur with some form of rheumatic disease, the latter is sometimes revealed by the history and definite physical evidences in the joints. In other instances the primary disease can be only suspected and rarely a definite history of an earlier rheumatic affection is obtained. In these cases when a specific etiologic factor for the eye manifestation is not obtainable, most of the textbooks include "rheumatism" in discussing the etiology, or they may suggest a "rheumatic background." Some of these conditions are considered as being associated with an arthritic diathesis. Others are considered as manifestations of a metabolic disturbance (gout). Those which are thought to occur in patients with a "rheumatic background" are sometimes activated by exposure to cold, draughts, and dampness. The term "rheumatic," therefore, applied to an ocular manifestation does not necessarily indicate its etiology, since it may only be an associated reaction which is found in this type of patient with no known specific etiology.

Acute rheumatic fever in particular cannot be said to cause any typical eye manifestations. However, the eye may be affected during the course of either the pharyngeal or cardiac manifestations of the disease. These instances are rare, however, and should be considered as possible complications, rather than as manifestations themselves.

The Orbicularis Muscle.—Paralysis of the orbicularis occurs most frequently as a so-called rheumatic affection (Fuchs). The extraocular muscles also may become paralyzed as the result of the toxic condition. During the stage of chorea in acute rheumatic fever, the eyelids may take part in the jerky movements of the face and extremities which characterize the condition. These twitchings and jerky movements of the lids may be only choreiform in type, and the accompanying movements so mild, that they are sometimes attributed to an acquired habit on the part of the child affected.

Paralysis of the orbicularis is characterized by an inability to close the eye completely. This results in epiphora which may be present only in mild degree. In cases of long standing the lower lid falls away from the eyeball with the production of paralytic ectropion. As a result, the cornea is exposed, especially during sleep, and an ulcerative keratitis may develop. These paralyses, however, follow a favorable course and offer a good prognosis. When seen early enough, they respond favorably to treatment with the salicylates internally, and the use of massage and the galvanic current to the affected part.

Conjunctiva (Arthritic Conjunctivitis).—The conjunctivitis which occurs with chronic arthritic conditions is similar to that found at times in gout. It generally occurs in patients of middle and older age, in most of whom disturbances of metabolism may be an added factor. The conjunctivitis is characterized by a scant discharge but considerable hyperemia, and it runs a chronic course. The conjunctival vessels are dilated and various sized ecchymoses may occur. The lid margins are red, irritated, and sometimes covered with a thin film of serous secretion. Both eyes are usually affected.

The patient complains of a dry, stiff feeling of the eyeball, and difficulty in opening the eyes, especially on awakening in the mornings. This is accompanied by burning, itching, and a scratching sensation. The eyeballs feel heavy and stiff, being aggravated by dampness, cold weather, and with exacerbation in the condition of the joints.

The treatment of rheumatic or arthritic conjunctivitis requires special attention to the primary disease. Local treatment is symptomatic and only palliative. This should consist only of a mild alkaline eyewash daily, avoiding the use of stronger astringent and irritating solutions.

Scleritis and Episcleritis.—Inflammations of the sclera are not uncommon in patients who suffer with arthritis. The episcleritis and scleritis occurring in these patients present no particular characteristics to identify them as rheumatic in origin. The patient is usually one of older age, who is known to have been suffering with rheumatism. The inflammation may be found in the episcleral tissue over the recti muscles and may extend to the limbus of the cornea. It has a violet or purple color and is nodular in appearance. The condition is accompanied by pain which is rather dull and constant. One or both eyes may be affected. An attack of episcleritis may subside after a rather protracted course, only to recur at some later date.

Scleritis may prove to be more severe and may be complicated by corneal or uveal involvement. It may occur in one or both eyes and presents the appearance of a bluish area around the cornea. The periphery of the cornea itself may in some cases become involved as in brawny scleritis. In other instances the inflammation may extend posteriorly. The deeper structures may become involved by the edema and result in great pain, impaired vision, interference with motility, and vitreous opacities. As the disease subsides, the sclera becomes thin and atrophic, sometimes resulting in an ectasia behind the limbus of the cornea.

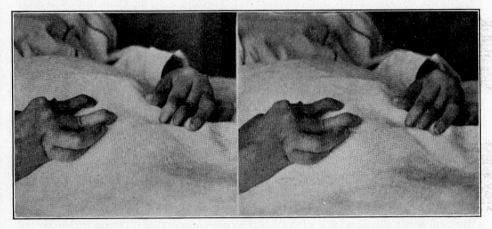

Fig. 137.—Hands of a patient with scleromalacia perforans. (From van der Hoeve: Arch. Ophth., January, 1934.)

In cases of osteo-arthritis, a grayish-blue discoloration of the sclera may be found in association with ochronosis, a bluish discoloration of the ears, and alkaptonuria. Brownish pigment spots may occur in the conjunctiva near the tendon insertions. The scleral ochronosis develops gradually and in association with the pigmentation of the ear cartilages. In advanced cases the cornea may also show superficial pigment spots on examination with the slit lamp. These occur near the temporal or nasal limbus. Smith,[8] who reported four of these cases and reviewed the literature on the subject, called attention to the fact that the pigmentation in the conjunctiva and cornea could be seen early in the patients with alkaptonuria who were past middle age. He also pointed out the fact that the first sign is often gray discoloration of the sclera with brown spots of pigment near the tendon insertions. The slit lamp examination shows the brown pigment to be subepithelial and arranged in small round and crescentic formations. The nose and finger joints may also be discolored in these cases.

The three important diagnostic features of the condition, however, are pigmentation of the sclera and ears, urine that becomes dark on exposure to air, and osteo-arthritis.

The treatment of episcleritis consists in the use of a mild, astringent eyewash daily, and the application of warm compresses to the affected eye for a period of ten minutes three or four times daily. Internally, the use of salicylates and epinephrine, in addition to active elimination and diaphoresis, is indicated.

Scleritis does not respond well to treatment. Active treatment of the rheumatic condition is indicated, with the salicylates being administered regularly. In addition, active elimination and diaphoresis are also indicated here. Locally, atropine sulfate, 1 per cent solution, should be instilled into the eye two or three times daily. An astringent eyewash and hot applications can be employed with relief from pain and congestion.

Scleromalacia Perforans is a degenerative condition of the sclera which has been described by van der Hoeve[9] as a clinical entity, and which occurs especially in patients suffering with rheumatic arthritis. Inflammation was said to play very little or no part whatsoever in the process, so that it was designated by the name "scleromalacia perforans." The condition was first noted by van der Hoeve in 1928 and was characterized by the presence of "holes in the sclera." These holes may coalesce with the formation of large gaps in which the uvea is either exposed or covered only by the conjunctiva. The degeneration of the sclera was found to occur with negative bacteriologic findings in patients with chronic rheumatic polyarthritis. The degeneration leads to the development of holes of various sizes in the sclera, over which the conjunctiva may be present or absent. When present, it may be atrophic. The cornea and uveal tract may become secondarily involved. Two cases by van der Hoeve were originally described, and later he reported two additional cases of Rochet. The first was in a woman, 55 years of age, who had suffered with chronic rheumatic polyarthritis for many years. The second case was an old woman with all the joints of the trunk and limbs ankylosed so that she was unable to move about. The third was also a woman, 54 years old, who suffered with ankylosis of almost every joint in the body. The disease began ten years earlier with an attack of acute rheumatism. In all three cases holes were present in the sclera with exposure of the uvea, although the latter was not prolapsed. This was explained by the fact that the tension of the eye remains normal and the uvea can, under certain conditions, stand the pressure without the support of the sclera, or that the exposed choroid permits enough fluid to pass out to prevent bulging. The holes which at first begin as small nodules, may occur in any part of the sclera from the corneal limbus to the equator. Secondary infection may occur, as in one of the cases originally described, with hypopyon and loss of vision. Both eyes are usually affected by the disease. The fourth case described occurred in a man of 69 years of age who had never had any symptoms of rheumatism, so that van der Hoeve concluded that it is possible for two types of scleromalacia to be distinguished, one occurring with rheumatism, and the other without.

Following von der Hoeve, other cases have been reported by Oast,[10] Verhoeff and King,[11] and Eggers,[12] as well as others.

Oast's case occurred in one eye of a man, 76 years of age, who had no symptoms of rheumatism or arthritic involvement. The condition here showed signs of some low-grade inflammation.

Verhoeff and King,[11] in reporting a case in which the eye was examined microscopically, also analyzed the reports of fourteen other cases. They found that the slightly elevated nodules involve the sclera and overlying tissue and develop simultaneously in one or both eyes. A moderate congestion may be present around or in the vicinity of the nodules. After a period of several months, one or more of the nodules may disappear, leaving a shallow but large cavity in the sclera. The conjunctiva may be absent or intact over the cavity. If the lesion occurs near the limbus of the cornea, it may perforate into the anterior chamber, producing a cystoid nodule resembling that following a trephine operation. The iris may or may not be prolapsed into this nodule. The condition may be complicated by synechiae, atrophy of the iris, cataract, and secondary infection. Verhoeff and King suggested the name of necroscleritis nodosa excavans.

The disease may occur in either sex, and principally in older patients. The visual acuity may be seriously affected, and the eye may even become blind. Severe and prolonged pain may be present in the eye.

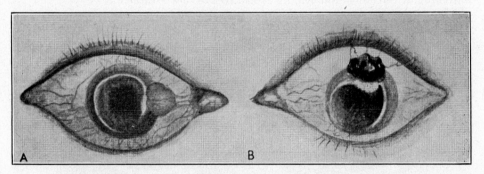

Fig. 138.—An unusual case of scleromalacia perforans. *A*, Right eye; *B*, left eye. (From van der Hoeve: Arch. Ophth., January, 1934.)

According to Verhoeff and King, the histologic changes showed that the primary ocular lesions consist of a sharply defined area of necrotic scleral tissue. Becoming surrounded by a wall of epithelioid cells and infiltrated slowly with pus cells, a sequestrum is formed which becomes disintegrated and densely infiltrated with necrotic material. The cavities in the sclera are due to the abscesses so formed. These perforate the sclera and discharge their contents externally. A thin layer of new formed fibrous tissue with pigment cells in its deepest portions remains at the site of the abscess. Destructive edema of the macula may result from the diffusion of toxins from the necrotic areas in the sclera through the vitreous. The histologic structure of the lesion excluded the possibility of tuberculosis or syphilis as a cause. Verhoeff and King also found that the nodules are essentially the same as the subcutaneous nodules occurring in rheumatoid arthritis.

Eggers' case[12] was described as ''necroscleritis nodosa and polyarthritis,[11] occurring in a 37-year-old white woman who complained of painful swollen joints of two years' duration. Both eyes were affected with swellings in the upper anterior portion of the sclera. A uveitis developed and bilateral massive hemorrhages of the vitreous. A sclerosing keratitis also developed in the right cornea.

In a report of three cases of rheumatoid arthritis with scleral involvement, Smoleroff[13] found the pathologic changes in the eye to be identical with those described by Verhoeff and King.

Treatment.—There is little information available concerning the treatment of this condition. Verhoeff suggested curettage of the scleral nodules to prevent edema of the macula and other intraocular complications.

Oast employed ultraviolet rays in the treatment of his case and obtained relief from the pain which had been present constantly from the onset. The old lesions began to disappear, and no new ones appeared. He used a Birch-Hirschfeld carbon lamp with a uviol filter and obtained satisfactory results after a few exposures.

Mills[14] recommended local treatment with a 20 per cent solution of zinc sulfate to arrest the lesion. Cocaine hydrochloride, 4 per cent, and epinephrine (1:1,000) are instilled four times. The application is then made with a wet swab and held there for twenty seconds. This is followed by washing with boric acid and the application of cold compresses. The treatment is repeated daily, with flattening of the lesion and healing after three to four treatments.

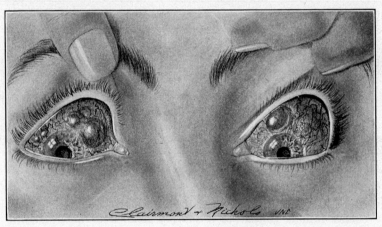

Fig. 139.—Necroscleritis nodosa associated with chronic rheumatoid polyarthritis. (Described by van der Hoeve as "scleromalacia perforans.") (From Eggers: Arch. Ophth., March, 1940.)

Tenonitis.—Tenonitis is an inflammation of the capsule of Tenon which is considered to occur in patients who suffer with rheumatic arthritis. The occurrence may be aggravated in such patients after exposure to cold and drafts. It is characterized by the appearance of redness, swelling, and chemosis under the conjunctiva of the affected eye. The condition may at first be confined to a particular area of the eyeball which is usually on the temporal side of the cornea. It may be accompanied by swelling of the eyelids, moderate pain, and occasionally a slight elevation in temperature. The onset may be rather sudden with a moderate edematous appearance of the bulbar conjunctiva and tenderness over this area, the pain being aggravated on rotation of the eyeball. The pain and edema may increase, and in time, considerable chemosis with interference of rotation of the eyeball is present. In more severe cases the inflammatory condition may extend deep into the orbit and cause a marked edema and chemosis of the entire eyeball and the eyelids. The condition may affect one or both eyes. The course of the inflammation is usually protracted and may remain unchanged for a number of weeks. The vision of the affected eye remains unimpaired. Episcleritis and scleritis are often found to accompany tenonitis.

Treatment.—This consists principally in the treatment of the primary condition and includes the use of salicylates, Colchicum, elimination, and diaphoresis. The administration of foreign proteins may be beneficial in some cases. The local treatment should include the application of warm boric acid compresses to the eye for a period of ten minutes three times daily, astringents, such as zinc sulfate, by instillation, and the occasional use of adrenalin. In cases with marked chemosis and edema of the conjunctiva and lids, which result in incomplete closure of the eyelids, the cornea should be protected from exposure which might result in the formation of corneal ulcers.

Rheumatic Iritis.—A form of toxic iritis occurs in patients who suffer with rheumatic arthritis which has a tendency to frequent recurrence and relapse. This has often been designated as rheumatic iritis and must be differentiated by the history and examination from other forms, such as gonorrheal iritis, and that which occurs in some of the acute infectious diseases. The onset is usually acute, while the course may be prolonged with marked impairment of the vision in the affected eye. The patient will usually give a history of having suffered with rheumatism sometime in the past. The iritis in these cases is also aggravated by exposure to cold, dampness, and draughts.

The objective symptoms on examination are found to be profuse lacrimation, photophobia, and a reddish injection around the cornea. The pupil is small when first seen, and on examination with the slit lamp, fine deposits may be found on the posterior surface of the cornea. There may also be posterior synechiae and very fine opacities in the vitreous, especially if the uveal tract has become involved to any extent. The iris itself may not show any noticeable discoloration, and there may be no signs of marked exudation. The patient complains of more or less pain, which radiates to the forehead and the face on the affected side. The pain is usually worse at night, and interferes with the patient's sleep. Examination of the blood reveals a negative Wassermann, and these cases also show no reaction to tuberculin tests. A rheumatic history or the history of pains in the joints is of particular value in establishing the condition as a rheumatic iritis.

Relapse may occur after full recovery has taken place. The condition may be complicated by increase in the intraocular tension, and the development of secondary glaucoma.

Treatment.—The patient should wear dark glasses. The local treatment consists in the instillation of atropin sulfate, 1 per cent, into the affected eye as soon as the case is first seen in order to dilate the pupil and prevent the formation of synechiae. This should be instilled three times daily. Relief from pain will be obtained from the use of atropine and the application of hot wet compresses to the affected eye for a period of fifteen to twenty minutes, three or four times daily. Ten grains of sodium salicylate should be given four times daily. The use of Colchicum and the iodides may also prove beneficial. The patient should avoid extremes of temperature as well as exposure to cold and dampness. Diaphoresis and attention to elimination will prove beneficial.

Choroiditis.—Rheumatic conditions may also be the cause of choroiditis, especially in those cases which have suffered with recurrent attacks of rheumatic iritis. The entire choroid is usually involved with the appearance of round yellowish areas in the fundus and moderate pigmentary changes. These spots are distinguished from exudates in that they are spots of atrophy and of a rather sharp outline later becoming white in color.

The treatment consists principally in the general treatment of the underlying rheumatic condition, the use of pilocarpine, mercury, iodides, and salicylates.

Undulant Fever (Brucellosis, Malta Fever)

Undulant fever is also known by several names which among others include brucellosis, Malta fever, Mediterranean fever, and Gibraltar fever. Although prevalent in North America, it originated in the Mediterranean countries of Europe and Asia.

An acute specific infectious disease, undulant fever occurs in epidemic form and is caused by the *Micrococcus melitensis* of Bruce or the *Bacillus abortus* of Bang. It was first described by Bruce after whom the organisms were named the Brucella. They were known to be present in goats, and later were found to be the cause of abortion and were isolated in cattle by Bang. Still later, they were found by Traum to be the cause of abortion in swine. In 1918 Evans showed that they were all identical by morphologic, biochemical, cultural, and agglutination tests. They have since been designated, therefore, by the generic name of Brucella, although the different species, *Bacillus melitensis* of Bruce, the *Bacillus abortus* of Bang, and *Bacillus suis* of Traum, are recognized.

The disease is usually contracted by those who work in slaughterhouses and by butchers, the organisms entering through the skin or the food being infected by contaminated hands. In others, the disease is produced by the ingestion of contaminated food, such as milk, butter, and cheese, which is made from the milk of infected goats and cows. Many animals may appear to be normal but are carriers of the disease. A raw milk supply may cause a large number of cases in a community, and the patients may have had no direct contact with cattle. The chief characteristic of the disease is a prolonged febrile course with irregular remissions and exacerbations. The *B. abortus* was first isolated by Keefer in 1924 from the blood of a patient who suffered with a long-continued fever. The bovine variety seems to be most pathogenic in human beings.

The incubation period is from about five days to three weeks, the average being about two weeks. There may be no prodromal symptoms during this period. The onset may be sudden and characterized by a chill and abrupt rise in temperature to 103° or 105° F., but usually there is a gradual onset with a temperature showing an increase at night and a drop to normal in the mornings. This is accompanied by sweating, chilly sensations, and progressive weakness. The patient nearly always feels better in the mornings, and the symptoms become more pronounced later in the day and evening. The temperature may reach as high as 106° F., although the patient might not appear to be as sick as this would indicate. In many, however, there are anorexia, constipation, gradual loss of weight, restlessness, and a typhoid state. The patient may suffer with polyarthritis which usually affects the larger joints and is characterized by a transient swelling and redness. The spleen is enlarged in a few cases, and abdominal pain may be present in moderate degree. Blood examination reveals a secondary anemia and a leucopenia. The leucocytes scarcely ever total more than 5,000, and there is a relative lymphocytosis. During the earlier stages of the disease, the organisms may be found in the blood culture. The infection may be widely disseminated by the blood stream and lymphatics, so that almost any organ may be the location of a local lesion. The tonsils have been found to harbor the organisms, while the genitourinary tract has frequently been found to be the site of a transitory infection. Abortion is frequent among pregnant women, and the organisms have been isolated from the fetus, placenta, and vaginal discharge.

The course of the disease may run for many months with recurrences of the fever which may last for periods of two to three weeks at a time. Any of the symptoms may either appear for the first time or reappear during the exacerbations. The disease may exhibit many different manifestations, and several varieties have been described. These include a latent type in which a long period will intervene between a definite infection and appearance of the fever. In such cases the organism has been isolated without any history or symptoms of the disease. In a second mild variety the patients are ambulatory but complain of fatigue and malaise especially in the evening, while they still continue at work. A third type, which is common, is characterized by prolonged fever with remissions and may last for several months. The fourth type includes those cases with undulating fever which is characterized by remissions and exacerbations at regular intervals. This type is commonly caused by the *Brucella melitensis*. The fifth type includes those cases which are chronic and exhibit either continuous or recurring forms of temperature which may last for more than a year. The third and fourth types may also become chronic and change into the fifth type, lasting for several years. The sixth is a rare, acute, or fulminating type which is usually fatal in this country. In any of these types one particular lesion only may be outstanding and dominate the clinical picture. As the result the true condition may fail to be recognized, and the diagnosis can be made only, if at all suspected, by recovery of the organism or by laboratory tests.

Green,[15] who published a detailed article on the subject, emphasized the importance of competent laboratory aid and described three tests to perform in these suspected cases. First, an opsonocytophagic test, in which 5 c.c. of the patient's blood are mixed with 20 per cent sodium citrate (0.2 c.c.). With this is mixed a standard strain of Brucella which has been incubated for forty-eight hours. The mixture is then incubated at 37° C. for one hour, after which ordinary blood smears are made and stained. Fifty white cells are examined to determine the number of organisms picked up by each. An opsonocytophagic index is calculated from this according to a method described by Foshay, which reveals the index number in most cases to parallel roughly the degree of the patient's resistance.

The blood agglutination test is said to be of value only if it is positive. In most of the chronic cases it is negative. It is not a test for the presence of organisms, but only for the determination of specific agglutinins in the blood. It has been pointed out that in patients who present a clinical picture of brucellosis, a partial agglutination with *B. abortus* is just as significant as is agglutination in higher dilutions of the serum. The test is carried out in the usual way with an agglutination titer of 1 in 160 or higher, for a positive diagnosis.

The cutaneous test consists in the intradermal injection in the forearm of a small quantity of killed bacillary suspension or Huddleson's brucellin.

Within twenty-four hours or sooner the reaction begins and is characterized by a quickly spreading area of redness with an indurated center. This is accompanied by heat, pain, and itching. Occasional sloughing of the superficial tissue may occur. A reaction which continues to the third day is considered to be positive. The patient may show variable effects of the test. A few may feel better in general, while in a great many, the symptoms may become intensified. About 25 per cent will show no reaction. Positive reaction to any of the tests does not prove an active brucellosis but indicates only that the patient has or in the past has had the disease. The cutaneous test is said to be the most sensitive and of greatest value in the detection of the condition which is inactive and presents few or poorly defined symptoms.

Eye Manifestations.—Green[15] reported on four of his own cases and twenty-seven other cases gathered from the literature. In all the clinical diagnosis was confirmed by laboratory tests and by the exclusion of other infections that might have caused the condition. From the description of these it is concluded that some ocular lesions formerly attributed to other conditions may be caused by brucellosis.

The external ocular muscles, the cornea, the uveal tract, the retina, and the optic nerve have all been affected. In an ocular condition such as uveitis with an obscure or undetermined etiology, the possibility of brucellosis should be seriously considered, and the laboratory tests described should be made to determine its presence or absence.

Pathologic examinations of human eyes affected with brucellosis have been lacking because of the fact that most of the lesions fail to destroy the eye to the extent that enucleation is necessary. However, an investigation of the eyes of guinea pigs which died of melitensis was reported by Orloff.[16] This described circumcorneal injection as the first manifestation in the eye. The cornea showed slight central clouding while the iris showed some hyperemia and the pupil was filled with a grayish exudate. On microscopic examination the cornea in cases of slight involvement showed extensive desquamation of the central epithelium, degeneration of the epithelium, and the formation of vacuoles in the nuclei at the periphery. Vacuoles and lesions of the endothelial cells were found to correspond to the cloudy center. In more pronounced cases the findings were similar to those seen in interstitial keratitis of syphilis. Many posterior synechiae and diffuse infiltration of the iris were found. The ciliary body was most commonly affected with infiltration of lymphoid and epithelioid cells. The vitreous was found to be fluid; the lens showed evidences of inflammatory cataract. The choroid was affected by hyperemia and infiltration and migration of subretinal pigment with round cells and fibrin in the posterior uveal tract. The ocular findings seemed to be very similar both pathologically and clinically to those occurring in ocular tuberculosis.

It is not possible to describe clinical eye manifestations which are typical or characteristic of brucellosis. From a survey of the cases gathered by Green, it is possible for almost any ocular condition to be found in the course of the disease. It is, therefore, necessary to enumerate these manifestations as described in the twenty-seven cases reported.

It should be remembered that these manifestations may occur at any time during the course of the disease and may improve as well as show recurrences. In some cases the patient may complain of failing vision, and this subjective symptom may lead to further examination which reveals objective signs. In most of the cases only one eye is affected, although the ocular condition may be bilateral. The visual acuity may be only slightly diminished or it may be greatly impaired and entirely lost. In a few cases the vision is regained after having been greatly impaired during the course of the involvement.

Other subjective symptoms which might be complained of are photophobia, lacrimation, and diplopia. These are usually due to the presence of actual involvement of certain of the ocular structures.

It is usually difficult to attribute the etiology of an ocular condition to brucellosis. This is especially true in those patients with eye manifestations who present no obvious clinical signs or symptoms of brucellosis. It is therefore important in cases of obscure origin to obtain a detailed history and to think of this disease as a possible etiologic factor. Very few, if any, patients with ocular involvement are found to exhibit any symptoms of active brucellosis. Careful questioning may bring out the history of drinking raw milk or of some contact with infected animals. When the systemic disease is suspected in a patient with ocular involvement, the diagnosis must be confirmed by serologic and laboratory tests. These may present evidence of past infection with Brucella or that the patient is suffering with the chronic form of the disease.

Paralysis of the Extraocular Muscles.—The extraocular muscles have been found to suffer a paralysis either unilateral or bilateral in a number of cases. The external recti seem to be the most commonly affected. This is characterized by an inability to rotate the eyes outward and may occur in both eyes simultaneously; more commonly, first one eye is affected and the second at a later date. The paralysis usually occurs as the result of meningitis or encephalomeningitis complicating the condition. In one case paralysis of the sixth, seventh, and tenth pair of nerves was reported. The oculomotor nerve may also be involved. In most of the cases the paralysis was found to improve.

Pupils.—The pupils were found to be affected in several ways. In one case they were dilated, while in several they were unequal in size, and in most instances the reaction to light was either weak or absent.

Conjunctiva and Cornea.—The external eye has been described as red and irritable, with the presence of conjunctivitis, usually associated with iritis or keratitis. In the first case described by Green, the patient first suffered with an inflammation of the right eye which was diagnosed as phlyctenular conjunctivitis. The cornea was clear. This condition improved only to recur at a much later date when the margin of the cornea showed a lesion extending from 3 to 4 o'clock. This recovered but was followed by several attacks later on in the course of the disease which finally led to the development of a marginal corneal ulcer, involving about one-sixth of the circumference. It appears that the cornea is the least involved of all the ocular structures, although in one or two cases, the condition was found to resemble parenchymatous keratitis. Hypopyon has also been found to occur.

Iritis and Iridocyclitis.—The iris and ciliary body are commonly affected by inflammation, resulting in the presence of iritis and iridocyclitis. The characteristic symptoms are photophobia, synechiae, and deposits on the posterior cornea. The inflammation may be either acute, subacute, or chronic, and vascularization of the iris may occur. In some cases the pupil may be bound down and cause serious impairment of the vision. Deposits of fine pigment may be found on the anterior capsule of the lens.

Examination with the ophthalmoscope will reveal the condition of the vitreous and fundus. In many cases with iritis and iridocyclitis the deposits on the cornea and anterior capsule of the lens can be observed, and the vitreous may be found to be cloudy.

The fundus oculi may reveal the presence of small hemorrhages, greenish-yellow exudates, edema of the retina, discoloration of the macula, and the presence of central retinochoroiditis. In one instance massive hemorrhages of the retina were described.

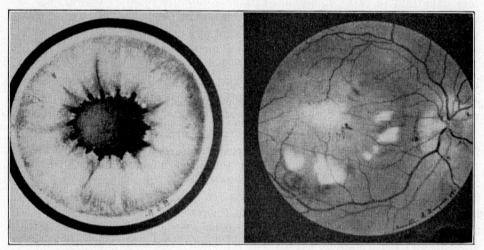

Fig. 140.—Left, Iritis in brucellosis. Right, Choroiditis in brucellosis. (From Woods and Guyton: Tr. Am. Acad. Ophth. [1943], March-April, 1944.)

Uveitis.—Woods and Guyton[17] described fifteen cases of uveitis as "probably" due to brucellosis. They also emphasized the fact that the etiology could not be established with certainty in any case. Moreover, the ocular picture was in no way characteristic. Seven of the fifteen patients revealed the presence of a simple recurrent iritis. One patient showed definite nodules on the iris, another showed questionable deep nodules, and a third showed Koeppe nodules. The uveitis affected both eyes in twelve patients and only one eye in three. The changes affected the choroid alone in three patients with one or more moderately circumscribed exudates which were elevated and with little surrounding reaction or edema. In five patients there was a generalized uveitis, and in eight the condition appeared to be granulomatous with thickening of the iris, posterior synechia and epithelial cells deposited on Descemet's membrane. Seven of the cases were of the nongranulomatous type with no nodules on the iris and only small lymphocytic keratitic deposits.

Optic Nerve.—The optic nerve may be affected by optic neuritis, retrobulbar neuritis, papilledema, and optic atrophy. The optic neuritis is characterized by the typical blurring of the disc margins and moderate edema around the disc. It may affect one or both eyes with impairment of the visual acuity. The condition improves in most instances, but may result in more or less permanent impairment of vision.

Papilledema is usually found to be bilateral and a choking of several diopters may be present. This has been reported in a number of cases, and in some of these the condition subsided with little or no impairment of the vision, while in others it was followed by optic atrophy. The papilledema may be found occasionally in undulant fever in the absence of other definite signs and symptoms. According to Rutherford[18] the central nervous system may occasionally be infected with melitensis, either with or without ocular complications.

Optic atrophy may occur following optic neuritis, neuroretinitis, papilledema, and retinochoroiditis. It is usually characterized by the appearance of a grayish-white color of the disc. The margins of the disc are slightly blurred, and the excavation usually is shallow. The alterations found in the visual fields in these cases consisted principally of a concentric contraction of the form and color fields.

Secondary glaucoma may occur as a complication, especially following hemorrhage into the vitreous and after recurrent cases of iritis and iridocyclitis.

Treatment.—The treatment of undulant fever includes prophylaxis, general and local treatment. Prophylaxis consists in removal of possible sources of infection and transmission. Gloves should be worn by those who are employed in the handling of infected cattle, goats, or pigs, and those who handle these meats in slaughterhouses. Thorough cleansing of the hands and the prevention of lacerations is important. Laboratory workers who handle cultures of brucella should take the same precautions and also wear masks to prevent infection through the respiratory tract. In sections of the country where the disease is known to be present in cattle, the milk should be pasteurized before it is consumed or made into butter or cheese. Herds supplying the milk should be tested for brucella infections.

The general treatment of the disease depends principally on its manifestations. If the disease is active, the patient should have rest in bed, plenty of fluids, and control of the fever. Attention should be given to restlessness, insomnia, and any of the other symptoms presented. There is no specific form of therapy which can be employed. Chemotherapy, fever therapy, and specific serums and vaccines have been employed with varying results.

Green employed Foshay's antimelitensis serum effectively in the acute stages of the disease. This was found to be beneficial also in choroiditis, uveitis, and keratitis where the clinical symptoms were confirmed by laboratory tests.

The local treatment of the ocular condition depends, of course, on the nature of the manifestation. Most of these seem to improve with improvement in the general condition of the patient. In some instances with severe optic neuritis and papilledema, the condition finally showed satisfactory improvement with no particular form of treatment. Cases of keratitis, iritis, and iridocyclitis should all be treated by the instillation of one drop of atropine sulfate, 1 per cent, into the affected eye three times daily. Black glasses should be worn by the patient, and the use of the eyes should be restricted absolutely. Hot, wet compresses of boric acid can be applied to the affected eyes for ten minutes, three times a day. In Green's case of marginal corneal ulcer, he employed ultraviolet radiation with the Hildreth lamp and kept the eye atropinized for two and a half weeks, with complete healing of the lesion and no recurrences. He also administered Foshay's vaccine which was said to be followed by marked improvement.

A well-developed case of kerato-iritis, in which the agglutination test for *Brucella abortus* and *Brucella melitensis* was negative, was reported by Green[19] in a young woman 24 years of age. The skin test and opsonocytophagic tests were positive and a presumptive diagnosis of brucellosis was made. The patient had previously received a number of other forms of treatment, all of which were ineffective. There was a vascular keratitis in the right eye with a plastic iritis. The left eye developed total posterior synechia, with iris hombe and secondary glaucoma. Carefully regulated courses of Foshay vaccine (*Brucella abortus* vaccine) were then administered beginning with a dose of $\frac{1}{20}$ c.c. of T-1 and gradually increased over a period of time. These injections were given three times a week and resulted in a clearing of both corneas and a great diminution in vascularization. Green emphasized the prompt and energetic treatment with a brucella vaccine as a means of checking the progress of the disease and preventing blindness in those patients in whom other etiology can be excluded.

Glanders

Glanders is a disease occurring among horses, but it may rarely occur in human beings as the result of inoculation of a wound with infected material. It is caused by the *Bacillus mallei,* and the incubation period is from three days to four weeks. Those who are employed with horses, such as hostlers, farmers, and stableboys, may become infected. The onset of the disease may be either acute or chronic. In the acute form it is ushered in with headache, malaise, nausea, and vomiting. Pain may be general. The patient may also suffer chills and increased temperature. After a few days, small abscesses with intense local reaction appear on the skin, and a lymphangitis, accompanied by hard nodules, develops. The mucous membrane of the respiratory tract may also be affected. The lesions undergo necrosis and suppuration.

In the chronic form the disease has an insidious onset and general symptoms are absent. There are noduar swellings on the skin which suppurate, then become necrotic with the formation of indolent ulcers which produce a sticky discharge. These ulcers may be multiple and are common on the mucous membrane of the nose and nasopharynx.

The diagnosis of the condition might be difficult, since the ulcers and nodules may resemble a syphilitic or tuberculous infection. If the *B. mallei* is found in the discharge, the diagnosis is definitely established. The course of the disease varies. Acute cases usually terminate fatally, while the chronic cases may last for a number of years.

Eye Manifestations.—Glanders manifests itself in the eyes chiefly in the form of a conjunctivitis called conjunctival glanders. The disease has been reported primarily in the conjunctiva and existed in association with enlargement of the preauricular glands. The mucous membrane of the nose and pharynx may be involved at the same time. Although the conjunctival infection is rare, the condition may be severe in type. Ulcers and granulomas similar to those found in other parts occur on the conjunctiva.

Treatment.—The treatment of glanders itself is described as being principally symptomatic and local treatment by surgery and thermocautery.

For the conjunctival ulceration galvanocautery has been recommended. A mild eyewash may be prescribed, such as boric acid or mercurophen or metaphen solution, flushing the eye at least three times daily. In some cases the condition may eventually clear up after a number of months.

Tularemia

Tularemia is an acute, specific, infectious disease caused by the *Bacterium tularense*. It is usually transmitted to man from rabbits, squirrels, mice, or other rodents. It might also be transmitted by the bites of intermediary insects, as fleas or ticks. It is frequently contracted by man, however, in the handling or skinning of the small infected animals. The disease is recognized as an oculoglandular syndrome which is characterized by a glandular swelling accompanied by a nodular form of conjunctivitis.

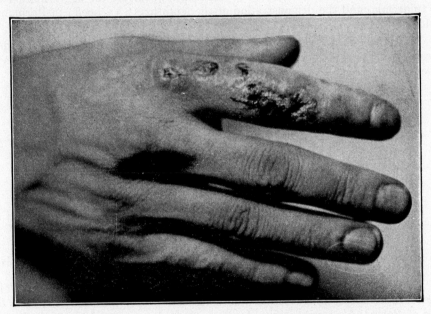

Fig. 141.—Lesion of tularemia on right index finger. (Courtesy of Dr. Walter M. Simpson, from Sutton and Sutton: Diseases of the Skin.)

The incubation period is from one to seven days, with the average about three days. The onset is usually sudden with a chill and fever, headache, malaise, general pains, prostration, and vomiting. This is accompanied by almost simultaneous swelling and tenderness of the glands of the neck on the affected side. These include the preauricular, parotid, submaxillary, and cervical glands. In most cases of the oculoglandular type the eye lesion appears early and is accompanied by a congestion of the conjunctiva, photophobia, and lacrimation. In other instances the primary lesion may occur on the hands or fingers, which spread by way of the lymphatics to the regional nodes. In some cases, there is a pronounced general adenopathy while in only a few others, there may be no conspicuous glandular enlargement, but a marked systemic reaction of the typhoid type. The disease has terminated fatally in some cases.

The *Bacterium tularense (Brucella tularensis)* is a gram-negative, nonmotile organism which can be grown on coagulated egg yolk medium, but no growth is obtained on agar. The first case of oculoglandular tularemia in man was recognized in 1914 and confirmed on laboratory examination by Wherry and Lamb. A number of cases have been reported since that time, and this number has been increased in recent years.

The history and clinical features of the disease are rather characteristic and the diagnosis of the condition should not be unusually difficult. This can be aided by a positive agglutination test since it has been shown that the patient's serum in tularemia will agglutinate the bacillus. This test is usually positive in the second week of the disease. Guinea pig inoculation may also produce the systemic symptoms.

This disease has often been confused with the oculoglandular syndrome of Parinaud, or what has often been termed Parinaud's conjunctivitis (See page 346). The two conditions are now separated, however, by the agglutination test for tularemia, and the demonstration of the leptothrix (Verhoeff) in Parinaud's oculoglandular condition.

In the past the disease has also been considered as a manifestation of tuberculosis, and the tubercle bacillus has been demonstrated in examinations of some lesions.

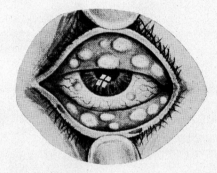

Fig. 142.—Conjunctival tularensis.   (After Vail, from Duke-Elder: Text-Book of Ophthalmology.)

Hurst[20] described twenty-three cases of oculoglandular disease, two of which cases were definitely diagnosed as tularemia and clearly differentiated from the cases of Parinaud's conjunctivitis by their clinical course and the agglutination reaction.

Eye Manifestations.—Tularemia affecting the eye is described as conjunctival tularensis. It has been called "the first American disease of the eye" by Duke-Elder, and "the only widespread disease of the human body discovered through the agency of ophthalmology."

The disease usually affects one eye, but it may occasionally occur in both. The primary seat of the infection is the conjunctiva. The vision of the eye is not necessarily seriously affected. The lids may be swollen and reddened, and the tarsal and palpebral conjunctiva reddened. Hurst[20] stated that in about 1 per cent of 6,274 cases the conjunctiva was the primary seat of the infection. Photophobia and lacrimation may be complained of.

The typical lesion is the occurrence, shortly after the onset, of small areas varying in size from 1 mm. to 5 mm. on the tarsal and palpebral conjunctiva. They occur mostly on the lower lid, but the upper may also be involved. The lesions are discrete and yellowish-colored ulcers spread over the conjunctiva.

They may number up to eight or ten in a single case. As the condition progresses, the ulcer becomes necrotic and, later, nodular. They have been described as "yellowish polka dots in a piece of red calico." (Vail, quoted by Hurst.)

The glandular involvement is usually observed at the same time, and this may progress to suppuration which requires incision and drainage. The patient is quite ill with a temperature which runs a somewhat prolonged course. The conjunctival involvement continues during this time and may not begin to subside for one to two months. Involvement of the cornea is rare, although several cases with corneal ulcer and also iritis have been reported. When the condition subsides, the conjunctival ulcers and nodules gradually disappear. The conjunctiva itself may remain somewhat thickened for some time, but no scarring results. The systemic and glandular manifestations may continue on for a longer period of time while they gradually subside.

Francis,[21] in reviewing the subject of tularemia in detail, analyzed seventy-eight American cases of the oculoglandular condition. Wild rabbits caused the disease in fifty-six of the patients by contamination with the hand and in two patients by blood spurting into the eye. Other cases were caused variously by tick tissue conveyed to the eyes by the fingers, a fly, ground hog bile entering the eye, a tree squirrel and a dog.

Dacryocystitis occurred in five patients and was purulent in three. The conjunctival secretion was purulent in five, chalazion was present in two, chemosis in ten, and epiphora in one. Ulcers were present on the tarsal conjunctiva in forty-three patients and on the bulbar conjunctiva in eight. Conjunctival nodules without ulceration on the tarsus were present in six and on the bulbar conjunctiva in one.

Six showed corneal ulcers with resultant scarring in three. Impairment of vision from perforation and prolapse of the iris occurred in one patient. Unilateral optic atrophy was found in one patient and bilateral optic atrophy with blindness in another.

Treatment.—Little is known concerning any specific treatment for tularemia itself. Vaccines and antiserums have been employed without significant results. For the ocular condition, a mild wash of boric acid solution is preferable; the use of warm compresses to the affected eye may also be employed. Strong antiseptics are not indicated.

A case reported by Cramer[22] in a boy aged 16 was treated with 15 c.c. of antitularemia serum intravenously. He received three injections, with local treatment consisting of applications of moist heat, boric acid, and applications of 1 per cent silver nitrate. The condition of the eye improved slowly with the use of the local treatment, but the general condition of the patient remained unchanged for some time.

Pascheff's Conjunctivitis

Another oculoglandular disease which is characterized by an infectious necrotic conjunctivitis is known as Pascheff's conjunctivitis. The disease was first described by Pascheff and is caused by a microorganism called *Microbacillus polymorphicus necroticans*. When inoculated into guinea pigs or rabbits, it causes coagulative necrosis in the spleen and death of the animals. The organism is nonmotile and gram-negative, resembling both a coccus and a bacillus in shape.

The condition is characterized by swelling of the glands of the neck on the affected side (preauricular, parotid, and submaxillary glands). The patient may also suffer with elevation of temperature and malaise. The inflammation of the affected gland may go on to suppuration, and run a course of several months.

Eye Manifestations.—The disease is characterized principally by the eye manifestation which is accompanied by the glandular condition. The conjunctiva resembles very much that which is seen with Parinaud's conjunctivitis (see page 384). The two conditions can be definitely differentiated by laboratory examination which will reveal the causative organism. In Pascheff's disease one eye is usually affected. The lids are swollen and red. Photophobia and lacrimation and itching are complained of. The tarsal conjunctiva of both lids, as well as the fornices, will reveal a number of small, white spots elevated on a reddened and infiltrated conjunctival surface. The small elevations which resemble a phlyctenule in appearance undergo ulceration and cicatrization. They may disappear after several weeks and may be followed by the appearance of others. There is no specific treatment known, and the condition must be treated symptomatically.

References

Erysipelas

1. Bellows, John: Ocular Complications of Erysipelas, Arch. Ophth. **11:** 678, 1934.

Gonorrhea

2. Sorsby, A., and Hoffa, E. L.: The Sulfonamides in Ophthalmia Neonatorum, Brit. M. J. **1:** 353, 1944.
3. Keyes, John E. L.: Penicillin in Ophthalmology, J. A. M. A. **126:** 610, 1944.

Leprosy

4. Prendergast, John J.: Ocular Leprosy in the United States, Arch. Ophth. **23:** 112, 1940.

Anthrax

5. Ross, A. S., and Shipman, J. A.: Malignant Anthrax Edema, Am. J. Ophth. **18:** 641, 1935.

Tetanus

6. Sattler, R.: Penetrating Injury to the Eyeball Followed by Acute Tetanus, Arch. Ophth. **47:** 64, 1918.
7. Zentmayer, William: Personal communication.

Polyarthritis

8. Smith, James W.: Ochronosis of the Sclera and Cornea Complicating Alkaptonuria, J. A. M. A. **120:** 1282-1288, 1942.
9. van der Hoeve, J.: Scleromalacia Perforans, Arch. Ophth. **11:** 111, 1934.
10. Oast, Samuel P.: Scleromalacia Perforans, Arch. Ophth. **17:** 698, 1937.
11. Verhoeff, F. H., and King, Merrill J.: Scleromalacia Perforans, Arch. Ophth. **20:** 1013, 1938.
12. Eggers, Harry: Necroscleritis Nodosa Associated With Chronic Rheumatoid Polyarthritis: Report of Case, Arch. Ophth. **23:** 501, 1940.
13. Smoleroff, Jules W.: Scleral Disease in Rheumatoid Arthritis: Report of Three Cases, in One of Which Both Eyes Were Studied Post Mortem, Arch. Ophth. **29:** 98, 1943.
14. Mills, Lloyd: In Discussion of Verhoeff and King's Paper, Arch. Ophth. **20:** 1034, 1938.

Undulant Fever

15. Green, John: Ocular Manifestations in Brucellosis (Undulant Fever), Arch. Ophth. 21: 51, 1939.
16. Orloff, K. C.: Melitokokkia (Maltafieber) und Auge, Klin. Monatsbl. f. Augenh. 81: 582, 1928.
17. Woods, Allen C., and Guyton, Jack S.: Role of Sarcoidosis and of Brucellosis in Uveitis, Tr. Am. Acad. Ophth. (1943) 48: 248, March-April, 1944; also Arch. Ophth. 31: 469, 1944.
18. Rutherford, C. W.: Papilledema in Undulant Fever, J. A. M. A. 104: 1490, 1935.
19. Green, John: Severe Kerato-iritis Due to Brucellosis, Am. J. Ophth. 26: 491, 1943.

Tularemia

20. Hurst, V. Reeves: Oculo-Glandular Diseases With Special Reference to Tularemia and Parinaud's Conjunctivitis, Tr. Am. Acad. Ophth. 43: 363, 1938.
21. Francis, Edward: Oculoglandular Tularemia, Arch. Ophth. 28: 711, 1942.
22. Cramer, Irving I.: Oculoglandular Tularemia, Arch. Ophth. 20: 88, 1938.

CHAPTER VIII

INFECTIONS AND INFECTIOUS DISEASES—Cont'd

Syphilis (Lues)

Syphilis is an acute and chronic disease due to a specific organism of the spirochete species called the *Treponema pallidum*. This is a delicate spiral organism about 10 microns in length and has a number of turns in its course. It is very labile and can be killed by weak disinfectants, soap and water. It can be transmitted by inoculation from one animal to another and is usually found in the local tissue lesions. They can be demonstrated by mixing some of the tissue fluid with Gunther's India ink on a glass slide and allowing it to dry. The Treponema can be observed as fine white spirals on a black background under the oil immersion and are also readily detected in the tissues when examined with dark-field illumination.

Although the usual and most common manner of inoculation is by sexual intercourse, transmission of the organism from one person to another may take place in many different ways. Moreover, all groups and classes of people may be infected, very often in an innocent way. This may occur through the medium of drinking cups, musical instruments, surgical instruments, contaminated hands, towels, handkerchiefs, kissing, and many others. Usually a slight break in the epithelium at the point of inoculation permits the Treponema to penetrate. This may even occur without any local reaction which is recognized by the patient or the reaction may be so slight that it receives no consideration from the patient at the time. At a later date, he, therefore, may honestly disclaim any knowledge of an infection taking place. This is particularly true among women, since the primary lesion within the vagina or on the cervix uteri may fail to attract any attention. Young nursing infants have been known to be infected by a syphilitic lesion on the nipple of a wet nurse.

The primary lesion of syphilis is rather characteristic and consists of a hard nodule with a cartilaginous firmness and is called a chancre or hard sore. This is to be differentiated from the nonsyphilitic chancroid which is a soft sore. The surface of the papule ulcerates, with a depression which is sharp and crater-like in appearance.

The lesion is characterized by an infiltration of leucocytes, lymphocytes, and plasma cells in the perivascular tissues of the smallest blood vessels and lymphatics. Later on, endovasculitis affects the intima and causes an obliteration of the lumen. A connective tissue formation with the presence of spindle cells, epithelial cells, and giant cells takes place. A large number of Treponema may be found in the lesion. These invade the blood stream and may be carried through the circulation. They may also reach the regional lymph glands, especially those of the inguinal region, by way of the lymphatics. The lymph glands may become hard and swollen, returning later to normal size. Suppuration and necrosis may take place with softening and discharge of the necrotic material. The spread of the virus leads to the widespread disseminated or secondary lesions, and later to tertiary lesions of a granulomatous variety which occur in some patients.

In the primary stage the incubation period is from ten to sixty days, with an average of about twenty-one days during which time very few or no symptoms may be noted. Chancre may occur on any site outside of the genital region and has frequently been found on the fingers, tongue, lip, tonsil, nipple, and eyelids. A number of cases have been reported where the eyelid was the site of the initial lesion. Very little pain or irritation may accompany the chancre which may heal slowly even without treatment and eventually leave little or no sign of its presence. When the infection becomes general, however, symptoms such as chilliness, fever and malaise may be complained of and lymphatic enlargement may also take place. Pains in the bones, joints, and muscles may also be complained of, the spleen and liver may be enlarged, and jaundice of the skin and conjunctiva might be observed. The period prior to the onset of these general symptoms and following the presence of the chancre is sometimes known as a secondary incubation period.

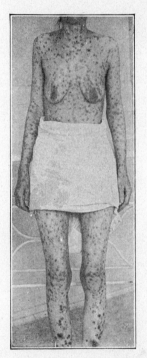

Fig. 143.—Papulopustular syphilodermas in a neglected case of syphilis. (Courtesy of Dr. Otto Leslie Castle, from Sutton and Sutton: Diseases of the Skin.)

The secondary signs and symptoms are the result of general toxic reaction and acute lesions in many organs including the eye, and also diffuse skin eruptions which now take place. The latter usually occur without pain and are unaccompanied by itching. The early eruption is usually of a macular or roseolar type, which in moist areas is known as a mucous patch and is very infectious. The eruption is usually found over the chest and abdomen and may vary in intensity from a diffuse rash to well-defined roselike macules. It is caused by dilatation of the capillaries which are supposed to contain large numbers of Treponema. The character of the eruption may be varied, and while it appears to be macular at first, it may later be slightly elevated and present a copper-brown color. The latter is caused by more marked pericapillary and capillary infiltration which remains for a longer period and is frequently followed by a well-defined area of pigmentation in the skin. The subsequent eruptions are papular in character and may be as small as a pinhead or as large as a pea in size. They are distinctly elevated, and the result of a more extensive lesion with pronounced vascular infiltration. They may

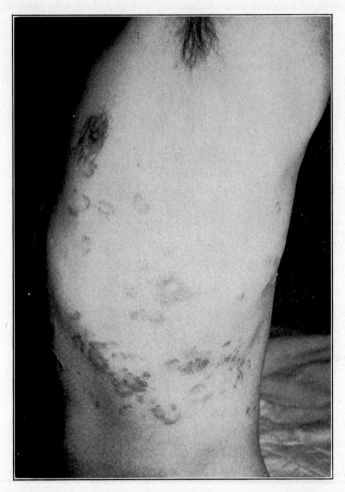

Fig. 144.—Secondary lesions on chest wall of patient with syphilitic optic neuritis in right eye and scleritis in the left eye. (I. S. Tassman, Graduate Hospital, University of Pennsylvania.)

be found on the body and also on the scalp, where they result in alopecia, on the palms of the hands and the soles of the feet, where they become dry, cracked, and ulcerated. The lesions all contain many Treponema, but they are not infectious unless they are ulcerated or macerated. When they occur on the mucous membranes, especially about the lip, mouth, and tongue, they are the source of transmitting the infection to extragenital parts in other patients. Chancre of the eyelid is usually transmitted, from this source. If infection of the papular eruption takes place, a pustule is produced, which is known as a pustular syphilide. It resembles very much the lesion in some of the other skin eruptions, such as acne, variola, or impetigo.

A later eruption which develops is a nodule which is bluish-red in color, and which leaves a depression because of destruction of tissue on healing. These are known as tubercles or tubercular syphilides. They may be numerous and coalesce over a large area and may also ulcerate. This nodular eruption usually precedes the tertiary lesion or gumma. The tertiary lesions in syphilis are produced in almost any organ or organs of the body by the distribution of the *Treponema pallidum* through the capillaries of the system. Any chronic lesion or symptoms should be considered as the possible result of syphilis until another cause has been determined. Constant headache and pain in the bones which is more severe at night should lead to the suspicion of syphilis as the cause. Local exostosis, periostitis of the long bones, and other destructive lesions of the bones may be caused by gummas. These may be difficult or impossible to recognize, but on x-ray examination, an absorption may be revealed which would indicate their presence. They may cause destructive lesions of the bones of the orbit, nose, and face, leading to deformities which are characteristic. Occurring in the orbit, they may cause proptosis of the eyeball and other changes in the eye. When they occur in the cranial cavity, secondary manifestation in the eye may be found. The eye, in addition to the heart, liver, bones, aorta, and skin, is very often involved as the result of a localized syphilitic reaction about the small blood vessels.

Congenital Syphilis.—The fetus is infected with syphilis by the mother. This may occur by way of the placenta years after her initial lesion. The possibility for infection to the fetus is increased, however, when the infection of the mother has been recent. A child may or may not show characteristic signs of syphilis at the time of birth, but the Wassermann reaction will be found positive in the mother and child, even though the latter appears healthy. The signs of syphilis may appear in the child any time after birth, and even after puberty.

Certain characteristic features are sometimes present which distinguish cases of congenital syphilis. Such children often suffer with nasal discharge, a macular and papular rash commonly seen on the face and buttocks, which has a copper-brown color, indurated masses on the skin, and alopecia. In childhood these patients may show changes in the long bones, especially the femur, and defects in the teeth, such as notching of the central incisors, known as Hutchinson's teeth. Epilepsy, idiocy, and hydrocephalus may also be found. Ocular manifestations of congenital syphilis are not uncommon and occur in the form of keratitis, iritis and optic neuritis, either alone or in association with other lesions.

In making the diagnosis of syphilis, especially in the presence of a primary lesion, other similar conditions, such as chancroid, herpes, lymphogranuloma, epithelioma, and chalazion on the eyelid must be differentiated. Any sore which looks suspicious should be examined for the presence of the Treponema, and, in addition, the Wassermann or Kahn test should be repeated every month or six weeks if any doubt remains. The secondary lesions usually appear in about six or nine weeks, or even later. Many otherwise unsuspected cases are detected by the routine use of the serologic tests. When syphilis is strongly suspected in the presence of negative blood Wassermann reaction, a spinal fluid examination should then be indicated. The latter may be found positive when the former was negative. In conclusion, some patients may live for many years and reach well-advanced age with no clinical evidences of syphilis except a positive serologic test. On the other hand, diseases of the cardiovascular system, central nervous system, and the eye are very commonly encountered as a result of this disease.

Eye Manifestations.—It has been estimated that about 2 per cent of all eye diseases are caused by syphilis. Moreover, numerous surveys have revealed that syphilis accounted for blindness in from 6 to 10 per cent of cases. This appears to be a fairly conservative estimate, and all data on the subject indicate without question the seriousness of syphilis as an etiologic factor in eye diseases.

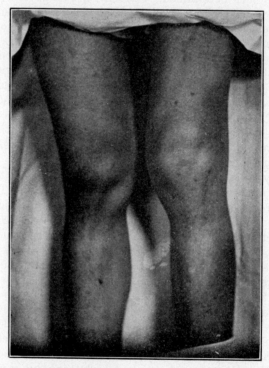

Fig. 145.—Enlarged knee joints (Clutton joints), in patient with congenital syphilis. (Courtesy of J. V. Klauder, Wills Hospital.)

The significance of this disease as a factor in causing eye lesions resulting in serious visual impairment and even blindness can be appreciated from a consideration of authoritative estimates such as those of Lewis,[1] who observed that in the syphilitic children of infected women, 50 to 75 per cent become afflicted with serious eye disease. Holloway[2] stated that in cases of congenital syphilis, ocular evidences of the disease are observed in 75 per cent. The early treatment of prenatal syphilis was emphasized by Goldberg[3] whose studies of 653 pregnant women provided evidence that the number of manifestations of late syphilis, especially those which cause blindness, can be reduced, and the occurrence of congenital syphilis in many children prevented by such early treatment. This was also stressed by Paley,[4] who, from a study of 617 pregnant women, showed that antisyphilitic treatment during the pregnancy reduced the incidence of syphilis complications in the offspring, regardless of the duration of the disease in the mother.

The results of a study of 100,000 case records by Berens and Goldberg[5] revealed some interesting data, especially with regard to the syphilitic manifestations in the eye. They found the percentage of positive Wassermann reactions in interstitial keratitis, 53.8 per cent; kerato-iritis, 50 per cent; Argyll-Robertson pupil, 41.7 per cent; optic neuritis and papillitis, 20 per cent; iritis and iridocyclitis, 15.4 per cent; uveitis, 14.2 per cent; and choroiditis, 12.4 per cent.

In general, however, these percentages run higher, with interstitial keratitis being considered to be positive in as many as 90 per cent, iridocyclitis 50 to 60 per cent, choroiditis 25 per cent, and ocular muscle palsies 50 per cent. Nearly all cases of primary optic atrophy are positive. In any case with eye lesions which might possibly be syphilitic, the Wassermann test should be performed.

Any of the structures of the eye may reveal manifestations of syphilis. In about 50 per cent of the cases, the condition is bilateral.

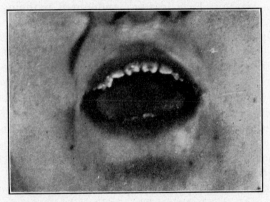

Fig. 146.—Hutchinson's (notched incisor) teeth, in patient with interstitial keratitis. (Courtesy of Dr. J. V. Klauder, Wills Hospital.)

The localization of syphilis in the eye is influenced by such factors as predisposition of the tissue and immunologic reaction. Special strains of the organism do not appear to be an important factor. The occurrence of eye lesions in man does not seem to depend on the earlier course of the disease. That is, an immunity which is known to occur experimentally in animals and which is thought to protect the eye when severe secondary lesions were previously present in other organs, does not seem to exist in man. Klauder[6] mentions the possibility of local tissue reaction as a factor in the defense mechanism of syphilis, since it may act as an "immunologic depot," the progress being held in check in other organs. Clinically, the disease may run its course at a given time in one organ, but later may become active in others. Late, active syphilis is considered usually to confine itself to one organ. Klauder found also that in 100 patients, studied at Wills Hospital Clinic, interstitial keratitis was invariably the only manifestation of active syphilis. However, in other studies the association of syphilitic lesions in different organs has been found to be present to a greater extent.

Trauma is apparently a prominent factor in the localization of syphilis in the eye. This is especially true with regard to the cornea in the production of interstitial keratitis and the occurrence of syphilitic iridocyclitis after ocular operations. According to Klauder[7] interstitial keratitis which occurs in an uninjured eye while the disease is still present in the injured eye can be regarded as the logical consequence of trauma, although the question of responsibility is solely a judicial one. However, this possibility is dependent on the interval separating the involvement of both eyes, since the late development of the condition in the uninjured eye would less likely be due to the traumatic condition. The spontaneous appearance of interstitial keratitis might ordinarily be expected at any time in patients with congenital syphilis.

Eye Lesions in Congenital Syphilis.—Various data have been presented from time to time for the presence of eye lesions in congenital syphilis. In reviewing this subject Klauder[6] referred to the study of 100 syphilitic infants and children by Green,[8] who reported that definite pathologic conditions in one or more of the ocular structures or some derangement of function was present in seventy-four. Fixed or unequal pupils were found in nine; strabismus in four; ptosis, one; nystagmus, three; keratitis or evidences of former keratitis in nineteen; fine vitreous haze in two; undoubted pathologic changes in the eyegrounds were present in fifty-two. The latter included nearly all forms of involvement. Optic neuritis was found in eight, and optic atrophy in eight. Peripheral and central punctate pigmentation which consists of tiny brown or brown-black dots scattered uniformly over the retina, were common. Green felt that the dark brown pigmentation is characteristic of congenital syphilis.

Eye lesions in congenital syphilis usually occur in an average of about 50 per cent. Keratitis is common. Retinochoroiditis may occur following keratitis. Iritis may occur, but is more common in acquired syphilis. Optic neuritis occurs in a fairly large number of cases. A haze in the vitreous may be present alone or in association with retinochoroiditis and is considered to denote the presence of congenital syphilis.

Syphilis of the Orbit.—Syphilis may rarely affect the bones of the orbit in the form of a chronic periostitis. This ordinarily occurs in adults and occasionally in children with hereditary syphilis. It occurs rarely as an acute condition with suppuration. In the third, or gummatous, stage there takes place a chronic increase in thickening of the orbital bones which results in a gradual contraction of the orbital cavity. This, in turn, produces a proptosis or exophthalmos, pressure on the orbital nerves, neuralgia, and paralyses of the ocular muscles.

Secondary involvement of the orbit is rare but may result from extension of syphilis from the sinuses. In congenital syphilis deformities of the face and nose may affect the shape of the orbit.

Gumma of the orbit may occur as a primary or secondary condition by extension from the nasal sinuses. Continued increase in the size of the gumma may lead to displacement of the eyeball, the direction depending on the location of the gumma.

The diagnosis of syphilitic involvement of the orbit can be made from the history, serologic tests, and x-ray examination. None of these may give any definite information, however, since the history may not be obtainable and the serologic tests are occasionally negative when syphilis is present. The roentgen studies sometimes reveal bony changes which are characteristic of the disease.

The treatment of orbital manifestations by antiluetic therapy will result in their improvement. Syphilitic growths and gummas will decrease in size and rather promptly clear up on the administration of general syphilitic treatment. The use of the iodides and mercury by inunction is very beneficial in these cases. Those conditions which are due to other causes will remain unaffected by this form of treatment.

Ocular Muscle Paralyses.—Paralysis affecting either the internal or external ocular muscles may occur during the course of syphilis. Paralysis of the sphincter of the iris and the ciliary muscle, known as ophthalmoplegia interna, may result in paralysis of the accommodation. This frequently occurs in cerebral syphilis and early in tabes and paresis. The paralysis of accommodation is accompanied by dilatation of the pupil (paralytic mydriasis).

Paralysis of accommodation will produce certain disturbances of the refractive state of the patient's eye. On attempting to read ordinary print at the reading point, the type will be blurred, so that reading and writing are difficult or impossible. If the patient had normal vision for distance and is not hyperopic, the vision for distance may be unaffected, but in the presence of hyperopia, the visual acuity for distance will be diminished. If the patient is myopic, the vision may be unaffected.

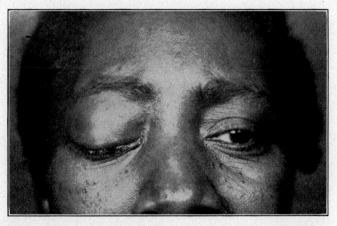

Fig. 147.—Gumma of right orbit. (I. S. Tassman, Willis Hospital.)

Syphilis, especially in its later stages, is a frequent cause of intracranial paralyses. The eye muscles may here be directly affected, or it may also occur in tabes and general paresis. Tabetic paralysis of the individual extraocular muscles may occur from a lesion in the nerve nuclei. The abducens and facial may be simultaneously affected because of the close location of the two nuclei. The paralyses in tabes may clear up for a period of time and recur again later, often becoming permanent.

Argyll-Robertson Pupil.—The Argyll-Robertson pupil occurs so rarely as the result of other conditions that its presence is almost pathognomonic of syphilis or neurosyphilis. It may be one of the earliest signs of tabes and is found in about 70 per cent of these patients. It occurs somewhat less in general paresis. The condition is characterized by a failure of the pupils to react to direct light stimulation, while the reaction to accommodation is present.

The size of the pupil is usually contracted or in a condition of miosis, although it is claimed by some authorities that miosis is not a necessary accompaniment. The pupils may be almost equal in size or one may be slightly larger than the other. The outline of the pupil may also be somewhat irregular. The lesion causing the condition affects the different pupillary fibers near the oculomotor nuclei.

Syphilitic Lesions of the Eyelids.—Chancre of the eyelids is not an uncommon condition and may occur in any one of a number of ways. It may be found on the upper or lower lid, usually at the canthi, but also in the intermarginal spaces and on the conjunctiva. Males and females may be equally affected, since the infection is usually accidental or the result of carelessness. The one affected may have no knowledge of the nature of the condition. The usual modes of transmission are by kissing, touch, contaminated towels and instruments, coughing saliva into the face of another, and in other ways. Chancre of the eyelids may be followed by severe secondary symptoms. The lesion is usually hard with a grayish-yellow, greasy base. Examination of some of the material under dark-field illumination will reveal the presence of spirochetes. The blood Wassermann test should also be performed. The sore may resemble a chalazion or epithelioma, but the differential diagnosis is usually not difficult.

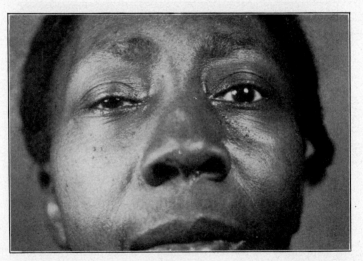

Fig. 148.—Same patient shown in Fig. 147 after receiving specific treatment.

The chancre usually increases in size and may ulcerate into the lid margin with involvement of the conjunctiva. Pain is usually absent or not seriously complained of, but there may be an accompanying swelling of the preauricular or submaxillary glands. The ulceration is usually covered by a glossy membrane, the removal of which will leave a bleeding, raw surface. The edges are slightly raised and well demarcated. A slight swelling of the lid and conjunctiva may be present.

Gummas of the lids occur occasionally in the form of indolent ulcers which may also involve the conjunctiva. They usually break down and reveal a smeary induration which may spread through the entire thickness of the lid.

In a few instances they are absorbed. Gumma of the lid may also resemble a chalazion or hordeolum but can be differentiated by the pronounced ulceration and also by serologic tests.

Treatment.—Antisyphilitic treatment should be instituted as soon as possible after a chancre or gumma of the eyelid is recognized. The general treatment should include the early use of arsenic, mercury, and bismuth, any or all of which must be continued over a long period of time even after the blood Wassermann tests have been negative. Local treatment may consist only of the use of a simple ointment, such as calomel ointment applied to the lesion. The use of active general antisyphilitic treatment will also produce a rapid improvement in the gummatous condition of the eyelid.

Syphilis of the Conjunctiva and Sclera.—The conjunctiva, in addition to being involved by a chancre either primarily or secondarily from the eyelid, may more commonly show manifestations of the secondary stage of syphilis.

A marked injection and chemosis might characterize a simple form of conjunctivitis which may accompany secondary skin manifestations.

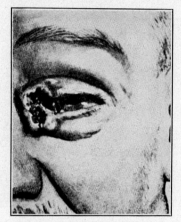

Fig. 149.—Chancre of the inner canthus with enlargement of preauricular and submaxillary glands. (From Ramsay: Clinical Ophthalmology for the General Practitioner, Oxford Medical Publications.)

A granular conjunctivitis which sometimes resembles trachoma may occur with a thickening of the tarsal conjunctiva of the upper and lower lids. This is diffuse red in color and is produced by papillary hypertrophy. It may be accompanied by pannus and the preauricular glands are usually involved. The condition rapidly clears after the patient receives antisyphilitic treatment. The conjunctiva is sometimes involved in cases with macular and papular syphilides. Ulcers of the conjunctiva as the result of syphilis are extremely rare but may occur as the result of contamination with infected material. The conjunctiva at the free lid margin is more apt to be affected in such cases, but the retrotarsal fold and bulbar conjunctiva may also show involvement. These ulcers, which may at first appear to be hard, later break down and result in a loss of tissue.

A diffuse scleritis which is more marked around the cornea may rarely occur as a complication of interstitial keratitis. Involvement of the sclera in syphilis may occur in the form of isolated nodules. These nodules may break down into the formation of ulcers. Syphilis does not ordinarily produce a typical scleritis which tends to recur, but a deep form of scleritis which may affect both eyes and last for a long period of time may be found in some younger patient with hereditary syphilis.

Gumma of the conjunctiva is comparatively rare. When present, it is usually found on the bulbar conjunctiva near the limbus and is about as large as a pea. They are hard, smooth, and have a pinkish color. Later they become white and break down with ulceration and necrosis because of the obliterative changes in the vessels. The preauricular glands may also be enlarged. These gummas of the conjunctiva increase in size and may involve the cornea and sclera by extension and may cause an iritis before specific treatment is started. With the latter, however, they will rapidly disappear. The condition of the conjunctiva in this stage may resemble such conjunctival infections as Parinaud's conjunctivitis and other granulomatous conditions which can be differentiated by the presence of a positive Wassermann reaction.

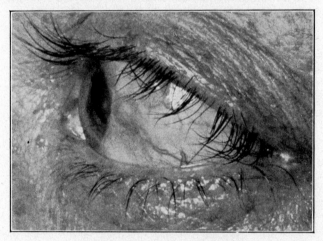

Fig. 150.—Scleritis of the left eye in same patient shown in Fig. 144. (I. S. Tassman, Graduate Hospital, University of Pennsylvania.)

Syphilitic Manifestations in the Cornea.—Involvement of the cornea in acquired syphilis very rarely, if ever, occurs. When this part of the eye is involved, it is nearly always the result of congenital syphilis. The latter is manifested principally by interstitial keratitis and also very occasionally by a form of sclerosing keratitis found in younger patients who may have hereditary syphilis. The sclerosing keratitis is rare in these patients and occurs mostly in females. Both eyes are often affected, and it may be found in association with scleritis. The corneal involvement usually begins as a triangular opacity from the site of a scleral nodule at the limbus. The base of the triangle is adjacent to the nodule while the apex extends forward, infiltrating the cornea toward the center. The opacities may also be irregular in shape, having a grayish color and becoming gradually denser with complete opacification of the area eventually taking place. There is practically very little or no vascularization present. After a while, regression takes place with some clearing at the apex of the opacity. The greater portion of the opacity remains, however, which is continuous with the scleral lesions and causes more or less permanent impairment of the vision in this area. Although this condition occurs in some cases with hereditary syphilis, it may be found more commonly in other conditions, such as tuberculosis and in older patients with rheumatic and gouty affections.

Acquired syphilis with corneal involvement is very uncommon. Gumma of the cornea scarcely ever occurs, and interstitial keratitis is a very rare occurrence, although it is sometimes difficult to account for its presence in an adult in any other way. Metastatic corneal abscesses, however, have been found as the result of acquired syphilis.

Keratitis Pustuliformis Profunda (Acute Metastatic Syphilitic Corneal Abscess).—This condition was first described by Fuchs in 1915, and might be designated also as acute metastatic syphilitic corneal abscess or purulent syphilitic keratitis profunda with hypopyon. The condition is comparatively rare, although a number of cases have been reported in the literature since Fuchs' description which did not include the etiology of the condition. Later cases treated with antisyphilitic therapy responded favorably. This led to the recognition of its syphilitic origin and the designation of the condition as acute metastatic syphilitic abscess which was first employed by Bryn after the successful treatment of four cases. In addition to cases studied histologically by E. Fuchs and Igersheimer, a complete clinical and histopathologic study with the report of a case was made by Bertha A. Klien.[9] This report confirms earlier observations that the characteristic features of the disease are presented about the third or fourth week after the onset.

The condition which occurs in the absence of external injury is characterized by a keratitis which is coordinate with a hypopyon iritis. The cornea reveals yellowish and rather sharply defined infiltrates in the deep layers. A clear or partly opaque area may separate this from the limbus. The iritis shows a gradual transition from a low-grade infiltrative type to the purulent exudative form. The clinical signs of the condition are early pain, photophobia, redness, and lacrimation in the affected eye. The vision is reduced and diminishes with the progress of the condition. Iritis is present and a hypopyon gradually forms which may fill the anterior chamber. Deep vascular infiltration may take place. Abscesses occur deep in the cornea, but Descemet's membrane remains intact. The intraocular tension may be increased late in the disease, and glaucoma may result as a complication. Involvement of the optic nerve and retina may occur as late complications.

The infection is produced by metastatic involvement of the eye by large numbers of spirochetes. The typical lesions which are found in the central portions of the cornea are said to be caused by the presence of spirochetes, but the avenue of invasion has not been explained.

Treatment of this condition consists in use of general antisyphilitic therapy as soon as the condition is recognized. This is followed by spectacular results. This would indicate the need for an early diagnosis with immediate Wassermann test in the presence of an early suspected infection. If permitted to progress without recognizing the syphilitic origin and instituting immediate treatment, the eye will be lost.

Interstitial Keratitis.—Sometimes known as parenchymatous keratitis, this condition is recognized as a manifestation of congenital or hereditary syphilis in nearly all cases. In rare instances it may be considered as an acquired condition. There is no satisfactory explanation as to why the cornea of children with congenital syphilis is more predisposed to interstitial keratitis than in cases of acquired syphilis. Although the children of syphilitic parents are commonly affected, it does not necessarily occur in the third generation or the children of those affected with the disease.

It is one of the late symptoms of hereditary syphilis, the nature of the connection being poorly understood. The spirochetes are not found in the cornea in the course of this disease, and the relationship is looked upon as an indirect involvement. It has been described as a manifestation of an allergy to syphilitic virus. In patients who are doing well in the course of a syphilitic infection, recurring interstitial keratitis has been described as a sensitization of the cornea caused by the early infection and now suffering from an allergy to the virus products in the system.

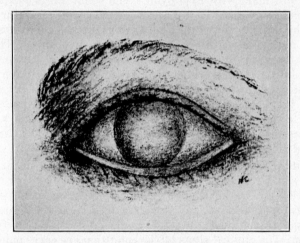

Fig. 151.—General haziness of cornea in early interstitial keratitis.

Interstitial keratitis occurs most commonly in patients between 5 and 20 years of age, although it may be found up to the age of 40. It also seems to occur more often in women than in men. The patients who are affected nearly always reveal other manifestations of hereditary syphilis. These include an elliptical shape of the cornea, deafness, deformities of the nose and face, nasal ozena, highly arched palate and cicatrices of the pharynx, enlargement of lymph glands, Hutchinson's teeth (notching of the central incisors), deformities of the long bones, and swelling or inflammation of the knee joints. The presence of any of these findings and a positive blood Wassermann will prove the diagnosis. This may also be confirmed by the additional history of syphilis in one of the parents. It should be remembered, however, that a small percentage of these cases are due to tuberculosis. If the patient has brothers or sisters, they should also be examined for evidences of the disease.

Both eyes are usually affected, and when only one is involved, the second eye invariably becomes affected sooner or later. The clinical symptoms which characterize the onset of the condition are pain, redness of the conjunctiva, especially around the cornea, intense lacrimation, and photophobia. The photophobia is so great that the patient assumes a characteristic appearance. The eyelids which may be slightly swollen are closed almost tight, and the head is lowered, so that the patient's chin almost rests on the chest, in an effort to avoid direct light. In attempting to examine the eyes in severe acute cases,

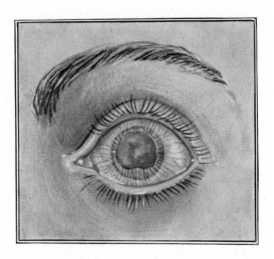

Fig. 152.—Interstitial keratitis, showing general active infiltration of the cornea and vascularization around the entire periphery

it is practically impossible to force the patient to open the eyelids. In some cases the symptoms are more mild. The condition may be associated with iritis, iridocyclitis, and uveitis.

Objectively, the disease may present several varieties. In one the opacification begins in the center of the cornea in the form of maculae, while in others, the maculae may be found peripherally and are rather dense, gradually encroaching on the center. The central opacity also becomes more dense and may remain permanently. Ulceration does not take place. In some cases the infiltration occurs in the lower portions of the cornea in a triangular area, resembling somewhat the appearance found in the cornea resulting from iridocyclitis. The vessels around the cornea are congested.

One of the characteristic findings in interstitial keratitis is the vascularization which takes place in most cases. When little vascularization occurs, the cornea takes on the appearance which has been described as "ground glass." However, when the vascularization is pronounced, the cornea presents a uniform reddish appearance. In other instances the vascularization varies in intensity around the cornea which in dense areas gives the appearance sometimes described as "salmon patches." The vessels in interstitial keratitis are found in the deep layers of the cornea. These can be observed in detail on examination with the slit lamp and are found to extend from the limbus toward the center of the cornea although they rarely reach the center. When a considerable number of vessels are present, they give this part of the cornea an elevated appearance, or the opaque portion may appear to be depressed.

The lesions are formed by unicellular leucocytes which accumulate in the middle and deep layers. The infiltration increases in the deeper layers as it approaches Descemet's membrane. A round-cell infiltration of the endothelium occurs, while the superficial layers and Bowman's membrane may not be involved.

The disease runs a chronic course and may last for several months. After the acute period most of the severe symptoms subside quickly, but subsequent clearing of the cornea takes place very slowly and gradually. Some of the milder cases may clear up in a shorter period of time, but the more severe cases may not clear to their fullest extent for more than a year. While the opacities may clear up in a few cases almost entirely, they remain permanently in the more severe cases. The vision of the affected eye is, therefore, impaired to a corresponding degree. In very old cases in which there are now no signs of active inflammation, the vision is reduced and the opacities of various degrees can be seen throughout the cornea on oblique illumination, ophthalmoscopic, and slit lamp examination. Recurrences of the disease are not very common, but occasionally take place.

The role of trauma in the causation of interstitial keratitis has already been mentioned. A number of cases have been reported to appear after trauma, and it is quite possible for interstitial keratitis to occur following traumatism to the eye which may activate the condition.

Treatment.—In discussing the treatment of interstitial keratitis it might be well to mention first the possibility of the occurrence of the Herxheimer reaction and the appearance of ocular lesions after the initial use of large doses of arsenicals in the treatment of syphilis. New lesions might appear, or previous lesions might be activated in this way. The initial treatment in acute cases should, therefore, consist of either small doses of arsenicals or intramuscular injections of bismuth. This may be supplemented by the use of mercury.

Alternating courses of arsphenamine and a bismuth compound may be given throughout the course of the disease. When the disease does not respond well, it might be necessary to modify the form of treatment. Different arsenical and bismuth preparations may be substituted. Foreign proteins and fever therapy are useful in helping to overcome the acute symptoms of inflammation.

The general condition of the patient should also receive attention from the standpoint of hygiene, diet, etc. A good diet and fresh air are important in supplementing the specific treatment. In young children tonics may be prescribed, and the use of cod-liver oil, potassium or sodium iodide, and iron preparations will prove beneficial. The use of thyroid extract has also been recommended in these cases. The constitutional treatment should be continued throughout the course of the disease.

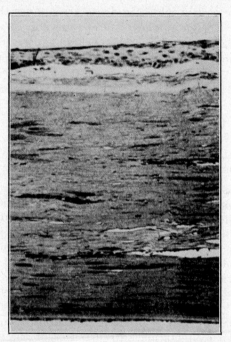

Fig. 153.—Interstitial keratitis. Vascular cornea and scar tissue in the stroma. Lymphocytic infiltration in central portion. (From Rones: Arch. Ophth., July, 1941.)

The local treatment of interstitial keratitis should be active from the start. The local measures employed are not expected to cure or arrest the condition, but they may serve to shorten the duration, prevent complications, and promote healing during the regressive period especially.

During the progressive stage, the eyes should be protected from exposure to light by the constant use of black glasses. The use of atropine sulfate, 1 per cent solution, should be started at once by the instillation of one drop into the affected eye, three times daily. This will dilate the pupil and relieve any accompanying iritis, while at the same time its use is apparently beneficial to the cornea. This is supplemented by the application of hot, wet compresses to the affected eye for a period of fifteen minutes, four times daily. This also serves to relieve the symptoms of irritation and promotes healing. In the stage of regression, dionin twice daily and yellow oxide of mercury may be prescribed.

Lastly, it should be remembered that active antisyphilitic treatment of the expectant mother may serve as a prophylaxis in the prevention of syphilis in the child, and thereby reduce the possibility for the subsequent appearance of interstitial keratitis.

Syphilitic Iritis and Iridocyclitis.—Syphilis of the iris may result in the appearance of several different manifestations. First, most of the cases of syphilitic iritis in adults are the result of acquired syphilis. A few cases occur in children either in association with interstitial keratitis or alone as the result of hereditary syphilis. The results of intrauterine syphilitic iritis may also be found occasionally in the eyes of newborn infants as evidenced by the presence of synechiae, occluded pupils, and atrophy of the iris.

Syphilitic iritis occurs in males more frequently than in females and is ordinarily a manifestation of the secondary stage of the disease, although it may occur more rarely in the tertiary stage as iridocyclitis. The earliest signs may occur during the first weeks of the disease and not long after the appearance of the initial lesion. This manifestation occurs on the lesser circle of the iris in the form of red spots resembling the macular lesion in the skin and are known as roseolae. These roseolae, which have been attributed to hyperemia in the vessels of the lesser circle of the iris, are transient in character. However, when their presence is noted, a thorough history should be obtained and serologic tests for syphilis are indicated. When roseolae recur in the later stage, they are usually accompanied by signs of inflammation, such as exudation on the capsule of the lens, cloudy aqueous, and synechiae of the iris.

Syphilitic iritis is often characterized by the presence of small nodules on the iris. This form, known as iritis papulosa, is easily diagnosed since the small nodules are readily observed usually near the pupillary margin, although occasionally they may be present at the ciliary border. They are yellowish in color and are about the size of a pinhead or slightly larger. They do not break down or suppurate but will disappear after a time, especially when the case is under treatment. Synechiae and atrophy of the affected area of the iris will result. Iritis papulosa usually occurs early in the secondary stage of the disease and the nodules are, therefore, considered as papules in relationship to the papular eruption on the skin. Accompanying lesions may be found in the mucous membranes of the mouth and pharynx.

The inflammation is characterized in addition by marked pericorneal injection, deposits on the posterior cornea, an irregularity of the pupil due to adhesions and posterior synechiae, and exudate in the pupillary space and on the anterior capsule of the lens. The iris itself is congested and swollen and is covered with a profuse fibrinous exudate which gives it a cloudy or muddy appearance. This exudate also causes the iris to adhere to the capsule of the lens and, when more pronounced, it may fill most of the pupil.

The principal subjective symptoms complained of are severe pain in the eye which is usually worse at night, headache, photophobia, and lacrimation. Usually one eye alone is affected, but in almost one-half of the cases both eyes may be involved, although not at the same time. Most of the cases occur during the early secondary stage and are accompanied in many instances by the typical skin rash. The condition may, however, occur late in the disease. In the latter instances recurrences are more common and the prognosis is more serious. Many of the cases occurring early clear up under treatment without serious or permanent damage to the eye. Recurrent iritis and iridocyclitis may also occur because of insufficient antisyphilitic treatment, or the first attack may appear as a manifestation of the Herxheimer reaction after a large dose of an arsenical preparation.

Gumma of the Ciliary Body.—Gummas occur infrequently, but they may develop in the ciliary body and more rarely in the iris. They can sometimes be seen on the iris, but on close examination these are found to be situated in the angle of the anterior chamber and spring from the ciliary body. They usually develop when the syphilitic choroiditis is a primary manifestation. Granulomatous masses may occur in certain areas which become necrotic and may involve the entire angle of the anterior chamber. A severe iridocyclitis with profuse exudation is usually present, and the sclera may also be involved. Unless active treatment is instituted, the condition will progress with complete loss of vision in the affected eye.

Syphilitic Choroiditis.—The choroid may be involved in syphilis either alone as a choroiditis or together with the retina as a chorioretinitis in from 10 to 15 per cent of cases. In congenital syphilis choroiditis is a much more common manifestation occurring in as many as 75 per cent of cases. None of the choroidal manifestations of syphilis present a characteristic or typical picture. The lesions in hereditary syphilis in the choroid may not show many differences from those of acquired syphilis. Moreover, the vessels may not reveal any characteristic changes and these may be very slight or entirely absent.

In many cases the choroid is involved together with the iris and ciliary body and the condition is actually a syphilitic uveitis. The history of the case may reveal the etiology, but in many instances, especially in females, this will be lacking. The Wassermann test must be depended on in most cases to confirm the diagnosis, although occasionally, even with a positive Wassermann, uveitis which appears to be typical of syphilis may be due to another cause. On the other hand many cases may reveal other associated lesions of syphilis, such as arthritis, periostitis, healed skin lesions, healed chancre, and others. In late cases of syphilis, moreover, the Wassermann reaction and other serological tests cannot be depended on in a percentage of cases for a positive diagnosis.

Choroiditis may occur during the early months of syphilitic infection, when it appears as a diffuse grayish change in the choroid analogous to the roseolar rash. It leaves small speck-like areas of atrophy, when it disappears after treatment.

The most common and characteristic form of choroiditis in syphilis was described early by Förster and is known as Förster's choroiditis. This is found in the secondary stage of syphilis, although it may occur late in the disease. There may be many small areas involved, and these sometimes become confluent with the formation of a few large areas having many different shapes. They are a type of inflammatory exudate and have a dirty yellow color. They are found around the macula and disc, but the posterior of the fundus is also involved. A proliferation of pigment is a characteristic feature of the lesion, this being due to involvement of retina which nearly always takes place. The pigmentation may also assume a variety of forms, sometimes appearing in masses, while at other times it occurs in discrete patches or deposits which are shaped like bone corpuscles in a circular formation and resemble very much that which occurs in pigmentary degeneration of the retina. Late in the disease, connective tissue is sometimes found lying beneath the retinal vessels.

The condition may begin in one eye, but is usually bilateral. It is characterized by failing vision, clouding of the vitreous, and sometimes slight clouding of the optic disc. A ring scotoma or other scotomas may be found in the visual fields, their size and appearance depending upon the location and extent of the lesion. The condition may last for a long time leaving patches of atrophy and sclerosis of the vessels in the areas of choroid involved. Occasionally, the condition may subside more quickly with little impairment resulting. Retinal atrophy may also occur late in the disease with a great reduction in the size of the visual field and also marked pigmentary degeneration. Night blindness in these cases may be a subjective symptom and optic atrophy may occur especially in congenital cases, with great reduction in the visual acuity.

Syphilitic choroiditis may also occur rarely in a later stage of the acquired disease in a more localized form. This may be found in almost any part of the fundus and also near the optic disc or the macula. In the latter instance a central choroiditis is present with impairment or loss of central vision while the former condition occurring near the disc may resemble the typical picture of chorioretinitis juxta-papillaris.

Choroiditis or chorioretinitis, as a manifestation of hereditary syphilis, may also occur in many different forms and either alone or in association with such other manifestations as interstitial keratitis. The most common form which is characteristic is the condition known as "pepper and salt fundus." Here the fundus in general is covered with numerous spots of fine pigment with yellowish spots lying between these. These are distributed especially in the periphery. The retinal vessels are narrowed, and the optic disc may become atrophic.

Pigment spots in the choroid, as manifestations of hereditary syphilis, may be found either singly or in larger numbers without other objective evidences. There may be only one or two isolated spots of pigment in the periphery of the fundus which are nearly as large as the disc. In other instances the lesions may be characterized by a number of atrophic white areas in the periphery of the fundus, or there may be only one or two areas, sometimes seen in the neighborhood of the macula, which are white in color and reveal some pigment within or around the edges.

Gummas of the choroid are rare, but they may occur by extension from the ciliary body. The choriocapillaris may be the seat of granulomatous masses or nodules which may undergo necrosis and involve a considerable area.

Syphilitic Uveitis.—*Treatment* of syphilitic iritis, iridocyclitis, and choroiditis can be described as the treatment of syphilitic uveitis. This includes both the local treatment of the particular eye manifestation and the general treatment of the internal disease. In most instances the general treatment will require the cooperation of the syphilologist with the ophthalmologist, and both forms of treatment should be started as early as possible.

In all forms of syphilitic uveitis the local treatment should begin at once with the use of mydriatics in order to maintain an open pupil and prevent the formation of synechiae. The best drug for this purpose is atropine sulfate (1 per cent solution). One drop should be instilled into the affected eye three times daily. If the pupil fails to respond or if it is already bound down, the strength of the solution may be increased to 2 per cent until a satisfactory result in this respect is obtained. In the cases of iritis and iridocyclitis especially, the need for the use of atropine in the eye is urgent and immediate. The effect is not only to dilate the pupil, but also to place the eye at rest by paralyzing the intraocular muscles. Even when the pupil is dilated, the use of the atropine should be continued in order to maintain an open pupil. One of the greatest dangers in this condition is the impairment of vision in the affected eye, because of the formation of synechiae produced by the products of inflammation. In most cases atropine is well tolerated, but in a few instances, its use over a long period of time may produce a dermatitis around the skin of the eyelids, especially the lower. This is caused not alone by the atropine, but also by irritation by the lacrimation which usually takes place and which is often profuse. When the use of atropine occasionally seems to be contraindicated, it may be replaced by scopolamine ($\frac{1}{4}$ to 1 per cent), duboisine ($\frac{1}{4}$ to 1 per cent), or paredrine (3 to 5 per cent). When it is desired to increase the action of atropine, this may be accomplished by the additional use of cocaine, adrenalin, or paredrine, either by instillation or, in severe and obstinate cases, by subconjunctival injection. The sympathomimetic drugs have been found to have a synergistic action with atropine.

Since the eyes in these cases are extremely sensitive to light, black glasses should be constantly worn and strong light should be avoided by the patient. For the pain which is invariably complained of from the beginning, the best results are obtained from the use of hot wet compresses to the eye. This is best accomplished by the application of gauze pads which have been dipped in a hot solution of boric acid or ordinary hot water. The applications are continued for fifteen or twenty minutes at a time and repeated about four times daily. This has the effect of relieving the pain by making the eye more comfortable and producing a relaxation in the congested vessels. If the congestion is intense, leeches can be employed just beyond the outer canthus of the eye to reduce the amount of blood and limit the inflammatory process. In some cases it might be necessary to resort to the use of local anesthetics in the eye, such as holocaine (1 per cent) or butyn (2 per cent) which will serve to relieve the local pain temporarily. Internally, the use of aspirin and salicylates is beneficial.

The general treatment of the case should also be started as early as possible and carried out in conjunction with the local treatment. The form of specific treatment employed will depend on the requirements of the individual case and the stage of the disease. It is only necessary to state here in general, that the treatment should be adequate and continued over a period long enough to obtain complete relief from symptoms and until the serology is considered to be normal. This means that the improvement of the local inflammation is not an indication for interrupting or discontinuing the specific general treatment, for in most cases this must be continued for a year or more after the iridocyclitis or uveitis has subsided. The importance of adequate treatment has long been recognized as a factor in the prevention of iridorecurrence.

The therapy usually consists in courses of arsphenamine, bismuth compounds, and mercury, while the iodides are given by mouth. In cases of chorioretinitis the use of foreign proteins and fever therapy is beneficial and can be employed either alone or in association with chemotherapy. The foreign proteins employed for the production of fever include injections of sterile milk, malarial parasites, and typhoid-paratyphoid vaccine. In addition, heat cabinets, hot baths, electric blankets, and diathermy are employed. The characteristics in the course of the disease and therapeutic response in the individual case should determine the procedure and the variations in the method of treatment employed.

Good results with artificial fever therapy by the use of the Kettering hypertherm in nearly all forms of ocular syphilis were obtained by Culler and Simpson.[10] With a simplified air-conditioned cabinet, the air temperature, relative humidity, and air velocity could be adequately controlled. This was said to have the advantage of maintaining the body temperature at a desired level. The patients were given ten weekly treatments of five hours each at a rectal temperature of from 105 to 106° F. Chemotherapy was combined by giving each patient thirty injections of 0.2 Gm. of bismarsen. Each of the ten fever treatments was followed by an injection, and twenty injections of the drug were given at weekly intervals.

Klauder and Dublin* studied syphilitic uveitis in a series of cases at Wills Hospital, with reference to diagnosis, the Herxheimer reaction, and results of treatment with various agents including penicillin. They discuss these considerations and also the Herxheimer reaction of the ocular lesion as evidence of syphilitic causation. The intensification of the inflammatory process (constituting the Herxheimer reaction) was evaluated by examination with the corneal microscope and slit lamp before and after antisyphilitic treatment. The Herxheimer reaction as observed by biomicroscopy has not been previously studied as a diagnostic aid.

Klauder and Dublin examined first a group of thirty-six patients with anterior uveal inflammation without clinical evidence of syphilis. The Wassermann reaction was positive in some and negative in others. In some, the uveitis was regarded as nonsyphilitic and was associated with other pathologic processes causing uveitis, as, for example, sarcoid. They concluded that the reaction cannot be regarded as an absolute criterion in differential diagnosis of syphilitic inflammation of the anterior uveal tract.

In seventeen patients with iritis associated with lesions of early syphilis who were treated exclusively with penicillin, the Herxheimer flare was not uniformly observed. In two patients the reaction was pronounced after increasing doses of penicillin to 50,000 units. In another the intensification of inflammation was noted by slit-lamp examination eighteen hours after an initial injection of 10,000 units of penicillin, following which additional doses of 10,000 units every four hours had been given at the time of slit-lamp examinations. They felt that in mild or moderately inflamed lesions of the anterior uveal tract, this focal flare is not harmful. A potential harm is the end result of continued energetic antisyphilitic treatment which produces too rapid retrogres-

*Arch. Ophth. 35, April, 1946.

sion, causing additional damage by fibrosis in healing too rapidly. They referred to this as the "therapeutic paradox."

In patients treated with chemotherapy, disappearance of active signs of inflammation as evaluated by slit-lamp examination occurred in from two to five weeks; in exceptional cases, from five to seven weeks. Fever therapy was found to help in initiating the treatment of some severe cases. However, initial reduced doses of bismuth prior to arsenical injections served the same purpose.

Penicillin Therapy.—In seventeen patients the uveitis associated with late secondary syphilis was treated exclusively with penicillin, with the exception of the local ophthalmologic treatment. Sodium penicillin was injected intramuscularly every four hours. The total dose was 2,400,000 units administered in eight days. These authors explained that this dose and duration of its administration will not necessarily be finally accepted as the proper treatment for secondary syphilis. Initial doses depended on the severity of the condition and varied from 5,000 to 10,000 units for the first four to six injections. Later doses were increased to a maximum of from 50,000 to 60,000 units. In all patients, the penicillin exerted a prompt effect. The ocular inflammation disappeared in from eight to fourteen days after the first injection in all but two patients. No subsequent antisyphilitic treatment was administered and no recurrence of ocular inflammation has been observed to date. However, these patients are still under observation, the maximum period of which has been twenty months.

Syphilitic Retinitis.—The retina alone rarely shows manifestations of syphilis, for in most of the cases, the retinitis is associated with inflammation of the optic nerve head, as a neuroretinitis or with the choroid as chorioretinitis. The retina is usually involved secondary to syphilitic choroiditis, but the involvement may occur primarily in the retina and the choroid may occasionally remain unaffected. It may also follow syphilitic iritis and iridocyclitis.

Syphilitic inflammation of the retina primarily is concerned with the blood vessels in which an obstruction of their lumen takes place from an endarteritis.

The characteristic manifestation is a diffuse syphilitic retinitis or neuroretinitis which is more common in the secondary stage of the disease. This is characterized by a diffuse grayish cloudy appearance of the entire fundus with a swelling which is more marked around the macula and the optic disc. The margins of the optic disc may show a marked blurring and dense gray spots around the macula. The vitreous also shows an early clouding, but as this and the fundus cloudiness subsides, a change takes place later in the pigment epithelium which results in a migration of the pigment into the retina. This occurs mostly in the periphery of the retina and the pigment has the typical bone-corpuscle appearance characteristic of retinitis pigmentosa. This also is practically the same as that occurring in syphilitic choroiditis described by Förster.

The vision of the patient is impaired, and the loss of sight may be greatly reduced, especially the central vision. A ring scotoma may be present, and night blindness may occur later.

A more rare form of retinal manifestation sometimes occurs from a localized involvement of the retinal vessels. As the result of vascular obstruction, retinal and pre-retinal hemorrhages may occur. The inflammation may be localized in the macular region or close to the larger retinal vessels in the form of a large white exudate. This leads later to the formation of proliferating tissue and retinal detachment may result.

A central retinitis also occurs in the secondary stage which is characterized by the formation of numerous white spots around the macular region. Both eyes are usually involved, and the vision is affected with a central scotoma. The retina may be faintly cloudy, but otherwise no ophthalmoscopic evidences may be present. Recurrences may occur resulting in marked impairment of the central vision.

Primary gumma of the retina is a rare condition. When these lesions occur, they are usually the result of secondary involvement from the choroid and ciliary body.

Treatment of syphilitic retinal manifestations must be directed against the internal disease. Better results are obtained in this condition from the use of mercury and the iodides which absorb the exudates and aid in clearing up the condition of the retina and vitreous.

There is very little that can be accomplished from any local treatment, but the use of diaphoretics and aids to elimination are beneficial.

Syphilis of the Optic Nerve.—The optic nerve may be involved in syphilis by an optic neuritis or papilledema, gummas, and primary optic atrophy. It should be stated here, however, that syphilis of the optic nerve in nearly all instances is a manifestation of syphilis of the central nervous system, or neuro-syphilis. The latter includes several conditions, such as syphilitic meningitis, paralytic dementia, and tabes dorsalis which should probably be described under diseases of the nervous system. Their eye manifestations, however, which are characterized principally by pathology of the optic nerve and the resultant signs and symptoms, are also considered here as manifestations of syphilis of the optic nerve.

Syphilitic Optic Neuritis and Papilledema (Acute Syphilitic Meningitis and Meningo-Encephalitis).—This is usually a conspicuous manifestation of an acute meningitis and meningo-encephalitis, which is an evidence of neuro-syphilis, and usually occurs most commonly in the secondary stage of the infection, either before, during, or just after the secondary exanthem; less frequently, after an acute exacerbation in children with congenital syphilis, and also in latent tertiary syphilis. A neurorecidive form of syphilitic meningitis which is believed by many to be due to insufficient treatment of early syphilis, is also characterized by optic neuritis accompanied by paralysis of the oculomotor, abducens, trochlear, and facial nerves.

Although acute syphilitic meningitis and meningoencephalitis are diseases of the central nervous system, a brief description must be given here. It may occur at almost any age, but more commonly in young adults, especially males. It usually appears during the first year of the infection and may begin suddenly or gradually. Headache is an early and very constant symptom and may be accompanied by nausea and vomiting. A moderate fever may be present up to 103° F. There may be rigidity of the neck and a Kernig sign may also be present. Convulsions may occur occasionally in children. Delirium or coma may be present early, and mental disturbances are common.

The optic nerve is usually affected by a papillitis or papilledema. Drake,[11] who reported a case and presented an analysis of fifty cases from the literature, found the optic nerve to be affected in sixteen cases. Both nerves were involved by swelling in fourteen. There may be a swelling of the nerve head to the extent of two to five diopters. The pupils are often found to be unequal and irregular in outline. An Argyll-Robertson pupil is sometimes found, but often the reaction to light stimulation is sluggish. The blood Wassermann reaction is positive in about 85 per cent of cases, while the cerebrospinal fluid is positive in nearly all.

The vision may be only slightly affected in mild cases, but in others the impairment may be very great. The visual fields may show a concentric contraction for form and color, an enlargement of the blind spot, central, cecocentral, or paracentral scotomas, or a nerve bundle defect.

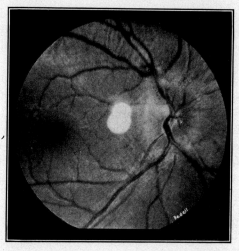

Fig. 154.—Syphilitic optic neuritis of the right eye in a man aged 41. Elevated gray disc, marked visual loss, and field constriction; prompt response to mercury and iodide. (From Bedell: J.A.M.A., March 18, 1939.)

Treatment of this form of optic neuritis is directed toward the causative condition rather than the ocular manifestation. This includes early and intensive courses of mercury or bismuth injections combined with the administration of iodides in large doses. The use of arsenic may be started guardedly after several weeks and continued once a week for a period of two months. A course of treatment is followed by a rest period of about two months, during which smaller doses of iodide alone may be employed. This form of treatment should be continued until a negative Wassermann of blood and spinal fluid is obtained repeatedly after several years.

Gumma of the Optic Nerve.—This is a rare condition, but it may occur in the intracranial part of the nerve or the optic disc. In the former the chiasm is likely to be involved either directly, or by extension from the gummatous meningitis occurring in this region. The condition results in an optic neuritis and atrophy of a descending variety.

The optic disc when rarely affected by a gumma may reveal a great deal of swelling with involvement of the surrounding retina. The vitreous may also be involved, and an iridocyclitis may also be present.

The treatment consists here also of active antisyphilitic therapy which, when started early enough and before destruction of the nerve fibers occurs, will improve the condition and save some vision of the affected eye.

Primary Optic Atrophy.—It is almost impossible to consider primary optic atrophy as a syphilitic eye manifestation without consideration of such forms of neurosyphilis as tabes and dementia paralytica with which it is associated as a late manifestation. In a few cases, however, it has been described as a syphilitic manifestation without other evidences of disease of the central nervous system.

Syphilitic optic atrophy occurs to the extent of about 1 per cent of eye affections. It occurs in about eight per cent of cases of acquired neurosyphilis and is more frequent in tabes than in any other form. It appears late in the course of the disease, usually after ten years, and also during middle age and later. Although the condition is considered to be due to an inflammation in the optic nerve, no evidences are found on ophthalmoscopic examination prior to the onset of atrophy.

Although the course of syphilitic optic atrophy is rather uniform and characteristic, the symptoms and visual field changes may show many variations and inconsistencies. An outstanding characteristic is that this is very often the first sign of tabes manifested. The visual impairment with the development of atrophy is, moreover, the only sign and, in some cases, may precede other neurologic signs of the disease by several years. On the other hand, in a few instances, it may occur somewhat later in association with other signs.

The optic atrophy is always bilateral, but it usually occurs first in one eye and is soon followed by involvement of the second eye. As a result the condition is usually a little more advanced in one eye than in the other. In most of the cases it progresses gradually with an accompanying decrease in the visual acuity. The optic disc is at first pale in color and this later becomes white, sometimes almost chalky-white, and at other times a grayish white. Another important feature is that the margins of the disc are always sharply outlined and clearly defined. The excavation in the disc is usually central, but it may be very deep and reveal the lamina cribrosa as bluish dots at the bottom. There may be no other visible ophthalmoscopic evidences present with the possible exception of a narrowing of the retinal arteries. The absence of any inflammatory signs about the vessels and the sharp outline of the disc serve to differentiate a primary from a postneuritic atrophy.

Although most of these cases progress to almost absolute blindness, the loss of vision is not necessarily in proportion to the amount of atrophy. In some cases there may be almost complete atrophy, and yet a fair amount of vision still remaining. The failure of vision is usually noticed at first by subjective disturbances, such as the appearance of shimmering, color, and light phenomena. The dark adaptation of the patient may become poor in the early stage, and before noticeable ophthalmoscopic changes are present. The visual field changes may show a variety of characteristics, chief of which might be said to be a general or concentric contraction of the peripheral form and color fields. Usually the red and green fields are affected first while blue and white follow. The central vision is usually retained until the last. Variations in the character of the visual fields include the rare occurrence of scotomas in different areas, while the peripheral field is still good. Another rare finding with a contracted peripheral field is the presence of a central or cecocentral scotoma, indicating involvement of the papillomacular bundle in particular. Other defects in the visual fields, such as homonymous hemianopia and quadranopia, may be found occasionally. Binasal hemianopia is a rare finding, but it has been reported in a few instances. Drake[12] reported a case with primary optic atrophy in tabes in a man 36 years of age and reviewed six cases from the literature. He found that the cases associated with binasal hemianopia usually show rapid progression of the optic atrophy to complete blindness.

In the presence of a primary optic atrophy, other signs of tabes which may be present should be examined for. These include the Argyll-Robertson pupil, absence of knee jerks, incoordination, ataxia, and anesthesia, especially that affecting the fifth nerve.

Treatment.—The results obtained in the treatment of syphilitic optic atrophy are very discouraging from the standpoint of improving the vision. Once the nerve has become atrophic, regeneration is impossible. Whatever form of treatment is employed, the best that can possibly be expected, if the case is seen early enough, is to check the progress of the condition temporarily and delay the further loss of vision over a period of years. In a series of 552 case records at the Wills Hospital examined by Lehrfeld and Gross[13] blindness occurred in less than three years in 74 per cent in those who received no treatment. Within five years, blindness occurred in all. This was in contrast to those who received antisyphilitic treatment in which blindness occurred in less than three years in 24 per cent, whereas all became blind in eight years. The usual treatment includes the use of mercury, iodides, and bismuth principally. The use of arsenic is considered to be questionable and not without recognized risk. When it is employed, careful and frequent observations of the visual field are necessary.

Fever therapy by use of the Kettering hypertherm[10] and the intravenous injection of typhoid or malaria may be employed with beneficial results in the treatment of the disease. In most instances, however, the condition of the optic nerve shows little or no change, and the vision and visual fields are unimproved.

In an analysis of 250 patients, Moore, Hahn, Woods and Sloan[14] found that the course of the untreated disease is extremely variable. The condition nearly always becomes bilateral and 90 per cent of untreated patients are blind within twelve years. The development of syphilitic primary optic atrophy, however, can be prevented by the adequate routine treatment of early syphilis. They found no benefit from routine therapy for syphilitic optic atrophy with the trivalent arsenicals and bismuth. However, fever therapy with the use of malaria was found by them to be the only efficacious method. This form of treatment was not employed by them in patients with the most rapidly developing disease. If visual failure progressed with malarial treatment, they concluded that no other form of treatment would prove of any value. It was therefore recommended, after early diagnosis, for immediate use in the hope of arresting the condition.

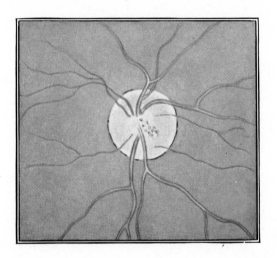

Fig. 155.—Primary optic atrophy, showing pallor, sharply defined disc margins, deep central excavation, and absence of retinal changes around the disc.

Improvement of the nutrition of the optic nerve by increasing the circulation has been claimed to provide at least temporary improvement in some cases. This is attempted by the retrobulbar injection of drugs, such as acetylcholine, in order to produce a vasodilatation by action on the vasomotor system.

Yaws (Frambesia)

Yaws is a specific infectious disease which is caused by a *Treponema pertenue,* very much like the organism of syphilis. The disease may occur in Asia, Africa, Australia, and America, and is transmitted by direct contact although not a venereal disease. The organism enters through the skin causing a papule which soon becomes moist and develops a dry crust. Other lesions appear which may coalesce and form larger ones. They often occur on the breast and buttocks of women. The primary lesions are accompanied by malaise, headache, irregular fever, and general muscle pains. The lymph glands may also become enlarged. The symptoms subside and the lesion may granulate or gradually heal. The disease may become generalized with a recurrence of symptoms and secondary lesions which may last for weeks before they disappear. Gummatous-like nodules may be found in a third stage affecting chiefly the skin, muscles, and bones. These nodules in the skin will ulcerate with considerable destruction of tissue.

Eye Manifestations.—The eye may be secondarily affected in yaws, principally during the secondary and tertiary stages of the disease. The granulations which occur on other parts may also be found on the skin of the eyelids. This is usually accompanied by a conjunctivitis with a discharge which does not necessarily contain the organism. During the third stage of the disease, the conjunctivitis is again present and the nodular lesions may be found on the margins of the eyelids, although not primarily on the conjunctiva. With ulceration of the gummatous nodules, the skin of the lids and the face about the eyelids will cause retraction resulting in ectropion and subsequent exposure keratitis.

The treatment consists in the use of neoarsphenamine. The first dose is 0.3 Gm. This is usually followed by improvement, but succeeding doses of 0.6 Gm. each may be administered at intervals of three to five days for about six doses. The granulomatous lesions also show improvement with the use of potassium iodide. The prognosis for recovery with this treatment is good.

Plague

Plague is an acute specific infectious disease transmitted to man by fleas from rats or rodents and caused by the *B. pestis.* It presents two forms, the bubonic, which is characterized principally by lymphadenopathy, and a pneumonic, in which there is a diffuse pneumonia. The onset is sudden with chills, temperature, headache, and prostration. The tongue is swollen and furrowed, and gastrointestinal symptoms are prominent. The spleen and liver may be enlarged. In the bubonic form the lymph glands of the groin, axilla, and neck become enlarged within twenty-four hours. Suppuration of the glands may sometimes take place. In the pneumonic form signs of bronchopneumonia are also present and there is cough and expectoration of a watery or blood-stained sputum. The infection may get into the blood stream with the occurrence of a septicemia which terminates fatally very early. In a mild form, however, the patient is ambulatory and the symptoms may be less severe. There is always suppuration of the buboes, and in more severe cases hemorrhages, or at least petechiae and ecchymoses, may occur in the skin and mucous membranes.

Eye Manifestations.—Various manifestations may occur in the eye in plague, although with no definite regularity. Some of the ocular lesions, as those in the conjunctiva, may be part of the infective process, and due to the presence of the organisms, while in others, they may be due to the action of the toxins. Congestion of the conjunctiva and conjunctivitis are among the earliest manifestations and occur in nearly every case. They may be accompanied by a chemosis and edema in some cases, while in others subconjunctival hemorrhages are present. Cauge,[15] who described the ocular symptoms during an epidemic of plague in Algiers, believes that in some cases the conjunctiva is the portal of entry for the organism.

The sclera may show involvement which may result in the formation of staphyloma.

The cornea also commonly reveals various forms of keratitis with iritis and iridocyclitis being frequently found.

The uveal tract is involved next in frequency to the conjunctiva and cornea. According to Cauge, it occurs in about 2 per cent of the cases and is a serious complication characterized by the appearance of an iridochoroiditis. The occurrence of this manifestation will lead to loss of vision or even loss of the eye, and it is said to indicate a virulent infection with regard to the general disease, and a lack of resistance in the patient. Clinically, there is no characteristic or particular appearance of the iridochoroiditis, but the iris may show pustules and small abscesses.

The retina may manifest an exudative retinitis, which may result in detachment. Optic neuritis may be present, but this is a rare finding.

The treatment consists in the local treatment of the ocular condition according to the type of manifestation, and also the use of a specific vaccine for the disease itself. The antiplague vaccine has been employed extensively and is said to produce a moderate immunity for a period of time, but is ineffective in extensive infections. Its use has not been followed by satisfactory results in the severe cases of uveal tract involvement. The conjunctivitis may be treated in the usual way by the use of a mild eyewash, while the presence of keratitis and iritis indicates the use of atropine sulfate in the eye and the application of hot, wet compresses.

Relapsing Fever

Relapsing fever or spirillosis is an acute infectious disease caused by the *Spirillum recurrentis* or *Spirillum obermeieri*. It occurs in Europe, Africa, Asia, and North America, but in each of these countries, the spirillum shows slight variations. It is transmitted by lice and ticks (ornithodoros) which are prevalent in filth and unsanitary surroundings.

The disease is more common among women and is ushered in with general malaise and muscle pain. This is followed during the first week by a sudden chill and rise in temperature. Headache, joint and muscle pains, nausea, and vomiting are common symptoms. The spleen is enlarged and the temperature reaches 105° F. or over. A crisis occurs which is followed in a week by another paroxysm. Skin eruptions, purpura, urticaria, herpes may occur, while cough, laryngitis, adenitis, and glossitis may also be present. The purpura may be accompanied by hemorrhages in the various organs resulting from the effect of the toxins on the blood vessels. The disease has a higher mortality among the very low classes, but recovery usually takes place from the first paroxysm, although the prognosis becomes more grave with successive ones.

Eye Manifestations.—In this disease the commonest eye manifestation is uveitis, or some form of involvement of the uveal tract. This occurs as the result of the toxic nature of the disease. It may occur in from 2 to 12 per cent of the cases in the form of a plastic iritis (Fuchs). In this form it may appear some weeks or months after the last paroxysm of fever and may be acute with marked exudation, formation of synechiae, and even hypopyon, or it may run a more prolonged uncomplicated course as a chronic iritis. This may continue for several months before recovery gradually takes place. The vitreous also may show infiltration evidenced by the presence of opacities and the ciliary body may be simultaneously involved. In about 2 per cent of cases, the condition is bilateral.

In some instances the choroid is the site of a metastatic choroiditis and in some the entire uveal tract may be involved.

The retina may reveal the presence of hemorrhages which result from the changes occurring in the retinal vessels from the altered composition of the blood.

Hamilton[16] studied ninety-two cases at the seventh Australian General Hospital and reported on nine cases. Twenty-eight of the patients were from the Western African Desert area (Libya) and sixty-three from Syria. One came from Greece and Crete. As the result of clinical findings, Hamilton felt that the Western Desert fever is louse borne, while the Syrian fever is tick borne. This also served to explain the disparity in ocular complications in the two groups. All of the patients suffering with iridocyclitis contracted it in the Western Libyan Desert (about 20 per cent). In only two was the spirochete isolated. In four patients with uveitis, there were, respectively, five, three, three and five relapses before the cyclitis appeared. In all the patients the ocular complication was unilateral and no case of optic neuritis was observed. One patient was observed with the complication of facial paralysis. Headaches are a troublesome complication. The iridocyclitis is without pain but encephalitis may be troublesome.

The treatment of the disease is specific with the use of arsphenamine. The intravenous dose of 0.25 Gm. every day for several doses causes the organism to disappear from the blood and the temperature becomes normal. The patient should be kept at rest in bed, and recurrences avoided. The local treatment depends principally on the nature of the eye manifestation and the uveitis requires principally the usual instillations of atropine sulfate, hot wet applications, and rest for the affected eyes.

Hamilton,[16] in discussing treatment of this condition, stated that no one was impressed with the results obtained from the salvarsan group in affecting the course of this disease. He described the treatment employed by the Trans-Jordan Frontier Force as follows: 3 c.c. bismuth oxychloride intramuscularly every five to seven days for three injections; tablets of stovarsol (4 gr.), 4 to 6 tablets daily in courses of three days starting on the day of injection; mistura potassium iodide, 500 mg. daily of ascorbic acid and 60,000 units of vitamin A daily during the fever (from 100 to 200 mg. of ascorbic acid and 30,000 units of vitamin A were given when each patient was afebrile).

Weil's Disease

Weil's disease is an acute infectious jaundice, otherwise known as spirochetosis icterohaemorrhagica, or spirochetal jaundice. It is an acute, specific epidemic hepatitis, with the principal sign of jaundice, caused by the *Leptospira icterohaemorrhagiae*. It occurs in the wild rat and is transmitted to man by way of the skin or the gastrointestinal tract. The onset of the disease is characterized by chills, fever, and prostration which is soon followed by the presence of jaundice. After lasting about ten days, the period of fever is followed by a second which ends either by crisis or rapid lysis. The liver and spleen may be enlarged, hemorrhages occur in the skin and mucous membranes, herpes labialis are present, and there is an anemia and leucocytosis. The spirochetes may be found in the blood and urine either on dark-field illumination or by guinea pig inoculation.

Eye Manifestations.—Early in the disease, the bulbar conjunctiva and conjunctiva of the lower lid especially, show a hyperemia which is present in nearly every case. A characteristic of the condition which indicates its nature, is the simultaneous appearance of a yellowish discoloration or jaundice of the sclera. The blood vessels of the conjunctiva are also congested in the periphery and around the cornea. They may present varicosities, and in some cases subconjunctival hemorrhages may be present. A slight discharge may occur because of a catarrhal conjunctivitis which is accompanied by moderate photophobia and lacrimation. The conjunctival manifestation usually clears as the disease itself subsides, but may reappear with a relapse of the infection.

In a number of cases the conjunctivitis is associated with a mild form of iritis and iridocyclitis. This is accompanied by moderate pain, lacrimation, and photophobia, which in exceptional cases is more severe and may be accompanied by hypopyon. It is a metastatic manifestation and usually subsides with recovery from the internal disease.

The posterior uveal tract is rarely involved by typical manifestation, although the retina and optic nerve may become involved. In the retina the vessels may be congested and tortuous, and small hemorrhages may be found. In association with the latter, or even occurring alone in an occasional case, the optic nerve head may reveal an optic neuritis.

The treatment is symptomatic and it depends on the nature of the eye manifestation presented. The conjunctivitis occurring in the early stage of the disease requires only a mild eyewash of boric acid to which a few drops of adrenalin have been added. When iritis or iridocyclitis occurs, the local treatment is the same as that described for this condition occurring in other diseases.

Rat-Bite Fever

This is a specific infection which occurs following the bite of an infected rat and is caused by the *Spirochaeta morsus muris*. During an attack it may be found either in the blood, in the local lesion, or in the enlarged glands. The initial bite is followed by an incubation period which may range from several days to a month. By the time of onset, the bite wound might be healed. Sudden chills and temperature develop, which are accompanied by headache, sweating, malaise, muscle pains, and signs of general infection. The local lesion becomes swollen, reddened, painful, and tender, but pus is not present. The attack subsides with a remission of a few days which is followed by another paroxysm lasting about two days. These attacks may be accompanied by a red, papular discrete rash which varies in size and has a bluish tint. It occurs mainly on the body and limbs. A leucocytosis with eosinophilia and lymphopenia is present and marked anemia may develop.

Eye Manifestations.—In addition to such manifestations as conjunctivitis and mild uveal involvement which may occur rarely as a secondary metastatic condition, the eyelid is often the site of the primary local lesion in rat-bite fever. In these cases the lid is swollen, red, and tender, and it is necessary to obtain the history of a bite in order to determine the etiology. In some instances the impression made in the lid by the teeth of the rat can be recognized. There may be an accompanying conjunctivitis, but the eye itself is normal in other respects. Children are frequently the victims, especially where they may be left alone in places which are infected.

A case of rat-bite fever resulting from rat bite of the left eyelid in a Negro boy, aged 6, reported by Swab,[17] was accompanied by swelling of the left side of the face and extreme swelling of the lid with closure of the eye. Two depressed marks in the skin of the lids were recognized as resembling the teeth of a rat. There was an accompanying swelling of the anterior cervical glands on the left side. The patient improved under treatment with neoarsphenamine, and at the time of discharge in sixteen days, he revealed only a slight edema of the lids.

Treatment.—The local lesion at the site of the bite should not be incised. Pus is not found in the swollen lids, but rather an edema. The treatment, which is specific, consists in the use of arsenic either in the form of salvarsan, arsphenamine, or neoarsphenamine in doses of 0.1 to 0.6 Gm. Two or three injections may produce a cure, whereas in some cases, as many as eight or ten may be required.

References

Syphilis

1. Lewis, Park: Interstitial Keratitis, a Modern Anachronism, Am. J. Ophth. **17**: 444, 1934.
2. Holloway, T. B.: Why Have Ocular Diseases? Am. Health Cong. Series, Vol. 4.
3. Goldberg, J. A.: Prevention of Congenital Syphilis, New York State J. Med. **34**: 290, 1934.
4. Paley, S. S.: Syphilis in Pregnancy, New York State J. Med. **37**: 585, 1937.
5. Berens, Conrad, and Goldberg, J. A.: Syphilis in Relation to the Prevention of Blindness. A Study of 100,000 Case Records, Tr. Sect. on Ophth. A. M. A., 1937.
6. Klauder, Joseph V.: Ocular Syphilis: Factors Influencing the Localization of Syphilis in the Eye, Arch. Ophth. **7**: 268, 1932.
7. Klauder, Joseph V.: Ocular Syphilis: Interstitial Keratitis and Trauma. Clinical, Experimental, and Medicolegal Aspects, Arch. Ophth. **10**: 302, 1933.
8. Green, John: The Eye in Hereditary Syphilis, Am. J. Dis. Child. **20**: 29, 1920.
9. Klien, Bertha A.: Acute Metastatic Syphilitic Corneal Abscess. A Clinical and Histopathologic Study, Arch. Ophth. **14**: 612, 1935.
10. Culler, Arthur M., and Simpson, Walter M.: Artificial Fever Therapy in Cases of Ocular Syphilis, Arch. Ophth. **15**: 624, 1936.

11. Drake, Ralph L.: Ocular Syphilis, Arch. Ophth. **9**: 234, 1933.
12. Drake, Ralph L.: Ocular Syphilis. Binasal Hemianopia Associated With Primary Optic Atrophy in Tabes Dorsalis, Arch. Ophth. **12**: 583, 1934.
13. Lehrfeld, Louis, and Gross, Elmer R.: A Statistical Investigation of Syphilitic Atrophy of the Optic Nerve, Arch. Ophth. **18**: 666, 1937.
14. Moore, J. E., Hahn, R. D., Woods, A. C., and Sloan L.: The Treatment of Syphilitic Primary Optic Atrophy, Am. J. Ophth. **25**: 777, 1942.

Plague

15. Cauge: The Ocular Symptoms of Bubonic Plague, Arch. d'ophth. **49**: 5, 1932.

Relapsing Fever

16. Hamilton, J. B.: Ocular Complications in Relapsing Fever, Brit. J. Ophth. **27**: 68, 1943.

Rat-Bite Fever

17. Swab, C. M.: Rat Bite of the Eyelids Resulting in Rat-Bite Fever, Am. J. Ophth. **13**: 884, 1930.

tubercle. These are seen in very young patients who have not developed an allergy, or in those with miliary tuberculosis in which allergy was destroyed by a massive infection. A more acute, confluent and caseating lesion occurs in those who are allergic. It is presumed that this is well localized and shows no extension when both allergy and immunity are pronounced, whereas it is spreading, extensive and exudative, when the allergy is pronounced but immunity is low.

The Mantoux test may be an important aid in the diagnosis of ocular tuberculosis. In all suspected cases this intracutaneous tuberculin test should be performed in order to determine the presence of a cutaneous sensitivity or a state of allergy in the patient. Its use has practically replaced the subcutaneous and Calmette conjunctival test with which the danger of activating local and constitutional reactions was found to be too great. Although the results of the Mantoux test cannot be interpreted as a positive indicator, it should always be employed and considered in association with the history, clinical eye picture, physical signs, x-ray examination, and other evidences.

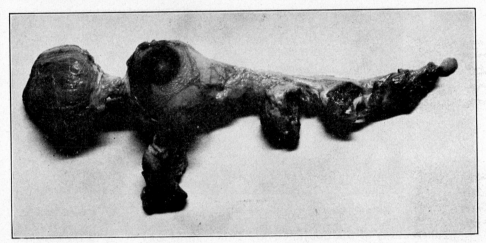

Fig. 156.—Tuberculoma of the recti muscles. Patient with pulmonary tuberculosis. (Courtesy of Dr. E. B. Spaeth.)

Several varieties of tuberculin are employed. These include Koch's old tuberculin (O.T.), new tuberculin (T.R.), Denys' bouillon filtrate, purified protein derivative of the tubercle bacillus (P. P. D.), and others employed in European countries. The method of administration is probably more important than the preparation employed. Adler and Meyer[1] recommended the use of a purified protein derivative (P. P. D.) prepared by Seibert, Aaronson, Reichel, Clark, and Long, because of its potency and because its strength varies little in different batches. The test dilutions should be made up fresh at least once a month, and refrigerated. They suggested starting with a subminimal dose (0.000001 mg.). This is increased tenfold with each negative reaction until positive. The results are recorded quantitatively as +1, +2, +3, +4, according to the size and severity of the reaction. The dose employed is also stated. Woods and Randolph[2] described the results of the Mantoux test in 180 clinical cases of ocular tuberculosis. Their results showed ninety-six or 53.4 per cent reacted to 0.001 mg. of tuberculin, seventy-five, or 41.6 per cent reacted cutaneously only to 0.01 mg., and nine, or 5 per cent only to 0.1 or 1 mg., or were insensitive. In ten additional cases with histopathologically proved ocular tuberculosis, the figures were somewhat similar. Woods and Randolph pointed out that a high degree of cutaneous reactivity should not necessarily be expected in patients with ocular tuberculosis and that a low degree of cutaneous reactivity is not positive evidence against the presence of ocular tuberculosis.

Orbital Tuberculosis.—Tuberculosis of the orbit as a primary condition is very uncommon. Involvement is usually secondary to tubercles of the lacrimal gland or results from tuberculous periostitis. Difficulties in diagnosis of orbital involvement are often encountered. Usually the outer wall is affected by an indurated mass. This may undergo swelling with subsequent degeneration and abscess formation. The abscess may break through the skin and result in fistula through the bone.

A tuberculoma may occur in the lacrimal gland or lacrimal sac which resembles a tumorous growth and should be excised. It consists of chronic inflammatory tissue which undergoes necrosis and caseation.

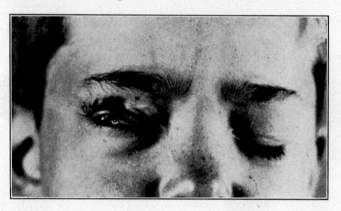

Fig. 157.—Tuberculous osteomyelitis of orbit. (Courtesy of Dr. E. B. Spaeth.)

Tuberculosis of the Conjunctiva.—Tuberculosis may occur in the conjunctiva either as a primary or secondary condition and may present a variety of manifestations. It may be a primary infection as the result of tubercle bacilli entering directly by contact with exogenous infected material. This may occur especially in the presence of an abrasion or injury of the conjunctiva. Secondary infections may occur as the result of contamination of the part by some act of the tuberculous patient, and also by endogenous involvement from metastasis through the blood stream. Secondary involvement of the conjunctiva may also occur in rare cases by direct extension from adjacent parts, such as from the lacrimal apparatus and from the skin of the face or nose in lupus.

The lesion is usually considered as a tubercle and occurs commonly in young people up to the age of 30 or 40 years. It may follow two main courses, the one which undergoes ulceration, and the other hyperplasia. The various manifestations have been described in several ways, nearly all of which resolve themselves into the following groups which may be found either alone or combined.

The first is an ulcerative variety which is characterized by the occurrence of small miliary ulcers which affect the palpebral and bulbar conjunctiva.

These small single ulcers may occasionally coalesce into larger ones. They cause no pain, but are chronic in nature and fail to heal.

The second is a nodular variety which presents yellowish or grayish-yellow nodules under the conjunctiva. These are very small at first and resemble the appearance of trachoma. They become larger and are accompanied by follicles and granulation which contain tubercle bacilli. A necrosis takes place in the central portion with caseation.

The third variety, which is sometimes considered as a later stage of the second, reveals hypertrophied granulation tissue accompanied by edema and reaction of the lids. This is found on the tarsal and palpebral conjunctiva, arising usually in the fornices. The granulation tissue outgrowths are often described as resembling a "cock's comb" in appearance.

The fourth variety is the polypoid type which occurs as a pedunculated tumor which resembles a papilloma or fibroma growing from the tarsal conjunctiva. It may attain a fair size and protrude over the lid margin.

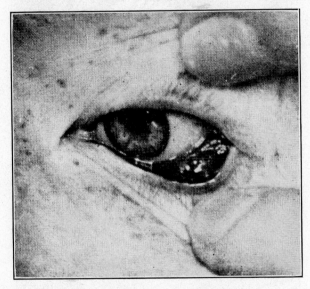

Fig. 158.—Conjunctival lesion in tuberculosis. (From Samuelson: Arch. Ophth., June, 1936.)

Scrapings from any of these lesions should reveal the presence of tubercle bacilli and confirm the diagnosis of the condition. In many instances, however, the appearance might resemble that of trachoma, vernal conjunctivitis, Parinaud's conjunctivitis, and others. Some of the cases may follow a short course and eventually clear up under treatment, while others are more chronic and fail to respond.

Other manifestations of conjunctival tuberculosis occurring in the form of tuberculides are described (Duke-Elder) as attenuated lesions with the histologic structure of miliary tubercles, but which rarely, if ever, contain tubercle bacilli. They present multiple, evanescent lesions on the skin and mucous membranes, which disappear without leaving any signs and are considered as a probable manifestation of an allergic sensitivity. These include two principal varieties, i.e., lichen scrofulosum and Boeck's sarcoid.

Lichen Scrofulosum.—This condition occurs either alone or in association with tuberculous scleritis or uveitis. It is characterized by the presence of globular nodules on the bulbar conjunctiva which may change almost daily from one place to another and are not accompanied by signs of inflammation. They have been found to be an allergic manifestation and usually occur in association with lichen scrofulosum of the skin and other tuberculous lesions, tuberculous parenchymatous keratitis, and as a response to ocular tuberculin reaction.

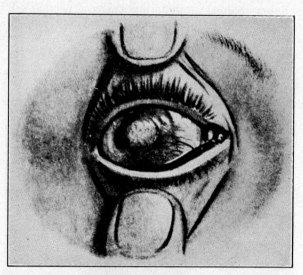

Fig. 159.—Tuberculous lesion of bulbar conjunctiva. (From Ramsay: Clinical Ophthalmology for the General Practitioner, Oxford Medical Publications.)

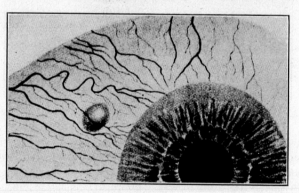

Fig. 160.—Lichen scrofulosum. (From Lowenstein: Ztschr. f. Augenh.) (Duke-Elder.)

The histologic structure is described as typical of a miliary tubercle, and they have also been considered to have a close relationship to the phlyctenule.

Boeck's Sarcoid.—Lesions on the lids and bulbar conjunctiva in the form of nodules have been found in a number of instances in tuberculous patients who revealed similar lesions in the skin, mucous membranes, and bones. The nodules are usually multiple and may be present for months. The tubercle bacillus has not been demonstrated in the lesion. However, these were considered by Igersheimer[3] to be without doubt tuberculoid tissue in its typical form. The iris may also be involved, with the presence of an iritis. The tissue has been described histologically as tuberculous granulation without necrosis.

It is a form of lymphogranuloma. The tubercles often contain giant cells within which are sometimes found a type of inclusion body known as "Schaumann bodies." These latter, when present, serve to differentiate the sarcoid lesion from the hard tubercles occurring in tuberculosis.

Sarcoid lesions may be accompanied by glandular enlargement, and the pathology may be found on microscopic examination of the lymph glands. Lesions might be found in the lungs on roentgenologic examination and these usually consist of a diffuse infiltration of the hilus and lower portions of the lungs.

In many cases the nodules are found in the skin, and these vary in size and consistency. They may also occur in the liver and spleen.

The exact cause of sarcoid is not known, but since the pathologic lesions resemble hard tubercles and because active tuberculosis has been demonstrated in some cases, the condition has been considered to be of a tuberculous nature. Caseation and necrosis characteristic of tuberculosis are rarely every found in this condition, however. A positive diagnosis can be made only by laboratory examination of a lymph gland and the demonstration of the characteristic lesion.

In the eye the nodules in sarcoid may occur on the lids, conjunctiva, episclera, and the orbit. The important ocular condition occurring in sarcoid is uveitis. The characteristic clinical picture has been described in detail by Woods and Guyton.[4] This consists of a nodular iritis resembling that which occurs in tuberculosis. In sarcoid, however, the nodules become larger, are pink in color and have a tendency to become vascularized. They are not accompanied by pain. In some cases the nodules may be scarcely visible, but the inflammatory reaction is quite marked. Posterior synechiae may be present in either form and a generalized uveitis may develop. This will be accompanied by a cloudy media, secondary clouding of the lens, deposits on the cornea and changes in the posterior uveal tract. In progressively severe cases, secondary glaucoma may develop and loss of the eye may follow. In the great majority, however, the condition follows a more favorable course. Hyalinization of the nodules occurs with disappearance of the inflammatory signs. The entire process may improve without sequelae.

In the report of Woods and Guyton, fifteen cases of sarcoid showed no significant sex distribution, but there appeared to be some predilection for Negroes. The age of the patients also showed no particular significance. The uveitis is, in most cases, bilateral and usually chronic, with nodules on the iris being found in some, while in others the entire uveal tract is involved. The nodules are normally larger than those found in tuberculous iritis and are more regular and more vascularized. They disappear without leaving any scar, whereas in tuberculous iritis, healing occurs with scarring and atrophy of the iris. In the absence of nodules, the cases may show corneal involvement with deposits and deep keratitis. The corneal deposits may be of fair size and of the "mutton-fat" variety.

All of the fifteen patients described by Woods and Guyton revealed systemic manifestations of sarcoidosis with the lesion occurring most frequently in the lungs. Glandular enlargement was also a common feature. Any of the glands might become involved. Histologic diagnosis of sarcoid can be made on biopsy of a lymph gland even though the gland may appear to be normal.

In seven of these patients the globulin was elevated over 3.0 per cent. Three of the fifteen patients reacted to 0.01 mg. of tuberculin, while five were completely insensitive.

The occurrence of Boeck's sarcoid in children is rare. Thornhill and Thornhill[5] reported nodular iritis in a 9-year-old Negro girl, the diagnosis being made by physical and roentgenographic examination. There was enlargement of the lymph nodes in the chest and mottling in the periphery of the lungs. The condition was differentiated from tuberculous iritis and syphilitic iritis by tuberculin and Wassermann tests, sputum examinations, innoculation of guinea pigs and microscopic study of a lymph node.

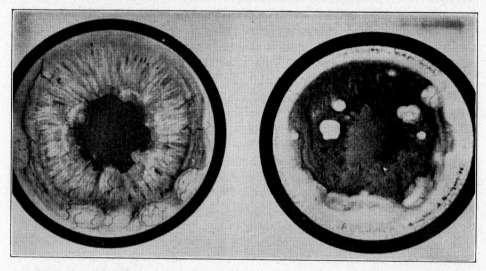

Fig. 161.—Iris nodules in sarcoid uveitis. Left, Active stage. Right, Subsiding stage in a different patient. (From Woods and Guyton: Tr. Am. Acad. Ophth. [1943], March-April, 1944.)

The patient ran a temperature of from 98.5 to 100.4° F. The vision in the affected eye was impaired with the presence of a corneal haze and descemetitis. The pupil was contracted and there were posterior synechiae present. Large cystic nodules were present on the iris and small pinhead yellowish granules on the nasal side. Pigmented deposits were found on the anterior surface of the lens. The posterior surface of the cornea showed some vascularization.

The general condition of the patient apparently improved with a high vitamin diet containing cod-liver oil, ascorbic acid, thiamine chloride and brewer's yeast. Atropine sulfate (0.5 per cent) was employed in the affected eye, but the ocular condition showed little improvement.

Lupus of the Conjunctiva.—Lupus of the eyelids and conjunctiva is some-times described as a rare tuberculous manifestation which may occur as an ulcer with granulations on the conjunctiva or may spread from the skin of the face and nose. The bottom of the conjunctival ulcers is covered with gran-ulations which contain tubercle bacilli (Fuchs).

Klauder and De Long[6] described three cases of lupus erythematosus of the conjunctiva and eyelids with typical lesions of the disease elsewhere. The lesions were characterized by a redness of the conjunctiva and lid, accom-panied by a mucoid discharge. Well-defined and depressed areas of atrophy were present. These authors stated that there appears to be, in some cases at least, an intimate relationship between tuberculosis and lupus erythematosus, but the specific etiology of the condition is not known. They felt that it should be included among cutaneous diseases that have an ocular expression.

Phlyctenular Conjunctivitis.—This condition, which is often associated with corneal involvement when it is designated as phlyctenular keratoconjunctivitis, is sometimes considered to be associated with tuberculosis. In many cases a tuberculous sensitivity has been found, and the lesion is now considered to be an allergic reaction to tuberculoprotein. Most of the patients are children and young people who present a scrofulous appearance and glandular affections. Many have also been shown to suffer with active tuberculous lesions. The phlyctenule itself is a small, round nodule or elevation with a slight pink color surrounded by a small area of hyperemia. The lesions occur more often near or on the limbus of the cornea and may ulcerate. This clears up slowly and usually leaves no sign of its presence. The rest of the conjunc-tiva is unaffected, although more than one may be present at the same time, and they also have a tendency to recur at almost any time. In some rare instances a fairly large number may be found around the limbus of the cornea. These may coalesce and form a ring ulcer. The latter is a more serious con-dition and may lead to perforation. In the average case the local symptoms are moderate photophobia, lacrimation, and itching. When the cornea is in-volved, however, the condition is more troublesome and lasts longer. Here scrofulous ulcers are formed by destruction of the epithelium which has been infiltrated by the nodules formed on Bowman's membrane. The latter may also be destroyed together with the substantia propria followed by vasculariza-tion and the formation of connective tissue (scrofulous pannus). The irrita-tion, pain, lacrimation, and photophobia are severe and blepharospasm may also be present.

In some cases the ulcers may suppurate with the collection of pus between layers of the cornea or in the anterior chamber. Perforation of the cornea may occur in extreme cases. The general condition of these young patients may also show signs of constitutional weakness. If the presence of tuberculosis cannot be definitely established, it can be reasonably assumed from their gen-eral physical condition that they are potential cases. Usually they are found to be underweight, poorly nourished, with a history of existing on an improper diet. Eruptions may be found on other parts of the body, the extremities are usually cold, and purulent infections may be present in the nose, ear, or elsewhere.

Treatment.—The treatment of tuberculous manifestations of the conjunc-tiva includes both general, or constitutional, and local treatment. This applies to the treatment of such affections in the cornea and all other structures of the eye, as well as those occurring in the conjunctiva. The local treatment depends on the type of conjunctival manifestation. In nearly all of these the patient will be benefited by the use of black glasses and the regular cleansing of the eyes with warm boric acid solution. This is especially true in cases of phlyctenular conjunctivitis, and when photophobia is a marked symptom, the patient should be kept in a darkened room. When the cornea is also involved, one drop of atropine sulfate, 1 per cent solution, should be instilled three times a day following the application of hot wet compresses.

In some of the milder cases the use of powdered calomel or iodoform powder and the ointment of yellow oxide of mercury (1 per cent) may prove effective. In some of the more severe cases x-ray or ultraviolet light has been found to be effective, while in some, excision of the entire granulomatous lesion followed by application of the cautery is indicated. The use of tuberculin in conjunctival affections is not very effective.

The general treatment should be directed toward the improvement of the physical condition and increasing the resistance of the patient. The nourishment should be substantial, avoiding sweets, pies, and pastry. Fresh air and plenty of sleep and rest are essential. Internally, the use of tonics, such as iron, calcium and cod-liver oil, is indicated.

Tuberculosis of the Sclera.—Involvement of the sclera in tuberculosis is not common, but it may occur in one of two forms. The first is a sclerokeratitis which is progressive and associated with a primary lesion in the cornea near the limbus. The latter is infiltrated with diffuse nodules which are poorly outlined while the surrounding sclera shows areas of inflammation. The infiltration of the cornea slowly increases and an associated uveitis of the anterior part of the eyeball adds to the severity of the condition. Although it is not typically characteristic, the pathology has been considered to be of tuberculous origin. Pain is a troublesome subjective symptom and marked impairment of vision or loss of the eye may result after running a prolonged course.

The second variety which is uncommon but somewhat more typical is a scleritis characterized by the formation of a hard, yellow nodule or tubercle which results nearly always from endogenous sources by way of the blood stream. In some instances it may also occur by direct extension from a primary lesion in the conjunctiva or ciliary body. The conjunctiva above the fixed tubercle in the sclera can move freely. After a while, ulceration and caseation of the nodule occur. The treatment consists in excision and the use of tuberculin.

Tuberculosis of the Cornea.—Tuberculous infections of the cornea do not ordinarily occur as the result of direct invasion by the tubercle bacillus but rather as the result of extension of the process from the conjunctiva and also in association with tuberculosis of the sclera and uveal tract. It may also become involved as a secondary infection from the anterior chamber by lesions in the iris and, lastly, as an allergic reaction to tuberculoprotein.

The clinical diagnosis depends principally on the appearance of the condition and on the response to the use of tuberculin. Although the cornea is rarely involved primarily, such cases have been reported and are described as being either infiltrative or ulcerative in form, the latter being more common. The ulcerative type is characterized by the formation of nodules which break down and ulcerate, the ulcer running a long chronic course over a period of months with little tendency to heal. It is accompanied by the formation of superficial and deep vascularization. The process may involve other structures of the eye by extension or may result in perforation of the cornea. The infiltrative type is also characterized by the presence of a nodule near the limbus which gradually extends through the cornea, leaving a gray superficial opacity.

Tuberculous Interstitial Keratitis.—An interstitial keratitis occurs occasionally as the result of an allergic reaction in tuberculosis, similar in appearance to that seen with syphilis. In many cases syphilis may also be present, and the etiologic diagnosis is difficult. In tuberculosis, the condition also runs a prolonged course, but it usually involves one eye and may be limited to only a portion of the cornea which reveals a dense nodular infiltration. This is accompanied by vascularization in the middle and deeper layers. Healing takes place slowly and results in formation of a permanent opacity. The condition is accompanied often by involvement of the neighboring glands.

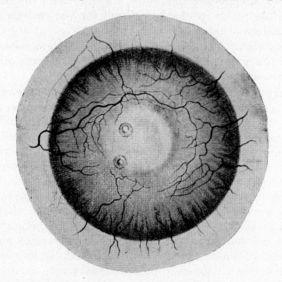

Fig. 162.—Tuberculous interstitial keratitis. (From Duke-Elder: Text-Book of Ophthalmology.)

Treatment consists in both local and general measures. The local treatment is the same as that described for syphilitic interstitial keratitis. (See Syphilis.) The general treatment includes complete rest, a wholesome and nourishing diet, fresh air, and sunlight. The internal administration of cod-liver oil and general tonics should supplement these measures.

Tuberculous Abscess of the Posterior Cornea.—The cornea may suffer from a metastatic inflammation in its deeper layers as the result of tuberculosis, similar to that occurring in syphilis. (See Syphilis.) The abscess ruptures through Descemet's membrane with subsequent involvement of the anterior chamber. The condition is considered to result secondary to, or associated with, iritis and may extend to and involve the anterior capsule of the lens.

Tuberculosis of the Uveal Tract (Iritis and Iridocyclitis).—Inflammation of the iris and ciliary body occurs in tuberculosis in the form of tuberculous iritis and iridocyclitis. It may also be described as tuberculosis of the anterior uveal tract. Statistics vary greatly with regard to the incidence of uveal involvement in general, but it can be safely said that tuberculosis of the uveal tract is the most frequent form of ocular tuberculosis. It is nearly always secondary to a tuberculous lesion elsewhere in the body and develops when a tuberculous nodule breaks down and on entering the blood stream, makes its way to the eye. Here it becomes lodged very often in the anastomosis of vessels around the ciliary border of the iris which accounts for the frequent involvement of these structures. It is, therefore, considered as metastatic involvement. The primary focus as a rule is a quiescent or a healed lesion which may be present in the lungs or mediastinal glands. As has been previously stated, ocular tuberculosis scarcely ever occurs in the presence of active tuberculosis elsewhere. An exception to this rule may be found to occur in young patients with miliary tuberculosis. Here, the eye manifestation in the form of bilateral iritis or iridocyclitis may occur early in the disease. Other cases of tuberculous uveitis are considered to be due to an allergic sensitization. The various degrees of allergy and immunity, together with the particular way in which an individual reacts, probably account for the various and many-sided clinical manifestations of tuberculosis of the uvea.

From the results of histologic examinations of these cases, they were divided by Igersheimer[3] into three main groups: 1, Acute and subacute; 2, chronic and recurrent; and 3, special types.

Acute miliary tuberculosis of the iris is not a common clinical occurrence. Numerous small yellowish-gray nodules near the ciliary border can be observed and studied on slit lamp examination. These are associated with a rather severe iritis which is characterized by pain, photophobia, and pericorneal injection. Sometimes the iritis appears first in a diffuse form which may reveal no specific characteristics, but which is followed by the later appearance of the nodules. The patient is usually very sick and may succumb to the disease. In other instances the nodules become confluent and the posterior segment of the eye may be involved, with nodules appearing in the choroid. They are usually situated at the posterior pole near the disc, although they may occur elsewhere. They are small gray areas with blurred margins and may measure as much as 2 mm. in diameter. Several small nodules may coalesce to form larger ones. These can be observed on ophthalmoscopic examination, but only one or two may be present. In most cases the eye is lost, even if the patient survives. In rare instances where healing does occur, the affected area is covered with pigment and resembles the picture of disseminated choroiditis. Tubercle bacilli are often, although not always, found in these cases.

A chronic variety of tuberculomas of the iris is found in which the iris is covered by many nodular growths which may or may not be accompanied by inflammatory evidences. In the latter instance the patient suffers little or no pain. In other instances, however, a severe exudative iritis occurs which may be complicated by the formation of a hypopyon. These cases may result in the loss of the eye, while in others, the condition may terminate by resolution and absorption of the nodules. A scar or atrophy of the iris which is characterized by the presence of a small white patch in the affected area may result.

Chronic Tuberculous Iridocyclitis.—In chronic tuberculosis, the ciliary body may be involved simultaneously with the iris. The condition may start very mildly and reveal only a moderate pericorneal injection with some deposits which have been described as ''mutton-fat'' in appearance, and are found on the posterior surface of the cornea. A few small nodules may also be present on the pupillary border of the iris. In some instances the onset is characterized by a more severe plastic iritis. These cases continue on more or less quietly and may travel to the posterior part of the eye with involvement of the vitreous and retinal vessels. The latter show a perivasculitis with the occurrence of hemorrhages. Chronic iridocyclitis is frequently complicated by an increased intraocular tension. Finoff[7] described these cases as a separate syndrome when they presented the following symptoms: 1, keratitic precipitates of the mutton-fat variety; 2, evanescent grayish nodules (Gilbert-Koeppe nodules) which are present at the pupillary margin of the iris; 3, increased intraocular tension; 4, vitreous exudates; 5, one or more yellowish tubercles in the choroid. The disease usually runs a long course over a period of months or years, but a few cases may recover to some extent after a few months.

Exudative Uveitis.—Two forms of tuberculous exudative iridocyclitis include the acute plastic variety and the chronic exudative iridocyclitis. Both are allergic in nature and nonspecific. The acute form usually is found in younger patients up to the age of about 30 years, and usually affects one eye. It may last several weeks or months and is characterized by pain, photophobia, the presence of a plastic exudate on the iris and posterior synechiae. Fine, hazy opacities may be found in the vitreous and small Koeppe nodules on the pupillary margin of the iris. Nodules may be present late and a patch of exudate may be found in the choroid. This usually occurs in the periphery or sometimes near the optic disc. It may be the same size as the disc or even larger. The condition usually subsides leaving a patch of atrophy surrounded by pigment in the affected area of the choroid.

The chronic variety usually affects older people of middle age and is usually bilateral. They run a chronic course and very few are ever examined pathologically, so that the tubercle bacillus is not demonstrated in the lesion. According to Igersheimer, no nodules but scattered epithelioid cells, lymphocytes, and plasma cells are found in the anterior uvea, while in other parts of the eye, small, hidden nests of epitheliod cells may be found which would indicate the nature of the condition. Clinically, exudation is marked, with the iris bound down to the anterior capsule of the lens until the pupil is almost entirely occluded. Numerous large mutton-fat deposits are found on the posterior surface of the cornea. If the vitreous can be observed through the small pupil, it will be found to be very hazy. The choroid and retina may also show an exudative lesion. This condition shows a great tendency to relapse and usually results in marked impairment of the vision or even in total blindness.

Tuberculosis of the Posterior Uvea.—The posterior uvea may also be involved in several different ways. These include involvement of the choroid in the form of choroiditis with the formation of one or more small tuberculomas. This usually occurs in younger patients up to the age of about 30. Both eyes are usually affected, and the condition is often accompanied by iridocyclitis. Round, grayish-yellow nodules are scattered around the choroid. The retina above is affected and breaks down with the formation of white pigmented atrophic areas in the fundus when the inflammation subsides.

Another variety of posterior uveitis occurs with involvement of the anterior segment in the form of a chronic, low-grade process which may run a prolonged course over a period of years. The symptoms are mild and on objective examination, fine opacities may be seen in the vitreous, a few fine deposits on the posterior cornea, and possibly one or two on the posterior lens.

Occasionally, a nodule may be present on the iris, but this is rare. With the exception of a gradual impairment of vision in the affected eye, subjective symptoms are not complained of. Later on the condition may be complicated by cataract formation and occlusion of the pupil by the products of inflammation.

The entire uveal tract may be involved rarely by an acute inflammation which spreads quickly throughout the various structures with ultimate loss of the eye. This is a diffuse proliferative type of uveitis which is characterized by a generalized inflammation of the iris and anterior chamber. There is posterior involvement of the choroid and retina by a round mass which proliferates forward into the vitreous. This becomes almost filled with the low-grade inflammatory or necrotic material and can be seen through the pupil with the unaided eye as a grayish mass occupying the posterior eyeball. This is sometimes called "pseudoglioma" since the appearance resembles that seen in glioma.

Tubercle of the Choroid.—A tubercle may occur in the choroid either at the posterior pole, near the disc and macula, or at the equator. Such a tubercle is described as solitary or conglomerate and is a comparatively rare manifestation. It usually begins as a small, round, grayish-white mass, which is poorly outlined. Gradually growing larger, it may reach a fair size and resemble an intraocular tumor which projects forward as a round white body. Ordinarily, a white irregular zone of inflammation can be seen to surround the mass itself. The retina is stretched by the growth and may eventually become detached. In some few cases, the tubercle may extend along the choroid as it develops without bulging forward. The vitreous is hazy and contains floating opacities while the anterior segment of the eye may reveal a mild anterior uveitis. The retina may become involved and a proliferating retinitis may take place. In some cases, the tubercle will regress after some months and leave a white scar with some pigment in the area affected. A fresh tubercle may recur later alongside the site of the original lesion. A more extensive inflammation may then take place with the occurrence of an exudative iridocyclitis, and all of its accompanying manifestations. The sclera may also become involved with perforation and subsequent loss of the eye.

Treatment of Tuberculous Uveitis.—Since there are many forms in which tuberculous uveitis may manifest itself, the treatment must vary in different cases. In general, it may be said that the active manifestations, particularly those affecting the anterior uvea, may require more active local treatment than those which affect the posterior uvea. Local treatment must be employed where indicated in an effort to relieve and perhaps limit the severity of the ocular manifestation rather than to cure the condition. In addition to the local treatment it is necessary in cases of tuberculous uveitis to employ general treatment intended to improve the physical condition and resistance of the patient, and also to consider the use of tuberculin in certain cases for the purpose of desensitization.

The local treatment may be described as that employed for any case of iritis and iridocyclitis. It differs very little if any from that described in the local treatment of syphilitic iritis and iridocyclitis. The use of mydriatics is of first importance and the best of these drugs is atropine sulphate, 1 per cent solution, or in the form of an ointment. The solution should be instilled into the affected eye in every case as early as possible about three

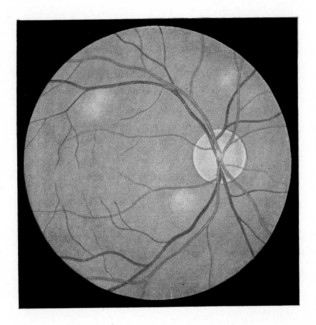

Fig. 163.—Miliary tuberculosis of the choroid. (After Koellner, from Troncoso: Internal Diseases of the Eye and Atlas of Ophthalmoscopy, F. A. Davis Co.)

times daily. Atropine is always employed for the purpose of dilating and maintaining an open pupil, and thereby preventing or overcoming the formation of synechiae. This is an important indication in all forms of iritis and iridocyclitis. It is also important here to place the eye at rest. This is also accomplished by relaxing the ciliary muscle and intraocular muscles by the use of atropine. The eyes should also be protected from light by the use of black glasses. When atropine is no longer tolerated and shows evidences of undesirable effects, other mydriatics, such as scopolamine, duboisine, or paredrine, may be substituted. In very obstinate cases when the pupil fails to dilate with any of the ordinary mydriatics, a small pack in the form of a little pledget of cotton may be soaked in atropine and adrenalin and placed under the closed upper eyelid for a few minutes. Adrenalin or other sympathomimetic drugs may be employed with atropine for their synergistic action, either as a pack or by subconjunctival injection. For example, a mixture of 2 minims each of atropine sulfate, 1 per cent, and adrenaline, 1:10,000 in about 10 minims of saline solution may be injected subconjunctivally in an effort to dilate the pupil. Paredrine, 3 or 5 per cent, may also be employed effectively in some cases with atropine, either by instillation or subconjunctival injection.

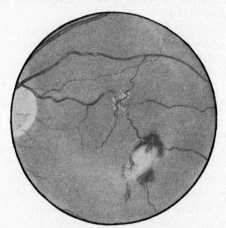

Fig. 164.—Conglomerate tubercle of the choroid. (After Reese, from Troncoso: Internal Diseases of the Eye and Atlas of Ophthalmoscopy, F. A. Davis Co.)

The use of heat in the treatment of tuberculosis of the anterior uvea is also of great value. It can be employed, as already described, by applications of ordinary hot water or boric acid solution, or by one of the various methods of applying dry heat. The beneficial effects are obtained by increasing the local blood supply, while at the same time, it relieves pain and has a soothing effect on the eye. Persistent pain, however, which is only complained of rarely in tuberculous iritis and iridocyclitis may require the occasional use of local anesthetics.

Other forms of local treatment which can be employed in tuberculous uveitis include x-ray, ultraviolet light, radium, and autohemotherapy.

Complications, especially the increase in intraocular tension and the occurrence of secondary glaucoma, may require surgical treatment. The presence of progressive hypopyon may indicate the need for paracentesis of the anterior chamber. This procedure may also be employed in order to decrease the intraocular tension in some cases where other operative procedures are not indicated and also for flushing the anterior chamber with normal saline solution. It also stimulates the formation of fresh aqueous in the anterior chamber. This is of value in some cases of tuberculous lesions of the anterior uvea, since it provides new immune bodies in the affected part and is followed by a decrease of the inflammatory condition. Other operative procedures for the reduction of the intraocular tension include iridectomy, iridotomy, and transfixion of the iris. The choice of the procedure to be employed will depend on the nature of the individual case and the judgment of the surgeon in charge.

The general treatment of the patient is directed toward increasing the power of resistance to the disease, improving the state of immunity, and lowering the sensitivity or allergic state.

To accomplish the first two, it is necessary to provide plenty of rest, good food, fresh air, and sunshine. Rest is of prime importance with regard to the eye and should be enforced just as in other tuberculous conditions. The diet of the patient should be nourishing and can be supplemented by the use of cod-liver oil and an adequate supply of the vitamins. While the general physical condition of the patient is being improved by these measures, the state of the immunity is also improved.

The use of tuberculin in the treatment of uveal tuberculosis is of great value. Its use is intended to provide a desensitization of the patient to tuberculoprotein. Several different preparations of tuberculin are obtainable, the names of which have been previously mentioned. Regardless of which preparation is employed, it should be remembered that its use is not intended as a cure but rather as an aid in lowering the sensitivity while the immunity is being improved, so that the patient is in better condition to overcome the manifestations of the disease. However, several other important considerations with regard to the use of tuberculin must be constantly kept in mind. The first of these is that its use should be avoided in the presence of active tuberculosis in another organ, as for example, in active pulmonary tuberculosis. In starting the treatment only minimum doses should be employed. In giving repeated doses the site of the injection should be observed for a local reaction, and the eyes should be constantly observed for signs of focal reaction. The dose should always be lowered in the presence of a local reaction and decreased to a point of safety with signs of focal reaction. When these signs have disappeared, it may again be gradually increased, but always keeping it below the reaction point of the patient. The general belief at the present time is that an ocular reaction is very undesirable, and dangerous, but there are some who believe it necessary to employ tuberculin in sufficient dose to produce just a slight focal reaction.

Woods and Randolph,[2] who used Denys' bouillon filtrate in the treatment of 175 cases, started with an initial dose of 0.0001 mg. The dose was increased and repeated every four days until 0.9 Gm. was given. Injections were then given once a week. One hundred forty-three of these patients received only one course of tuberculin according to what they described as the "perifocal concept" of treatment, whereby the tuberculin was supposed to cause repeated minor perifocal reactions which result in a local immunity and encapsulation of the lesion. Thirty-two patients, on the other hand, received the treatment more or less constantly for a period of at least two years on the basis of what was described as the "desensitization concept." According to this theory, the tuberculin is said to act by desensitizing the ocular structures, thereby removing the factors which cause the inflammatory and destructive phases of the lesion. These authors obtained the best results with those patients who were treated according to the desensitization concept and recommended this procedure, with tuberculin being administered for at least two years, to be discontinued only when the skin reaction fails almost entirely and the eye manifestation has been entirely quiet and apparently encapsulated for at least a year.

A contraindication in the use of tuberculin because of the danger of specific toxic damage has been pointed out by Werdenberg,[8] in cases of malignant, exudative forms of ocular tuberculosis. These cases require conservative general and local treatment.

Favorable results in the treatment of recurrent tuberculous iritis was obtained in two patients by Brown, Irons and Rosenthal,[9] who employed inhalation of the fumes from suspensions of dead tubercle bacilli (BCG) in salt solution. In one patient a reduction of cutaneous sensitivity to tuberculin and freedom from iritis were obtained. This lasted for twenty-six months. In the second patient, there was no recurrence for seventeen months.

The suspension of dead tubercle bacilli (BCG) was supplied in a small 500 c.c. Florence flask which contained about 200 c.c. of a suspension of bacilli in salt solution. The vapors were inhaled by the patient through a small funnel for ten seconds on the first two days, thirty seconds on the next two days, and for sixty seconds on the next four days. The flask was heated to 40° C. on the following day and the patient took one whiff; the breathing time was gradually increased on succeeding days to sixty seconds. The heat of the flask was again increased to 100° C. and the inhalation time also gradually increased from ten seconds to two minutes. Although the results reported in these two cases appeared favorable by this new method of densensitization, no further observations are available to determine the efficacy of the treatment.

Uveoparotitis or Uveoparotid Fever (Heerfordt's Disease)

The syndrome of uveoparotid fever, first described by Heerfordt in 1909, consists of a bilateral parotitis and uveitis, often associated with paralyses of the cranial nerves, especially the seventh nerve. The parotitis occurs usually without pain and without suppuration, progressing to a stage of spontaneous resolution. The other symptoms are said to occur less frequently, and include malaise, rheumatic pains, skin eruptions, slight fever, polyuria, dry mouth, facial palsy, paresthesias, and gastric disturbances. The course is chronic and the onset of symptoms irregular. The disease may begin with the parotid swelling occurring somewhat earlier than the uveitis in some cases, while in others the uveitis may be found to occur early. In most instances there is only a short interval between the occurrence of the two manifestations. The disease is more common in young people up to about 30 years of age, and it is usually considered to be of tuberculous origin.

Eye Manifestations.—As indicated by the name, the important eye lesion is the uveitis. In many cases this appears to occur as a nodular type resembling that which is found in tuberculosis. The condition is usually bilateral. Objective signs which may be present are ciliary congestion, synechiae, deposits on the posterior surface of the cornea, and the anterior surface of the lens, as well as opacities in the vitreous.

Among the other ocular findings are keratitis, optic neuritis, cataract, and glaucoma, all of which have been reported.

Because of the appearance of the ocular manifestations, the condition in many cases has been considered to be due to tuberculosis or associated with tuberculosis. Opinions as to etiology seem to be divided. In a few cases the tubercle bacillus has been found in the parotid gland and submaxillary glands on biopsy, and a generalized tuberculosis has also been found in some cases which have come to autopsy. The condition has been called uveoparotid tuberculosis by Garland and Thompson.[10] Cogan[11] reported a case in a woman, 29 years old, who had bilateral parotitis, uveitis, fever, and complete facial palsy on the right side. A diagnosis of tuberculosis was based on the symptoms.

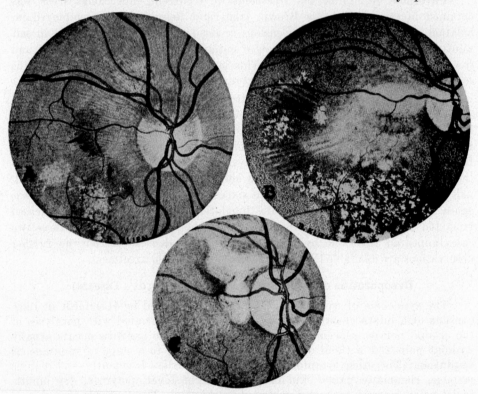

Fig. 165.—Chorioretinitis juxtapapillaris. *A*, Direct view of fundus, Oct. 3, 1929. *B*, The fundus on Jan. 4, 1930. *C*, Same fundus on April 30, 1931. (From Abraham: Arch. Ophth., October, 1932.)

Folger,[12] in reporting a case occurring in a 34-year-old woman, published a comprehensive review of the subject. In an analysis of forty-four cases it was found that tuberculosis was considered responsible for the condition by many authors, although no positive proof could be found. There is considerable evidence in some instances, but in others this is lacking. At the present time there is no definitely accepted etiology.

Besides tuberculosis, uveoparotitis may have to be differentiated from other conditions such as mumps, syphilis, and Mikulicz's disease. Mumps can be eliminated in most cases by the history of having had this disease at an earlier date. Moreover, uveoparotitis is more chronic in nature, while in mumps, the facial paralysis is absent, and the parotid swelling in the latter would nearly always precede the onset of iritis or uveitis. Orchitis also is absent as a complication in uveoparotitis.

The condition has at times been considered to be a variation of Mikulicz's disease. The latter condition, however, is characterized by a symmetrical swelling without inflammation of the lacrimal glands, although this may occur in association with systemic symptoms which have led to the term Mikulicz's syndrome.[13]

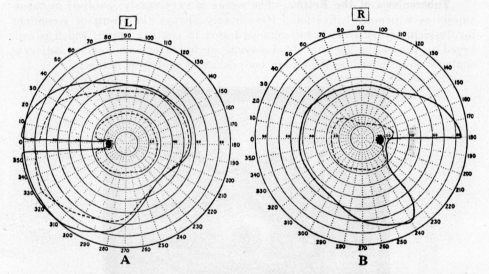

Fig. 166.—Visual fields in chorioretinitis juxtapapillaris, showing, *A*, radiating horizontal scotoma temporal side of blind spot corresponding to lesion on nasal side of optic disc and, *B*, the typical wedge-shaped defect in temporal field corresponding to lesion at upper inner side of optic disc. (From Traquair: An Introduction to Clinical Perimetry.)

Treatment.—The treatment of uveoparotitis is usually symptomatic. The ocular condition may clear with resolution of the disease and cause little interference with the vision. Folger, in his case, employed atropine, ethylmorphine hydrochloride, and hot compresses for the eyes and obtained satisfactory results. Very few deposits remained on the back of the cornea and anterior lens, and the vision was 20/20 in each eye.

In general, the local treatment should include that usually employed in cases of iridocyclitis and uveitis.

Chorioretinitis Juxtapapillaris (Jensen's Disease).—This is an inflammatory condition described by Jensen, the most probable cause of which is considered to be tuberculosis. The typical lesion consists of an inflammatory mass which borders the margin of the disc and which usually involves only a portion of the nasal margin. On clearing, signs of the lesion remain in this marginal area. The visual field shows a characteristic sector-like defect which is continuous with the blind spot and the base of which extends into the periphery. This is due to the fact that the fibers extending into the periphery of the retina are injured in addition to those which go to the ganglion cells. The cases nearly all show disturbances of vision, and in about 70 per cent the vision is permanently impaired. The inflammation is considered by some to begin in the retinal vessels and extend to the choroid. In a case which was studied histologically by Abraham[14] the condition was found to be a chronic inflammatory process which is primary in the choroid and involving the plexus of vessels forming the circle of Zinn. The changes in the retina are secondary.

The area of exudate may vary in size from one to two disc diameters and is usually gray or grayish white in color. It is irregular in shape and outline, the latter fading out indistinctly. One or two small hemorrhages may be present. The vitreous is hazy, and a few precipitates may be present on the posterior cornea.

Tuberculosis of the Retina.—The retina is very rarely involved in tuberculosis as a primary affection. It is nearly always the result of secondary involvement either from a tuberculous lesion in another organ, which is conveyed to the retina by the blood stream, or by extension from an adjacent ocular structure, such as the ciliary body, choroid, and optic nerve.

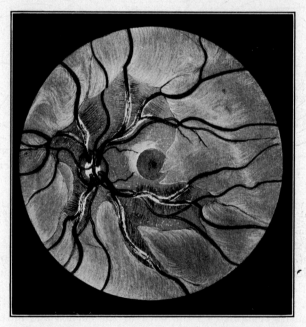

Fig. 167.—Progressive tuberculous periphlebitis with early flat retinal detachment (Eales' disease). Patient, aged 30 years, with early pulmonary tuberculosis, positive skin sensitivity tests, and several years of tuberculin therapy. Complete blindness with secondary glaucoma and loss of eye. (Courtesy of Dr. E. B. Spaeth.)

Tubercles of the retina are very rare, and it is very unusual to find miliary tubercles in the retina in the course of a generalized miliary tuberculosis, although they are found in the choroid. A conglomerate tubercle in the retina without involvement of the choroid is also a very rare condition.

Tuberculous retinitis occurs very rarely also, although a few cases have been reported. This is characterized by the appearance of numerous yellowish-white exudative lesions or, in some instances, by a larger area of exudation accompanied by congestion and dilatation of the vessels and occasional hemorrhages.

Tuberculous Retinal Periphlebitis.—This condition is characterized by the occurrence of numerous and repeated, or recurrent hemorrhages in the retina and often in the vitreous. A case was reported by Goldstein and Wexler[15] in which the tuberculous lesions involved the retina and optic nerve following an earlier inflammation in the anterior uveal tract. They were, therefore, led to believe that this was the site of the primary affection. The disease usually occurs in young people and is sometimes known as Eales' disease, although the latter is considered to result also from other causes. The lesion is a tubercle usually along the course of the veins, occupying the wall of the vein and the perivascular space. Other tubercles may occur in the choroid and other structures of the eye in cases with miliary tuberculosis. The tubercle bacillus has been found to be present. Two schools of thought seem to exist with regard to the mode of occurrence. The one holds that the condition is dependent on a pre-existing iridocyclitis or involvement of the anterior uvea from which it spreads by direct infection, as in Goldstein's and Wexler's case, while the second attributes the condition to involvement of the affected veins by way of the blood stream. The exact cause, however, is as yet not definitely determined.

On examination with the ophthalmoscope grayish-white patches covering the retinal vessels may be seen early in the disease. The veins are very large and their perivascular sheaths are prominent. Later, the veins become engorged and distorted, with their lumen occluded in places. Hemorrhages of various sizes may be seen in close proximity to the veins. They may be so large and extensive that they rupture into the vitreous. Smaller hemorrhages and white exudative spots may be seen in the fundus near the retinal vessels in the milder cases. Both eyes are usually affected, although not necessarily to the same extent. When the hemorrhages are small, they may clear up in a short time, but others may occur at a later date. The disease, therefore, runs a prolonged course with various degrees of visual impairment. It may be complicated by the formation of proliferating connective tissue (proliferating retinitis), secondary glaucoma, and detachment of the retina.

The treatment consists principally of the general methods of treatment outlined for tuberculous conditions and possibly the internal administration of calcium.

Vitreous Hemorrhages.—Hemorrhages into the vitreous may occur in tuberculosis as well as in other conditions when they rupture through the internal limiting membrane. When such a hemorrhage is massive, it may occupy the entire vitreous. The fundus reflex is, therefore, abolished, and on examination with the ophthalmoscope the pupil appears black. Such hemorrhages are very slow to absorb, if they do at all, and the vision of the eye is correspondingly impaired. Organization eventually takes place with the formation of a proliferating retinitis. The condition may be complicated by detachment of the retina or the occurrence of secondary glaucoma. With the former the intraocular tension may be lower, whereas it will be increased with the latter.

Tuberculosis of the Optic Nerve.—Manifestations of tuberculosis in the optic nerve are generally rare. However, the nerve or its sheath may become affected as a secondary involvement, either by direct extension from a tuberculous process in an adjacent structure of the eye and orbit, from tuberculous disease in the brain, and also by metastasis through the blood stream.

In a case of tuberculosis of the uveal tract or retina, the optic nerve may become involved by the direct spread of granulomatous masses or tubercles, especially in miliary tuberculosis, such as was previously described in the production of tuberculous periphlebitis. The optic nerve and its sheath may become infiltrated with tubercles and the inflammation may affect any portion of the nerve within the orbit.

It is rare for involvement of the optic nerve to occur by extension from a tuberculous inflammation of the orbit. Such a process first involves the sheath of the nerve which it penetrates to involve the nerve fibers themselves. The sheath and the optic nerve itself may also be involved as the result of extension of a tuberculous meningitis which may produce tuberculous granulations and caseation with destruction of the nerve fibers. The ocular symptoms depend principally on the location of the lesion at the time, but the vision on the affected side would be destroyed.

A diagnosis of tuberculous inflammation of the optic nerve, as a metastatic manifestation in the absence of a demonstrable tuberculous lesion, cannot be definitely made. However, in addition to the occurrence of miliary tubercles with infiltration by giant cells, epitheliod cells, and lymphocytes in the course of a generalized miliary tuberculosis, the optic nerve may be the site of solitary and conglomerate tubercles. Cases of this kind have been established by the result of pathologic examination since the clinical diagnosis is usually difficult, especially if the lesion affects the nerve behind the globe. The presence of an active tuberculosis in another organ may be diagnosed, but in its absence, the reaction to tuberculin and the clinical appearance of the lesion must be depended on. This is characterized by the presence of a large white mass which can be observed on or close to the disc and which is surrounded by an area of edema and possible hemorrhages. The mass may project forward into the vitreous which may also appear cloudy. With further progress the details of the fundus can no longer be observed, but instead a grayish reflex will be found to appear behind the pupillary space. Pain may be a troublesome symptom, with the formation of connective tissue and detachment of the retina, so that eventual enucleation of the affected eye may become necessary.

References

Tuberculosis

1. Adler, Francis Heed, and Meyer, George P.: Tuberculosis of the Uveal Tract. A Review of the Literature, Arch. Ophth. **18:** 275, 1937.
2. Woods, Alan C., and Randolph, M. Elliot: Treatment of Ocular Tuberculosis, Arch. Ophth. **18:** 510, 1937.
3. Igersheimer, Josef: Pathology of Tuberculosis of the Anterior Uvea, Arch. Ophth. **11:** 119, 1934.
4. Woods, Alan C., and Guyton, Jack S.: The Role of Sarcoid and Brucellosis in Uveitis, Tr. Am. Acad. Ophth. (1943) March-April, 1944, p. 248.
5. Thornhill, P. S., and Thornhill, E. H.: Boeck's Sarcoid With Nodular Iritis in a Child, Am. J. Dis. Child. **64:** 262, 1942.
6. Klauder, Joseph V., and De Long, Perce: Lupus Erythematosus of the Conjunctiva, Eyelids and Lid Margins, Arch. Ophth. **7:** 856, 1932.
7. Finoff, William C.: A Syndrome in Uveal Tuberculosis, Arch. Ophth. **9:** 13, 1933.
8. Werdenberg, E.: Useful and Harmful Therapeutics in Tuberculosis, Arch. Ophth. **13:** 303, 1935.
9. Brown, E. V. L., Irons, Ernest E., and Rosenthal, S. R.: Results of Desensitization in Tuberculous Iritis, Arch. Ophth. **28:** 1028, 1942.
10. Garland, H. G., and Thompson, J. G.: Uveo-Parotid Tuberculosis, Quart. J. Med. **2:** 157, 1933; Lancet **2:** 743, 1934.
11. Cogan, D. G.: Uveoparotid Fever, Am. J. Ophth. **18:** 637, 1935.
12. Folger, Howard Price: Uveoparotitis (Heerfordt), Arch. Ophth. **15:** 1098, 1936.
13. Leucutia, T., and Price, A. E.: Mikulicz's Disease and Mikulicz's Syndrome, Treatment by Irradiation, Am. J. Roentgenol. **24:** 491, 1930.
14. Abraham, Samuel V.: Chorioretinitis Juxtapapillaris (Jensen) First Histologic Report, Arch. Ophth. **8:** 503, 1932.
15. Goldstein, Isadore, and Wexler, David: Acute Tuberculous Periphlebitis of the Retina and Optic Nerve, Arch. Ophth. **3:** 552, 1930.

CHAPTER X

VIRUS INFECTIONS

The viruses include a group of disease agents which have certain definite common properties: They possess the ability to be filtered; they are cell parasites and do not multiply outside living cells; and most of them produce cytoplasmic or nuclear inclusion bodies in affected cells. Thygeson,[1] in an exhaustive study of viruses and virus disease, described their properties and the diseases which they cause or are suspected of causing. He divides these agents into two groups: the larger virus and the larger virus particles. The larger virus can be seen under the ordinary compound microscope with good oil immersion lenses and proper illumination. The larger virus particles, which are generally known as elementary bodies, can be seen when properly stained. In such diseases as trachoma, psittacosis, inclusion blennorrhea and lymphogranuloma venereum, the elementary bodies will stain with simple stains such as Giemsa stain. The others require a mordant or prolonged staining. This may greatly increase the size of a virus particle so that it can be made visible with the resolving power of the microscope whereas it was invisible before prolonged staining. Among the diseases produced by these elementary bodies are included variola, vaccinia, varicella, herpes zoster, herpes simplex, molluscum contagiosum and others.

Although the primary changes of virus diseases result from their direct action on the cells, secondary effects may also indirectly occur. This is illustrated in trachoma which directly affects the epithelium of the conjunctiva and cornea, while secondary changes are produced in the subepithelium with the production of folliculosis, necrosis and finally scar tissue formation. It also seems probable that remote changes are produced in virus disease by some soluble toxins similar to those which produce remote changes in bacterial disease. Although no such soluble toxins have as yet been definitely demonstrated, certain of the viruses, such as those of lymphogranuloma venereum and vaccinia, produce soluble antigens which react with specific antisera.

The viruses vary greatly in their ability to induce immunity. Those of trachoma and molluscum contagiosum, which affect only epithelium and are local in action, confer no demonstrable immunity. Others such as those of variola and vaccinia produce permanent immunity. A third group such as herpes simplex, the common cold and the virus of foot and mouth disease confers a transient immunity.

The virus diseases are all very infectious because of their ability to multiply in living cells. They are also communicated with ease in many instances as illustrated by smallpox and measles. On the other hand, herpes zoster virus is one which is scarcely ever transmitted.

Herpes Simplex

According to Thygeson, all herpetic eruptions other than herpes zoster are due to the same virus, irrespective of localization. Herpes cornea occurs most often in the form of dendritic keratitis, but it may also occur as a disciform keratitis. The condition has been said to occur in epidemic form, but this is evidently not true of herpetic keratitis. The ocular infection may occur as a result of contamination of the eye by the virus from an outside source, the virus may reach the eye endogenously by way of the blood stream, or it may be transmitted to the eye from herpetic lesions on other parts of the body. The first mentioned is apparently the most probable source. The virus has been demonstrated in saliva from persons in apparently good health, and the most

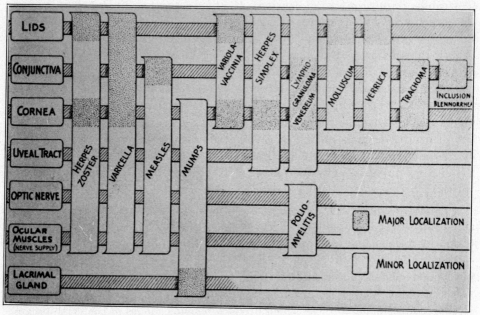

Fig. 168.—Ocular structures affected in important virus diseases. (From Thygeson: Arch. Ophth., March, 1943.)

common method of spread is probably by droplet infection. Although herpes virus has been demonstrated in the blood stream, there is little of other evidence that it occurs by endogenous transmission. It is possible that the lesion may spread to the eye from elsewhere on the body. It could reach the eye by auto-inoculation from another lesion or from saliva containing virus from another person with a latent oral infection. The keratitis may be produced immediately on the virus entering the eye or it may remain quiescent until activated by some predisposing factor such as trauma or upper respiratory infection.

Hamilton[2] felt that 63 per cent of the keratitis in Australians in the Middle East was due to the virus of herpes simplex and the majority occurred after a true or artificial pyrexia or a gross change of climate. He emphasized the fact that these cases must be separated from those of bacterial origin. This type usually appears in malaria, relapsing fever, influenza or coryza. In his experience, iritis does not occur with herpes simplex virus and for this reason he omits the use of atropine in the treatment of the condition. Since it follows pyrexia, he feels that the use of local heat or foreign protein is also contraindicated in the treatment.

The treatment of herpetic infection is principally curettage and cauterization of the affected cornea. Iodine and similar agents are employed. Vitamin B_1, sulfanilamide, vaccination with smallpox vaccine and injections of mocassin snake venom have all been recommended, but no specific treatment is available. Hamilton advises the use of ice compresses and painting of the corneal epithelium with a 2 per cent solution of silver nitrate following the instillation of cocaine and adrenalin. He follows the painting with the instillation of unguentum butyn and metaphen (Abbott).

Smallpox (Variola)

Smallpox is an acute infectious disease caused by a specific, filtrable virus. The onset of the disease is accompanied by headache, pain in the back, and a characteristic vesicular eruption. It occurs in epidemic form, and the virus can be transmitted directly from one person to another by washings from the nasopharynx, the fluid of the vesicles, and the dried exudate of the scabs. Inclusion bodies in the cytoplasm of the epithelium of the skin are present, but it is not known definitely whether these represent the virus itself or the result of cellular reaction to the virus. The symptoms include chills and fever of severe intensity, severe headache, pains in the extremities and back, especially in the lumbar region. The entire face and body of the patient may be covered by eruption. Secondary lesions occur which can be accounted for by bacterial septicemia. The disease must be differentiated from measles, scarlet fever, chicken pox, dengue, and meningococcal meningitis.

The treatment is principally prophylactic which consists in vaccination of children during their first year and repeating this at intervals of five to ten years. This practice has almost entirely eradicated the disease in certain areas. The active treatment is mostly symptomatic.

Eye Manifestations.—Before vaccination, about 35 per cent of blindness was due to smallpox, but now smallpox has been almost entirely eliminated as a causative factor. The following structures may be involved in the following ways: Hyperemia of the conjunctiva may be present. Pustules can occur on the conjunctiva, the lacrimal passages, and on the skin of the lids. The cornea may become involved as a secondary affection. Ulcus serpens of the cornea, which is seen most frequently in this disease, usually occurs at the stage of desiccation and in convalescence. These ulcers cause an extensive and deep involvement of a large portion of the cornea. When they become infected, which is not infrequently, they result in loss of sight.

The presence of ulcus serpens can be differentiated from smallpox pustule by the time of occurrence. The ulcus serpens develops only after the stage of eruption and the establishment of immunity. Pustules which occur late are usually found on the conjunctiva, but they may lie near the limbus and encroach on the margin of the cornea. Ulcus serpens has been attributed to an outside infection of the cornea. It cannot be due to the etiologic factor of smallpox since it does not occur until immunity has been established.

Variolous ulcers are found in children and adults and may affect both eyes, causing blindness. Iritis from general infection may occur late. Other manifestations in the eye include choroiditis, retinitis, optic atrophy, inflammation of the lacrimal apparatus, and inflammation of the bones of the orbit.

Of 726 opacities of the cornea, including leucomas and nebulae, Wright[3] found that fifty-nine of these followed smallpox. Of 143 anterior staphylomas (ectatic corneal scars), sixteen followed smallpox. With universal vaccination, the cause of blindness due to smallpox could be eliminated.

Vaccinia

The eye may be infected by the virus of vaccination as the result of contamination. The sufferers are usually children who have been recently vaccinated on some other part of the body from which the virus is transmitted, through carelessness, to the eye. Sometimes the infection is transmitted from one patient to another. The commonest site of this accidental inoculation is the skin of the lids, then the conjunctiva, and lastly the cornea. The infection may spread from the lid to the other structures although any of these structures may be directly inoculated. Even though a fairly large number of cases have been reported, the incidence of inoculation is comparatively small considering the large number of vaccinations performed.

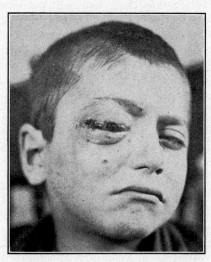

Fig. 169.—Accidental vaccination of conjunctiva. (From Sezer: Arch. Ophth., July, 1938.)

The common lesion is a papule on the lid which appears several days after vaccination. Ulceration takes place at the site of the lesion with induration of the lids around the ulcers. The ulcers usually heal after several weeks, but with the disappearance of the scab, a depressed scar may remain. In many cases the preauricular and submaxillary glands are enlarged and tender.

In 1920 Bedell[4] reported a case involving the lids and cornea and listed ninety-three cases collected in the literature at that time. The cornea becomes involved in about one-third of the cases. A number of cases have been reported since that time. In 1938 Sezer[5] reported an accidental vaccination in which an 8-year-old boy was inoculated on the skin of the lid and palpebral conjunctiva of the right eye by contamination with the vaccinations of his brothers. More recently, two cases were reported by Atkinson and Scullard[6] in which the patients were little girls, aged five years and three and a half years. Each had been vaccinated a few days earlier. According to these authors, who reported the condition in detail, corneal involvement resembles a keratitis disciformis and is centrally located, being accompanied by a serous iritis.

The diagnosis can readily be made in the presence of a characteristic involvement and with the history of a recent vaccination. Often, however, the doctor is kept in ignorance of the latter so that the condition is at first mistaken for a stye or hordeolum and might not be recognized until ulceration takes place and a recent vaccination is mentioned. Atkinson and Scullard recommended the use of the complement fixation for diagnosis and the agglutination tests described by Gordon.[7] The result of the former is obtained on the first day and may be checked by the agglutination test on the following day. Both reactions appear to be specific for vaccinia and variola.

Vaccinia and variola are generally considered to be caused by a single virus. Vaccinia has been modified by passage through the calf. Vaccinia virus shows a marked affinity for epithelium, and inclusion bodies, known as Guarnieri bodies, are found in the cytoplasm of the affected cells.

The virus of vaccinia produces an immunity which may last for an indefinite period but which is not necessarily permanent. This usually appears about the sixth day after inoculation and becomes complete in about two weeks. The cornea, however, has not been found to enjoy this same immunity in all cases. In cases where vaccinial infection of the eye is suspected in the absence of other cutaneous lesions, the laboratory studies may prove to be of value. A satisfactory test would be the inoculation of rabbit cornea with the development of a keratitis in which the Guarnieri (inclusion) bodies could be demonstrated.

Treatment.—This includes the use of immune sera to check and render the action of the virus inactive. This has been employed by some to produce immunity and prevent corneal involvement. In order to render the vaccine virus inactive, the local use of potassium permanganate up to 1:100,000, in contact with the virus for one hour, has been recommended. A 1:2,000 dilution of ascorbic acid was also said to inactivate the infective dose of the virus. Atkinson and Scullard,[6] as a result of their investigation, recommended potassium permanganate, tincture of iodine, metaphen or mercury bichloride to be applied to the lesion as soon as this is diagnosed. Ascorbic acid may be administered generally and locally. As a result of the eye inoculation, corneal opacities and symblepharon may result. The latter may be treated by surgical means after the condition has completely healed.

Chicken Pox (Varicella)

Chicken pox is an acute specific infection which is very contagious and is characterized principally by the presence over the body of a diffuse vesicular eruption. The exact cause of the condition is not known, but it is considered to be due to a filtrable virus. The systemic symptoms accompanying the eruption are usually negligible, although in some there may be moderate malaise and elevation of temperature. With the spread of the skin eruption over the body, macules, vesicles, and pustules may be present at the same time. The condition commonly affects children, although adults are also often affected. The patients usually recover, and mortality is very low except from serious secondary infections which might occur.

It is now generally believed that varicella can arise from cases of herpes zoster and without contact with varicella. The virus of these two diseases are similar in many ways. The period of incubation is about twelve to fourteen days. The cutaneous lesions of both are histologically similar, the inclusion bodies of the virus are similar, the elementary bodies have been found to have similar staining properties, lasting immunity is common to both, and the generalized condition is similar. (See Herpes zoster.)

Eye Manifestations.—In an ordinary case of chicken pox, eye manifestations are not usually very pronounced, but lacrimation and moderate injection of the bulbar conjunctiva may be present at the onset, especially in children. The eyelids, conjunctiva, and cornea may all be the seat of vesicular involvement. Usually these present no serious difficulty when they occur on the eyelids or conjunctiva. On the cornea, however, they may cause considerable annoyance. The vesicles on the eyelids and less frequently on the conjunctiva usually accompany those present on the rest of the body.

A case of late corneal involvement was reported by Packard[8] in which the lesion occurred three weeks after the disease. On the posterior surface of the cornea there was a flat, brownish-yellow mass with a free spongy surface. It was considered that the deep corneal involvement occurred late because the nonvascularity of the structure makes transmission of the virus difficult. In severe cases iritis and occasionally optic neuritis may occur secondarily. If the vesicles of the lids are interfered with or fingered and the scab removed, scarring and secondary infection may occur, possibly leading to gangrene of the lids.

Treatment.—The treatment of manifestations of varicella in the eye is only symptomatic and does not include anything more than washing the eyes with a solution, such as boric acid two or three times a day. If vesicles occur on the conjunctiva, they should not be disturbed. Scratching of the vesicles on the eyelids should be prevented in order to avoid scar formation and secondary infections.

Mumps (Parotitis)

Mumps is an acute infectious disease supposedly due to a filtrable virus and is characterized by a long incubation period (eighteen to twenty-one days), an inflammation and swelling of the parotid glands, and the frequent development of lesions in the testes, ovaries, mammae, pancreas, and meninges. The virus is said to enter through the mouth while the disease develops insidiously with a small, painful swelling in front of one or both ears, which rapidly increases in size to involve the whole parotid region. Some cases begin with headache, malaise, fever, and chilliness, or other mild early symptoms. In addition to the general symptoms at the onset, there is a moderate fever and a bradycardia and a slight increase in leucocytes with a relative lymphocytosis. The spleen may be enlarged and palpable.

The disease is rather common among children up to the age of 15 or 16 years, but it may also occur among adults. It may occur in epidemic form and is highly contagious during any period of the year. It may affect people of either sex and is usually spread by crowding and association in schools and public places.

Eye Manifestations.—The local swelling in mumps may extend over the cheek accompanied by considerable enlargement of the surrounding lymph glands and the presence of edema which may cause swelling of the eyelids and involvement of the lacrimal gland. Pain may radiate to the eyes as well as the ears and occipital region.

The eyes themselves are rarely involved in mumps. However, dacryadenitis, analogous to the parotitis is most frequent.

Extraocular muscle palsies, affecting especially those supplied by the third nerve and the sixth nerve, similar to those seen following diphtheritic infection, may occur.

A dilatation of the conjunctival and episcleral vessels without secretion may produce an edema of the bulbar conjunctiva.

Other complications which may affect the eyes are keratitis, iritis which is usually not severe, iridocyclitis, cycloplegia, retrobulbar neuritis, optic neuro-retinitis, encephalitic optic neuritis and atrophy, papilledema, and paralysis of accommodation.

Treatment.—The treatment of the ocular manifestations depends principally on the nature and location of the involvement. The edema of the eyelids and enlargement of the lacrimal gland, when present, may gradually subside with recovery from the parotitis. When conjunctivitis is present, a mild eyewash such as boric acid solution and cold compresses may be employed. Keratitis and iritis should be treated with the application of hot compresses to the affected eyes and the instillation of atropine sulfate solution (1 per cent) twice daily.

Measles (Rubeola)

Measles is a contagious infection which usually occurs in epidemic form principally among children, although adults may be affected. It is charac-terized by an initial coryza and a buccal exanthema followed by a maculo-papular eruption which terminates in desquamation. The exact causative organism is still unproved, but it is suspected to be a filtrable virus. This is now generally believed to be the causative agent, but as yet little is known about the properties of the virus. The portal of entry of the virus is no doubt through the nasopharynx. The initial pathology of the disease involves the conjunctiva of the eye together with the pharynx, larynx, and bronchi. Sec-ondary lesions occur in the skin and mucous membranes. In the mucous mem-brane of the mouth the diagnostic lesions known as Koplik's spots are found. These occur as early as the first day of the disease. With the initial coryza ushering in the condition, the temperature may be around 102 or 103° F. The disease must be differentiated from scarlet fever and smallpox.

Eye Manifestations.—These can prove to be rather serious and are usually present at the onset of the disease. At this time there is a definite catarrhal conjunctivitis characterized by an injection and redness of the bulbar conjunctiva, lacrimation, and photophobia. In some cases there may be a moderate puffiness of the eyelids. If neglected, the conjunctivitis may become purulent in character. Very occasionally, Koplik's spots may also be found on the conjunctiva. The eyelids may also be affected by blepharitis and hordeola. In severe cases the cornea may become the seat of ulcus serpens and keratitis with resulting impairment of vision. Panophthalmitis rarely occurs but may result from perforation and infection of the eyeball. Optic neuritis and metastatic ophthalmia may occur as the result of toxins. Paralysis of the extraocular muscles is rare, but insufficiency or weakness of the accommodation of the eye may be a sequela which can last for some time after recovery.

Treatment.—The first requirement is the protection of the eyes from the onset by keeping the patient in a darkened room. Photophobia, lacrimation, and other disturbances from light are, therefore, eliminated. The use of the eyes should be restricted, particularly in those patients who are not very ill and who express a desire to read while confined. If the lids are swollen or redened, cold compresses can be applied for a period of about ten minutes two or three times a day. The eyes themselves may be flushed with some solution as boric acid, two or three times daily, for the conjunctivitis. If the latter shows signs of becoming purulent, solutions, such as metaphen or mercurophen 1:10,000 or 1:12,000, may be employed. These can be used by instillation, by flushing, or by means of an eyecup. Stronger antiseptic solutions are not indicated. If keratitis develops, one drop of atropine sulfate, 1 per cent solution, should be instilled two or three times a day. This will keep the eye at rest and has the quality of aiding the cornea in healing. Warm or hot boric acid compresses should be employed if the cornea becomes involved. On recovering from the disease, the patient should resume the use of the eyes for close work gradually, so that excessive strain on accommodation is avoided. Later, normal use of the eyes can be better sustained. The more rare and unusual complications, such as optic neuritis and panophthalmitis, must be treated according to their requirements in the individual case.

Herpes Zoster

The understanding of herpes zoster and herpes in its various forms does not seem at present to be altogether clear. Meakins, in his book, *Practice of Medicine,*[9] defines herpes zoster as an acute infection of the posterior root ganglia with signs in the segmental distribution involved. The cause of the condition is given here as a probable infection which may occur with other infections in the body, especially pneumonia. It may also follow noninfectious lesions of the posterior roots, as injuries or tumors. It occurs most often in those of middle age and in older patients. The condition has been described in epidemic form and as having a close relationship to chicken pox. In this regard, Duke-Elder[10] states that herpes zoster is related to herpes simplex and that the former occurs in two forms; an epidemic herpes zoster, and a symptomatic herpes zoster. Epidemic herpes zoster is described as an acute epidemic disease, caused by a filtrable virus, the chief focus of infection probably being in the gasserian ganglion (a posterior root ganglion). The specific virus is considered to have been demonstrated in the peripheral vesicles. For a number of reasons herpes zoster is considered to be closely related to varicella. The antibodies in the serum are identical in both; one often confers immunity against the other and both occur together in epidemics. The relationship is considered similar to that existing between smallpox and vaccinia.

Epidemic herpes zoster usually follows the distribution of the affected nerves and is always preceded by a neuralgia. It attacks the deep layers and may result in scarring. The condition may occur independent of any previous disease and may run a course of about four weeks. It seems to confer further immunity. This is contrasted to simple herpes, which usually follows some other infection and which affects the superficial layers with no subsequent scarring. With herpes simplex, moreover, recurrences may be frequent.

The vesicles occurring in herpes zoster contain a fluid which is clear at first and may later become purulent. They are accompanied by burning and severe shooting pains in the area involved. A postherpetic neuralgia may be a troublesome sequela.

The virus of herpes zoster was said to have been cultivated in tissue culture and on chorioallantoic membrane of the chick embryo, although this is not as yet generally accepted. The virus does produce a pronounced immunity, however, and agglutinins and complement-fixing bodies can be produced and demonstrated in the second week of the illness with fluid of the vesicles or dried crusts as antigens. The fact that both can also be obtained when convalescent serum from varicella has been used is one of several factors indicating the close similarity between varicella and herpes zoster (see Varicella).

Eye Manifestations (Herpes Zoster Ophthalmicus).—When the disease involves the areas supplied by the supraorbital and infraorbital branches of the fifth nerve, the condition is known as herpes zoster ophthalmicus. This is characterized by the appearance of the vesicles on one side of the face, above and below the eyelids, and following the distribution of the nerve. The area involved is usually sharply demarcated. The vesicles are about the size of a pinhead and slightly larger. They occur singly and in small groups, which develop to their entire extent almost at once. They contain a clear fluid at first, which may later become purulent. The subepithelial layer of the skin is involved and healing results in scarring about the lids and face. This is especially true if the patient picks on the vesicles.

From the onset the patient suffers severe pain which may be very difficult to relieve. There is severe burning and throbbing, while the pain extends up over the forehead and scalp. Cold air may aggravate the pain. This may continue for a period of three to four weeks and will diminish as the eruption subsides.

Ocular Complications.—When the vesicles occur on the cornea, they may result in ulceration which may lead to impairment of the vision in the affected eye. Carmody[11] in reporting a case with exophthalmos listed the complications under four types: i.e., (1) keratitis; (2) iridocyclitis; (3) muscular palsies; (4) optic neuritis. He stated that the globe was affected in about 50 per cent of the cases and in many of these the cornea is involved. Scleritis, superficial keratitis, and other forms of keratitis may occur. The iris may also be involved. The third nerve, sixth nerve, and the fourth nerve have all been affected with resulting paralysis of the ocular muscles. An associated paralysis in the nervous system may also occur. Exophthalmos has been rarely encountered as a complication, but Carmody reported a case in a 40-year-old Negro who showed a complete immobility of the globe and exophthalmos. Mydriasis and atrophy of the optic nerve may also occur as complications. Anesthesia, occasional neuralgic pain, and paresthesia may be present for a long time around the affected area.

Treatment.—A patient with an acute herpes zoster should be confined to bed and sedatives should be prescribed. For the vesiculation a mild ointment or oily salve may be employed as a dressing. The patient should be warned against picking at the vesicles and care should be exercised to prevent secondary infection. The pain may require the administration of morphine in very severe instances. Intramuscular injections of obstetrical pituitrin (0.5 to 1.0 c.c.) administered at 48-hour intervals has afforded relief in some cases after two or three injections.

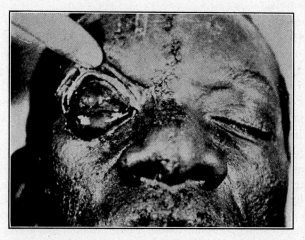

Fig. 170.—Herpes zoster ophthalmicus. (From Carmody: Arch. Ophth., November, 1937.)

For the accompanying swelling and edema of the eyelids, calamine ointment may be employed and the eyes flushed with a solution of boric acid. When the cornea is involved and keratitis occurs, atropine sulfate, 1 per cent solution, should be instilled about twice daily.

Other forms of treatment, such as vitamin B$_1$ and autohemotherapy, have also been employed. Walker and Walker[12] reported the use of diphtheria antitoxin which they injected for the pain in these cases with excellent results. They give 5,000 units of the antitoxin which is repeated in two days, if necessary. Usually, however, they found that the pain ceases and the inflammation rapidly disappears after the first dose. Gundersen[13] treated a fairly large number of patients by immunotransfusion, or convalescent blood. He used between 250 and 450 c.c. of blood and found that good results could be expected if administered before ocular infection is well established.

Foot and Mouth Disease (Epidemic Stomatitis)

Foot and mouth disease is a specific infectious disease affecting principally cattle, sheep, pigs, and occasionally it occurs in man. It is also contagious. The cause is a filtrable virus, and the lesions are vesicles which occur on the mucous membranes of the lips, mouth, pharynx, and on the skin of the hands, fingers, and toes.

After an incubation period of about four to ten days, the onset of the disease is sudden and characterized by symptoms of malaise, headache, fever, and vomiting. Diarrhea occurs early and later constipation. The mouth and lips become red and swollen, while a burning sensation is experienced in the mouth, hands, and feet. Small vesicles appear on the mucous membranes, which are yellowish in color. These contain a clear fluid which later becomes cloudy. The vesicles break down later, leaving an ulcer which becomes dry and scaly and heals without leaving a scar. The tongue is thickened, the mouth is sore, and chewing and swallowing are difficult and painful. The disease runs its course in several weeks and results in recovery.

Eye Manifestations.—These are ordinarily rare, although contact with infected animals may result in infection by the virus of the conjunctiva and also the cornea in association with the oral infection. The conjunctiva of the lids becomes swollen and reddened, with a rather profuse discharge. Small vesicles which resemble phlyctenules and are yellowish in color occur on the conjunctiva and at the corneal limbus. These break down with the formation of ulcers and an accompanying vascular infiltration around the limbus. The ulcers gradually heal as the entire condition subsides after a period of several weeks. No serious impairment of the vision should result.

Treatment.—These cases should first be isolated and the treatment instituted should be generally symptomatic. The eyes should be flushed frequently throughout the day with a solution of boric acid. Warm compresses can be applied for about ten minutes, three times daily. The ulcers on the conjunctiva can be touched with a weak solution of iodine and followed by irrigation with normal saline solution. Atropine sulfate, 1 per cent solution, should be instilled into the affected eye twice daily.

Lymphogranuloma Venereum

This disease, which is also known as lymphogranuloma inguinale, primarily involves the lymphatic system. It is caused by a filtrable virus. The principal lesion in the male is inguinal adenitis and in the female, enlargement of the external genitals, and ulceration of the vulva, peritoneum, anus and rectum. An intradermal test known as the Frei test will produce an inflammatory reaction which is specific in patients who have the disease or who have suffered with it in the past. The antigen is prepared from the pus of an unruptured abscess and although sometimes difficult to obtain, the test is of great value in establishing the diagnosis. It is a test for allergic reaction similar to the tuberculin test and is positive in nearly all cases.

Eye Manifestations.—The principal ocular manifestation is a conjunctivitis accompanied by preauricular adenopathy. This has been described as very similar to that occurring in Parinaud's conjunctivitis. In fact, Thygeson,[1] in his discussion of the disease, stated that, "Beyond all doubt the virus must now be included among the agents producing the so-called oculoglandular syndrome of Parinaud.'' (See Parinaud's conjunctivitis.)

The conjunctivitis usually occurs in one eye although it might be bilateral. The conjunctiva is reddened and areas of granulation are present. A moderate amount of secretion with swelling of the lids is also found. In addition to conjunctivitis, other ocular conditions that may occur are keratitis, episcleritis, uveitis and optic neuritis.

It might be necessary to differentiate this condition from granuloma inguinale. Extragenital lesions of the latter are rare, but they may occur in patients suffering with the disease. Weiner and associates[14] reported a case of a destructive ulcerative lesion of the eyelid in a patient with granuloma inguinale in whom the condition began as a hard edematous area and progressed to ulceration and destruction of the tissue. Histologic sections showed polymorphonuclear leucocytic cells containing Donovan bodies. The latter are peculiar organisms which are usually found in this condition, while the Frei test is negative.

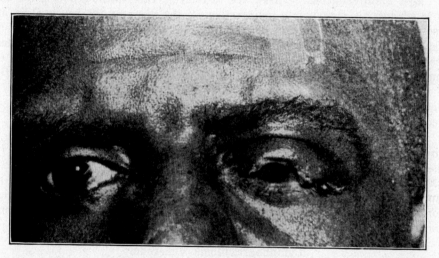

Fig. 171.—Granuloma inguinale ulcer of the eyelid. (From Weiner, Graynon, and Osherwitz: Am. J. Ophth., January, 1943.)

The treatment described by Weiner and co-workers for granuloma inguinale is injection of 1 per cent tartar-emetic solution, 10 c.c. biweekly for several months after the lesion cleared, to prevent relapse, which is not an uncommon occurrence with this disease.

The treatment of the ocular conjunctivitis of lymphogranuloma venereum consists principally in the use of sulfanilamide. It appears that the virus is very susceptible to this drug. The antigen used for diagnosis in the Frei test has also been employed for treatment with some success.

Molluscum Contagiosum

This is a disease in which the hands and face of young patients are affected by crops of small round tumors or nodules which are colorless and have a central point of umbilication. On pressure, a white sebaceous material containing molluscum bodies can be expressed from their center. The disease is caused by an infective filtrable virus and can be transmitted from person to person. The virus, like that of trachoma and inclusion blennorrhea, confers no immunity since it involves only epithelial cells and has no access to immunity-building tissues.

Eye Manifestations.—These consist usually of the occurrence of small tumors or nodules on the margins of the eyelids. The agent is usually carried here by the fingers. These tumors or nodules may be accompanied or followed by a catarrhal conjunctivitis. This is often follicular in type, involving the tarsal conjunctiva, and may resemble trachoma in its appearance. The tumor formations have also been reported as occurring on the bulbar conjunctiva, especially near the limbus.

The treatment consists in excision of the tumors or they may be incised and their contents curetted. Maceration by tears sometimes makes the clinical diagnosis of molluscum nodules difficult. In these instances the lesion can be excised and the diagnosis established by microscopic examination of sections. Material expressed from the center of a nodule can also be examined by staining with suitable elementary body stain.

Rocky Mountain Spotted Fever

This is an acute specific disease, sometimes known as tick fever, and is caused by a rickettsia which is transmitted to man by the wood tick. It is characterized chiefly by a macular eruption which becomes purpuric. It occurs in the western parts of North America and is ushered in with chills, anorexia, and malaise. The temperature of the patient is elevated to 104 or 105° F. The rash appears about the fourth or fifth day and is found on the chest, abdomen, forehead, and extremities. It may also occur on the mucous membranes. In severe cases the patient may suffer with insomnia, delirium, convulsions, and finally coma.

Eye Manifestations.—The eye is not particularly involved in this disease except during the onset and perhaps as a complicating condition in some of the later stages with nervous symptoms in severe cases. Intense headache may be complained of early in the infection, and this is accompanied by injection of the conjunctiva of the lids and bulbar conjunctiva. Photophobia is also a troublesome complaint. Clouding of the cornea and anterior chamber, iridocyclitis and keratitic precipitate may also occur.

The treatment of the condition is principally symptomatic. The eyes of the patient should be protected from light by the use of dark glasses and the patient should be kept in a darkened room. The conjunctivitis requires only the use of a warm boric acid eyewash.

Dengue

Dengue is an acute specific infectious disease which is also caused by an unknown filtrable virus transmitted among humans by a mosquito, *Aedes albopictus*. The disease is somewhat similar to yellow fever and is characterized by the presence of pain in the limbs, temperature, and a scarlatiniform rash. The onset is sudden, with chills, rigor, malaise, fever, and muscle and bone pains.

Eye Manifestations.—There are no characteristic eye manifestations in dengue, but the condition is usually accompanied by severe headache and pain in the eyes at the onset. In addition to a flushing of the skin and injection of the mouth and pharynx, the conjunctiva may reveal a diffuse injection. Movement of the eyes may be accompanied by discomfort, and tenderness is present on palpation of the eyeballs. Iritis may accompany the conjunctivitis during the course of the disease and keratitis, iridocyclitis and paralysis of the extraocular muscles have also been found to occur.

Typhus Fever (Brill's Disease)

This is an acute specific infectious disease otherwise known as Brill's disease, ship fever, camp fever, jail fever, and others. It is characterized by an acute onset, with chills, rigors, high fever, prostration, purpuric eruption over the neck, thorax, abdomen, and extremities, and with a crisis in about ten to fourteen days. The spleen may be enlarged; anorexia, vomiting, and delirium may occur. It is caused by the Rickettsia prowazeki which are minute, gram-negative, rod-shaped, and are transmitted through the skin of patients by lice.

Eye Manifestations.—The principal eye complications of typhus fever occur in the retina in the form of exudative and hemorrhagic retinitis. Small typhus nodules occur as perivascular infiltrations about the small vessels of the skin which lead to thromboses and occasionally necrosis. The small arteries and veins including those of the central nervous system are involved with proliferative lesions. Thromboses are not uncommon and may lead to the presence of the retinal lesions.

With the onset of the disease, the conjunctiva shows a marked injection and this may be found on the skin of the face, and around the eyelids. Small subconjunctival hemorrhages may occur later in the disease.

The photophobia is said to be very severe in this disease and may cause the patient to avoid ordinary daylight. Miosis may also occur and would indicate a poor prognosis.

Venable and Pollock[15] divided the more severe symptoms of typhus fever into two groups: those occurring during the febrile stage and those occurring during convalescence. In the first group were included discoloration of the iris and secondary cataract, changes around the retinal vessels (especially pigmentation), optic neuritis which might lead to optic atrophy and complete blindness, and ocular palsies involving the third and sixth nerves especially. In the second group, the complications include palpebral abscesses, orbital abscess which might lead to exophthalmos, corneal ulcers in the lower cornea usually occurring during the first week of convalescence, and optic atrophy.

Swineherd's Disease

Swineherd's disease, sometimes called pseudotyphoid meningitis, is an acute febrile disease which occurs among swine and is transmitted to man. It is strongly suspected of being caused by a filtrable virus, and it occurs more commonly in some of the countries of Western Europe. The characteristic symptoms manifest a typhoid state and include headache, abdominal pain, malaise, and skeletal pains. A second stage is characterized by meningeal symptoms.

Eye Manifestations.—The disease is ushered in with fever and headache which is commonly accompanied by a bilateral conjunctivitis similar to that seen with other acute infectious disease. Other ocular manifestations, such as iritis, iridocyclitis, or even a choroiditis, may be found as the result of metastatic involvement of the eye. The cerebrospinal fluid pressure may be increased during the secondary stage of the disease, and this may be accompanied by significant eye manifestations.

Epidemic Keratoconjunctivitis

Epidemic keratoconjunctivitis is a distinct clinical entity which is characterized principally by a sudden onset of acute conjunctivitis, glandular adenopathy and the occurrence of small infiltrates in the deeper epithelium or Bowman's membrane. As the name implies, it occurs in epidemic form and was recently very prevalent throughout the United States where a large number of cases were reported and studied. The etiology was found to be a filtrable virus which was isolated from scrapings of the conjunctiva by Sanders.[16] This was confirmed by Braley[17] who also described the disease in detail.

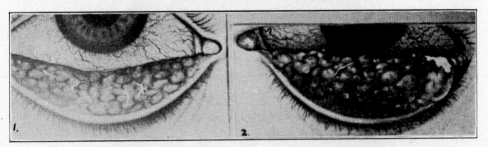

Fig. 172.—Epidemic keratoconjunctivitis (Berliner). *1.* Early stage of follicular formation. *2,* Folliculosis and exudation, later stage. (From Berliner: Am. J. Ophth., January, 1943.)

The acute stage of the disease begins rather suddenly with a conjunctivitis which causes the patient to complain of a foreign body sensation in the eye, lacrimation, itching and pain, especially on rotation of the eye. This is accompanied by an edema of the bulbar conjunctiva which may become quite marked. The conjunctival vessels become hyperemic. At this stage of the disease, the condition resembles any other form of conjunctivitis and cannot be definitely diagnosed. The edema and chemosis may become more marked and in two or three days after the onset a folliculosis occurs with subconjunctival infiltration of the lower lid especially. There is a papillary hypertrophy and hyperemia between the follicles. Tearing of the eyes may now be marked and the preauricular glands are tender. This may last for a week or slightly longer, after which time the edema and glandular swelling may subside. A thin pseudomembrane is also present at about this time on either the upper or lower lids. This was described by Braley to consist of epithelial cells with some monocular cells scattered throughout. No virus inclusion bodies were found.

As the acute stage subsides and folliculosis is still present, the cornea begins to show evidences of involvement accompanied by symptoms of blurred vision and photophobia. It is in this stage, in the presence of the corneal infiltration, that a definite diagnosis of epidemic keratoconjunctivitis can be made. This usually occurs about the beginning of the second week of the disease and is evidenced first by the presence of small superficial punctate spots. At first a number of very small, discrete, epithelial dots may be seen which increase in number and size to form definite opacities which are grayish in color and are found under the epithelium and on Bowman's membrane. They usually occupy the central portion of the cornea and can be observed on examination with the slit lamp. They may continue to increase in number with continued photophobia and noticeable impairment of vision. The duration of the opacities may be prolonged, but they decrease in number and clear up gradually without visible scarring. The vision usually improves also without permanent impairment.

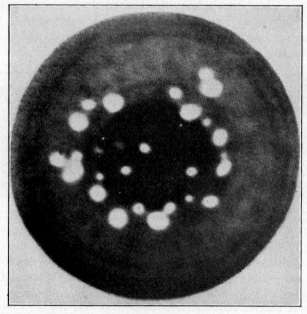

Fig. 173.—Epidemic keratoconjunctivitis (Berliner). Indirect illumination. Biomicroscopic view of corneal lesions in a severe case. (From Berliner: Am. J. Ophth., January, 1943.)

The treatment of this condition is principally symptomatic with varying results. Since the disease is contagious, the patient should be isolated. Most of the cases respond poorly to any treatment. Sulfathiazole in solution and ointment was found to be of very little or no benefit. The same was true of sulfadiazine and penicillin ointments. Pontocaine instillations have been employed for the pain. Adrenalin has also been employed by instillation as well as in mild lotions. While most of the patients are under observation it is difficult to determine just which form of treatment provides any benefit. In many patients the application of ice compresses seemed to afford relief.

Braley administered convalescent plasma to forty-seven patients and found that good results were obtained in those in whom the plasma was given before the fifth day. After that, the results are unpredictable.

References

1. Thygeson, P.: Viruses and Virus Diseases of the Eye. I. Properties and Nature of Viruses, Arch. Ophth. **29:** 285, 1943; II. Viruses of Ocular Importance, Arch. Ophth. **29:** 488, 1943; III. Viruses of Ocular Importance, Arch. Ophth. **29:** 635, 1943.
2. Hamilton, J. B.: Notes on Forms of Keratitis Presumably Due to Virus of Herpes Simplex, Brit. J. Ophth. **27:** 80, 1943.

Smallpox

3. Wright, R. E.: J. Madras Univ. **7:** 1, 1935.

Vaccinia

4. Bedell, A. J.: Am. J. Ophth. **3:** 103, 1920.
5. Sezer, F. N.: Accidental Vaccination of the Conjunctiva, Arch. Ophth. **20:** 89, 1938.
6. Atkinson, Walter, and Scullard, Garner: Vaccinia With Ocular Involvement, Arch. Ophth. **23:** 584, 1940.
7. Gordon, M. H.: Studies on the Viruses of Vaccinia and Variola, Medical Research Council, Special Report series No. 98, London, H. M. Stationery Office, 1925.

Chicken Pox

8. Packard, R.: Varicella of the Cornea, Brit. J. Ophth. **20:** 15, 1938.

Herpes Zoster

9. Meakins, Jonathan Campbell: The Practice of Medicine, St. Louis, 1938, The C. V. Mosby Co.
10. Duke-Elder, W. Stewart: Text-Book of Ophthalmology, Vol. II, St. Louis, 1938, The C. V. Mosby Co.
11. Carmody, R. F.: Herpes Zoster Ophthalmicus Complicated by Ophthalmoplegia and Exophthalmos, Arch. Ophth. **18:** 707, 1937.
12. Walker, J. R., and Walker, B. F.: A Specific Treatment for Herpes Zoster, Arch. Ophth. **20:** 304, 1938.
13. Gundersen, Trygve: Convalescent Blood for Treatment of Herpes Zoster Ophthalmicus, Arch. Ophth. **24:** 132, 1940.

Lymphogranuloma Venereum

14. Weiner, A. L., Gaynon, I. E., and Osherwitz, M. S.: Granuloma Inguinale of the Eyelid, Am. J. Ophth. **26:** 13, 1943.

Typhus Fever

15. Venable, H. P., and Pollock, F. J.: Rickettsias in Ophthalmology, Arch. Ophth. **30:** 362, 1943.

Epidemic Keratoconjunctivitis

16. Sanders, Murray: Epidemic Keratoconjunctivitis. Isolation and Identification of a Filtrable Virus, J. Exper. Med. **77:** 71, 1943.
17. Braley, A. E.: Epidemic Keratoconjunctivitis, Tr. Am. Acad. Ophth. **48:** 153, 1943.

CHAPTER XI

FUNGUS INFECTIONS

Parinaud's Conjunctivitis (Conjunctivoglandular Syndrome of Parinaud)

The oculoglandular syndrome of Parinaud (Parinaud's conjunctivitis) (leptothricosis) was first described by Parinaud in 1889, as a disease characterized by the formation of granulations in the conjunctiva of the eyes which is associated with inflammatory enlargement of the preauricular gland. The glandular swelling may appear simultaneous with the ocular condition or it may occur later. The systemic symptoms are usually mild. Parinaud's description of the condition in general was not given in detail, and the etiology of the condition remained obscure until Verhoeff,[1] in 1913, demonstrated a minute leptothrix in the conjunctival lesion. Since it occurred in great numbers and no other demonstrable organisms were found in any case studied, Verhoeff regarded this as the cause of the condition and suggested the term leptothricosis conjunctivae. Since that time, he has demonstrated the organism in a large number of cases, and it has also been recovered from the preauricular glands (Wherry and Ray).

The incubation period of the disease is about four days. The source of infection is still unknown. Parinaud originally believed that it was transmitted from animals, but Verhoeff believes that the infection comes from the mouths of cats. This is based on the fact that most of his cases gave a history of close association with cats, and that they occurred mostly in the winter months when cats are indoors. The condition may occur at any time of the year, however, and usually affects children and young people. It seems to affect males more than females, and is more common in some sections than others. The course of the disease is somewhat long and protracted and may last for a period of several months. Healing has taken place spontaneously, however, by resolution. A case was also reported by Harner,[2] in 1934, which was said to be transmitted to the patient from a cat which had acquired lesions of the paws, face, and eyes from contact with ground squirrels in Southern California. The leptothrix of Verhoeff was identified, and the condition was differentiated from tularemia and tuberculosis.

Blood examination in some of the cases has shown a moderate eosinophilia, but this does not seem to be a characteristic finding. Hurst,[3] in a report of twenty-three cases of oculoglandular disease, states that the blood examination in the leptothrix cases showed 9 per cent of eosinophiles in one instance, 8 per cent in another, and 4 per cent in a third.

In two cases reported by Lamb[4] in which Verhoeff's leptothrix was present, an eosinophilia of 4 per cent was found.

Gifford,[5] who also demonstrated the organism in the conjunctival lesion following Verhoeff and who also reported several cases, suggested the name "Conjunctivoglandular syndrome of Parinaud" in order to avoid confusing this condition with Parinaud's syndrome, which is a neurologic condition.

Eye Manifestations.—The clinical appearance of the ocular manifestations has changed very little from that first described by Parinaud. It is more common for only one eye to be involved. More rarely, the condition may be bilateral. The conjunctiva is the seat of the affection which may be more or less generalized. This is characterized by a redness of the conjunctiva on which are found vegetative growths or granulations. These are red or yellowish in color and semi-transparent or opaque. They become slightly larger than a pinhead in size and may be accompanied by several smaller yellowish growths. The eyelids become swollen and hard, and a moderate secretion is present. The glands of the neck become enlarged and swollen almost simultaneously, the preauricular being more commonly affected. The inflammation of the glands may go on to suppuration. The patient may suffer with constitutional symptoms which can be either mild or severe. Chills and fever are common, and the temperature may reach 105° F.

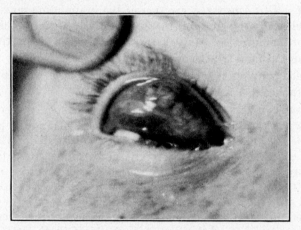

Fig. 174.—"Parinaud's disease," conjunctival granuloma with preauricular adenopathy. (Courtesy of Dr. V. R. Hurst.)

The condition has often been confused with conjunctival tularensis (see Tularemia), and the terms applied to either condition interchangeably. In recent years, however, the two conditions have been distinctly separated, tularensis being diagnosed essentially by the agglutination test, whereas Parinaud's conjunctivitis is definitely established by demonstrating the leptothrix in the conjunctival vegetation. The staining process of leptothrix is somewhat difficult according to Verhoeff, and in some cases may not be demonstrated. Verhoeff inoculated the conjunctiva of rabbits and of guinea pigs with the organisms and produced lesions which were clinically and histologically similar to those of the disease in human beings.

In Hurst's cases,[3] in which histologic studies were made, the clinical signs were the same in those cases in which the leptothrix was found and those in which it was not demonstrated.

Pascheff's conjunctivitis resembles Parinaud's conjunctivitis, and the condition must be diagnosed by laboratory examination. The former condition is caused by *Microbacillus polymorphicus necroticans*. It may also resemble tuberculous conjunctivitis in its clinical appearance.

The cornea and other structures of the eye are rarely, if ever, involved in this condition. It is almost solely an affection of the conjunctiva and may be accompanied only by swelling of the lids. Cases have been reported of leptothrix in the canaliculi and tear ducts, but Verhoeff-King[1a] stated that their examination showed these to be a branching form of leptothrix rather than the nonbranching variety.

One of the extragenital lesions of lymphogranuloma venereum, a virus disease, has been described as a conjunctivitis with preauricular adenopathy similar to Parinaud's conjunctivitis. A number of these cases were reported, the first of which was said to have been the result of accidental laboratory infection with the virus. Thygeson stated that, "Beyond doubt the virus must now be included among the agents producing the so-called oculoglandular syndrome of Parinaud."[6]   (See Lymphogranuloma venereum.)

Treatment.—This consists of excision of the granulating mass from the conjunctiva and cleansing by flushing the eye regularly with a mild solution such as boric acid or mercurophen (1:10,000). The presence of constitutional symptoms may require general treatment as indicated.

If the accompanying inflammation of the glands goes on to suppuration, incision and drainage may be required.

Other fungus infections of the eye are less commonly encountered. Occasionally, however, an infection of this type is reported and it is possible that some may come under observation without being recognized. These conditions are nearly all characterized by the formation of granulomatous tissue and nodules, which may be present over a long period of time, and in some instances, cause suppuration. The group includes a large number of individual fungi, each of which may show slight variations from the others. They may even be present in the conjunctiva and mucous membrane under normal conditions. Under pathologic conditions the diagnosis depends on the recognition of the causative organism and a knowledge of its characteristics. They are the cause of affections of the respiratory tract, and, in the lungs, they may cause a chronic inflammatory condition resembling tuberculosis.

Actinomycosis

Actinomycosis is a ray fungus which may affect the lungs, sinuses, scalp, and occasionally the viscera. It usually occurs as a secondary infection from the mouth or from some adjacent area. It produces a granulomatous condition with chronic ulceration and sometimes abscess formation. It is accompanied by considerable fibrosis. The actinomycetes occurring in the sputum, pus, or material obtained from the sinuses can be recognized by the unaided eye. The disease runs a rapid, serious course, and usually involves the surrounding tissues.

Eye Manifestations.—Ocular involvement by actinomycosis is comparatively rare, but a number of cases of secondary involvement are on record in which the disease occurred mainly in the orbit. In most instances the seat of the primary lesion was never definitely determined. This is due to the fact that the disease process which spreads through the tissues by extension, may have been healed in the primary structure at the time the orbit became involved. The involvement of the orbit presents a serious problem in the management and treatment of the condition. In all probability extension takes place into the orbit, in most cases, through the sphenoid fissure. Cases have been reported as occurring by extension from the nasal sinuses.

Beigelman[7] reported a case of actinomycosis of the orbit in a man 45 years of age, which began with a swelling and infection of the right parotid gland. The eyelids and orbit showed involvement about four months later. After two years, the patient developed a meningitis and brain abscess which resulted in death.

The orbital involvement is characterized clinically by presence of exophthalmos and edema of the lids with the appearance of isolated swellings or nodules. The visual acuity may remain unimpaired unless the optic nerve becomes involved. This may occur later as the result of pressure or inflammation resulting in optic neuritis.

The exophthalmos is caused by the gradually increasing granulomatous process behind the eyeball. The direction of the displacement of the eyeball depends on the location of the granulomatous condition. The exophthalmos increases gradually, and the nodules in the eyelids may rupture through the skin and result in sinus formation. As a result of the mechanical obstruction of the orbit by the mass which is increasing in size, the rotation of the eyeball becomes limited and later fixed.

The extraocular muscles themselves may become involved, as well as some of the cranial nerves. Ptosis of the upper lid has occurred as a result of secondary involvement of the oculomotor nerves.

The optic nerve may become involved as the result of pressure with subsequent atrophy, and also from inflammatory involvement resulting in optic neuritis. The earliest signs of such a complication are an increased congestion in the vessels observed on examination with the ophthalmoscope. This is followed by visual impairment of varying degree. As a result of the marked exophthalmos and accompanying interference with closure of the lids, the cornea may become involved from exposure. However, in a number of cases, the vision remained unaffected, and involvement of the optic nerve was absent in spite of the marked exophthalmos. This was explained by Beigelman by the tendency of the process to become a localized fibromatosis, so that the fungus activity is walled off and the optic nerve escapes involvement.

Actinomyces in the lacrimal canaliculus may produce concretions which cause epiphora and a dacryocystitis. This is characterized by swelling in the region of the lacrimal sac and a drop of yellowish pus may be seen when slight pressure is made over this region. Such cases, however, are comparatively rare and can be cured by removal of the mycotic concretion.

According to Hagerdoorn,[8] the superior or inferior canaliculus may be involved. When the inferior canaliculus is involved, the early signs may be slight or absent, and on syringing the tear sac, there is found no interference with the passage of the fluid.

Epiphora is absent when the upper canaliculus alone is affected. Later on, however, the swelling over this point will be observed, which may resemble a chalazion or small tumor. When the canaliculus is slit, the yellowish concretions may be found. Hagedoorn was able to isolate the organism by treating the removed concretion with a drop of 96 per cent alcohol which killed the bacteria. The alcohol was evaporated and an emulsion of this material was made in sterile physiologic salt solution. This was mixed with a dextrose agar which was liquified by warming. After lowering the temperature again to solidify the agar, a few drops of the emulsion were added to the tube and mixed with dextrose agar by rolling the tube between the hands. After placing in an incubator at 37° C., a pure culture was obtained which grew beneath the surface of the agar.

Treatment.—The prognosis of the condition is serious, since treatment is of little value and is mostly palliative. Massive doses of the iodides are commonly employed. X-ray has also been advocated and used with doubtful benefit. The only relief is from surgical procedures and this is only of temporary benefit. This consists in incision and drainage of abscesses, and curetting of sinuses and fistules. More radical surgical procedures are almost futile, since the condition will, in all probability, recur and because of the strong possibility of extension of the process to the brain and nervous system.

Streptothricosis

Streptothricosis is a rare infection which affects the respiratory tract with the occurrence of bronchopneumonia, abscess formation, gangrene, and bronchiectasis. The infection may spread into other parts by metastasis through the blood stream.

The fungus is to be differentiated from the leptothrix by its branching ends which give it the appearance under the microscope of the bare branches of a tree. Leptothrix is an unbranched, thread-like fungus. In addition, the streptothrix is anaerobic and gram-positive, grown by slab culture on peptone glycerine agar.

Eye Manifestations.—The affection in the eye is characterized most commonly by the occurrence of concretions in the lacrimal canaliculus. This may result in a conjunctivitis. Streptothricosis of the conjunctiva, which is rare, is characterized by the presence of granulomatous nodules which represent accumulations of streptothrix about the size of a pinhead and may be found on the palpebral conjunctiva, the bulbar conjunctiva, either at the angles or near the cornea, and is usually accompanied by a stubborn conjunctivitis or occasionally by the formation of a yellowish membrane. The organism may be found in the granulomatous material and is mixed up with epithelioid, lymphoid, polymorphonuclear, and giant cells. The infection may exist for some time with gradual improvement.

Corneal involvement is rare in streptothricosis. When it occurs, it causes a dry necrotic patch of ulceration which is surrounded by a yellow furrow of nodular demarcation. The ulceration may result in perforation, hypopyon, and iritis. The fungus may be found in the sequestrum which is desquamated.

Treatment.—The treatment of streptothricosis conjunctiva is removal of the granulomatous nodules wherever possible by excision. The lacrimal apparatus also should be examined and any obstruction by accumulations of streptothrix should be removed.

Streptothrix ulcers of the cornea should indicate the removal of the sequestrum by excision and cauterization of the ulcer.

The eye should be irrigated several times daily with a mild astringent eyewash.

Aspergillosis

The aspergillus is a moldlike fungus which occasionally causes chronic pulmonary disease and which is characterized by a rather mild ulcerative bronchitis and the presence of peribronchial nodules which may result in extensive granulomatosis and gangrene. The symptoms include cough and and blood-tinged sputum and may simulate tuberculosis. The molds can be found in the sputum, and by contamination this may be the source of infection elsewhere.

Eye Manifestations.—The ocular lesion caused by the aspergillus is rare but is characterized by ulceration of the cornea. It is produced by contamination from the saliva or by infection by the spores from an outside source following trauma or injury to the eye. The cornea is the seat of superficial necrotic ulceration which is gray in color and with its outline well demarcated by a yellow border. The outline of the ulcer becomes deeper with the involved area gradually sloughing off leaving an ulcerative infiltration. This is followed by gradual healing after running a slow, chronic course. It may be accompanied by pain of varying degrees, and iritis, hypopyon, or perforation of the cornea may result. More rarely, the lesion may occur near the limbus where it is accompanied by vascularization.

The infection very rarely invades the sclera or penetrates into the eyeball with involvement of the posterior chamber.

Treatment.—This requires cauterization of the site of the ulcer after excision of the sequestrum. This results in healing and subsequent formation of a leucoma which may be rather dense and cause considerable visual impairment in the affected eye.

Rhinosporidiosis

This is a comparatively rare disease caused by infection with the fungus, rhinosporidium. The common site of infection is the mucous membrane of the anterior nares of the nose. It may, however, also be found in the larynx, pharynx, lacrimal sac, and penis. It seems to occur more frequently in the male than in the female. The exact mode of infection is not known.

The condition is characterized by the presence of polypoid growths on the membrane involved. The growths are soft and reveal small white areas on their surface which are the mature sporangia.

Eye Manifestations.—The ocular infection by rhinosporidium presents a clinical appearance similar to that found in the nasopharynx and other structures. The conjunctiva is most commonly affected, although the lacrimal sac may also be involved. The palpebral or bulbar conjunctiva reveals the presence of the polypoid growths which consists of granulomatous tissue. The growth can be removed with a very slight amount of bleeding.

Several cases of rhinosporidiosis of the conjunctiva and also of the lacrimal sac have been reported. Barnshaw and Read[9] described a case in a young man, aged 17, who revealed a vascular papillomatous growth under the upper lid springing from the palpebral conjunctiva. The appearance resembled that of "granulomatous tissue from a ruptured chalazion." The diagnosis of rhinosporidiosis was made on histologic examination of the granuloma which was removed.

Treatment.—The treatment ordinarily consists of excision of the growth from its attachment to the conjunctiva. When this is done thoroughly, the condition will clear up. No special local medication is indicated.

When the lacrimal sac is infected, surgical removal of the sac is indicated.

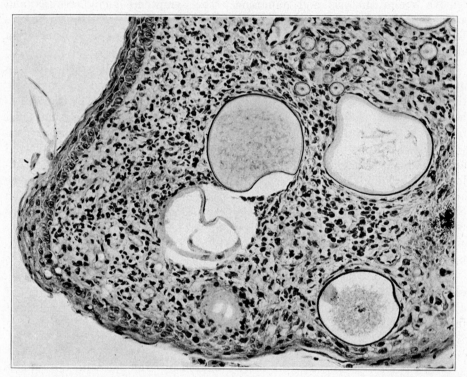

Fig. 175.—Rhinosporidiosis of conjunctiva. Section of conjunctiva showing small organisms in the trophic stage as well as developing sporangia. ×120. (From Barnshaw and Read: Arch. Ophth., August, 1940.)

Blastomycosis

This is a fairly common form of mycotic infection, when the spores occur in the lungs. They usually arrive here by inhalation or through the blood stream from cutaneous infection. The lesion may travel from the lung to other structures through the blood stream. This infection includes a number of different yeast-like organisms. It resembles tuberculosis very much, except that more suppuration takes place with the formation of small isolated abscesses at first which later form large cavities. The blastomycetes are found in the sputum and confirm the diagnosis. The general infection is serious, and the prognosis is grave, with no specific treatment being available.

Eye Manifestations.—Infection of the eye with blastomycosis is rare, but the skin of the eyelids and the conjunctiva may be affected from infection of the face and lungs. It is probably caused by contamination from the infected sputum which contains the fungus in large quantities.

Blastomycosis of the conjunctiva is characterized by the appearance of granulomatous masses which are found in the conjunctiva and subconjunctival tissue. It is raised and pinkish color in appearance and may spread around the cornea, growing rather rapidly. It may also occur at either canthus. The growths are made up of large mononuclear cells, lymphocytes, and giant cells. The fungus is found in the mononuclear and giant cells.

In one or two instances, the cornea has become involved by ulcers which also reveal the fungus. This can be diagnosed on microscopic examination.

Treatment.—There is little known in the way of treatment for blastomycosis, but massive doses of the iodides, x-ray, and radium have all been tried.

Thrush (Parasitic Stomatitis)

The condition commonly known as thrush is due to an infection by the *Oidium albicans.* It is very common in poorly nourished and artificially fed infants. The principal seat of infection is the buccal membrane. It may also extend down the esophagus to the stomach. It may more rarely affect the larynx, trachea, and bronchi. It occurs also in debilitated adults and in the vagina of pregnant women.

The general condition is characterized by the loss of appetite, restlessness, difficulty in swallowing, and diarrhea. The mucous membrane which is involved may reveal patches of white deposit resembling a veil in appearance. They are slightly raised and difficult to remove. Large numbers of lymphomycetes may be found on microscopic examination of the deposits.

Eye Manifestations.—The eyelids are the chief site of infection, the conjunctiva being less commonly involved. In the latter the condition may resemble a pseudomembranous conjunctivitis. The deposits may also be found very occasionally in the cornea. The ocular involvement usually occurs in children who suffer with infections of the mouth and respiratory tract.

Treatment.—There is no definite treatment to employ with the exception of extreme cleanliness, oral hygiene, and the use of a mild antiseptic wash. The general condition of the patient should be improved along hygienic and nutritive lines.

Trichophyton (Ringworm)

Ringworm due to *tinea circinata* and *tinea tonsurans* may occur on the skin of the face and adjacent to the conjunctiva. Occasionally, the conjunctiva itself may become involved secondarily, and the fungus has also been found in the conjunctival sac independent of skin involvement. It causes a chronic form of conjunctivitis. When the condition occurs in the scalp, the cornea, as well as the conjunctiva, has been said to be affected. Cases of keratitis due to trichophyton are very rare, however.

References

Parinaud's Conjunctivitis

1. Verhoeff, F. H.: Arch. Ophth. **42**: 345, 1913.
1a. Verhoeff, F. H., and King, Merrill, J.: Leptothricosis Conjunctivae (Parinaud's Conjunctivitis), Arch. Ophth. **9**: 701, 1933.

2. Harner, C. E.: Parinaud's Conjunctivitis, Am. J. Ophth. 17: 629, 1934.
3. Hurst, V. Reeves: Oculo-Glandular Diseases With Special Reference to Tularemia and Parinaud's Conjunctivitis, Tr. Am. Acad. Ophth., 1938.
4. Lamb, H. D.: The Histopathology of Parinaud's Conjunctivitis, Am. J. Ophth. 19: 571, 1936.
5. Gifford, Sanford R., and Dillon, E. E.: The Conjunctivoglandular Syndrome of Parinaud: Report of a Case Showing a Thread Mold in Sections, Arch. Ophth. 12: 518, 1934.
6. Thygeson, P.: Viruses and Virus Diseases of Eye. II. Viruses of Ocular Importance, Arch. Ophth. 29: 635, 1943.

Actinomycosis

7. Biegelman, M. N.: Actinomycosis of the Orbit, Arch. Ophth. 10: 664, 1933.
8. Hagedoorn, A.: Concretions in a Lacrymal Canaliculus Caused by Actinomyces, Arch. Ophth. 23: 689, 1940.

Rhinosporidiosis

9. Barnshaw, Harold D., and Read, William T., Jr.: Rhinosporidiosis of the Conjunctiva, Arch. Ophth. 24: 357, 1937.

CHAPTER XII

OCULAR PARASITES AND PARASITIC INFECTIONS

There are three main groups of parasites which invade the eye; namely, the nematodes, the tapeworms, and the fly larvae. Tapeworms (*Taenia solium* and *Taenia echinococcus*) are in a larval cystic form with short protruding necks. Fly larvae are spindle shaped and segmented. Nematodes are of smooth cuticle, unsegmented, and coiling, and are the class most frequently found.

The nematode group is subdivided into several classes; the *Filaria loa*, *Trichinae*, and *Filaria bancrofti* are the most important ones. The *Filaria loa* is peculiar to Africa, the west coast in particular, ranging some 600 miles inland. The larvae develop in the stomach of the mangrove fly and migrate after ten days to the head, and then into the skin of the human victim. It will not infect rabbits, monkeys, or guinea pigs. The adult is 3 to 15 cm. long. It is filiform and cylindric, whitish, semi-transparent, and has a coiled tail. It moves quickly, causing itching and irritation of the parts involved, and benign Calabar swellings appear. These are described as smooth, slightly raised tumors, temporary in character and occurring on the head, arms, or legs.

Filaria loa can be diagnosed by recognition of the microfilariae which are present in the circulating blood only in the daytime, by determining its cycle of appearance and its location as indicated by the location of the Calabar swellings, and by the absence of edema of the extremities which is typical of other forms of filariasis. The adult worm may be found under the skin of the finger, back, breast, scrotum, penis, eyelid, conjunctiva, and mucosa of the tongue. The embryos in the human host are believed to escape from the adult worm and pass through the lymph spaces into the blood stream where they are known as *Microfilariae diurnae*.

Filaria bancrofti are similar in effect to the *Filaria loa*. They are transmitted by the culex fatigans mosquito and develop in the lymphatics of the host. This may be followed by a lymphangitis or chronic lymphatic obstruction. The adult is 200 microns long, and the microfilariae are present in the peripheral blood only at night.

Filaria in the Eye.—Although parasites are found usually in the extraocular tissues or the conjunctival sac, penetration into the eyeball or anterior chamber is comparatively rare. Such instances have been reported, however.

A case of filaria loa subconjunctivalis was reported as occurring in a white male, aged 48, by Cregar and Burchell.[1] The patient himself saw the parasite under the bulbar conjunctiva while looking for a supposed foreign body in the eye. Examination of the blood of the patient revealed many microfilariae, one to four being encountered in each drop of blood. The total number of white cells was 16,750, with lymphocytes 34 per cent, monocytes 3 per cent, polymorphonuclear leucocytes 50 per cent, 47 per cent of which were segmented, and eosinophiles 13 per cent. The worm, three inches long, was removed through an opening made in the conjunctiva under local anesthesia.

Invasion of the anterior chamber of the eye is rare, but such a case of *Filaria loa* described by Gabrielides[2] involved the ciliary body and necessitated subsequent enucleation of the eye.

The larva of the intestinal roundworm ascaris was reported in the lens of an eye by Calhoun.[3] The iris and ciliary body were involved early in this case, and secondary glaucoma occurred. An unsuccessful attempt at removal of the larva was made, but the eye was said to have recovered. It was believed that the larva was later absorbed.

An adult type of nematode worm was seen in the anterior chamber of the right eye of a patient by Jones et al.[4] The worm was removed and although lost, it was considered to be a *Filaria bancrofti*. The patient was a woman, aged 42, who had never been in the tropics. She gave a history of being bitten by a tick, the bite being swollen and painful for six days. She was also bitten by mosquitoes and had a swollen face for several days. Among the ocular symptoms in this case were herpes oculi, iritis, and increased intraocular tension.

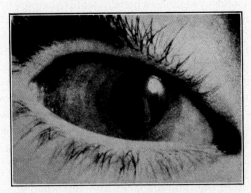

Fig. 176.—Larva of Ascaris lying behind the iris and on the anterior surface of the lens. (From Calhoun: Arch. Ophth., December, 1937.)

Other cases of *Filaria bancrofti* in the eye have been reported by Wright,[5] Fernando,[6] and Nayar and Pillat.[7]

Symptoms of parasitic infection of the eye may cover a wide range of conditions. The subjective symptoms may include such common complaints as itching, sensation of foreign body in the eye, feeling of irritation, pain, epiphora or lacrimation, and photophobia. In at least one case, the patient was able to see the parasite under the conjunctiva of his eye.

Objectively, the eyelids may be unaffected, or they may be slightly reddened. A parasite visible in the eye may produce manifestations which vary according to its location. These include edema and chemosis of the conjunctiva, keratitis, iritis, iridocyclitis, dislocation of the lens, and secondary glaucoma. Lastly, the parasite may be seen in the structures of the eye on examination with the ophthalmoscope and with the slit lamp.

Infection of the eye by a genus of microfilaria which was observed in Mexico and Guatemala was described by Quevedo as ocular *onchocerciasis*.[8]

The general infection was characterized by the presence of fibrotic nodules localized more or less superficially under the hairy skin, ribs, crest of the ilium and near the flat bones. The fibrotic nodules contain the adult parasite, *Onchocerca caecutiens*. The microfilariae are liberated from the mother and emerge from the nodule to spread over the surface of the body. Transmission is by Simulium flies as intermediaries. Since the only real damage that onchoceriasis produces is manifested in the vision, Quevedo felt that the condition should be considered as a disease of the eyes.

The ocular changes of onchocerciasis are produced by the presence of microfilariae in the eye. The symptoms appear fairly soon after the formation of the nodule. The course of the infection is insidious. It begins with irritation, congestion, lacrimation and photophobia. This may be present for a long time but when several nodules are present in the head, the course of the ocular condition may be more rapid. Iritis, ciliary congestion, turbidity of the aqueous, and a small, slightly mobile pupil with posterior synechia will develop. In advanced cases, the anterior uvea, posterior uvea, or both may be involved.

If a biopsy specimen of the conjunctiva is taken in early suspected cases and the tissue placed in physiologic salt solution under the microscope, the microfilariae can be observed in a few minutes moving about actively.

A keratitis develops which is characteristic of onchocerciasis. Small whitish opacities occur near the limbus on either side. They are usually round, about 0.25 or 0.5 mm. in diameter, and usually located in the most superficial part of the substantia propria but occasionally deeper. They result from the inflammatory reaction produced by the body of the dead microfilariae in the cornea. With the slit lamp, Quevedo was able to follow the behavior and evolution of the microfilariae in the cornea. The opacities resulting from the inflammation may become very numerous and are characterized as punctate keratitis of onchocerciasis.

Another change in the cornea sometimes observed is coffee-colored pigment on both sides of the horizontal meridian near the limbus. It is seen with the slit lamp to be localized superficially in the substantia propria and is composed of thousands of tiny spots of pigment. Although the microfilariae disappear for one reason or another, the pigment remains in the cornea for a long time.

Either superficial or deep vascularization may also occur, usually in advanced cases when the transparency of the cornea is affected. This vascular reaction was said to resemble the pannus of trachoma, but it is localized on the nasal and temporal sides just below the center.

Small exudates may occur on Descemet's membrane and whitish deposits of leucocytes may rarely occur on the endothelium. The microfilariae can be seen to be floating free in the anterior chamber and may disappear behind the iris. A plastic iritis may be present and posterior synechia with occlusion of the pupil can occur. Secondary glaucoma is a possible complication. In the posterior segment, chorioretinitis and optic atrophy may occur.

There is no specific treatment known for the disease but the nodules should be excised. Since these are said to be the source of the microfilariae, they should be removed early. When patients are seen in the early stage of the disease, without apparent tumors, a search for tumors should be made with great care.

Eye Manifestations in Trichinosis.—Trichinae are found in pork and other meats and are ingested through the alimentary canal. The general symptoms are headache, fever, abdominal discomfort, and malaise. Its chief ocular manifestations are chemosis and edema of the conjunctiva. Diban[9] reported the occurrence of trichinosis in a group of thirty-seven persons living on a farm. These patients had all eaten pork in which trichinae were found on microscopic examination. The cases occurred in from fourteen to twenty-eight days after ingestion of the pork.

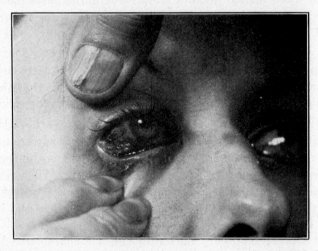

Fig. 177.—Conjunctival edema in trichinosis. (Courtesy of Dr. L. B. Lehrfeld, Wills Hospital.)

The earliest sign of the condition in the eye was edema of the eyelids, extending also over the face. This was observed in thirty of Diban's cases on the first day of illness and in a few on the third and fourth days. Limitation of motion of the eyeball and exophthalmos were observed in four patients. Subconjunctival hemorrhages and distention of the conjunctival vessels were seen in many. Fundus changes were not pronounced and, when seen, were only transient. Four patients complained of blurred vision, and the ophthalmoscope revealed a hyperemia of the disc which cleared up within a week. In three patients edema of the retina and striated hemorrhages were seen in the fundi.

Lehrfeld and Breisacher[10] reported a case of trichinosis affecting the eyes of a young woman patient at Wills Hospital in which the symptoms were edema of the eyelids and of the bulbar conjunctiva. When first seen, the lower bulbar conjunctiva of each eye was intensely chemotic and protruded between the lids preventing complete closure. The conjunctival vessels were slightly injected, and the entire conjunctiva had a yellowish, waxy appearance. The cornea, irides, pupils, and fundi were normal. The diagnosis of trichinosis was suspected and confirmed after laboratory examination. A section of the gastrocnemius muscle was excised and examined in the laboratory with the report that well-developed cysts of the larva of *Trichinella spiralis* were observed. These indicated the presence of an old infestation by the parasite. The patient also gave a more or less dubious history of recent ingestion of raw pork.

The blood count in cases of ocular manifestation of trichinosis is important. Most of these cases show a leucocytosis with a high eosinophilia. In Lehrfeld's case, six blood examinations revealed an average leucocyte count of 11,533. The average number of eosinophiles was 23 per cent.

In ten cases examined and treated by Andes et al.,[11] the eosinophile content of the blood was found to rise continually during the day, being highest in the evening.

The clinical course of the disease is usually mild, and the chemosis and swelling subside, leaving only a slight injection of the conjunctiva which remains for a while.

Treatment.—Attempts have been made to remove most of the parasites described in the eye. In many cases this was successful, but in a number of these, the worm was lost either during or after removal. This procedure seems to prove more satisfactory with those located in the conjunctiva or anterior chamber of the eye. When located in the lens, the latter can be removed. Involvement of the ciliary body and secondary glaucoma presents serious complications.

Such manifestations as iritis, iridocyclitis, and increased intraocular tension must be treated accordingly. With the latter, miotics should be employed and surgical treatment instituted whenever indicated. In other cases atropine should be instilled, and the eye treated according to the indications.

Various forms of antiparasitic treatment have been described, such as placing a grain of salt in the conjunctival sac to remove the worm. In one case described, a cure was said to have been obtained by subcutaneous injections of sulfarsphenamine in two series of treatments, the one employing doses of 0.4 Gm. each, and the second using doses of 1.08 Gm. each. Cregar and Burchell employed friadin intramuscularly. They stated that it had no effect on the numbers of microfilariae found.

There is no specific treatment for trichinosis available. Lehrfeld employed complete rest in bed, boric acid flush for the eyes several times daily, and purging with magnesium sulfate. He stated also that the use of neoarsphenamine intravenously has been advocated with varying results, but did not consider this advisable for use in his case which was of a mild nature. X-ray therapy has been employed by some with satisfactory results. Andes et al.[11] in the treatment of their cases administered 2.5 to 3 c.c. tetrachlorethylene by mouth, followed by magnesium sulfate. In almost all of their cases, this resulted in very early relief from practically all symptoms.

Hydatid Cysts in the Eye.—These are the result of collections of larvae of the *Taenia echinococcus* in the tissues of man. The eggs are usually ingested, and by way of the alimentary tract, they reach the blood stream and are carried to other organs. Hydatid cyst may occur in the appendages or in the other structures of the eye, although the conjunctiva is not often affected. They are usually unattended by severe local inflammation.

Eye Manifestations of Cysticercus Cellulosae.—The larvae of the large flatworm *Taenia solium* develop in the tissues of man after being ingested with pork as eggs, which are conveyed to the part by the lymphatics and blood stream. They are oval and translucent bodies with a head and elongated portion or caudal vesicle representing the neck.

A number of cases of cysticercus have been reported as occurring in various parts of the eye. It usually appears at the inner angle and near the fornix or the cornea in the form of a round circumscribed nodular swelling. They may be found mostly in children and young people. The cyst can be felt under the swelling and, in some cases, can be moved about, while in others, it is firmly attached to the sclera or to an ocular muscle. The head of the worm can occasionally be seen when the walls of the cyst are very thin. These encapsulated cysts can be removed by dissection after separating the conjunctiva.

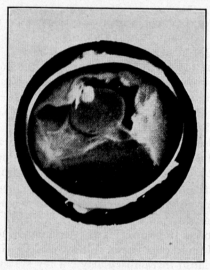

Fig. 178.—Intraocular cysticercus. (After D. J. Wood, from Duke-Elder: Text-Book of Ophthalmology.)

The cysts caused by cysticercus are also occasionally found on the iris or lodged in the anterior chamber. The ciliary body and choroid may also be invaded by way of the circulation. From here it may rupture through into the vitreous, or it may reach the vitreous by way of one of the vessels. When this happens, the cysticercus should be removed in order to prevent loss of the eye. This can be attempted by means of a posterior sclerotomy. Ordinarily, the vitreous is occupied by a mass which is bluish white in appearance and may in early cases be observed on examination. Sometimes the movements of the parasite can be observed, but this is rare, for it is soon surrounded by a membrane with which it becomes enveloped and the diagnosis of the condition is rendered difficult.

Detachment of the retina may occur from a subretinal cysticercus. The detachment appears to be solid rather than wavy, and the enveloped cyst which lies beneath may occasionally cause the detachment as a whole to move. Cysts in the structures of the eye similar to those produced by the cysticercus may also be produced by the echinococcus. Both of these parasites may also occasionally form cysts of the orbit.

Myiasis.—The larvae of flies may infest the eyes of certain peoples, especially in Eastern Europe and Central America. This occurs as the result of close contact with infected animals where these insects are prevalent. They may occur in the conjunctiva where they attach themselves in the conjunctival sac and are difficult to remove. A conjunctivitis is produced which causes considerable itching and burning with lacrimation, redness, and thickening. The maggots can be observed on close examination and are found to be long, narrow, and movable crawling bodies. They can be rendered immobile by the instillation of cocaine into the conjunctival sac and when their hold is relaxed, they can be removed.

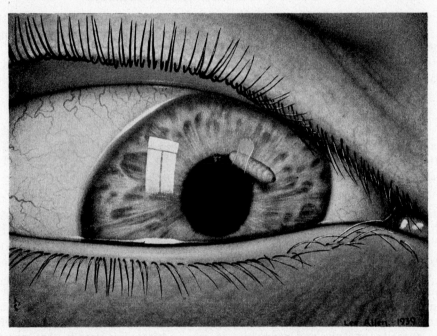

Fig. 179.—Hypoderma larva in anterior chamber. (From O'Brien and Allen: Am. J. Ophth., September, 1939.)

In some cases the cornea may become involved by the formation of ulcers. In other instances the larvae in certain patients may penetrate the lacrimal passages and the orbit or inner eyeball itself. This is accompanied by severe signs of inflammation and pain with the rapid loss of the eye.

Attempts should be made to destroy and remove the parasites before they enter the inner eye. For this purpose, the use of aqua chloroform, carbolic solution, and potassium permanganate has been recommended.

A case of myiasis of the eye caused by the larva of sheep gadfly was re-reported by H. R. Sniderman.[12] A man who suddenly felt something strike his left eye shortly afterward felt a burning, itching, and foreign body in the eye. This was accompanied by a congestion of the tarsal and bulbar conjunctiva caused by a number of small wormlike bodies attached to the conjunctiva. These were removed after the instillation of a local anesthetic and the use of 2 per cent silver nitrate solution.

Another case of conjunctival myiasis was reported by Hedges and Humphries in 1942.[13] This occurred in a patient in Virginia who was struck in the right eye by a fly. Two hours later he felt as if there were something alive and crawling in the conjunctival sac. He complained of itching and lacrimation. Examination revealed the cul-de-sac to be full of minute larvae running about over the cornea and deep into the conjunctival folds. It was thought that the larva on examination was the *Oestrus ovis*. The larvae were nearly all removed by hand and the eye bathed continuously with mineral oil. Ice compresses were employed for the congestion and edema. No intraocular infestation occurred and the patient recovered without permanent damage to the eye.

Another unusual case of the larvae of the warble or heel fly of cattle in the anterior chamber of the eye was reported by O'Brien and Allen.[14] The organism was described as 0.5 by 2.5 mm. in size and cigar shaped. It entered the anterior chamber from the vitreous. The patient, who was a 6-year-old boy, had a nail run into his foot 10 days previously in a barnyard.

Malaria

Malaria is a specific infectious disease which has an acute onset and is characterized by the occurrence, at regular intervals, of chills and fever. The latter may also be of a continuous type and have marked remissions. The disease may prove very serious and terminate fatally.

Malaria is common to European countries and certain sections of the United States. It is also more prevalent in the warmer countries and where a heavier rainfall produces stagnant pools and swamps. There are a number of clinical forms of this disease and varying signs and symptoms, but the disease is caused by the plasmodium which occurs in three varieties, each of which may cause distinct clinical symptoms. The *Plasmodium vivax* is the cause of tertian malaria, *Plasmodium malariae* is the cause of quartan malaria, and *Plasmodium falciparum* is the cause of estivo-autumnal malaria. They are introduced through the skin of the patient by the female mosquito, anopheles. The parasites mature and reproduce in man. After inoculation, they are attached to the erythrocytes which they eventually penetrate. Here they grow until they occupy the entire erythrocyte, when they divide into a number of divisions, each with a small nucleus. They then rupture into the blood stream after which each division or rosette attaches itself to another erythrocyte and again reproduces. Their multiplication, however, is limited by the phagocytic power of the leucocytes and the cells of the reticulo-endothelial system. They also lodge in the spleen, liver, and bone marrow. This asexual cycle occupies a definite period for each variety of the parasite—forty-eight hours for the tertian, seventy-two hours for the quartan, and twenty-four hours for the estivo-autumnal.

The disease can be readily diagnosed in an acute case. This is definitely established by identification of the parasite in the circulating blood, or by splenic puncture. This should be done before therapy is begun in a suspected case. Since the active treatment of the disease consists in the administration of quinine, it will be difficult to determine whether the absence of the parasite is due to the treatment, or whether some other disease is present. Malaria should be differentiated from other tropical diseases as yellow fever, dengue, relapsing fever, septicemias, typhoid fever, and bacillary dysentery.

Eye Manifestations.—Perhaps the commonest form of eye involvement in active cases of malaria is the occurrence of corneal ulcers. Retinal hemorrhages are also noted, especially in the presence of anemia. The ocular conditions often seen in patients suffering from malaria are not necessarily due to malaria but to other infections which might be present. It seems that the diseases in the eye which are described are more common in chronic malaria than in the acute cases. The former is that manifestation of the disease which occurs most often in European countries in which the parasites exist in various internal organs for a long period of time, after having disappeared from the blood stream. In these cases the involvement may affect any part of the eye, namely, the media, the retina, the choroid, the optic nerve, and the motor apparatus. According to Goldfeder and Moldavskaja,[15] this form of the disease can be definitely diagnosed by a melanoflocculation reaction described by Henry. In the study of several dozen cases they found that the latent form of malaria was the cause of periodical swelling of the lids, simple and intermittent blepharitis, conjunctivitis, superficial and deep keratitis, uveitis, neuritis, retrobulbar neuritis, retinitis, edema of the disc, arterial emboli, thrombosis of the retinal veins, and hemorrhages into the retina and vitreous. They also found it to cause accommodative asthenopia, paresis of accommodation, and paresis of the extraocular muscles.

What was described by these authors as a pathognomonic sign of malarial disease of the eyes is the presence of bluish-gray stripes which form a peculiarly shaped network in the retina around the macular region and in the periphery. These "stripes" are described as long and thread-like, lying both over and beneath the retinal vessels. In the reported cases all of the ocular manifestations cleared up following treatment for malaria, whether a history of previous infection was obtained or not.

In the eyes of 100 Chinese patients suffering from malaria, A. Montegi and associates[16] found ocular symptoms not resulting from malaria in 45 of the 100 patients on admission to the hospital. The visual acuity, pupils, accommodation, and fields of vision were not impaired in malaria. Fundus changes were found in fifty-four patients. These included grayish-white edema of the retina, small petechial arterial extravasations, tortuous and distended veins and arteries, and "reddened" discs. These changes occurred in nine cases of quartan, twenty-four of tertian, and in seventeen of what is called tropical malaria. The hemorrhages were absorbed with no trace of pigmentation remaining, and retinal edema disappeared promptly. Optic neuritis was observed in two cases. Yellowish discoloration was coupled with a low hemoglobin which was said to be due to "decay of red blood corpuscles."

A study of the blood picture seems to be of some help in the differentiation of malaria of the eye, particularly from tuberculosis and syphilis. In the study of a large series of cases by Marcus,[17] it was found that there is a rather similar blood picture in malarial and syphilitic diseases. This is characterized by pathologic polychromasia, thrombopenia, at times a leucopenia, and a shift of Schilling's curve to the right. The differential points are as follows: in malaria there is a monocytosis with a normal number of eosinophiles, while in syphilis of the eye there is monopenia and eosinophilia.

Trypanosomiasis

Two clinical varieties of trypanosomiasis are to be found which are caused by flagellate protozoa known as trypanosoma and schizotrypanum. Trypanosomes are also of two types and are found in Africa; they are almost identical and are transmitted by the tsetse fly. One is the *Trypanosoma gambiense* which causes a more chronic infection, while the other is *Trypanosoma rhodesiense*. The former also is the cause of severe epidemics. A South American variety is caused by the schizotrypanum which is transmitted by an insect, known as triatoma, inoculation taking place either by way of a scratch and abrasion, or as the result of a bite.

African sleeping sickness or African trypanosomiasis is caused by the gambiense and occurs mostly in Central Africa and Western Mongolia. The rhodesiense variety is common to Rhodesia, East Africa, and Southern Kenya. The trypanosomes are spindle shaped and have a large oval nucleus which contains a red dot located at one end of the cell. A flat flagellum tapers out from this and has a free anterior extremity. They are very mobile, being found in the blood and spinal fluid, and stain with Giemsa.

The disease, which is rather insidious in onset, has an incubation period of two to four weeks (gambiense) or about twelve to fourteen days (rhodesiense). It is characterized by either a localized or a diffuse edema accompanied by asthenia, a transient rash, irregular temperature, enlargement of the spleen and lymph glands. In the later stages central nervous system involvement is manifested. These symptoms may include headache, mental dullness, progressive somnolence, general weakness, and more severe signs, such as localized paralyses, convulsions, head retraction, opisthotonos, coma, and death. Anemia is a prominent finding in the advanced stage. An early diagnosis is important, the condition resembling typhoid fever, relapsing fever and malaria, from which it must be differentiated. The blood, cerebrospinal fluid, and glandular smears should be examined for the parasite. The prognosis is fairly good with treatment when the disease is recognized in an early stage. When not recognized early, the mortality from the disease is extremely high.

The treatment consists in the early use of arsenicals, especially atoxyl, tryparsamide, and germanin. Preparations of antimony, as tartar emetic or double salt of antimony tartrate, are also employed. Tryparsamide is given in the chronic stages in doses of 0.5 to 3 grains. It is administered on alternate days for four injections and followed by a second course after an interval of one month. This may be repeated fifteen to twenty times. During the course of the treatment, the patient must be carefully observed for signs of amblyopia, optic atrophy, and liver involvement.

Schizotrypanosomiasis is sometimes known as Brazilian trypanosomiasis or Chagas' disease, and occurs mainly in South American countries, such as Brazil, Peru, Venezuela, and Panama. The parasite is found in the blood cells in which it multiplies and which it destroys. It has a nucleus and blepharoplast and resembles a leishmania. In the blood the trypanosomes are free, have an undulating membrane, and a free flagellum. The disease may be acute or chronic. The former may also become chronic, but otherwise it runs a course of two to four weeks and usually results fatally. Children are often affected with high temperature and a pseudoedema of the tissues. The lymph glands, spleen, liver, and thyroid are enlarged. The chronic form mostly affects adults and presents symptoms according to the localization of the trypanosomes. These include, cardiac, thyroid, nervous, ovarian, and other types of symptoms.

The diagnosis of the disease also depends principally on finding the parasite in the blood and spinal fluid. The treatment includes the use of those drugs employed for African sleeping sickness and isolation of the affected population. .

Eye Manifestations.—The principal eye manifestations occurring in trypanosomiasis are keratitis, iritis, and iridocyclitis. In Brazilian trypanosomiasis or Chagas' disease, the face and eyelids are swollen and have an edematous appearance closely resembling that of myxedema. The cornea also may be involved, with an acute keratitis being a characteristic finding.

Trypanosome Keratitis.—In trypanosomiasis gambiense this has been described as a form of interstitial keratitis. It is not very common but has been found in parts of Africa in as many as 30 per cent of patients suffering with the disease. It is usually bilateral and is characterized by the presence of congestion of the vessels around the cornea, moderate photophobia, and perhaps some iridocyclitis.

The cornea itself reveals a rather diffuse involvement which is characterized by the development of an opacity in all the layers and which is accompanied by vascularization. The condition is probably the result of direct infection rather than an allergic manifestation and usually clears up on early treatment of the internal disease by the drugs previously mentioned. In such cases, or when treatment is not started early enough in the course of the disease, permanent scarring of the cornea may result with consequent impairment of the vision.

Experimental production of keratitis in animals has demonstrated the direct local involvement by the infection rather than the development of the condition as the result of allergy or from the effect of toxins. The treponema has been demonstrated in the cornea of dogs who suffered with a keratitis of this kind and which cleared up on treatment with arsenicals.

The anatomic changes in trypanosomiasis occur principally in the lymph glands. The submaxillary, mesenteric, and inguinal glands especially are enlarged. A hyperplasia of lymphoid tissue takes place with the presence of trypanosomes in almost any organ as well as in the central nervous system. In chronic cases the spinal fluid may be increased and a leptomeningitis can occur. As a result, iritis, iridocyclitis, and chorioretinitis may be associated or occur as a complication in the chronic type of case.

Leishmanial Conjunctivitis and Leishmanial Keratitis.—These ocular conditions are similar to the manifestations occurring in trypanosomiasis, but the internal disease is caused by a slightly different variety of protozoa producing two types of infection.

Leishmania tropica, which is transmitted by a sand fly, is common in the Mediterranean region, Africa, Arabia, Syria, India, and other Eastern countries. It is the cause of cutaneous leishmaniasis or what is also called Oriental sore, Aleppo sore, Aleppo boil, and Delhi boil. It occurs in dog and man and is characterized by the presence of single or multiple ulcers which begin as papules covered by scales which gradually enlarge. A serous exudation then occurs with development of the ulcer. These ulcers may granulate for a long period of time and may cause considerable destruction of tissue. In the conjunctiva a hyperemia and thickening may be found which are often associated with involvement of the cornea. These show evidences of infiltration resulting in scarring and vascularization. In the countries where the disease is prevalent, the parasites have been recovered from the cornea. The condition is commonly described as a form of interstitial keratitis.

Another form of Leishmaniasis is kala-azar, a disease which is caused by *Leishmania donovani* and which is found in the leucocytes or free in the circulating blood. It is distributed in the endothelial cells of the organs, especially the spleen, lymph glands, liver, and bone marrow (reticulo-endothelial system). This form of the disease is also more prevalent in the countries of the far east and is a systemic infection affecting infants and children as well as adults. A cutaneous manifestation may also be found, with the occurrence of nodules affecting the skin and which may also be found on the lids. The eye may also show other manifestations resulting from such complications as hemorrhage, anemia, mastoid disease, and emaciation.

The keratitis sometimes occurring in leishmaniasis is accompanied by pain, photophobia, lacrimation, and corneal infiltration of all layers. The latter may begin with a small superficial lesion in the center which may quickly involve the entire structure. An abscess may form in the central portion and rupture eventually with perforation and involvement of the anterior chamber. This may take place within three to four weeks with resulting loss of vision or even loss of the eye.

The treatment consists in the general treatment of the disease itself and also local treatment for the keratitis. The former includes the use of antimony either in the form of tartar emetic or sodium or potassium antimony tartrate. This is given intravenously in 2 per cent solution in doses of 2 c.c. and increased by 1 c.c. every other day until 5 c.c. have been injected. This is continued as a maximum dose until 4 grams of the drug have been administered (Meakins).

Local treatment of the keratitis consists in the use of atropine sulfate solution instilled into the eye three times daily. A mild antiseptic eyewash may also be employed. The use of the cautery is effectual in these cases, but it should be started early and will result in the formation of opacity and impairment of vision. However, it may prevent loss of the eye from the infection.

A detailed description of the keratitis in leishmaniasis occurring in South America was published by de Andrade in 1942.[18] He stated that the inflammatory corneal process is "not a consequence of nutritive disturbances or the like, but is rather a direct manifestation of leishmaniasis occasioned by the presence in loco of the parasite in the parenchyma of the cornea." He felt that the pathogenesis of interstitial leishmaniasic keratitis presents a perfect analogy with tuberculous, leprous, and syphilitic keratitis when they appear with the same clinical aspect.

Biomicroscopic examination of interstitial leishmaniasic keratitis showed slightly diffuse infiltration. There was noted a slight exudation between the upper corneal layers by a confluence of movable corpuscles, or leucocytes, with a proliferation of fixed cells on a smaller scale. In the zone of infiltration there were small, more or less confluent patches which resembled plastic deposits irregular in outline. They were denser in the center and rarer in the periphery. Through these the nerves intertwined, visibly swollen and brilliant, resembling silklike filaments. A vascular network was prominent at the edge and advanced in the direction of the infiltration.

The white patches which reflect the initial infiltration showed a tendency to invade the entire thickness of the cornea, but the deepest layers and endothelium were almost entirely intact. The aqueous humor was not involved in any way.

Interstitial keratitis of leishmaniasis recedes more rapidly than that of hereditary syphilis, especially if the lesions are not too deep. The well-defined spots and the exudation gradually disappear under specific and local treatment without the damage resulting from syphilitic or tuberculous keratitis.

The vascularization is less intense and passes through a slowly regressive process. The uveal tract is not seriously involved. The ulcerosis type of leishmaniasic keratitis was described by de Andrade as much more frequent and showed a direct relation to other lesions in the vicinity of the eye. In no cases did he observe the "typical phlyctena," considered by some to be the principal phenomenon, closely followed by a deep and general infiltration in the cornea. The ulceration of the cornea was similar to other common ulcerative lesions in the cornea and presented no distinctive characteristics. Staining the area with methylene blue showed, with the corneal microscope, a strongly infiltrated zone with an accumulation of cellular elements in a state of degeneration. Surrounding the ulceration were superficial and deep vessels in which the completely paralyzed red cells formed solid columns. This vascularization was less extensive than in the interstitial variety. However, the pericorneal vascularization was much more intense in the ulcerous form and was also accompanied by intense inflammatory phenomena. The lesions may regress slowly but often penetrate to Descemet's membrane and may even perforate.

The treatment described by de Andrade as specific is the intravenous injection of antimony and potassium tartrate, a 2 per cent solution of the tartrate in double-distilled water or in physiologic whey. Two cubic centimeters are given in the initial injection, and in the grave forms this may be increased to 12 or 15 cg. Smaller doses repeated at shorter intervals are recommended in certain cases, but the treatment should be regular and intensive to avoid development of resistance to the drug by the organism. Treatment should also be continued for some time after cure in order to prevent recurrence of the disease. Occasional reaction to the intravenous treatment is characterized by headache, arthralgia, fever, diarrhea, tremor, violent coughing and anginal sensations. These manifestations disappear with reduction of the dose of the tartrate and the administration of epinephrine and calcium chloride.

For the cicatrization of the ulcerous tegumentary lesions, including those of the eyelids, ultraviolet irradiation is said to give excellent results.

Toxoplasmic Encephalomyelitis

This is a disease which was first described as occurring in infants as a severe disseminated encephalomyelitis. The symptoms and signs indicated widespread involvement of the central nervous system, frequent internal hydrocephalus, convulsions at birth or soon thereafter, roentgenographic evidences of cerebral calcification and the regular occurrence of lesions in the eyes. It was later observed as a milder form of encephalitis among older children and also adults as a generalized infection with pulmonary involvement. The disease apparently has a wide geographic distribution and most of the cases recently reported have occurred in the eastern part of the United States.

The human toxoplasmosis is a protozoan infection, the source of which was said to be rodents and birds, although no specific evidence of the mode of transmission is available. The onset of symptoms, either at or soon after birth, led to the belief that the infection is present before birth and that congenital defects, such as occasional microphthalmos in association with others, were an indication of interference with normal development during intrauterine life. The parasite is believed to reach the brain and other organs from the placenta by way of the fetal circulation.

Although not many cases are on record at the present writing, a number have been reported in the literature in the last two or three years. It appears, however, that many more cases exist and are encountered than are recognized. The disease is apparently not uncommon.

Suspected cases have been described in the past in which it was suggested that they were caused by Toxoplasma, but it has been only since 1939 that more conclusive evidence of the cause has been established and the cases better identified. In 1941 Sabin,[19] who also did some earlier work on the subject reported two cases of toxoplasmic encephalitis occurring in boys 6 and 8 years of age during October, 1939. Investigation provided definite etiologic relationship of the Toxoplasma in at least one of the cases and suggestive evidence in the other. One patient died thirty days after onset and the other was said to have completely recovered in ten days. In both cases the diagnosis was made not alone on the clinical symptoms, but also by laboratory tests and after death of the patient. The disease can be transmitted to animals such as the guinea pig and the identity of the Toxoplasma established by comparative biologic and immunologic studies.

In both patients the outstanding clinical symptoms were generalized convulsions, disorientation, fever, pleocytosis without signs of meningeal irritation such as Kernig's sign or rigidity. There were no evidences of cranial nerve involvement.

The chief pathologic changes are found in the nervous system. These consist of microscopic necrotic and granulomatous foci, around which were found structures similar in morphology to Toxoplasma.

In 1940 Pinkerton and Weinman[20] reported a case occurring in a 22-year-old Peruvian in whom they demonstrated lesions and toxoplasmosis in the central nervous system, heart, spleen, liver, bone marrow, lymph nodes, adrenals and kidneys. Later, Pinkerton and Henderson[21] described two cases of acute febrile, exanthematous disease in adults due to Toxoplasma. Intracellular Toxoplasma organisms were found in the tissues in both patients. The clinical picture, however, was different from that described as occurring in infants. These cases closely resembled Rocky Mountain spotted fever and endemic typhus. The patients exhibited an atypical pulmonary involvement resembling a pneumonia of unknown etiology. A maculopapular eruption covered the entire body except the palms of the hands, soles of the feet, and scalp.

Cowen, Wolf, and Paige[22] reported a total of fifteen cases of the infantile form of the disease and described the clinical condition in detail. Eight of the patients were females and seven were males. The symptoms and clinical features of the disease were alike in nearly all. These included convulsions in nine of the fifteen patients. These convulsions persisted in most of the patients who survived. Clinical or roentgenologic evidence of internal hydrocephalus was found in seven patients, and in two it was discovered at autopsy. Six of the patients showed enlargement of the head during the first month of life. Because of the wide distribution of the lesions in the central nervous system, there may be a variety of nervous symptoms present, such as head retraction, opisthotonos, twitchings and tremors of the extremities, spastic contractions, difficulty in sucking and swallowing. In older children who survived the disease, mental retardation, speech difficulties and behavior problems were present.

Other signs and symptoms encountered include enlargement of the spleen and liver, occasional jaundice, gastrointestinal disturbances such as vomiting and diarrhea, and a diffuse maculopapular skin eruption. The temperature in general is not characteristic. There was a tendency toward a normal temperature with variations to slightly below or slightly above normal.

Examination of the blood and spinal fluid is apparently not characteristic. In four instances the spinal fluid showed pleocytosis. Lymphocytes seemed to predominate. The blood examination revealed either a slight leucopenia or a normal count. No significance could be attached to the blood count.

The disease is usually fatal in the early months of life but some patients survive and even reach adult life. In these patients, the toxoplasmic lesions heal with the protozoa either disappearing or remaining in a quiescent state.

Eye Manifestations.—Ocular involvement in this disease appears to be an early and prominent accompanying feature. In some patients, it was the most prominent manifestation, characterized principally by the presence of focal lesions of chorioretinitis which are severe, extensive and nearly always bilateral. Both eyes are usually affected in some way by the disease. The macular region is especially susceptible, but the lesions are also found in the periphery of the fundus. Most of the lesions found are quiescent or healed when the patient comes under observation. Active lesions are more rarely encountered. In one patient seen fairly early by Cowen and associates,[22] the lesion occurred in the macular area and was acute. This was described as being "homogenous, somewhat raised, reddish brown and approximately in the position of the fovea. A somewhat more advanced lesion in the macular area of the other eye of the same patient was also an indefinitely marginated zone of edema of the same color, having a diffuse marginal band of grayish-brown pigment and a central whitish area of chorioretinal atrophy bordered by brown and deeply situated black pigment.''

The acute lesions seem to be characterized by localized edema with indefinite demarcations. The entire macular region is usually involved. Later, chorioretinal atrophy takes place with deposits of pigment. The advanced lesions become more sharply outlined with a subsiding of the edema. Proliferation also occurs later. These chorioretinal lesions are usually multiple and as many as twelve have been found in one eye.

The older lesions may be round, oval or irregular with fairly sharp outlines. They may vary in size from 1 to 6 disc diameters. They are either slightly elevated or concave and yellowish white or reddish brown and white in color. Brownish-black or black pigment usually stipples the borders. The retina between lesions and its vasculature is usually unaffected. The media is nearly always clear but when proliferation occurs in the late stages, this may extend forward into the vitreous.

It has been stated that the infection probably reaches the eyes by way of the fetal circulation from the placenta. Toxoplasmas have been found in the retinal lesions of eyes examined and were most common in the more severely affected areas. They occurred also, however, in relatively normal parts of the retina but usually near the inflammatory foci. They were found singly and in groups—free, intracellularly, or as cysts. In one of the early cases reported by Janku,[23] he found what he described as "parasitic cysts" in the lesion of the right eye which he considered to be some form of sporozoon. These were later considered to be Toxoplasmas.

The pathologic changes of early lesions have been described as focal areas of swelling and edema of the retinal tissue with distortion and varying degrees of necrosis and inflammation. All layers were involved by the congestion and edema but it was more intense in the three inner layers. The necrosis involved all the retinal layers and occurred in the more central parts of the lesion. In some instances, however, only the inner layers were degenerated. Amorphous cytoplasmic and nuclear debris replaced the normal structures. At the margins of the necrotic areas, there was perivascular and diffuse infiltration by lymphocytes, plasma cells and occasional eosinophiles and lipoid-laden phagocytes. Polymorphonuclear leucocytes were observed in some of the lesions. There was endothelial hyperplasia of the capillaries. The internal limiting membrane showed small amounts of exudate on its free surface. These were often associated with ingrowth of fibroblasts and capillaries into the vitreous. The retinal structure was distorted where partial degeneration had occurred at the margin of the necrotic areas. The cells of the nuclear layer were often displaced, and the retinal pigment layer was at times hypertrophied. Free pigment and cells were displaced into the inner retinal layers. Most of the nerve cells of the ganglionic layer had disappeared. In the stratum opticum and inner molecular layers, the edema was often intense.

In parts of the choroid close to the retinal lesions, there were areas of moderate infiltration. Congestion and infiltration by plasma cells, lymphocytes and eosinophiles occurred in the choriocapillary layer. Some showed endothelial hyperplasia. Mild or moderate infiltration of the leptomeningeal sheaths of the optic nerve was similar to that seen in the choroid.

In more chronic lesions, the inflammation was found to be less pronounced and astrocytosis and capillary hyperplasia were fairly prominent. There was also extensive outgrowth of granulation tissue into the vitreous.

Although the most common and frequent ocular signs were those seen in the eyegrounds, other eye manifestations of the disease are regularly present. Microphthalmos, either unilateral or bilateral, is quite common. This has been attributed to an interference with normal development of the eye in the presence of the infection before birth. Other ocular conditions which are found include strabismus, nystagmus and nystagmoid movements, narrowed palpebral fissures, exophthalmos, nevus flammeus of the lids and brow, deviations of the head and eyes to one side, impaired ocular movements, posterior cortical cataract, lenticonus and remnants of pupillary membrane.

The optic nerve heads are usually atrophic as the result of destruction of the macula and other parts of the retina.

Children who have survived the disease will suffer with greatly reduced vision or even blindness. They may reveal any of the ocular signs mentioned and if a diagnosis of the general condition has not been made when such cases first come to the attention of the ophthalmologist, toxoplasmosis should be considered as a possibility. This is especially true in infants, since toxoplasmic chorioretinitis occurs in nearly all cases of toxoplasmic encephalomyelitis and is considered to be of great diagnostic aid in the clinical recognition of the disease. The history of convulsions in infants together with hydrocephalus, mental retardation, speech difficulties, defective vision and intracerebral calcification should lead to further consideration and measures to recognize the presence of this condition as the etiologic factor.

Toxoplasmic involvement of the eye, especially in the form of late chorioretinitis in infants and young children, may resemble a number of other ocular conditions and must be differentiated. These include principally pseudoglioma, syphilitic and tuberculous choroidal foci, cerebromacular degeneration or amaurotic family idiocy (Tay-Sachs disease), tuberous sclerosis, acute metastatic chorioretinitis, intraocular tumors, intraocular injuries occurring at birth and some congenital developmental defects.

Pseudoglioma describes almost any extensive, old inflammatory condition of the eye which in appearance resembles a glioma. In the presence of a white area or mass in the pupil which might have resulted from an extensive chorio-retinitis in the eye of an infant or young child, the condition is commonly called Pseudoglioma. It usually exhibits proliferation of connective tissue and would be difficult to differentiate from toxoplasmic chorioretinitis. In all such cases, therefore, the history and other clinical features of the condition should receive careful study and the possibility of toxooplasmic infection should be strongly considered.

Syphilitic and tuberculous lesions should not be difficult to differentiate. The former are rare in infancy and early childhood and usually occur in the form of congenital syphilis. Tuberculous foci in the choroid usually occur in the late stages of disseminated, miliary tuberculosis and are small, dark yellow areas irregularly distributed in the choroid.

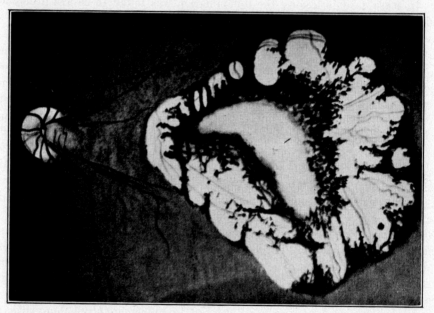

Fig. 180.—Toxoplasmic encephalomyelitis. (From Koch and Others: Arch. Ophth., January, 1943.)

Tay-Sachs disease is also easy to differentiate. This condition is always bilateral and nearly all cases present the characteristic cherry-red spot in the macula with a pronounced optic atrophy.

Tuberous sclerosis usually involves one eye and is rarely found in infants and young children. It is characterized by the presence of a mulberry-like or nodular mass in the retina, at or near the disc. It is only when cerebral symptoms are simultaneously present that the differentiation from toxoplasmo-sis may be more difficult.

An acute severe metastatic chorioretinitis occurring during the course of or after one of the severe infections may resemble toxoplasmic chorioretinitis. These lesions, however, are usually smaller and widespread in the fundus to-gether with some degree of involvement of the anterior uvea. The history or presence of a definitely recognized general infection of specific nature will also serve to differentiate the condition.

Among the intraocular tumors, retinoblastoma may somewhat resemble the appearance of toxoplasmic chorioretinitis. In cases which have progressed, the yellowish-white reflex is seen in the pupil. If seen early, the lesions appear as small, round yellowish-white nodules in the retina and increase in size to large masses growing forward into the vitreous. Very little pigmentation and atrophy occur.

Intraocular injuries at birth resulting from abnormal or difficult labor may produce extensive hemorrhages into the vitreous with subsequent proliferation of connective tissue and loss of vision. These, however, should provide no serious difficulty in differentiation.

Such developmental defects as coloboma of the optic nerve head, choroid, retina and macula are easily distinguished from toxoplasmic lesions, principally because of the absence of any inflammatory signs.

In any inflammatory condition where the ophthalmoscopic picture cannot be definitely diagnosed etiologically, the clinical signs and general symptoms of toxoplasmosis may help to differentiate the ocular condition. This was well stated by Koch and associates[24] who said: "Symptoms and signs beginning at birth or early in life, a subacute or chronic course, evidence of widespread involvement of the nervous system, convulsive seizures, internal hydrocephalus and the occurrence of intracerebral calcification all point to the presence of infantile toxoplasmic encephalomyelitis, of which toxoplasmic chorioretinitis is an outstanding feature. Antitoxoplasmic activity of the serum tends to confirm this diagnosis."

References

1. Cregar, John S., and Burchell, Edgar B.: Filaria Subconjunctivalis, Arch. Ophth. **14:** 435, 1935.
2. Gabrielides, C. A.: Filaria in the Anterior Chamber of the Eye, Ann. d'Ocul. **175:** 581, 1938.
3. Calhoun, F. Phinzy: Intraocular Invasion by the Larva of the Ascaris, Arch. Ophth. **18:** 963, 1937.
4. Jones, Lesher T., Jordan, Lewis W., and Sullivan, Nicholas P.: Intraocular Nematode Worms, Arch. Ophth. **20:** 1006, 1938.
5. Wright, R. E.: Adult Filaria Bancrofti in the Anterior Chamber, Brit. J. Ophth. **18:** 646, 1934.
6. Fernando, S. E.: Ocular Filariasis (Adult Wuchereria Bancrofti in the Anterior Chamber of the Human Eye), J. Trop. Med. & Hyg. **38:** 17, 1934.
7. Nayar, K. K., and Pillat, A. K.: A Case of Filariasis Oculi, Brit. J. Ophth. **16:** 549, 1932.
8. Quevedo Arturo: Ocular Onchocerciasis, Am. J. Ophth. **24:** 1185, 1941.
9. Diban, A. P.: Ocular Complications in Trichinosis, Sovet. vestnik oftal. **3:** 228, 1933.
10. Lehrfeld, Louis, and Breisacher, Carl F.: A Case of Trichinosis Presenting Chemosis of the Bulbar Conjunctiva, J. A. M. A. **115:** 1794, 1940.
11. Andes, Jerome E., Greene, Robert A., and Breazeale, Edward L.: Early Mild Infestation With the Parasite Trichinella Spiralis, J. A. M. A. **114:** 2271, 1940.
12. Sniderman, Harold R.: Larval Conjunctivitis (Report of a Case Due to Oestrus Ovis), Am. J. Ophth. **22:** 1253, 1939.
13. Hedges, H. S., and Humphries, M. K., Jr.: Conjunctival Myiasis Due to Oestrus Ovis: Report of a Case, Arch. Ophth. **28:** 251, 1942.
14. O'Brien, C. S., and Allen, J. H.: Ophthalmomyiasis Interna Anterior (Report of Hypodermalarval in the Anterior Chamber), Am. J. Ophth. **22:** 996, 1939.
15. Goldfeder, A. E., and Moldavskaja, V. D.: Malaria and the Eye, Arch. Ophth. **17:** 228, 1937.

16. Montegi, A., et al.: Ophthalmologic Observations on One Hundred Patients With Malaria, Klin. Monatsbl. f. Augenh. 92: 797, 1934.
17. Marcus, I. M.: Value of Hematologic Data in the Etiology of Ocular Diseases, Vestnik oftal. 11: 646, 1937.
18. de Andrade, Cesario: Interstitial and Ulcerous Keratitis in Leishmaniasis, Arch. Ophth. 27: 1193, 1942.
19. Sabin, Albert R.: Toxoplasmic Encephalitis in Children, J. A. M. A. 116: 801, 1941; Toxoplasmic Neutralizing Antibody in Human Beings and Morbid Conditions Associated With It, Proc. Soc. Exper. Biol. & Med. 51: 6, 1942.
20. Pinkerton, H., and Weinman, D.: Toxoplasmic Infection in Man, Arch. Path. 30: 374-392, 1940.
21. Pinkerton, H., and Henderson, R. G.: Adult Toxoplasmosis—A Previously Unrecognized Entity Simulating the Typhus-Spotted Fever Group, J. A. M. A. 116: 807, 1941.
22. Cowen, David, Wolf, Abner, and Paige, Beryl: Toxoplasmic Encephalomyelitis—Clinical Diagnosis of Infantile or Congenital Toxoplasmosis; Survival Beyond Infancy, Arch. Neurol. & Psychiat. 48: 689, 1942.
23. Janku, J.: Parasites in Coloboma of the Macula, Čäsop. lék. Čěsk. 62: 1021, 1054, 1081, 1111, and 1138, 1923.
24. Koch, Ferdinand L. P., Wolf, Abner, Cowen, David, and Paige, Beryl H.: Toxoplasmic Encephalomyelitis. VII. Significance of Ocular Lesions in the Diagnosis of Infantile or Congenital Toxoplasmosis, Arch. Ophth. 29: 1, 1943.

CHAPTER XIII

FOCAL INFECTIONS

A great many ocular manifestations are seen with an obscure etiology. These include principally infections of different degrees which occur in the various structures of the eye and are considered often, in the absence of a definite etiologic factor, to be due to the presence of a focus of infection in another organ or part of the body. In most cases this is also impossible to prove, and the decision is usually arrived at by conjecture. In some cases it is possible to demonstrate the presence of more than one focus. Inflammations of the uveal tract in particular, which may be either exudative or purulent, and usually localized, are often accounted for by the presence of a focus of infection. In some instances an acute infection in the eye may be directly connected with the presence of a focus in another part, when purulent material from both is available for bacteriologic examination and is found to be identical. In other cases it is assumed that the ocular manifestation was directly caused by a primary focus elsewhere, because of the fact that the eye condition began to improve only with treatment or removal of the suspected primary focus of infection.

The most common forms of focal infection are the streptococcal and tuberculous. The former are usually derived from the teeth, tonsils, or other organs, and the latter from the lungs and mediastinal glands.

Among the possible foci which may lead to the appearance of eye manifestations may be included principally the teeth, tonsils, nasal accessory sinuses, middle ear, respiratory tract, and lungs, the prostate gland and urethra, the intestinal tract, and colon.

The more common of these, from the ophthalmologic standpoint, are the teeth, tonsils, and nasal sinuses. The upper respiratory tract may not be considered strictly as a possible focus of infection, but rather as a site which is involved early, or sometime during the course of many of the acute infectious diseases.

The lungs and mediastinal glands are also considered as possible foci of infection in cases of latent or quiescent tuberculosis in which the eye manifestation may occur as previously explained in the form of an allergic reaction.

The Prostate Gland and Urethra.—These structures are often the seat of gonorrheal infection and may result in involvement of the ocular structures during the acute stages of the disease or shortly afterward, as previously described; recurrent attacks of milder inflammation may occur even years after the first infection was present. In these cases the eye lesion usually occurs in the form of a low-grade or mild iritis or iridocyclitis which is considered to be an allergic manifestation. Such cases resulting from infection in the prostate or deep urethra, however, are not necessarily due to the presence of the gonococcus. Cases of iritis and iridocyclitis of this kind have often been found to be the result of the association of streptococcus and gonococcus, and in numerous instances the presence of the streptococcus alone has been considered responsible. Prostatic infection should be strongly suspected, especially in those cases of uveal involvement occurring in men of middle age or older. Most of these were found by Pelouze[1] to be due to streptococcal infection secondary to infection of the teeth and tonsils, and rarely associated with gonococcal infection. The successful treatment of these cases includes the proper treatment of the prostatic infection by a competent urologist.

In addition to the prostate gland and the urethra, the urinary tract may also occasionally be a focus of infection of the eye by the *Bacillus coli.*

Chronic cystitis has been reported as the cause of vesicular keratitis and optic neuritis with the presence of exudates and hemorrhages in the retina.

The eye manifestations arising from diseases of the female generative organs will be discussed in a later chapter, and it will suffice to state here that the latter rarely act as a focus for infection of the eye. However, chronic inflammations of the uterus and the endometrium may be responsible for the presence of scleritis or a low-grade nonsuppurative form of iridocyclitis or uveitis occurring in women.

The Intestinal Tract and Colon.—The intestinal tract and colon cannot be considered as common foci of ocular inflammation. When such infection does happen, it is probably the result of extension to the bowel of a streptococcic infection from the mouth. In the past cases of iritis and iridocyclitis were considered to arise from infection of the intestinal tract as the result of the bacterial infection or from their toxic products. A chronic mucous colitis, cholecystitis, and even appendicitis may serve as a focus of infection for cases of iritis and iridocyclitis especially.

Lastly, attention might be called to the fact that among older people, the gastrointestinal tract may serve as a focus of infection because of the accumulation of toxins resulting from chronic constipation. The latter, being common in these patients because of poor elimination caused by relaxation and flabbiness of the abdominal muscles as well as the reduced contractile ability of the intestines, results in absorption and dissemination of the toxins to other structures. This may be an important factor in those who are operated on for cataract extraction and other intraocular operations.

Dental Infection

Almost any variety of dental affection may be a cause of disease of the eye. Foremost among these, however, especially as a possible focus, is the presence of infections in and about the teeth in forms of apical and periapical abscesses, infected roots, and impacted infected teeth. Thus Wilmer[2] groups these as: 1, apical and periapical abscesses; 2, pyorrhea alveolaris; 3, septic, broken roots; 4, maxillary or mandibular infection remaining after extraction of diseased teeth; 5, impacted, infected teeth; 6, pulp stones; and 7, degenerating pulp of an anomalous extra root from a nutritive disturbance following traumatism. According to Steinbügler,[3] the most dangerous forms of dental infection are those of the pulp, pulpless teeth, and apical abscesses. These are usually free from symptoms and, therefore, unsuspected. They are located in the osseous tissue and drainage takes place into the circulation. He listed the dental causes as: 1, pyorrhea alveolaris; 2, caries; and 3, apical and periapical infection, usually in the form of granulomas of the roots. Gillet[4] named infected vital pulps, apical areas, peridontoclasia areas, and impacted teeth as the four most common foci of the mouth to be considered.

Various estimates have been given for the frequency of ocular lesions resulting from dental infection, but it is safe to state that a fairly large number of eye infections occur in this way, even in the presence of other foci. The condition of the teeth should always receive careful consideration and examination, especially roentgen examination. Even when the latter is negative, the teeth cannot always be eliminated as a possible focus. Moreover, it should be unnecessary to state that the absence of pain is without diagnostic significance.

The method of infection of the eye from the teeth is not definitely determined, but several ways have been described, nearly any of which may account for different cases. These include transmission of organisms from the dental focus to the eye by way of the lymph channels and blood stream, extension through the upper jaw into the orbit or extension along the periosteum to the malar bone and involvement of the orbit.

The organism most commonly found as the cause of dental infection resulting in eye manifestations is the *Streptococcus viridans* and *hemolyticus*. Others may be found, however, including the *Staphylococcus aureus* and *albus, pneumococcus*, and *Bacillus pyocyaneus*. The laboratory proof of pathologic microorganisms in the affected eyes of those suffering from dental infection is not always found, but from the result of innumerable clinical observations, the close relationship between the two conditions must be recognized.

Eye Manifestations.—These may occur either in one or both eyes, although the former is more common. It has been already stated that almost any form of eye manifestation may occur. However, the uveal tract, including the iris, ciliary body, vitreous, and choroid, is most frequently involved by secondary inflammation.

It should be stated also that reflex disturbances may result from the presence of impacted teeth, the most common manifestation being the presence of almost constant pain in and around the eye and orbit. Visual disturbances and even amblyopia have been known to occur without visible evidences in the fundus of the eye. Other manifestations include blepharospasm, asthenopia, and occasional paralysis of the extraocular muscles.

Inflammatory manifestations of dental infection may occur in the conjunctiva as a conjunctivitis, either alone or in association with orbital cellulitis. The latter has been frequently reported as the result of dental infection. Orbital abscess may also occur from infection of the antrum produced by infection of the teeth.

Episcleritis is a rare manifestation of dental infection, although it has been reported on several occasions and its presence should suggest the possibility of a connection with some disease of the teeth.

Corneal involvement resulting from diseased teeth is somewhat more frequent. This is manifested by the presence of herpes and phlyctenules which are found especially in children, vesicular keratitis, dendritic ulcers, kerato-iritis, and even interstitial keratitis has been reported.

The uveal tract is the site most frequently affected by ocular lesions which result from diseased teeth. Iritis and iridocyclitis have been reported by different authors to occur from this source in from 10 to as many as 40 per cent of cases. The primary condition in most cases was found to be either periapical or apical abscesses, and also pyorrhea alveolaris. In some cases a focus is also found to be present in the nose and accessory sinuses at the same time.

The choroid is also frequently affected in the form of an exudative choroiditis. Because of its close connection with the choroid, involvement of the retina is nearly always associated. In three cases caused by diseased teeth, Wilmer[2] found one to manifest an extensive choroidal exudate which displaced the retina. With extraction of two infected teeth and treatment of the associated pyorrhea alveolaris, the ocular condition cleared up entirely. In another case, he found an extensive bilateral chorioretinitis of long standing with reduced visual and central field defects, all of which were considered to be due to the presence of several large apical abscesses. Extraction of the infected teeth and dental treatment were followed by improvement of the central and peripheral vision in both eyes.

Postoperative infection from the presence of diseased teeth is also not infrequent. This usually occurs in the form of mild iridocyclitis and hypopyon as manifested in Wilmer's third case which occurred four days after a descission of a lens capsule.

The author has also seen infection following cataract operation which was characterized by the presence of a mild iridocyclitis and hypopyon in the eye six days after operation. Examination of the teeth revealed the presence of two infected broken roots, removal of which was immediately followed by recovery of the ocular infection.

The optic nerve occasionally reveals the presence of an optic neuritis as the result of dental infection. The vision in the affected eye is reduced, and the blind spot is enlarged. Most of the cases of retrobulbar neuritis occurring with diseased sinuses and tonsils and associated dental disease are probably due to infection of the former, although the diseased teeth may contribute to the ocular manifestation.

Tonsil Infection

The tonsils merit serious consideration as a focus of infection in inflammations and infections of the eyes. A frequent and serious variety is streptococcal infection which may also be secondary to or associated with a focus in the teeth. Staphylococci are also found to be the microorganism responsible. The mode of transmission to the eye is probably by way of the blood stream. Chronically diseased or embedded and infected tonsils are always to be regarded as a likely source for endogenous infection of the ocular structures.

Eye Manifestations.—Statistics vary with regard to the frequency of occurrence of ocular disease resulting from the tonsils, but these range from as low as 6 per cent to as high as 26 per cent. The latter would appear to be extremely high, and in the opinion of the writer, the former is more nearly correct.

The ocular condition may manifest itself either in the form of a functional disorder or as a plastic or a purulent inflammation.

Functional disorders occur in the eyes as the endogenous effect of the bacterial toxins and include, principally, ocular asthenopia, weakness of accommodation, and weakness of convergence. These are usually all characterized by a tired feeling of the eyes, inability to perform any close work, such as reading, sewing, etc., for even a short period of time.

Conjunctivitis and corneal involvement are infrequent manifestations of a focus in the tonsils, although either one or both may occur in association with iritis and iridocyclitis. Conjunctivitis, when present, is usually of the recurrent catarrhal variety and is found in the presence of chronically infected tonsils. The margins of the lids are usually reddened, and the bulbar and palpebral conjunctiva is always moderately reddened and inflamed. A mild but annoying catarrhal discharge is present, which may clear up with the use of mild eye-washes only to recur after a short time.

The cornea is occasionally the site of a simple catarrhal ulcer, which may occur especially in children. It is usually benign in its course and situated near the margin.

Iritis and iridocyclitis are more common manifestations of tonsillar infection. The iritis is often the result of streptococcic infection in the tonsils and is sometimes called a streptococcic iritis. It may be found in association with inflammatory disease of the joints or with endocarditis. It may occur in the acute form, but more frequently as a chronic or recurrent iritis.

An acute attack of iritis, iridocyclitis, or even a full-blown uveitis may occur following trauma or intraocular operations in the presence of chronic infected tonsils, even in the absence of any such former attacks. A typical example of this occurred in the experience of the writer, wherein a uveitis characterized by sudden pain, marked pericorneal injection, dense infiltration of the vitreous, and marked reduction in vision in the right eye developed in a patient seven days after a muscle operation. In the absence of any other possible cause, the tonsils were found to be badly infected. With their removal and the use of an autogenous vaccine together with other local treatment, the condition began immediately to clear and went on to complete recovery.

Choroiditis and involvement of the posterior uvea may also occur as a manifestation of tonsillar infection. Although not common, this should be remembered, especially in the absence of other etiologic factors. The choroiditis is usually exudative in character and when found in the presence of diseased tonsils, the latter should be removed.

Endogenous panophthalmitis is extremely rare resulting from infection in the tonsils, but a case of this kind was reported by Van Fleet[5] in which it was necessary to enucleate the infected eye of a 2-year-old child. The conjunctival sac also revealed a discharge, the culture of which showed a growth of *Staphylococcus albus,* whereas that from the interior of the eyeball and the one from the tonsils revealed the same bacteriology, namely, profuse growths of *Staphylococcus albus* and short-chain hemolytic streptococcus pyogenes.

Optic neuritis of a congestive type may rarely occur as the result of tonsil infection. This may also be found in association with exudative choroiditis or chorioretinitis.

A slight papillitis and severe thrombosis of a branch of the central vein were reported by P. Knapp[6] in a woman aged 24, as the result of chronic tonsillitis. The tonsils were removed late, but this was followed by clearing of the retinal strands which were present.

Retrobulbar neuritis is a possibility from diseases of the tonsils, teeth, or both, but this is also extremely rare. However, acute disturbance of the central vision may occur in one or both eyes with inflammation of the optic nerve behind the globe for this reason. This is more apt to occur, however, when the nose or accessory sinuses are also infected.

Nose and Sinus Infections

Infections in the nose and nasal accessory sinuses are frequently manifested by ocular involvement. The latter may occur in almost any pathologic process affecting these structures. Ordinary recurrent "head colds" which usually indicate the presence of an infection in the sinuses may be accompanied by ocular manifestations. Subjective symptoms, such as frontal headache and pain in or behind the eyeballs, are almost constant complaints. An important differential factor with regard to such headaches is the fact that they may occur at almost any time and are often present on arising in the morning, and may not be relieved on lying down. Moreover, they have no direct relationship to the use of the eyes which is in contrast to headaches occurring as the result of primary ocular disturbances or primary asthenopia. They are usually localized in the frontal region and over the bridge of the nose and between the eyes.

Acute or chronic infections of one or more of the sinuses may reveal eye manifestations and a pansinusitis is very apt to be accompanied by some form of orbital or ocular involvement. However, chronic ethmoiditis and chronic sphenoiditis are probably the most common causes with the maxillary and frontal sinus infections following in rather close order. When it is considered that these sinuses lie in such close anatomic relationship to the orbit, with the sphenoidal sinus, for example, being separated in many cases by a wall only ¼ mm. thick, it will be readily understood why sinus disease is a common focus for lesions in the eyes.

Although sinus disease is very common, it is often difficult to determine the precise nature or condition of the sinuses, especially in the absence of an active purulent involvement, or when it is deep-seated, at the time of the ocular disease. The diagnosis must, therefore, be made by a laryngologist by clinical examination and such additional methods as x-ray examination, transillumination, and other available means.

Eye Manifestations: *Functional and Reflex Symptoms.*—In addition to those subjective symptoms previously described, as headache, pain in and behind the eyeballs, chronic sinusitis, especially, may produce certain disturbances of function in the eyes which are characterized by asthenopia, a tiredness of the eyes especially after a slight amount of reading, impaired accommodation, and weak convergence. The pain complained of behind the eyeballs is due to distention or congestion of the ethmoid cells or sphenoids. Infection of the antrum causes pain over the cheek bone radiating up to the eye, usually on the affected side. A not uncommon subjective complaint, especially with the onset of a severe acute "cold" or "sinus attack," is transient impairment of vision. This is usually of short duration and improves quickly as the acute attack subsides.

The Lacrimal Apparatus (Dacryocystitis).—The most common manifestation affecting the lacrimal apparatus as the result of disease of the nose or nasal mucous membrane occurs in the form of a chronic dacryocystitis. This usually results from an interference with the outflow of the tears and their drainage into the nose with subsequent inflammation and infection of the lacrimal sac. These tears at first collect in the conjunctival sac and flow over the cheek. In the different forms of acute and chronic coryza, the nasal inflammation may spread by extension to the nasal duct, the lumen of which might be closed by compression of the congested veins. Later, a cicatricial contraction of the mucous membrane will cause a more or less permanent constriction of the duct.

Ulceration of the mucous membrane of the nose, such as that which may occur in syphilis or scrofulous inflammation, may also lead to a chronic dacryocystitis.

Tumors, polyps, and other obstructions in the nose may also cause compression of the nasal duct and impede the drainage of tears with a subsequent chronic infection.

The diagnosis of dacryocystitis has been previously described.

The treatment of dacryocystitis which results from disease of the nose or nasal mucous membrane consists first in the treatment of the primary condition. If the latter is one that can be removed with relief of the compression on the duct, the dacryocystitis may clear up with mild treatment of the lacrimal sac by way of the canaliculus. The lacrimal syringe is employed to irrigate the sac with a solution, such as metaphen or mercurophen.

If the constriction of the duct cannot be removed by treatment of the nasal condition, the inflammation of the lacrimal sac becomes chronic and is characterized by the presence of a chronic purulent discharge which can be expressed from the canaliculus on the affected side by gentle steady pressure over the lower lid toward the inner canthus. The treatment of these cases consists in the surgical removal of the infected sac.

Occasionally, an acute lacrimal abscess may develop over the location of the sac during the course of a chronic dacryocystitis. This is characterized by the presence of an acute red swelling which is hot, tense, and painful. On examination, this will be found to fluctuate, and if permitted to remain, it may rupture spontaneously. Such an abscess should be incised and drained of the purulent material. A fistulous opening is thereby made with the lacrimal sac, which can be packed with gauze, and drainage permitted to continue until the fistulous opening is healed. It is then necessary to restore the permeability of the sac if possible, by removal of the constriction or surgical removal of the sac as already mentioned.

Conjunctivitis.—Acute and chronic forms of conjunctivitis are very common manifestations of disease in the nose and nasal sinuses. An acute conjunctivitis, characterized by redness and mild congestion of the bulbar and palpebral conjunctiva with "watering" of the eyes, invariably accompanies the onset of an acute coryza.

An acute or chronic catarrhal and sometimes mucopurulent conjunctivitis may occur during the course of any chronic sinusitis. The conjunctiva may also be affected, together with involvement of any of the other structures of the eye as the result of acute or chronic infection in the sinuses. This is characterized usually by redness and swelling caused by edema of the bulbar conjunctiva, and is seen nearly always in association with other ocular manifestations resulting from disease in the frontal sinus.

Inflammation of the Uveal Tract.—Disease of the nasal accessory sinuses is the cause of deep keratitis, iritis, iridocyclitis, and choroiditis in a small percentage of cases. These range anywhere from 2 to 8 per cent with various authors. Purulent infections in the frontal, ethmoid, or maxillary sinuses are the most frequent causes from this source.

Iritis and iridocyclitis may occur alone as the result of infections in the nasal sinuses, or they may occur in association with a scleritis or conjunctivitis. Choroiditis is a rare complication of sinus infection.

Optic Neuritis and Retrobulbar Neuritis.—Involvement of the optic nerve is an important consideration as the result of nasal sinus infection. In the course of such a consideration, it is not possible in the present state of our knowledge to make any definite statements as to the frequency of optic nerve involvement resulting from disease of the sinuses. In the past optic neuritis and retrobulbar neuritis were probably considered to be caused in this way much more than at present. Although opinions are still greatly divided, the tendency in recent years has been to subordinate the nasal sinuses as a cause of this condition. Volumes have been written and are still being written with regard to the etiology, but it is not necessary here to deal with the opinions of all of these. It is sufficient to state that sinus disease, especially of the ethmoids and sphenoids, is still recognized as a factor in the production of optic neuritis or retrobulbar neuritis, and a careful investigation of the sinuses by a competent laryngologist, employing all the necessary means, is indicated in nearly all such cases. It is even contended by some that such consideration should be given even in the presence of other possible causes. On the other hand there are those who contend that the optic nerve involvement is the manifestation of some other disease such as multiple sclerosis, even in the presence of sinus disease.

That the optic nerve may be involved by direct extension from the sinuses has been proved by the close anatomic relationship found between the structures in these cases. Moreover, the nerve may become involved as the result of an infection in the orbit having its origin in the sinuses, or it may occur from edema and pressure on the nerve resulting from the swelling in the sphenoid sinus.

Eagleton[9] described cases with optic nerve involvement and blindness resulting from fulminating cavernous sinus phlebitis arising from a pimple on the nose and nasal sinusitis, sudden blindness with whitness of the fundus from subacute cavernous thrombophlebitis, and exophthalmos with blindness and retinal vascular obliteration caused by nasal operation with subsequent contraction of the pupil.

The clinical symptoms of inflammation of the optic nerve depend mostly on the location and extent of the lesion. The presence of optic neuritis is characterized by early reduction and loss of the central vision of the affected eye. When the optic disc itself is involved, the neuritis will present evidences which can be observed on ophthalmoscopic examination. These include swelling of the nerve head similar to that which characterizes papillitis. The disc margins are blurred and cannot be outlined, so that it blends with the surrounding retina. The retinal veins are congested, and isolated small hemorrhages may be found on or near the disc. A moderate amount of edema and one or two exudates may be found in the retina about the disc. On examination of the visual fields, a central or paracentral scotoma is found to be present.

As the swelling of the nerve subsides, the vision may improve to some extent, but, in the average case, the condition is followed by atrophy with a corresponding impairment of the vision. The excavation of the disc becomes shallow and filled in with connective tissue and products of inflammation, with the development of the postneuritic atrophy. The retinal arteries close to the disc also reveal a thickening of the perivascular sheaths at this stage, due to the fibrosis which occurs as the result of the inflammation.

Retrobulbar neuritis, which is due to inflammation of the nerve behind the eyeball, may, on the other hand, reveal no evidences whatever, on ophthalmoscopic examination. The optic disc may appear almost normal and the only signs of the condition to be found are the loss of vision and the central visual field defect in the form of a central or cecocentral scotoma. The peripheral fields may show some contraction, especially later. The visual defect may last for some time, but a gradual clearing usually takes place after several weeks, with perhaps some slight pallor remaining.

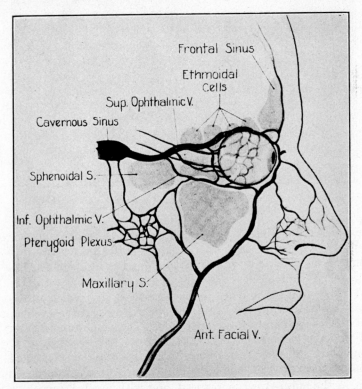

Fig. 181.—Schematic drawing showing relation of the venous circulation of the orbital cavity to the surrounding accessory sinuses, the brain, and the cavernous sinus. (From Cohen: Arch. Ophth., March, 1936.)

The treatment of optic neuritis or retrobulbar neuritis which is considered to be due in any case to sinus disease depends, of course, on the treatment of the primary condition. As previously stated, the sinuses should, in any case, be carefully studied in order to establish the etiologic factor. If it is then decided that such an infection is present in the absence of any other known cause, the operative treatment of such a sinus condition will merit the serious consideration of both the ophthalmologist and laryngologist, and can with all justification be decided on.

Orbital Involvement.—Inflammation of the sinuses may frequently involve the orbit. This results most often from disease in the ethmoid cells, since these are separated from the orbit by the lamina papyracea, which is a very thin wall of bone.

Purulent material which is present in the sinuses may produce an orbital cellulitis, suppuration in the orbit in the form of a subperiosteal or orbital abscess, retrobulbar phlegmon, and other complications. In most of the orbital affections the optic nerve is also involved in the form of an optic neuritis or retrobulbar neuritis.

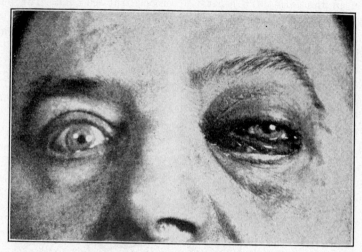

Fig. 182.—Inflammatory exophthalmos with edema, chemosis, and displacement of eyeball. (From Cohen: Arch. Ophth., March, 1936.)

The exophthalmos which is usually the most prominent symptom in orbital involvement from sinus disease was designated by Cohen[7] as "inflammatory exophthalmos" in which the venous circulation has an important part. The infection is carried to and from the orbit by the veins which are without valves. A marked congestion takes place in the orbital cavity which is accompanied by chemosis of the conjunctiva, swelling and redness of the eyelids, and protrusion of the eyeball on the affected side. The condition is nearly always unilateral, and the patient suffers severe headache, the temperature is elevated, and he may show signs of prostration. When the infection is marked, the eyeball becomes fixed in position, and often there is a paralysis of the ocular muscles. The vision in the affected eye is reduced, and with involvement of the interior of the eyeball, panophthalmitis may result. If the cranial cavity is involved by extension, a purulent meningitis or brain abscess might occur. Thrombosis of the cavernous sinus is another serious complication.

Acute frontal sinusitis often presents a similar picture characterized by swelling, redness, and edema of the lids and conjunctiva on the affected side. The eyeball may be immobile because of the swelling, and the patient suffers severe pain, elevated temperature, and prostration.

When the course of an orbital abscess has reached its height, it might perforate through the skin of the eyelid with the discharge of pus. This is then followed by a regression of the symptoms and ultimate healing.

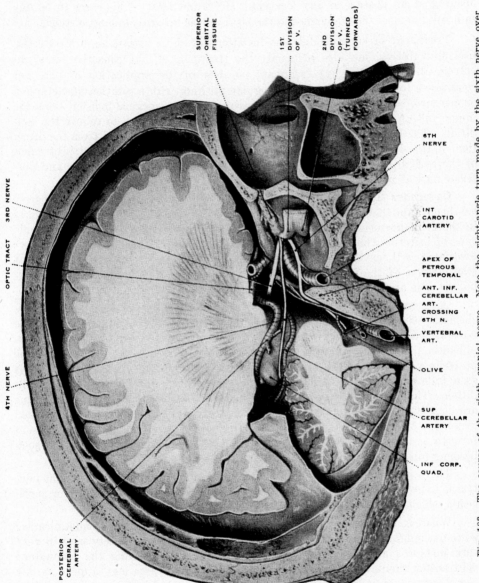

Fig. 183.—The course of the sixth cranial nerve. Note the right-angle turn made by the sixth nerve over the apex of the petrous portion of the temporal bone. (From Wolff: The Anatomy of the Eye and Orbit, The Blakiston Co.)

Gamble[8] described certain differences of orbital inflammation resulting from sinus disease in children as compared with that occurring in adults. These concerned primarily the small size, but active growth of the sinuses and the tendency to develop a blood stream infection from premature or even properly timed opening of an abscess in any location. He found most of his cases to be due to involvement of the ethmoids and the left eye was involved in most of them.

Treatment of such orbital manifestations of sinus disease, as orbital cellulitis and abscess, includes primarily the treatment of the causative sinus involvement. The local eye treatment consists in the application of hot, wet compresses to the affected eye and regular flushing with a solution of metaphen or mercurophen. In the presence of an orbital abscess, surgical incision along the inner wall of the orbit and drainage of the pus is necessary to relieve the condition. The location of an abscess in the orbit can be determined from the direction of the displaced eye. For example, a downward and forward protrusion of the eyeball would indicate the presence of the abscess in the upper and posterior part of the orbit.

Cavernous Sinus Infection.—The name of "protective retrobulbar space" has been applied by Eagleton[9] to the closed faciomembranous muscular space in the orbit posterior to the eyeball. This author calls attention to the specific type of infection characterized by those cases of orbital phlegmon almost always associated with cavernous sinus phlebitis in which the veins are the mode of transmission of the infection, and the vessels within the fasciomuscular retrobulbar cone are involved.

Cavernous sinus thrombophlebitis, characterized by swelling of the lids, chemosis, exophthalmos, and fixation of the eyeball may follow infections of the nose as well as those of the face and lip as the result of a diffuse thrombophlebitic phlegmon of the orbit. These infections reach the cavernous sinus posteriorly by way of the ophthalmic vein. The swelling of the lids which is soon followed by exophthalmos of any degree should call attention to the condition. The third, fourth, and sixth cranial nerves which pass through the sinus are usually affected with the presence of motor disturbances. There is a marked distention of the retinal veins, but only after other symptoms have been present for two or three days(Benedict[10]). The infection occurs on one side, but soon becomes bilateral, usually within forty-eight hours.

There is little or no tendency of the condition to improve, but on the contrary, it grows worse with the appearance of symptoms of meningitis or septicemia which results in early death.

Whereas these acute cases have their origin in the veins communicating with the ophthalmic vein, atypical infections of low-grade variety may in very rare instances arise posteriorly without necessarily involving the ophthalmic vein and without characteristic ocular signs. These cases may appear as late complications of sphenoid sinus disease or otitis media, the cavernous sinus becoming involved by way of the petrosal or posterior basal sinuses. Keegan and Ash[11] reported such a case of proved bilateral cavernous sinus thrombosis without characteristic exophthalmos or chemosis and with only unilateral third, fourth, and sixth nerve involvement. The left side revealed no external evidences and the inflammatory signs were of a low-grade variety. The left cavernous sinus was found on necropsy to be involved, while the right side was healed.

A meningeal abscess in the left temporal region was located, and the primary focus found to be an osteomyelitis of the base of the sphenoid bone.

Treatment of cavernous sinus thrombosis is limited and practically futile. Surgical procedures have been attempted, but with little hope of cure in nearly all cases. Eagleton[9] stated that a low-grade compensatory process may be cured spontaneously. He described evisceration of the orbit and removal of the outer edge of the superior orbital fissure, after which the sinus is located by a probe passed through the superior or inferior ophthalmic veins. The sinus is incised for removal of a septic clot, and a drain is inserted. The common carotid artery should first be ligated under local anesthesia.

Ear Infections (Petrositis).—Inflammation at the apex of the petrous portion of the temporal bone originating from infection of the middle ear with occasional swelling at this point occurs with pressure on the sixth nerve as it passes through Dorello's canal. This results in a paralysis of the external rectus muscle or abducens paralysis with pain in the trigeminal region on the affected side. This manifestation is known as Gradenigo's syndrome and is not uncommon because the nerve at this point changes its course almost at a right angle and lies in very close apposition to the petrous apex. A very slight swelling of these cells from inflammation may, therefore, produce pressure on the nerve as it passes here.

The condition may be present for a number of weeks in most cases during which time the external rotation of the eye on the affected side is limited and attempts to rotate the eye to this side are accompanied by diplopia. The pain in the region of the face supplied by the trigeminal nerve is caused by the associated involvement of the fifth nerve.

The prognosis for recovery is good in the average case, since function returns as the primary disease subsides.

Infections of the middle ear may also lead to involvement of the cavernous sinus by way of the petrosal sinuses. This was described by Eagleton[9] as a "more or less localized abscess surrounded by a limiting clot within a large venous radicle," and characterized by a low-grade compensatory thrombus progressing slowly. The exophthalmos and chemosis presented were described as being moderate or slight and transient in nature, since the venous congestion, which is the cause, quickly subsides. Eagleton also called attention to the fact that when symptoms of thrombophlebitis of a venous sinus are present around the ear, the appearance of chemosis or exophthalmos from pressure of a sandbag on the neck is diagnostic of cavernous sinus involvement.

Septicemia

Septicemia may result from almost any primary infection and may be due to a variety of organisms. Moreover, a patient who develops septicemia may be suffering with two or more primary diseases. It is, therefore, difficult and often impossible in these cases to determine whether the ocular pathology present is due to the septicemia or to one of the primary diseases. In many instances the eye lesions may be a manifestation of any one or all of the diseases, with which the patient suffers. This was clearly demonstrated by Friedenwald and Rones,[12] who described, among others, a case in which the medical diagnosis was hypertension, arteriosclerosis, chronic nephritis, syphilitic aortitis with aortic insufficiency, and streptococcus viridans septicemia. The ophthalmoscopic examination revealed a typical albuminic retinitis with extreme sclerotic changes in the retinal arteries and three yellowish elevations in the macular region of the right eye apparently beneath the retina. The streptococcus viridans septicemia was a terminal condition superimposed on a complicated disease background and, as Friedenwald and Rones pointed out, the inflammatory nodules in the choroid could be attributed to any of the primary conditions.

Eye Manifestations.—Septicemia alone may produce manifestations in almost any of the structures of the eye, but the more common are those which occur in the posterior uveal tract and which are presumed to be the result of infected emboli which are carried to the capillaries of the retina where they become lodged. Here they may lead to localized foci of inflammation or abscesses in the retina and choroid which characterize a septic retinitis described by Roth, and a septic choroiditis described by Friedenwald and Rones.

The latter described nine cases of chronic septic choroiditis due to a variety of organisms and diseases. The posterior segment of both eyes was involved by small metastatic localized abscesses which presented no typical clinical picture on ophthalmoscopic examination. Pathologically, they consisted of small lymphocytes in predominance, but large mononuclear cells resembling the transitional cells of the blood stream were also present in large numbers.

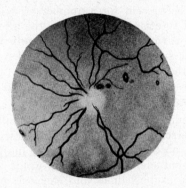

Fig. 184.—Retinitis septica of Roth. (After Doherty, from Duke-Elder: Text-Book of Ophthalmology.)

Periarterial inflammatory nodules similar to those described as occurring in periarteritis nodosa were also found in the choroid in septicemia, but the relationship to the other systemic diseases has not been definitely determined.

Septic retinitis described by Roth is a manifestation of systemic infections especially those resulting from endocarditis. It is presumed to be caused by the toxin of the infection rather than the result of infective emboli. On ophthalmoscopic examination, small, round, white patches which are often associated with small hemorrhages are observed near the disc. The hemorrhages may lie above or below the retinal vessels and resemble those which are found in the retina in leucemia, in that they have a white center. In cases of endocarditis the patches may disappear and then reappear later, while in other instances, they are transient in character. They are rarely found around the macula and were said by Roth to be due to hyaline or granular degeneration of the nerve fibers.

In other instances, acute localized abscesses may occur in the anterior or posterior segment of the eye which may spread to the other structures and soon involve the entire eyeball with panophthalmitis.

Lastly, metastatic involvement from a generalized septicemia may be manifest in the anterior uveal tract in the form of a purulent iridocyclitis with hypopyon, which is more or less chronic in nature and constantly recurs. This may go on for a long period of time and lead to degeneration of the eye and loss of vision. In other instances the posterior uveal tract may be involved by the infection which soon spreads to the vitreous with the development of endophthalmitis and ultimate loss of the eyeball. In the later stages, these cases often reveal the grayish reflex in the posterior eyeball resembling that which is seen in glioma and is often referred to as a pseudoglioma.

The prognosis and treatment of the eye manifestations of septicemia depend principally on the nature and course of the underlying condition. When benign in nature, the involvement may clear up almost entirely without serious impairment of vision or permanent damage to the ocular structures. In the more severe forms of ocular pathology characterized by the development of endophthalmitis, pseudoglioma, and panophthalmitis, the vision is permanently destroyed and the eyeball lost.

Uveitis With Associated Alopecia, Poliosis, Vitiligo, and Deafness (Vogt-Koyanagi Syndrome)

The presence of uveitis in association with alopecia, poliosis, vitiligo, and deafness is a rare condition of unknown origin, and one for which no specific treatment is available. It has also been designated as the Vogt-Koyanagi syndrome and is definitely accepted as a clinical entity. Parker[13] reviewed twenty-nine cases reported in the literature, including two of his own. The clinical picture was similar and striking in all. The condition is defined as a severe uveitis affecting both eyes and characterized by a rapid course, a grave prognosis and the association of alopecia, vitiligo, poliosis, and partial deafness.

The average age of the patients was 30 years with the youngest 10 and the oldest 52. Both eyes are usually involved simultaneously. It occurs almost equally in both sexes. In forty-five cases, twenty-five were males and twenty females. The visual acuity is greatly impaired but it may improve, the final result probably depending on the severity of the uveitis in the individual case. In all the reported cases it was reduced to the counting of fingers or perception of light, but 30 per cent of the patients recovered vision of $6/12$ or better. The uveitis has been thought by some to occur first and result in the change in the other pigmented structures by toxins which are formed. Others attributed all of the symptoms to one common cause. Syphilis and tuberculosis have at times been mentioned as the cause, but the former was found positive in only five cases and the latter has also failed to show any evidence of importance in connection with the etiology of the condition.

Alopecia and poliosis was present in all the cases reported. The loss of hair of the head usually occurs about two or three months after the appearance of the uveitis, although it has occurred as early as the third week. The bleaching of

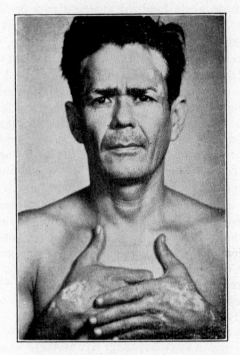

A.

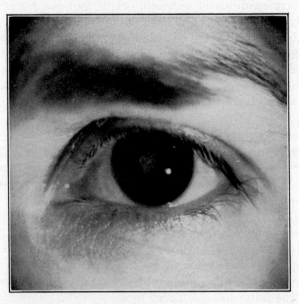

B.

Fig. 185.—*A*, Vogt-Koyanagi syndrome. Patient with uveitis, alopecia, poliosis, and deafness. Note the symmetric distribution of the lesions. *B*, Showing one eye of Carrasquillo's patient with atrophy of the iris, ragged pupillary margins, synechiae, cataractous lens, white cilia, and eyebrows. (From Carrasquillo: Arch. Ophth., September, 1942.)

the lashes and eyebrows is noted early but this is said to occur actually after the loss of hair. The new growth of hair is white but it was found to regain its normal color in 5 to 8 months.

The alopecia was described in general as due to an infection, a reflex neurosis or an endocrine disturbance. Alopecia areata or a patchy loss of hair is said to occur with the first two types while alopecia totalis or complete loss of hair characterizes the third.

Vitiligo was present in 70 per cent of the cases reported and was found to occur either at the same time or immediately after the appearance of the uveitis. It was seen in different parts of the body, especially the head, neck, shoulders, and lids. Although its appearance in this condition is significant, the nature of the cause is unknown.

Impaired hearing also occurs about the same time and was present in 69 per cent of the cases. In most of these it returned to normal. No satisfactory explanation for these symptoms is available.

The clinical appearance of this form of uveitis resembles that of bilateral sympathetic ophthalmia. No definite connection between the two has been established, however. Two cases referred to by Parker were examined microscopically. In one, Ogawa[14] concluded that the changes did not agree with those typical of sympathetic ophthalmia. In the other, Matsuoka[15] concluded that microscopically as well as clinically, the picture was the same as that of sympathetic ophthalmia. Several other investigators have attempted to explain the condition as a form of sympathetic ophthalmia, especially since most of the structures involved are rich in pigment. No conclusions, however, have been drawn on this basis. Carrasquillo[17] reported a very striking case together with a thorough review of the literature and a discussion of the theories concerning its origin and pathogenesis. From this and from his personal study he believed that a "neuropathic factor of sympathetic activity is operative in the production of the Vogt-Koyanagi syndrome."

The results of all forms of treatment have been found unsatisfactory. Parker treated his two cases with injections of foreign protein, large doses of salicylates and tuberculin without beneficial effect. The pupils failed to dilate with any of the mydriatics employed. An iridectomy was performed in one case and the iris was found to be adherent to the anterior capsule. Diphtheria antitoxin was administered by Luo (mentioned by Parker) in doses of 20,000 units daily for a week and once after the lapse of a week, with unsatisfactory result.

As Davies pointed out in reporting a case in a man 31 years of age, an attempt should be made to locate and eliminate a focus of infection.[16]

References

1. Pelouze, P. S.: Ophthalmologic Importance of Focal Infective Prostatitis, Arch. Ophth. 7: 372, 1932.
2. Wilmer, W. H.: The Relation of Teeth to Diseases of the Eye, Arch. Ophth. 4: 453, 1935.
3. Steinbügler, W. F. C.: Dental Infection in Disease of the Eye, Arch. Ophth. 4: 220, 1930.
4. Gillett, Henry W.: Infections of the Mouth and Their Relation to Diseases of the Eye, Arch. Ophth. 4: 228, 1930.
5. Van Fleet, J. F.: Endogenous Panophthalmitis Accompanying Tonsillitis, Arch. Ophth. 6: 426, 1931.

6. Knapp, P.: Periphlebitis and Endophlebitis Obliterans. Report of a Case, Klin. Monatsbl. f. Augenh. 93: 748, 1935.
7. Cohen, Martin: Inflammatory Exophthalmos in Catarrhal Disorders of the Accessory Sinuses, Arch. Ophth. 15: 457, 1936.
8. Gamble, Richard C.: Acute Inflammations of the Orbit in Children, Arch. Ophth. 10: 483, 1933.
9. Eagleton, Wells P.: Exophthalmos from Surgical Diseases, etc., Arch. Ophth. 14: 1, 1935.
10. Benedict, W. L.: Ophthalmologic Aspects of Cranial Sinus Thrombosis, Proc. Staff Meet. Mayo Clin. 5: 367, 1930.
11. Keegan, J. J., and Ash, W. E.: Bilateral Cavernous Sinus Thrombophlebitis Without Involvement of the Ophthalmic Vein, Arch. Ophth. 12: 72, 1934.
12. Friedenwald, Jonas A., and Rones, Benjamin: Ocular Lesions in Septicemia, Arch. Ophth. 5: 175, 1931.
13. Parker, W. R.: Severe Uveitis With Associated Alopecia, Poliosis, Vitiligo and Deafness, Arch. Ophth. 24: 439, 1940.
14. Ogawa, A.: Acta Soc. Ophth. Jap. 38: 38, 1934.
15. Matsuoka, H.: Zentralbl. f. d. ges. Ophth. 30: 520, 1933-1934.
16. Davies, W. S.: Uveitis With Associated Alopecia, Poliosis, Vitiligo, and Deafness, Arch. Ophth. 14: 239, 1935.
17. Carrasquillo, H. F.: Uveitis With Poliosis, Vitiligo, Alopecia and Dysacousia (Vogt-Koyanagi Syndrome), Arch. Ophth. 28: 385, 1942.

CHAPTER XIV

DRUG AND CHEMICAL INTOXICATIONS

Intoxications due to drugs and chemicals may occur in an acute or chronic form and in many instances produce eye manifestations. The latter may develop as the direct result of an acute intoxication and is illustrated by the contraction or dilatation of the pupils, paralysis, and spasm of accommodation, visible changes in the eye grounds and visual hallucinations occurring in aniline, nitrobenzol, or carbon monoxide poisoning. The eye symptoms also develop indirectly such as the retinal hemorrhages which result from the changes in the vascular structures caused by the intoxication. Often the eye manifestations are the result of an acute hemorrhagic or other form of nephritis which is caused by the accumulation of the poison in that organ.

Intoxication from poisonous gases often produces conjunctivitis, hyperemia of the conjunctiva, and often more or less reduction of the corneal sensitivity.

Direct eye manifestations, such as the miosis due to chronic nicotine or morphine, mydriasis in chronic belladonna, and the like, are not very common in chronic forms of intoxication. Symptoms, such as asthenopia, anemia, slight nystagmus, hemeralopia, discolorations, and the like, are not uncommon. Moreover, the symptoms resulting from chronic intoxication are sometimes aggravated by an added or intercurrent acute infection. Poisons which are different in their chemical structure often produce clinical pictures which are very similar, as illustrated by alcohol, tobacco, carbon disulfide, and lead.

Acetylcholine.—Acetylcholine is a white, hygroscopic crystalline powder which has a bitter, saline taste and is formed by a combination of acetic acid and cholin occurring in ergot. It possesses extremely poisonous properties. Cholin lowers intraocular pressure in small doses while larger doses raise the intraocular pressure.

Acetylcholine belongs to that group of drugs which have been designated pharmacologically as cholinergic drugs and have an effect in stimulating the parasympathetic system, and which are directly antagonistic to the adrenergic drugs which stimulate the sympathetic system. The action of acetylcholine is synergistic with such drugs as prostigmin and eserine which increase its effect, while such drugs as atropine or adrenalin would inhibit its effect. It is manufactured in the body in the interneuronic synapses and between the nerve and the cell. Clinically it is employed to lower blood pressure and as a vasodilator in such conditions as embolus of the central artery of the retina, increased intraocular tension, generalized vascular hypertension, and when it is desired to improve the local blood supply.

Employed to excess, it results in such symptoms as generalized flushing, sweating, and cardiac failure. In the eye it produces a contraction of the pupil, increase in the accommodation, and dilatation of the retinal vessels. A solution of mecholyl (acetylcholine) can be employed in the eye in concentrations up to 10 or 20 per cent with no general effect.

431

Aconitin.—Aconitin has the action of a local mydriatic and is used internally in certain neuralgias. Mydriasis resulting from aconite poisoning is only occasionally seen. Jerky movements of the eyelids have also been observed.

Alcohol.—The eye manifestations of alcoholic intoxication are numerous. In acute alcoholism the first symptoms appear after the early stages of excitement. These are characterized principally by incoordination of the pupil and impairment of the light reaction. Four cases of acute alcohol poisoning caused by ethyl alcohol were reported by Carroll and Goodhart,[1] which were characterized by total blindness in both eyes, normal reactions of the pupils to light and convergence, normal appearance of the fundus, and rapid recovery.

The manifestations of chronic alcoholic intoxication are probably more important. In the absence of other complications, the eye grounds may be quite normal in delirium tremens. The interstitial changes, effects on the nervous system, and changes in the vessel walls resulting in chronic alcoholism are of great significance in the production of the eye changes. The most prominent of these probably occurs in the form of an axial neuritis affecting the optic nerve, and which is designated as toxic or alcoholic amblyopia. It begins with symptoms of disturbed or fogged vision, usually affecting both eyes and gradually progressing. The vision may not be disturbed to the same extent, however, in the two eyes. At this stage, ophthalmoscopic evidences of the condition may still be lacking. The patients often complain of greater visual difficulty at twilight or in the dark (nyctalopia). A sensation of fluttering and spots before the eyes and colored after-images may also be complained of. At the same time the patient may manifest other nervous and gastrointestinal disturbances such as loss of appetite, loss of weight, nausea and vomiting, tremors of the extremities, and tongue. In most instances the patient gives the history of excessive use of tobacco as well as alcohol. Many of these cases are, therefore, regarded as a combination of tobacco-alcohol amblyopia, occurring in association with vitamin B and other dietary deficiencies. Five cases of toxic alcohol-tobacco amblyopia reported by Johnson[2] revealed the typical eye manifestations associated with vitamin B deficiency.

The decrease in central visual acuity is progressive and examination of the visual fields will reveal a central defect in the form of a central or centrocecal scotoma. This usually affects the form and color sense for red and green but, in more severe cases, may affect the perception of all central colors. At the same time the peripheral field of vision may be normal or only slightly affected. According to Traquair,[3] the character of the visual field is typical of this condition, while others, like Lillie,[4] claim that the same field picture is present as well in conditions such as multiple sclerosis and other intoxications. In the experience of the writer, similar visual field changes have also been found in cases of multiple sclerosis. Carroll,[5] in a report of fifty-five cases, found the centrocecal or cecotemporal characteristic of the scotoma to be striking. The centrocecal scotomas noted were much larger for red than for blue.

Examination with the ophthalmoscope reveals the outer half of the optic disc occupied by the papillomacular bundle to be pale and resembling the color of porcelain. The inner half is a dull red gray with margin slightly blurred and swollen. Anatomically, there occurs an interstitial inflammation and degeneration, especially affecting the papillomacular neurons and nerve fibers with inflammatory changes in veins and increased sclerosis of the vessels. The pallor of the optic disc is usually permanent, even though the vision may improve under treatment.

The changes in the retina and retinal vessels which are observed are not necessarily typical of this condition. They are characterized principally by the presence of angiosclerosis, hemorrhages, and exudates. These evidences are not unusual in amount and are not necessarily due to the intoxication, since they might also be found in any other group of patients of the same age and suffering with other conditions.

The prognosis is favorable with treatment of the condition when it is not of too long standing.

The treatment includes, first, the elimination of the use of alcohol and tobacco. This is replaced by an adequate diet, rest, and proper nourishment. In the past strychnine sulfate (gr. $\frac{1}{60}$-$\frac{1}{30}$) has been extensively prescribed. Vasodilators have also been employed.

More recently, however, the use of vitamin B complex in these cases has been found to be very effective. This can be supplied in capsule form or in the form of brewer's yeast. The vision usually improves to a considerable extent, and in some cases returns to normal.

Methyl Alcohol.—Methyl alcohol produces an acute intoxication and may cause complete blindness within twenty-four hours. It is ingested either by the mouth when mixed with other alcoholic drinks, or by inhalation of fumes into the lungs and through the skin. The two latter may occur among workers in certain occupations and industries in which it is necessary to handle the poison. In establishments where the fumes are plentiful, poor ventilation and aeration may add to the possibility of intoxication. Many cases of sudden or rapid loss of vision from methyl alcohol poisoning have been reported.

It is characterized also by the presence of such general symptoms as severe headache, abdominal pain, vomiting, delirium, convulsions, weak pulse, stupor, and death. The loss of sight is usually permanent when the patient recovers from the general effects of the poison. In more chronic cases when the poison is being ingested over a long period of time, the loss of vision may be gradual, and examination of the visual fields will reveal the presence of a central or paracentral scotoma and peripheral contraction.

On examination of the eyes the pupils are found to be dilated, and with the ophthalmoscope the optic nerve head reveals signs of a neuritis or papillitis with dilatation of the veins. The color of the disc may soon become pale or chalky-white. In more chronic cases the atrophy of the disc will follow the presence of a retrobulbar neuritis. In late stages the margins can be clearly outlined and the lamina cribrosa is plainly visible in the bottom of a deep excavation. Pathologically, there occurs an extensive degeneration of the ganglion cells and optic nerve fibers.

The prognosis is very poor for vision, and in chronic cases the pupils may remain permanently inactive; paralysis of the extraocular muscles and ptosis may develop.

Treatment of acute cases consists in the daily use of gastric lavage and attempts to eliminate the poison. Elimination and purgation by the use of hot drinks, hot packs, sweats, and pilocarpine are indicated. Large doses of alkaline solutions by mouth, the use of galvanism for stimulation of the optic nerve before atrophy occurs, and lumbar puncture have all been recommended.

Since methyl alcohol amblyopia is a form of toxic neuritis, the administration of large doses of thiamine chloride (vitamin B_1) may be beneficial.

Aniline.—Aniline is used in certain industries for coloring or dyeing and may cause eye manifestations of poisoning after absorption or inhalation. Intoxication is accompanied by headaches, general feeling of illness, tired feeling of the eyes, and some photophobia. Objectively, the patient may show a mydriasis, and occasionally pericorneal injection. On ophthalmoscopic examination, the disc is hazy; the retinal vessels are constricted, tortuous, and darker; the fundus is dark red in color, and some hemorrhages may be present in the retina. The visual fields may show a central scotoma and peripheral contraction.

The prognosis for recovery is good when contact with the chemical is removed. No further treatment than this is required.

Antipyrine.—Antipyrine may cause an urticaria about the eyelids and an increased secretion of the tears. Other manifestations are extremely rare, but transient amaurosis has also been noted.

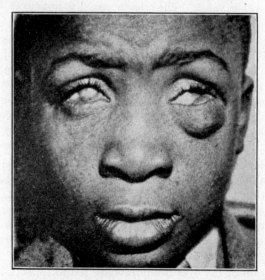

Fig. 186.—Opaque corneas and subconjunctival cyst due to arsenic poisoning. (From Hallum: Arch. Ophth., July, 1934.)

Apomorphine.—Pronounced anesthesia of the conjunctiva and cornea accompanied by a clouding of the cornea may occur very shortly after injection of apomorphine.

Arsenic.—The most prominent eye manifestations resulting from arsenic poisoning are those which occur from the use of preparations in the treatment of diseases such as syphilis. The normal optic nerve is very susceptible to damage in this way, while an already diseased nerve may suffer greater harm from their use. The eye symptoms may be the only signs of intoxication found and usually affect both eyes with rapid and complete loss of vision due to degeneration and atrophy of the nerve. It is, therefore, necessary in these cases to make frequent and repeated tests of the visual fields since a rapid concentric contraction of the peripheral field nearly always is present as an early sign. This is soon followed by an optic atrophy which can be observed on ophthalmoscopic examination. The visual acuity becomes progressively worse and may be totally and permanently lost.

Such general symptoms of intoxication as headache, dizziness, abdominal pain or colic, vomiting and nervous symptoms, may be present. Older patients are more frequently susceptible, and disease of the liver, kidneys, and cardiovascular system may prove a contraindication to the use of these drugs. Some preparations of arsenic are more dangerous in this respect than others. The trivalent compounds are considered to be comparatively more safe, but these may also produce blindness.

The continued use of arsenic in certain occupations and for treatment of certain other conditions may produce redness and scaliness of the skin of the lids, clouding of the cornea and vitreous, and a brownish discoloration of the skin similar to that occurring in Addison's disease.

An unusual case of bilateral corneal ulceration with a subconjunctival cyst in one eye was reported by Hallum.[6] The patient was a 7-year-old colored boy who lost the sight of both eyes following arsenic poisoning after eating peaches recently sprayed with an insecticide.

Atropine.—The use of belladonna or atropine is very extensive in the practice of medicine, and its action should be under constant observation. In excess, it causes a drying of the secretions, dry scratchy throat, rapid pulse, flushing of the face, digestive and nervous disturbances. It may also affect the heart and glands by the inhibitory action on the parasympathetic system. It is said to be synergistic in its action with the sympathomimetic drugs, such as adrenalin, ephedrine, paredrine and cocaine, and antagonistic to such drugs as acetylcholine, prostigmine, and eserine.

Instilled into the eye, atropine acts as a powerful mydriatic and cycloplegic and may also increase the intraocular tension. The same effects can also be obtained in a much weaker degree, by the internal administration of belladonna. When administered in excessive amounts over a long period of time, the internal use of belladonna may produce the same symptoms as atropine poisoning which are characterized by visual hallucinations, occurring especially at night or in the dark, mental and nervous disturbances, a dilated pupil with paralysis of the accommodation, congestion of the conjunctiva, hyperemia of the retina, and acute glaucoma.

The excessive use of atropine in the eyes may produce all of these acute symptoms and its instillation over a period of time may cause an irritation or a dermatitis around the skin of the lids.

The symptoms usually subside with the withdrawal of the drug and discontinuance of its use. This should be the first step in the treatment. To counteract the effect, morphine, pilocarpine, and eserine can be used.

Carbon Monoxide.—Carbon monoxide is a colorless, odorless, and tasteless gas which causes the bodies of those overcome to become very red, because of the carbon monoxide hemoglobin in the blood. Poisoning from carbon monoxide occurs commonly as the result of inhalation of gas fumes from the exhaust of automobiles with the motor running in closed garages. It may also occur from the inhalation of illuminating gas and gas fumes produced by furnace fires.

The symptoms are headache, vertigo, and rapid breathing. Apparently no part of the nervous system is immune to the poison. There is a predilection for the basal ganglia, causing lenticular softening, and also for the peripheral nerves. Parkinsonian syndromes and peripheral nerve palsies are frequent, and cortical involvement is characterized by mental deterioration and psychotic manifestations. Complete dementia may result.

The ocular symptoms include conjunctival injection, dilatation of the pupils, acute ophthalmoplegia, ptosis, progressive decrease and loss of central vision. Disturbances of the vision frequently affecting the color sense result from cortical involvement. The pupils and fundi may be normal, but hemianopia has been found after asphyxia with illuminating gas. Although the color vision is usually lost and peripheral vision is affected, Wechsler[7] reported a unique case in which the reverse occurred. In a 13-year-old boy who recovered from asphyxiation in a fire and who suffered cortical damage, the color vision remained normal while the vision was otherwise markedly impaired.

The treatment consists in removal from the source of the gas and supplying fresh air, oxygen, and giving artificial respiration when necessary. If the patient recovers, the eye symptoms usually clear up.

Carbonic Acid.—Accumulation of carbonic acid in the blood causes mydriasis because of sympathetic irritation. On ophthalmoscopic examination, the retinal vessels and fundus are found to be very dark in color because of the black color of the blood. Hemorrhages may also be present in the retina.

Carbon Disulfide.—Carbon disulfide is a chemical which is used rather extensively in certain industries, such as the manufacture of rayon materials and transparent paper. It is absorbed chiefly through inhalation, but also to a slight degree by the skin and alimentary tract.

The eye manifestations of carbon disulfide poisoning, which are usually associated with a peripheral neuritis, occupy a rather prominent position and include failing vision as an early and common sign. Photophobia and chromatopia (colored vision) are sometimes complained of before the loss of vision. The patient may see green, blue, or red. Nystagmus has occasionally been noted; the cornea may lose its sensibility. A variety of traumatic superficial punctate keratitis has been described in which the cornea becomes gray with small punctate elevations appearing under the epithelium which eventually break down. Healing takes place, however, with no permanent opacification.

The other eye signs are part of a systemic intoxication mostly affecting the central and peripheral nervous system. Impairment of accommodation, micropsia, macropsia, and monocular diplopia, with hysterical hemianesthesia and tubular fields, have been found. Amblyopia has been found in nearly 50 per cent of cases without necessarily revealing any fundus changes. A small, bilateral, central scotoma may be present which varies in intensity. There is also a slight peripheral depression of the visual field.

McDonald,[8] who examined 120 workers in a rayon industry, reported ocular complaints in about 75 per cent. These included diminished corneal reflex, pupillary disturbances, enlarged blind spot, visual field defects, optic disc changes, vascular changes, and nystagmus. The nystagmus was of a rotary type and was present on horizontal and upward gaze in about one-half the workers. Decreased corneal reflex was the most constant finding. The enlargement of the blind spot which had not been previously noted was found in ten cases who were considered to have a slight blurring of the margins of the optic disc.

Bromide of Potassium.—After the continued internal administration of potassium bromide, a conjunctivitis of a phlyctenular variety may occur. Large doses over a long period of time in the treatment of other illnesses may produce mydriasis in addition to the conjunctivitis.

Caffeine.—Caffeine is a weak mydriatic and has been said very rarely to produce an amblyopia similar to that caused by quinine.

Cannabis Indica.—Hashish causes symptoms similar to those of tobacco although more damaging. Visual hallucinations occur, disturbances of accommodation, mydriasis, fogged vision, and amblyopia. The amblyopia may affect only one eye, and the color vision may be unimpaired.

Chloral.—Chloral used as a narcotic causes a strong miosis, but after long-continued use, a mydriasis may occur. In some cases a skin eruption occurs which is accompanied by an irritation of the skin of the eyelids and a conjunctivitis. The vision is very rarely disturbed, although double vision and transient amaurosis have been observed.

Chloroform.—Death from the vapor of chloroform has occurred frequently. The fatal effect sometimes happens very quickly, in some cases from shock, syncope, or convulsions, while in others, from asphyxia. A very small dose at any time may prove fatal. When taken by mouth, the fatal effects of chloroform may be deferred.

In the early stages of narcosis the pupil is small, and the conjunctiva soon becomes insensible. Sudden dilatation of the pupils is a warning sign and in deep narcosis the pupils are dilated.

The treatment of poisoning after swallowing chloroform consists principally in the use of the stomach pump. When the poisoning results from inhalation of the vapor, the patient is given fresh air, artificial respiration, and carbon dioxide stimulation.

Chrysarobin.—Chrysarobin ointment rubbed into the skin may produce a conjunctivitis which is usually bilateral and sometimes associated with a keratitis. This is said by some to inhibit any secretion from the eyes, whereas chrysarobin which is accidentally introduced into the eye will produce a unilateral conjunctivitis characterized by intense lacrimation, photophobia, and blepharospasm.

Cocaine.—Subcutaneous injections of cocaine in ordinary concentrations may produce serious results in patients with an idiosyncrasy. Instillation of cocaine into the conjunctival sac may produce some local ill effects, but rarely if ever causes any general symptoms. On the other hand chronic cocaine poisoning may cause a large variety of symptoms, including eye manifestations.

Instilled into the conjunctival sac, cocaine in 4 per cent solution acts as an excellent local anesthetic. Its constant and repeated use in this way, however produces an edema of the corneal epithelium which is followed by clouding of the cornea and exfoliation. This may occur with the use of comparatively small quantities. It also acts to dilate the normal pupil and has a tendency to increase the intraocular tension. In cases of acute poisoning mydriasis is present and glaucoma has developed in the eye after long-continued cocainization of the nasal mucous membrane.

In chronic poisoning and among cocaine users, visual hallucinations are common. In addition, they may also suffer micropsia, double vision, and amblyopia.

There is no direct antidote for the drug, but drugs like mecholyl (acetylcholine), prostigmine, and eserine are antagonistic in their local action.

Cytisine.—*Cytisus laburnum* is a cathartic, diuretic, and emetic. Signs of poisoning are the presence of vomiting, cold sweat, weak pulse, and eye manifestations consisting of wide pupils, pallor of the optic nerve, and thinning of the retinal veins.

Digitalis.—In poisonous dose, digitalis may produce vomiting, purging, colic, headache, slow and irregular pulse, prostration, and coma. The eye manifestations are principally clouding and colored vision and mydriasis.

Dinitrophenol.—Dinitrophenol has been used extensively by women for the reduction of weight. As a result, many cases of cataract were reported in 1935 and later, among younger women in particular. These cases included two by Boardman,[9] three by Horner, Jones, and Boardman,[10] two by Cogan and Cogan,[11] one in a man aged 38, and the other in a woman aged 25; one case by Kniskern,[12] in a woman aged 37; one by Lazar[13] in a woman aged 44; one occurring in a woman aged 25, by Allen and Benson,[14] and others.

In nearly all of the cases, the cataract was bilateral and was discovered some time after the use of dinitrophenol. The development seems to occur from its continued use and is evidently an accumulative result. The condition could not be produced experimentally outside of the eye by exposure of the lens to dinitrophenol. It has been assumed that the change in the lens takes place as the result of unknown intermediary changes after the continued ingestion of the drug.

When the lens changes once have started, they usually continue rapidly to complete cataract formation. According to Horner[15] the earliest change consists of bilateral, faint gray, dustlike opacities just under the anterior capsule of the lens. The posterior subcapsular layers were described as showing a peculiar saucer-shaped granular metallic luster which he called a "cloth of gold" reflex. The vision at this stage may still be normal, but the lenticular changes soon progress very rapidly.

Treatment of this condition is operative extraction of the affected lens. Other forms of nonoperative treatment have proved to be ineffective.

Duboisine.—Duboisine is an alkaloid of *Duboisia myoporoides* and is similar to hyoscyamine. It is an efficient mydriatic, and in overdosage, it may cause an increase in the intraocular tension with the development of glaucoma. The local effect can be counteracted by the instillation of eserine.

Ergot.—Ergotine and other preparations of ergot cause a contraction of muscles and a constriction of the vessels. Continued and excessive use may, therefore, result in necrosis of the tissues. Poisoning may result in tetany.

Vascular spasm or contractures occurring with ergot poisoning may be observed in the retinal vessels on examination with the ophthalmoscope. A neuroretinitis may be present, and in some the disc may be pale in color.

Hemorrhages may occur in the retina as a result of continued cramp of the vessels. The resulting condition may resemble that seen in thromboangiitis obliterans.

The pupils are usually somewhat enlarged but react to light.

The development of cataract of the lens from ergot poisoning has long been recognized, and many cases have been observed. The condition has been attributed by some to a progressive impairment of nutrition due to long-continued cramps of the vessels and ciliary muscle, while others have considered it to be due to a toxic action on the capsular epithelium.

Eserine (Physostigmine).—Eserine is one of the most commonly used of miotics. It causes a marked contraction of the pupil accompanied by considerable ciliary spasm and sometimes pain. Its continued use in the eye over a long period of time may produce a marked irritation of the conjunctiva. It is employed in the treatment of glaucoma to reduce the intraocular tension.

Atropine is antagonistic in its action to eserine and is used to overcome the effect of the latter in cases of poisoning.

Ether.—Intoxication from absorption is very similar to that caused by alcohol. The eyes are fixed in position during ether narcosis and rather sudden dilatation of the pupils is a signal of danger. This is usually accompanied by pallor and venous congestion.

Eyelash Dyes.—Certain dyes which are placed on the market from time to time for beautifying the eyelashes cause eye symptoms among women, resulting from poisoning. In 1933, a number of cases of this kind were reported.[16] These included three cases by Horner characterized by a dermato-ophthalmitis due to the dye in lash-lure; a case of inflammation with chemosis and edema of the lids and conjunctiva from a chemical irritant was reported by Bourbon; a case of corneal ulceration following the use of lash-lure, which caused an intense edema of the lids with chemosis of the conjunctiva and epithelial involvement of the cornea and loss of vision (Farmer and Loomis); a case of conjunctivitis and dermatitis from lash-lure or eyelash dye (Jamieson).

In most cases of this kind the dye is applied without thought to any danger, but even with the utmost care, it will invariably affect the skin of the lids and conjunctiva. In my own experience the accidental spurting of an open tube containing a depilatory ointment caused a severe chemical burn of the cornea and conjunctiva in a young girl, with eventual loss of the eye.

Felix Mas (Aspidium).—The use of large doses of felix mas for the treatment of tapeworm has been followed by severe eye manifestations and blindness. The effect is similar to that produced by quinine poisoning. The intoxication may be manifested in the eyes often by a bilateral amaurosis which may be permanent and total, or it may manifest itself as a transient amblyopia one eye, and the fundus may show no evidences on ophthalmoscopic examina- with peripheral contraction of the visual field. This may also affect only one eye, and the fundus may show no evidences on ophthalmoscopic examination. In other instances the retinal vessels may be seen to be constricted, and an edema of the retina is present. In some cases the pupils are wide and fail to react. Several cases of bilateral optic atrophy with blindness have been reported.

Gelsemium.—Gelsemium is a powerful motor depressant and causes paralysis and loss of sensibility by its central action on the spinal cord. Poisoning produces vertigo, weakness, slow heart action, anesthesia, and paralysis of respiration. The eyes may manifest ptosis, diplopia, and dilated pupils.

Homatropine.—Homatropine is employed by instillation into the conjunctival sac and produces symptoms similar to those produced by atropine. Cases of poisoning in this way scarcely ever occur. Overdosage or long-continued use may result in prolonged mydriasis, paralysis of the accommodation, hysterical blindness, and attacks of glaucoma. The effect may be counteracted by the use of eserine or pilocarpine.

Hyoscyamine.—Hyoscyamine is the alkaloid of hyoscyamus which is ordinarily a feeble narcotic. In very large doses it causes vertigo, flushing, excitement, and a heavy feeling in the head.

The pupils become dilated; light flashes may appear before the eyes; diplopia and paralysis of the accommodation are present. Intoxication may lead to nervous symptoms such as delirium, hallucination, loss of speech, and loss of power in the limbs.

Iodine and Potassium Iodide.—Iodine causes pain and burning with catarrhal conjunctivitis. Cases of acute iodine poisoning have been observed with trigeminal neuralgia, characterized by pain and tenderness at the pressure points.

Chronic iodine poisoning as iodism may occur from the constant use of potassium iodide. This is characterized by irritation of the alimentary tract, headache in the region of the frontal sinuses, and an eruption of the skin which resembles that of measles or acne. Dryness and irritation of the throat are accompanied by a watery secretion from the eyes and nose and a redness of the eyelids.

The antidotes for iodine are starch and milk. The treatment should consist in producing vomiting by feeding with any starchy material such as flour and water, or milk. The further use of the drug should be discontinued.

Iodoform.—The local use of iodoform in surgical dressings has resulted in intoxications manifested in the eyes by narrow pupils and amblyopia without ophthalmoscopic evidences. Sprinkling a syphilitic abscess of the lid with iodoform has caused an erysipelatous-like swelling and blistering of one side of the face which healed when the drug was discontinued.

Lead Poisoning.—Lead poisoning may occur among workers in certain occupations, such as painting, plumbing, and others, where the lead may be ingested. It may also occur among children who handle toys or other playthings, or from drinking water which acts as a source of supply for the lead. Poisoning is characterized principally by the presence of severe gastrointestinal symptoms and colic accompanied by lead palsy. The latter is commonly manifested by the presence of wrist drop. Chronic or slow lead poisoning among workers produces a characteristic blue line or spots on the gums, a tendency to bleed easily, pallor of the skin, anemia, rapid pulse, obstinate constipation, and attacks of colic. Acute poisoning may produce an increased intracranial pressure with its accompanying symptoms. Late cases of poisoning may result in chronic nephritis.

The eye manifestations of lead poisoning are varied and numerous. In acute cases and in those with increased intracranial pressure as the result of edema and internal hydrocephaly, there may be paralyses of the ocular muscles and papilledema. Paralysis of the accommodation and unilateral or bilateral abducens or oculomotor paralyses may occur. Ptosis may also be observed.

On ophthalmoscopic examination the optic nerve head may reveal the presence of a unilateral optic neuritis. In other cases, there may be a disturbance of central vision from the presence of a one-sided retrobulbar neuritis. A so-called amblyopia may also occur without any visible ophthalmoscopic evidences. As previously stated, the presence of increased intracranial pressure will be evidenced ophthalmoscopically by a choked disc. With the occurrence of nephritis, a picture of albuminuric neuroretinitis may be presented, although albumin is not necessarily present in the urine.

Vascular changes in the retinal vessels may be observed with the ophthalmoscope. These are mainly a sclerosis and periarteritis, sometimes accompanied by the presence of hemorrhages. Secondary optic atrophy may result from any of the optic nerve affections.

The prognosis with regard to vision depends on the nature of the ocular involvement and on the extent of the poisoning. Recovery usually takes place in nearly all cases except those in which there has been considerable optic nerve atrophy and those in which serious kidney complications occur.

In the treatment of acute poisoning it is necessary to remove the toxic substance as soon as possible. This can be accomplished by lavage with sodium or magnesium sulfate. The salt of lead is thereby converted into insoluble sulfate. Milk, or milk and eggs, should be administered. An emetic or the stomach pump can be employed in the absence of vomiting.

In cases of chronic poisoning the patients should be removed from the source of ingestion. Aub, Minot, and Fairhill[17] recommended that the diet should contain a low calcium content, ammonium chloride (8 to 12 grams daily), or 10 doses of 20 to 25 cc. of phosphoric acid sweetened and diluted. In addition, 40 grams of bicarbonate of soda should be given to increase the secretion of lead. The use of milk and calcium lactate prevents lead symptoms among workers by storing the lead in the bones and thereby preventing its circulation and further damage.

Mercury (Hydrargyrum).—The mercurial compounds rarely cause eye symptoms. Acute poisoning by corrosive sublimate is similar to that of phosphorus poisoning. The principal eye manifestations are hemorrhages and degeneration of the retina. Transitory attacks of blindness have been caused by the use of gray salve. Workers in quicksilver may suffer a chronic intoxication resembling that of chronic lead poisoning.

Methylthionine Chloride (Methylene Blue).—Methylthionine chloride (methylene blue) is a dye which is sometimes used medicinally as an intestinal antiseptic and also as an analgesic in cases of neuralgia, sciatica, and other diseases. It is absorbed quickly from the intestinal tract and is excreted principally by the kidneys. Intravenous administration produces an increase in blood pressure. It is absorbed into the tissues in colorless form, but in the presence of oxygen it produces a blue coloring.

Gerber and Lambert[18] reported three cases in which the fundi were blue as a result of prolonged ingestion of methylthionine chloride. On ophthalmoscopic examination the fundus in all three cases revealed a greenish-blue color. This was considered by Gerber and Lambert to be due to the presence of the dye in the vitreous. This was observed at autopsy when they opened an eye of one of the patients who died. It was also noted that some of the other organs revealed the same color when removed and exposed to the air.

In one case the patient had been receiving six grains of methylthionine chloride by mouth, three times daily for a period of four years; the second received two grains by mouth three times daily for one and one-half years, while the third received two grains by mouth three times daily for about two years. None of the cases revealed any visual impairment or other pathology.

Morphine.—Morphine and opium are similar in their action, being employed therapeutically to relieve pain and to produce hypnosis and narcosis. A number of eye symptoms have been observed in morphine poisoning. First and most significant among these is a marked narrowing of the pupils. The subcutaneous injection of large doses of morphine is followed by contraction of the arteries observed in the retinal vessels. Visual disturbances occur and a condition similar to a toxic amblyopia may oppear, characterized by a pallor of the temporal side of the papilla. The visual field tests may reveal a concentric peripheral contraction or a hemianopia.

Barbital is employed frequently as a therapeutic substitute for morphine. Chronic intoxication from its constant use is not uncommon, and the ocular manifestations are similar to those caused by morphine.

Muscarine.—This is the poison of a fungus which sometimes contaminates certain foods such as mushrooms. The intoxication is characterized by a catarrhal condition of the gastrointestinal tract and disorders of the central nervous system. The principal ocular manifestation is a contraction of the pupils and paralysis of the accommodation.

Mustard Gas.—Mustard gas is a colorless, oily, heavy liquid with a faint odor resembling that of mustard. Its action is local and general, causing headache, nausea, and vomiting. The gas is very irritating to the skin and mucous membranes.

Eye manifestations of exposure to the gas are difficulty in opening the eyelids, swelling and edema of the lids and conjunctiva, and photophobia. There is a marked conjunctivitis due to chemical irritation.

In addition to the conjunctivitis, a chemical burn of the cornea may occur which is characterized by the presence of ulceration accompanied by marked photophobia and lacrimation.

The degree of ocular involvement depends principally on the period of exposure and the concentration of the vapor. The action is accumulative. The effect of the mustard vapor on the eyes becomes manifest after a period of from two to forty-eight hours following exposure. The action of the gas has been therefore completed before the patient receives any treatment. Prophylaxis is therefore an important detail in order to avoid contact. For this purpose gas masks are adjusted as soon as the faintest odor of the gas is suspected. Flushing with sodium bicarbonate and boric acid is recommended for the eyes of those who are knowingly exposed to the fumes.

Hughes,[19] in a review of mustard gas injuries to the eyes, described the treatment as largely symptomatic and prevention of complications. The patient should be reassured that he is not blind. Pontocaine 0.5 per cent can be instilled for anesthesia and examination.

The eyes should be irrigated for two minutes with sodium bicarbonate, 1.5 per cent; physiologic salt solution; boric acid, 2 per cent; or dichloramine, T 0.5 per cent in chlorinated paraffin.

Atropine, 1 per cent solution, should be instilled in cases with corneal involvement. In severe cases, either liquid paraffin, cod-liver oil with added sodium bicarbonate and dextrose or acroflavine in castor oil 1:15000 are recommended for use three times daily. The eyes should not be covered with eye pad or bandage.

Mild silver protein solution, 10 per cent, followed by boric acid irrigation three times daily and the use of zinc sulfate, 0.25 per cent, during convalescence are recommended.

Patients with severe cases may suffer relapses and after a period of years a degenerative ulceration of the cornea may occur. This was described by I. Mann[20] as a delayed mustard gas keratitis. The changes caused by the gas in general tended to self-limitation and spontaneous recovery, the final result being better than the condition originally suggested.

Naphthalene.—Although very few, if any, manifestations of naphthalene poisoning have been observed among humans, it has been used extensively for the experimental production of cataract in the eyes of animals. It produces a cataract in animals closely simulating the senile cataract occurring in humans. Opacities in the vitreous and retinal hemorrhages have also been observed.

Nitrobenzol.—Nitrobenzol or nitrobenzene is a product of coal tar and nitric acid and sometimes is used as a substitute for essential oil of almonds. The effects of the latter due to prussic acid come on immediately, however, while those of nitrobenzol appear in about two hours. Poisoning from nitrobenzol may cause a marked venous hyperemia of the retinal vessels with a darkening of the fundus that can be observed on ophthalmoscopic examination. The eye manifestations are similar to those caused by aniline. The visual fields may show a concentric contraction with reduction in vision Retinal hemorrhages and papilledema may occur.

Nitrous Oxide.—Nitrous oxide causes a widening of the retinal arteries and increased redness of the optic nerve head. A narrowing of the pupils occurs in a comatose state. The narcosis of nitrous oxide may bring pleasant visual hallucinations.

Optochin (Ethyl-hydro-cupreine).—Optochin is employed because it is considered to be specific for the pneumococcus. The manifestations of intoxication are similar to those caused by quinine, but optochin is more toxic to the visual neurons. Visual disturbances and cases of amblyopia have occurred from a toxic dose. There may be a considerable contraction of the peripheral field of vision and central scotoma may also occur.

Paradichlorobenzene.—Paradichlorobenzene is a by-product of the manufacture of trinitrophenol and is used to protect furs and clothing against moths. Paper wrappers and containers or moth bags to protect clothing are impregnated with the substance.

Although intoxication from inhalation of the fumes is a rare occurrence. Berliner[21] showed that when inhaled in sufficient quantities, it may produce toxic effects in humans and in animals. He reported two cases of cataract associated with jaundice and loss of weight in young women following inhalation and exposure to the fumes for a period of one and two years.

Picric Acid.—Poisoning from picric acid causes disturbances of color vision characterized by yellow vision and loss of vision for blue and violet.

Phosphorus.—Phosphorus poisoning causes early retinal hemorrhages which occur even before anatomic changes in the vessels are observed. Later, a degeneration occurs in the arteries and large patches are found in the retina itself which are visible to the ophthalmoscope and have the appearance of those seen in nephritic retinitis. Hemorrhages which occur in the optic nerve and brain may also cause eye symptoms.

Pilocarpine.—The instillation of pilocarpine into the conjunctival sac causes a contraction of the pupil. Taken internally, the miosis produced is very slight. It may cause an increased lacrimal secretion. Injections of strong solutions can cause an amblyopia, and cataract has also been said to occur.

Potassium Cyanide.—Potassium cyanide is employed by photographers and electrotype workers. Prussic acid poisoning has occurred from eating peach kernels and bitter almonds. The main symptoms are loss of reflexes, convulsive respirations, cold, clammy skin.

The eyes are fixed and glistening, and the pupils dilated and fixed. Hydrocyanic acid causes a clouding of the cornea. Potassium cyanide has caused enlargement and protrusion of the eyeballs. The upper eyelids become puffed and swollen. Transient hemianopia has occurred from the inhalation of prussic acid.

Quinine.—Eye disturbances resulting from large doses of quinine are not uncommon. Most of the cases occur among those who have suffered with malaria. Some individuals have an idiosyncrasy to quinine. The symptoms resulting are headache, ringing in the ears, deafness, delirium, stupor, and collapse.

The eye manifestations are diminished vision which is quite marked. The central vision may be affected, and there may be a concentric contraction of the peripheral fields with and without color disturbances. Hemeralopia may also occur. A final result may be optic atrophy.

Examination with the ophthalmoscope shows a pale nerve head and a narrowing of the retinal vessels. Considerable retinal exudation is present and may occur around the macula with the appearance of a cherry-red spot similar to that seen with embolus of the central artery of the retina.

The vision in quinine poisoning does not remain completely impaired, but the field of vision may be permanently affected. The temporary visual disturbances are probably caused by arterial spasm. A selective toxin action on certain nerve fibers or retinal elements has been advanced as the cause by Scardapane[22] who found a greater reduction in color fields with several cases showing a marked interlacing of the color fields and relatively slight damage to the macular region.

A patient with toxic amaurosois due to quinine who was successfully treated with intravenous administration of sodium nitrite was reported by Pelner and Saskin.[23] The patient had received 40 gr. of quinine for malaria and within four days the pupils were dilated and failed to react to light. A large area of edema extended from both optic nerve heads temporally and surrounded each macula. A cherry-red spot developed. The discs were pale and their margins blurred. The arteries were contracted and the veins dilated. Within two weeks after the intravenous administration of sodium nitrite solution there was a rapid improvement of vision to 20/30 in each eye, although the visual fields showed a 10- to 15-degree concentric contraction of the white field and slight pallor of the nerve heads remained.

Resorcin.—Conjunctival inflammation may result from the use of resorcinol ointment similar to that caused by chrysarobin.

Santonin.—Santonin poisoning is manifested in the eyes by the presence of yellow vision (xanthopsia). This occurs in about ten to fifteen minutes after taking the poison, while just before this, the individual sees violet. The spectrum shrinks with the violet, and one can no longer perceive the light rays in the retina. Besides yellow and violet, the patient also sees streaks and sparks. The pupils are normal and the central vision and the eye grounds are normal. The visual fields are unaffected, but the dark adaptation is retarded.

Silver.—After the long-continued use of silver, the eyelids and conjunctiva will become pigmented. The brownish color resulting is known as argyrosis.

The use of strong concentrations of silver nitrate in the eyes will cause a marked irritation characterized by secretion, redness, swelling, and edema of the conjunctiva and eyelids.

Snake Poisoning.—Snake poisoning may cause acute hemorrhagic diatheses, differing according to the kind of snake. Central or peripheral hemorrhages may cause disturbances of vision and of ocular movement. The optic nerve may be affected with partial loss of vision, or optic atrophy may result.

Strychnine.—Strychnine which is ordinarily used for the treatment of amblyopia does not cause any essential eye symptoms. The sense of sight may be stimulated, but in spite of intensive irritation of the vasomotor center, one does not find any marked effect on the pupils.

The spasms occurring in strychnine poisoning may also affect the muscles of the face and eyelids. Arterial cramps in acute strychnine poisoning may lead to nephritis with resulting evidences in the retina of the eye.

Sodium Salicylate.—The effects of large and continued doses of sodium salicylate resemble those produced by quinine. This is true also of the visual disturbances, especially those affecting the visual fields. These disturbances are of short duration, however, and soon clear up. In the absence of kidney involvement, the ophthalmoscopic examination is negative. Burning of the lids and edema with eruption on the skin have been observed. Reddening and edema of the conjunctiva and miosis have also occurred, but cleared up after discontinuing the use of the drug.

Sulfide of Hydrogen.—The eye manifestations of poisoning by hydrogen sulfide are mydriasis, exophthalmos, loss of corneal sensitivity and of the corneal reflexes.

Sulfonal.—The cumulative effect of the use of drugs in this group results in ptosis, visual disturbances and hallucinations, paralysis of the ocular muscles, and diplopia.

Thallium.—Thallium sulfate and acetate are found in preparations which are marketed as depilatories and cosmetics. Symptoms of thallium poisoning are characterized by symptoms of the gastrointestinal tract and peripheral nerves.

The eye manifestations of acute or chronic thallium poisoning are due mostly to involvement of the optic nerve and pathologic change in the pathway. This is characterized by the presence of an optic neuritis, retrobulbar neuritis, and subsequent optic atrophy. The visual fields will present a bilateral central scotoma, and the visual acuity may be permanently impaired.

Other eye manifestations observed are conjunctivitis, blepharitis, ptosis, strabismus, mydriasis, and cataract.

Experimental evidences were produced in animals by Swab[24] which showed pathologic change in every part of the visual pathway, including even the cortex of the occipital lobe.

Tobacco.—Nicotine and tobacco after long-continued use, either alone or in association with alcohol, may cause visual impairment. This occurs in the form of an amblyopia similar to that described for alcohol. It usually affects both eyes, and is equally common among men and women. The visual impairment is characterized by central blindness as the result of involvement of the papillomacular bundle in the optic nerve. The visual field defect is manifested by a central or cecocentral scotoma in each eye. In ordinary cases there may be no ophthalmoscopic evidences visible, but in later stages, a pallor of the temporal side of each nerve head may be observed. The condition is also characterized by the presence of other symptoms, such as loss of appetite, irritation of the mucous membranes, and disturbances of the central nervous system.

The treatment consists in the complete abstinence from the use of tobacco and removal from the influence of nicotine. Fresh air, a nourishing diet, and vitamin B should be supplied, and in marked cases, strychnine and vasodilators have been prescribed.

Trichlorethylene.—Trichlorethylene is used in certain industries for dissolving rubber, tar, pitch, and in certain cleansing fluids. It may produce poisoning by being absorbed through the skin and also by inhalation over a long period of time.

In the eye it may produce alterations in the pupil with loss of light reflex and affections of the optic nerve characterized principally by a bilateral retrobulbar neuritis with the loss of central vision. The condition is similar to a tobacco amblyopia, and with secondary optic atrophy occurring, it offers a poor prognosis.

Other Physico-Chemical Agents.—The eye may be affected by certain external influences and physico-chemical agents, such as direct exposure to extremes of sunlight and artificial light, direct exposure to extreme heat in certain occupations, x-rays, radium, and electricity.

Direct exposure to extremes of heat will produce a conjunctivitis characterized by a burning sensation of the eyes, redness and chemosis of the conjunctiva, and swelling of the eyelids. The cornea may suffer from the presence of a keratitis and among furnace workers in certain occupations, cataract has been known to occur.

Exposure to direct sunlight or arc lamps for a period of time, without the use of smoked glasses or goggles, may result in a conjunctivitis which is characterized by redness, swelling, and edema of the bulbar conjunctiva and puffiness of the eyelids. A temporary visual disturbance may result in the presence of a central scotoma or blind spot in the vision.

A solar retinitis has been known to occur after looking directly at the sun or observing an eclipse of the sun without smoked glasses. Although vision in mild cases is only temporarily affected, it may be permanently impaired.

Workers in certain occupations, such as electrowelders, and those who work with acetylene torches, are exposed to brilliant light from which the eyes should be protected by the use of goggles. In the absence of this protection, a severe conjunctivitis may result after a short exposure. The retina also may be affected by the ultraviolet and other rays which penetrate the eyes, which after a period of time may result in retinitis. The visual acuity for distance may not be permanently impaired, but visual defects with metamorphopsia will result.

Exposure to x-ray and radium may produce a retinitis characterized by the appearance of small white patches near the disc and some pigmentation of the periphery of the fundus. Radium has caused preretinal hemorrhages and overexposure to x-ray and radium may produce cataract.

Electric shock resulting from the passage of high voltage current through the body may produce cataract. Holloway[25] reported a case of bilateral complete cataracts which occurred in a 14-year-old boy, six months after an electric shock.

References

1. Carroll, Frank D., and Goodhart, Robert: Acute Alcoholic Amaurosis, Arch. Ophth. 20: 797, 1938.
2. Johnson, Lorand V.: Alcohol-Tobacco (Toxic) Amblyopia Treated With Thiamin Chloride, Arch. Ophth. 21: 602, 1939.
3. Traquair, H. M.: An Introduction to Clinical Perimetry, St. Louis, 1933, The C. V. Mosby Co.
4. Lillie, W. I.: Am. J. Ophth. 17: 110, 1934.
5. Carroll, Frank D.: Analysis of Fifty-Five Cases of Tobacco-Alcohol Amblyopia, Arch. Ophth. 14: 421, 1935.
6. Hallum, Alton V.: Involvement of the Cornea in Arsenic Poisoning, Arch. Ophth. 12: 93, 1934.
7. Wechsler, Israel S.: Partial Cortical Blindness With Preservation of Color Vision, Arch. Ophth. 9: 95, 1933.
8. McDonald, Robb: Carbon Disulphide Poisoning, Arch. Ophth. 20: 839, 1938.
9. Boardman, W. W.: Rapidly Developing Cataracts After Dinitrophenol, J. A. M. A. 105: 108, 1935.
10. Horner, W. D., Jones, R. B., and Boardman, W. W.: Cataracts Following Dinitrophenol. J. A. M. A. 105: 109, 1935.

11. Cogan, D. G., and Cogan, F. C.: Dinitrophenol Cataract, J. A. M. A. 105: 793, 1935.
12. Kniskern, J. A.: Cataracts Following Dinitrophenol, J. A. M. A. 105: 794, 1935.
13. Lazar, N. K.: Cataract Following the Use of Dinitrophenol, J. A. M. A. 105: 794, 1935.
14. Allen, T. D., and Benson, V. M.: Late Development of Cataract Following the Use of Dinitrophenol About a Year Before, J. A. M. A. 105: 795, 1935.
15. Horner, Warren D.: Cataract Following Dinitrophenol Treatment for Obesity, Arch. Ophth. 16: 447, 1936.
16. Horner, C. E.:
Bourbon, O. P.:
Farmer, A. G., and Loomis, E. C.: } J. A. M. A. 101: 1558-1560, 1933.
Jamieson, R. C.:
17. Aub, Minot, and Fairhill: J. A. M. A. 83: 588, 1924.
18. Gerber, Alexander, and Lambert, Robert K.: Blue Appearance of the Fundus Caused by Prolonged Ingestion of Methylthionine Chloride, Arch. Ophth. 16: 443, 1936.
19. Hughes, William F., Jr.: Mustard Gas Injuries to the Eyes, Arch. Ophth. 27: 582, 1942.
20. Mann, I.: Mustard Gas Lesions of the Eyes, Brit. M. J. 1: 353, 1942.
21. Berliner, Milton L.: Cataract Following the Inhalation of Paradichlorobenzene Vapor, Arch. Ophth. 22: 1023, 1939.
22. Scardapane, F.: Blindness and Amblyopia From Quinine, Sagga. di oftal. 5: 62, 1930.
23. Pelner, L., and Saskin, J.: Toxic Amaurosis Due to Quinine: Treatment With Sodium Nitrite Administered Intravenously, J. A. M. A. 119: 1175, 1942.
24. Swab, Charles Marion: Ocular Lesions Resulting From Thallium Acetate Poisoning as Determined by Experimental Research, Arch. Ophth. 12: 547, 1934.
25. Holloway, T. B.: Electric Cataract, Am. J. Ophth. 13: 595, 1930.

CHAPTER XV

DISEASES OF THE CARDIOVASCULAR SYSTEM

Diseases of the cardiovascular system here include the cardiac diseases which reveal prominent eye manifestations and diseases of the circulatory system, such as arteriosclerosis, vascular hypertension, certain diseases of the peripheral vessels, and renal disease. The close relationship which exists between nearly all of these conditions results in many cases in the presence of more than one at the same time. Then again, the prolonged presence of one condition often leads to the presence of another, as can be seen in the development of cardiac or coronary disease after an essential hypertension of long standing. Hypertensive vascular disease also leads eventually to renal disease and the two conditions are coexistent. In some cases the general vascular system may be more seriously affected by the disease while in others the vascular system of special structures, such as the brain or kidneys, may be the more seriously affected. The clinical picture presented therefore varies principally according to the organs or parts which are more seriously involved by the diseased process.

Since the retinal vessels are considered as terminal branches of the general vascular system, they are frequently affected by the same changes which affect other vessels, so that eye manifestations may be found in the presence of hypertension, arteriosclerosis, and kidney disease. For the same reason, the appearance and condition of the retina and the retinal vessels may be of important diagnostic and prognostic significance in some forms of cardiac disease and other diseases of the circulatory system.

Arteriosclerosis.—Since generalized arteriosclerosis is met with so frequently, especially in association with one or more of the related conditions mentioned, it is apparently responsible for many of the changes which occur in the organs affected. Clinically arteriosclerosis is often associated with intoxication and infection (including syphilis and nephritis), senility, and hypertension. The arteries are involved by a hyperplasia, fibrosis, and degeneration of their walls. As a result of the pathologic changes, the arteries lose their elasticity and become more or less rigid and tortuous. Weakening of the arterial wall may occur, leading to rupture. In the smaller vessels proliferation of the intima may so narrow the lumina as to cause complete obliteration. When the arteriosclerosis is secondary to hypertension, the smaller arteries and arterioles are involved. A hyperplasia of the intima and hypertrophy of the media are, therefore, more likely to be found here than degenerative changes.

Eye Manifestations.—Sclerosis of the retinal arteries occurs in association with generalized arteriosclerosis, but it may also occur in the retinal vessels alone. The structural changes resulting have been previously described in detail. These changes may be divided into two stages: 1. Arteriosclerosis of the retinal vessels alone, and 2. Arteriosclerosis of the vessels with additional changes in the retina itself.

The changes in the arteries include alterations in their course with increased tortuosity; alteration in caliber, either along the entire length or in certain portions which results in "beading," alterations in reflection, with increased distinctness of the central light streak, loss of translucency so that it is impossible to see an underlying vein at the point of crossing, whitish stripes on the side of the vessel indicative of degeneration of the walls or infiltration of perivascular lymph sheaths, and increased pallor of the arteries leading to a "silver-wire" appearance.

The retinal veins may show alterations similar to those of the arteries with added alternate contractures and dilatations resulting in "beading." An important sign is venous compression where a vein is crossed by a diseased artery. The thickened walls of the artery produce pressure on the underlying vein so that its caliber is restricted and an ampulliform dilatation is present beyond the point of crossing. Alterations in the form of varicosities may be found.

In arteriosclerosis of the retinal vessels the neural elements of the retina are not involved. The arteries appear narrower than usual in relation to the veins. The walls of the arteries and later the veins become visible due to atheromatous deposits and they appear as if ensheathed in a gray veil. The condition is a patchy one, affecting some vessels while others remain normal in appearance. In this stage of the process the blood supply of the retina may still be adequate so that the retina itself will show no changes and the vision is practically unaffected. The blood pressure is slightly elevated or normal, and the urine may show a faint trace of albumin. The blood chemistry is usually normal.

In the more advanced stages of the process, the blood supply to certain portions of the retina becomes inadequate, and now changes may be found in the retina itself. These are characterized by the appearance of grayish opacities near the optic disc or along the vessels, a brick-red congestion of the disc with blurred margins, and hemorrhages in the form of linear or streaked extravasations along the vessels in the nerve fiber layer, or round hemorrhages scattered over the fundus in the deeper layers.

The hemorrhages either absorb leaving areas of retinal atrophy covered with granular pigment, or organization occurs which results in the appearance of round, white plaques. Other white plaques may appear as the result of lipoid infiltration and degeneration from the lack of blood supply. They are common about the disc and macular region. This condition is also a patchy process with involvement of certain areas of one or both eyes, while other areas are unaffected. In this stage of the process the patients are more apt to show elevation of blood pressure and evidences of renal involvement.

Senile Arteriosclerosis.—The degeneration which takes place with oncoming age is manifested by a diffuse atherosclerosis. This usually becomes more pronounced at about the fifth decade of life. The degree of sclerosis may be far in advance of the changes in the organs and tissues. The blood pressure is usually normal. The ocular manifestations are therefore very minor or absent. Perhaps the only changes seen are those which affect the retinal vessels and these are characterized by a dull light streak and pallor. due to translucency. This is followed later by increased tortuosity, constric-

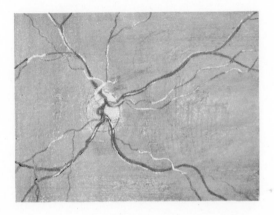

Fig. 187.—Drawing showing changes in advanced arteriosclerosis. Marked tortuosity of vessels and silver wire arteries. (From Tassman: Medical World, October, 1936.)

tion, copper-wire appearance, sheathing of the walls, and compression of the veins. In the absence of other complications such as hypertension and complete obstruction of the lumen of the vessels in well advanced cases, no other changes in the retina may be found.

Obstruction of the central vein of the retina or one of its branches may occur occasionally in advanced arteriosclerosis in older patients, especially those who suffer also with valvular heart disease. This is characterized by a sudden loss of a great part or all of the vision. Usually only one eye is affected. Ophthalmoscopic examination will reveal the presence of distended, tortuous veins and numerous large hemorrhages which cover the retina. Many of the larger hemorrhages occur close to the disc which may be obscured. Some of the hemorrhages may clear up after a while but others will appear. Secondary glaucoma may be a complication.

In many older patients with generalized arteriosclerosis, either moderate or advanced, cataract is prone to develop. This usually occurs in both eyes although it may progress more rapidly in one than in the other with a corresponding reduction of the vision. When the cataract has reached the stage of maturity it can be removed by operation, even in the presence of the arteriosclerosis.

Vascular Hypertension.—Hypertension may be present in several different forms. First, it may occur alone as essential hypertension without arteriosclerotic changes. Secondly, a persistent hypertension will result in a diffuse arteriosclerosis, or the hypertension may eventually develop in a patient with arteriosclerosis.

Hypertension is characterized essentially by a progressive and constant elevation of the blood pressure. The exact cause of the production of the increased blood pressure is not known but it is considered to be in the nature of a vascular response to some basic disorder, either toxic, glandular or other disturbance, which results in stimulation and increased vasomotor activity.

The earliest vascular response is a functional tonic contraction of the walls of the vessel. This may occur for a long period of time in the presence of an elevated blood pressure without sclerosis. On the other hand the presence of the underlying cause over a period of time causes the high blood pressure to persist with the result that further changes occur in the peripheral vessels and the development of a diffuse arteriosclerosis.

The increased systolic pressure gives an indication of the cardiac action while the diastolic pressure gives more of an indication of the state of the vessels. The higher the diastolic pressure, the more serious is the effect on vessels, with a grave outlook, while the high systolic pressure indicates only a good cardiac response.

Essential or benign hypertension may be present alone for some time and does not necessarily produce severe symptoms. It usually occurs in people of middle age and later life. After a time, however, the changes in the vessels lead to the presence of arteriosclerosis which is accompanied by more pronounced symptoms and signs. While the vascular signs of essential hypertension may be only negligible, it is often difficult to differentiate between the picture of diffuse atherosclerosis alone and that found in association with hypertension.

In simple hypertension one of the earliest signs is a spasm of the arterial walls. This leads after a while to further changes in the vessels.

In arteriosclerosis with hypertension the arteries are definitely constricted and narrowed. Another important change is the branching of the arteries at a more acute angle. In more advanced cases the retinal picture is one of arteriosclerotic retinopathy, which is characterized by the presence of hemorrhages, exudates, and other retinal lesions previously described. Both eyes are usually affected although not necessarily to the same degree. The vision may not be greatly impaired until the later stages of the disease.

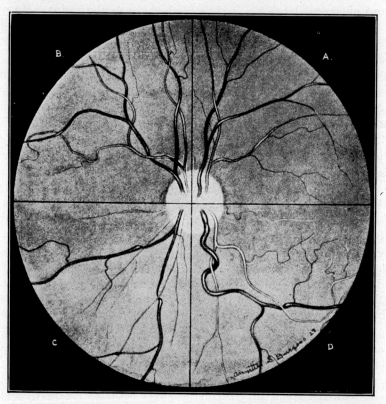

Fig. 188.—The vessels in arteriosclerosis and hypertension. *A*, Normal. *B*, Atherosclerosis without hypertension—beading, visibility of arteries, moderate arteriovenous compression, normal arterioles. *C*, Arteriosclerosis with hypertension—straight constricted arteries, branching at acute angles, variations in caliber, marked arteriovenous constriction. *D*, Arteriosclerosis—full, tortuous copper wire arteries, branching at right angles, moderate constriction, arterioles showing irregular tortuosity, fine caliber variations, visibility of walls and silver wire changes. (From Friedenwald: Tr. Ophth. Soc.)

Malignant hypertension may develop in some instances from a previous essential hypertension. More typically, however, it appears rather suddenly in younger patients as the result of a toxic condition. Both eyes are affected and it is characterized by diffuse and marked constriction of the retinal arteries. A swelling of the optic nerve head takes place which may be very marked and resembles the papilledema occurring with brain tumors. The swelling, however, is not dependent on a rise of intracranial pressure, although the latter condition may also be present. There is also present an edema of the disc and retina with numerous superficial hemorrhages and "cotton-wool" exudates. These are scattered about the fundus and together with a star-shaped figure in the macula, the picture resembles very much that which is seen in nephritic retinitis. Renal failure is not necessarily present, however, although in the terminal stage nephritis develops. The prognosis is very grave; the blood pressure may reach a systolic of 300 and a diastolic of 150, or over, and there is nitrogen retention. These cases are of a fulminating type and die within a period of about two years from uremia or convulsions. It is very difficult to differentiate clinically between the signs of glomerulonephritis and this variety of hypertension. The history of the case, however, may aid in separating the two conditions and ophthalmo-scopically, the retinal vessels reveal the presence of angiospasm and arterio-sclerotic changes of a former essential hypertension. (See Nephritis.)

Valvular Heart Disease.—Endocarditis is probably known best of the cardiac diseases because of the possible occurrence of a typical eye manifestation resulting from obstruction of the central retinal artery or one of its branches. This may be caused in younger patients by an embolus which is carried to the eye through the circulation. In older patients with arteriosclerosis the condition may result from thrombosis.

The obstruction of the central artery of the retina usually occurs in only one eye and is accompanied by the sudden loss of all vision. If only a branch of the central artery is occluded, the loss of vision is incomplete.

The ophthalmoscopic picture of embolism of the central artery of the retina is typical with the appearance of a "cherry-red" spot in the macula which is surrounded by a rather large white area. The retinal arteries are very narrow, and the optic disc is found to be pale in color which later becomes more pronounced. The red spot in the macula disappears slowly after a time.

The prognosis for recovery of vision in the affected eye is poor. Only in cases where a cilioretinal vessel is present, the blood supply may not be completely cut off. When only a branch of the central artery has been obstructed, the visual loss may be partial and will depend on the area of the retina supplied by the obstructed vessel.

The local treatment of these cases is rather limited. In addition to confining a cardiac patient of this kind to bed and enforcing complete rest, an attempt can be made to dislodge the embolus by the use of vasodilatation. If the patient is seen early, the chances for satisfactory results are much better. Such drugs as amyl nitrite, nitroglycerin, acetylcholine, and other vasodilators can be administered. If the case is not seen immediately, however, the chances for drug treatment to be effective are very remote.

Subacute bacterial endocarditis as it affects the eyes was described in detail by Dienst and Gartner[1] who referred to these manifestations as the "ocular syndrome of subacute bacterial endocarditis." This designation takes into consideration the neuritis, papillitis and choroiditis which were referred to as important features.

The disease itself is insidious in onset and after running a protracted course, usually terminates fatally. It is accompanied by anemia, progressive weakness and irregular elevations of temperature. A bacteremia occurs at times with a positive blood culture. Nonhemolytic streptococci of the viridans type occur in about 90 per cent, while in the remaining 10 per cent the influenza bacillus, *Micrococcus catarrhalis*, staphylococcus, meningococcus, and others occur.

Petechiae which vary in size from that of a pin point to a pinhead are commonly found in the conjunctiva. They occur in irregular groups and last for several days. Retinal hemorrhages are common and characteristic in appearance. The retina itself is somewhat cloudy. The hemorrhages may be flame shaped or round and elliptical. Then hemorrhages may contain a white center similar to those found in leucemia and septicemia. White spots also occur in the retina itself and are the same as those seen in cases of septicemia and which were first described by Roth (see Septic retinitis of Roth under Septicemia). These spots are often called "Roth spots." The hemorrhages and patches in endocarditis may disappear and reappear again.

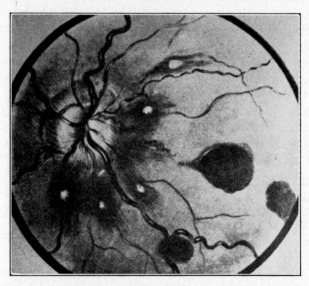

Fig. 189.—Drawing of the fundus in case of subacute bacterial endocarditis, showing retinal hemorrhages, some of which have a white center. (From Dienst and Gartner: Arch. Ophth., March, 1944.)

An inflammation of the optic nerve head occurs in some of the cases in the form of a papillitis which is also said to be of diagnostic significance. The margins of the disc are blurred and the disc itself is elevated and enlarged. The vision itself, however, may not be very much impaired.

Dienst and Gartner also found the choroid to be extensively involved with foci of dense infiltration of small round cells. These areas of infiltration occurred principally between the vessels and near the posterior pole.

The aqueous and vitreous may show infiltration with floating cells which can be observed on examination with the slit lamp.

Coronary Sclerosis.—Interference with the coronary circulation through one of the main vessels or a large branch may be caused by scarring such as occurs in syphilis or from an atheromatous plaque. A greatly diminished circulation caused by such interference may result in either local or distal occlusion by thrombosis. However, marked atheromatous changes may be present and cause considerable narrowing of the coronary lumen without the development of symptoms. This often occurs in older patients. Arteriosclerosis may be associated with cardiac disease and produce either diffuse symptoms or local manifestations following thrombosis or hemorrhage.

The ocular lesions occurring in cases of coronary sclerosis are similar to those found in generalized arteriosclerosis. The ocular condition may be present either with or without evidence in other organs, but even in the absence of such evidence, arteriosclerosis in the eye indicates its possible presence elsewhere. In cases of coronary arteriosclerosis the ocular lesion present is an associated sclerotic lesion. The principal findings on ophthalmoscopic examination are sclerosis of the retinal vessels and choroidal sclerosis, which may occur either separately or together.

Cohen[2] examined the eyes in twenty-six cases in which a diagnosis of coronary sclerosis was made. Ten of these revealed retinal arteriosclerosis while one presented choroidal sclerosis alone. Fifteen cases showed no positive signs of ocular sclerosis. The choroidal sclerosis is attributed to sclerotic lesions in the arteries, the veins being rarely affected. Degenerative changes in the intravascular stroma and pigment epithelium produced by the sclerotic process result in exposure of the choroidal vessels.

Cohen described the histologic changes in a case of choroidal sclerosis without evidence of retinal arteriosclerosis. These were limited to the focal area of the choroid on the temporal side and consisted of pigmentation, relative fibrosis and atrophy of the choroid, and sclerosis of the choroidal arteries. They resembled degenerative changes of the vascular coats without alteration of the thickness of the walls or encroachment of the lumen and differed from hyperplastic changes occurring in cases of essential hypertension or chronic glomerular nephritis.

Cerebral Arteriosclerosis.—The degree to which cerebral arteriosclerosis is present is not necessarily in proportion to that manifested in other parts. However, pathologically and clinically, it has been shown that the association between cerebral and retinal arteriolar sclerosis is very significant. It can be safely stated that the presence of arteriolar sclerosis as observed on ophthalmoscopic examination would indicate the presence of cerebral sclerosis.

The manifestations of cerebral arteriosclerosis are due to chronic progressive decrease in circulation, to the occurrence of sudden vascular lesions, usually of a thrombotic variety, and also to pressure on some portion of the optic chiasm or tracts produced by one of the cerebral vessels, usually in the circle of Willis. Atheromatous and other changes occurring in the cerebral arteries in the ordinary cases of senile arteriosclerosis result in impaired nutrition followed by senile mental changes.

Sudden loss of vision may occur as the result of embolus or thrombosis of a vessel with occlusion. If the occlusion is partial, some form of hemianopia will result, the type of which is determined by the location of the vessel affected.

Pressure resulting from arteriosclerotic changes in the cerebral vessels will also manifest itself usually by hemianopic defects in the visual fields. Tnese may be either homonymous, bitemporal, altitudinal and occasionally binasal hemianopia, depending on the location of the vessel involved and the portion of the optic chiasm or tract affected by the pressure.

Binasal hemianopia is probably the rarest type of visual field defect encountered and nearly always results from the presence of a vascular lesion.

Thromboangiitis Obliterans (Buerger's Disease).—Buerger's disease is a disease in which the deeper and larger arteries and veins are involved by pathologic changes resulting in the development of thrombi and occlusion of the lumina of the vessels. It is one of several diseases of the peripheral circulation which may be either of inflammatory or noninflammatory type. Others which might be included in this group and which present similar manifestations are arteriosclerosis obliterans and endarteritis obliterans. Arteriosclerosis obliterans occurs in those aged patients of either sex who suffer a generalized arteriosclerosis with definite impairment of the circulation and the consequent signs and symptoms already described. In endarteritis obliterans the smaller vessels are usually affected rather than the larger and deeper vessels as in Buerger's disease. The difference between the two appears to be in the pathology whereby the lumen of the vessel is occluded by the thrombus and the elastica lumina remains intact in Buerger's disease, whereas, the occlusion of the lumen in endarteritis obliterans is caused by the heaping up of the intimal cells.

The patient suffering with Buerger's disease is usually of middle age or older, although young people may also be affected. The symptoms include pain in scattered areas of the skin and subcutaneous tissues of the lower extremities. These areas may be very tender and may indicate the presence of thrombosis in the small superficial veins, due to phleboarteritis or a periphlebo-arteritis. Cramps occur in the muscles of the calf and foot, especially after walking. Numbness and coldness of the foot occur especially in colder weather. Both feet are usually involved, although not necessarily simultaneously. Later they become swollen and exhibit a deep purple-red color, although they are cold to the touch. Elevation results in a change of color to white and the feeling of fullness disappears. There is a marked reduction or absence of pulsation in the posterior tibial and dorsalis pedis arteries. Dry areas of gangrene may appear in time which are very painful. Sudden death sometimes occurs from coronary occlusion or from occlusion of a cerebral vessel.

The retinal vessels also may be affected by a so-called thromboangiitis obliterans in association with the same condition in the extremities. Such patients complain of headache and obscured vision as prodromal symptoms which are likely to be followed by sudden and complete blindness. The arteries and veins of the retina are involved by a perivasculitis and endovasculitis. The vessels eventually look like white strands or may be accompanied by pronounced white sheaths.

Periarteritis Nodosa.—This is a comparatively rare disease which affects chiefly the medium-sized and smaller arteries. The lesions comprise small nodules which are distributed along the course of the vessels. These vary in number and a great many may be present arranged in rows which soon produce an occlusion of the vessel or they may lead to minute aneurysms. By extension to the intima the lesion may produce destruction of the endothelium and thrombosis which may lead to local infarctions. Scar tissue is formed on recovery and the thrombi become organized. The cause of the disease is not definitely known but it is considered to be due to an associated infection.

The eye manifestations which have been described in association with periarteritis nodosa are numerous and may affect almost any of the ocular structures. Among these, the pupillary reaction to light may be reduced. Any of the vessels may be involved. Arterial lesions occur in the choroid which are considered to be infectious in nature. The disease may also affect the vessels in the greater arterial circle of the iris.

Goldstein and Wexler[3] described characteristic lesions of necrotizing type affecting the media with proliferation of the intima of the choroidal arteries. Later they reported a case[4] of bilateral atrophy of the optic nerve with considerable pigment disturbance in the fundus. Microscopic examination showed extensive disease of the ciliary and choroidal arteries of each eye. Periarteritis nodosa also involves the vessels of the kidneys, liver, mesentery, diaphragm, spleen, lungs, and heart.

According to Goldstein and Wexler, the arteries of the ciliary system are apparently most vulnerable. In nearly every instance the choroidal vessels are affected, and in some, the posterior ciliary arteries as well. Where the retinal artery has been found to be diseased, the change is limited in that portion behind the lamina cribrosa and not in the retinal arterioles.

Raynaud's Disease.—This is a local symmetrical asphyxia due to local and recurring interruption of the arterial circulation through a more or less extensive distal part of the extremities. The condition is usually bilateral and affects the fingers and hands. There is tingling of the fingers and toes and the hands and feet are cold and light lavender in color. Later this becomes white and blebs may appear which are filled with serum. Pain may be severe in the early stages, and in the asphyxial stage, the pulse to the part is weak or absent. The attack may vary in duration from an hour or two to several weeks. When more prolonged, gangrene may occur. The specific cause of the disease is not known but it frequently occurs in women although men are also affected.

The foremost manifestation of Raynaud's disease in the eyes is probably spasm of the retinal vessels of which a number of cases have been reported. This may affect any of the retinal vessels including the central retinal artery. When the latter is involved, the patient suffers almost complete loss of vision. The optic nerve becomes pale and atrophic. In other cases the vision may be only slightly impaired and the retinal arteries are found to be somewhat smaller than normal.

A case of bilateral spasm of the central retinal arteries was described by Dunphy[5] in a young girl with Raynaud's disease. The right eye was affected first and was followed not long after by the same condition in the left eye. The vision in the right eye improved somewhat after a period of time but that in the left eye was only light perception.

Another case of spasm of the central artery of the retina was reported by Anderson and Gray.[6] This occurred in a 39-year-old man who suffered with Raynaud's disease, and who suddenly lost the sight of the right eye. The vision in the left eye was normal, and the retinal arteries were smaller than average with the veins normal.

The description of the ophthalmoscopic picture in these cases of spasm of the central artery resembles very much that which is seen in embolus of the central retinal artery. A red spot is present in the macula of the affected eye, which is surrounded by a large white opaque area in the retina. The retinal arteries are very thin and small and, in some instances, they are bloodless. The prognosis for improvement in vision in the affected eye is not good, since the optic nerve head becomes pale and atrophy occurs, resulting in permanent blindness. The red spot in the macula eventually clears up and the retina in general appears more normal.

Attempts have been made to treat these cases by inhalations of amyl nitrite and other vasodilators just as in embolus of the central artery, but with little or no success in improvement of vision. Sympathectomy has also been performed as in Dunphy's case, with improvement in vision in the right eye to counting fingers at three feet. The left eye was unimproved.

Nephritis.—The present-day conception of nephritis or renal disease and its relationship to retinal lesions is based principally on the work of Volhard, Lohlein, Fahr, and others. The term nephritis does not refer to a disease but to a group of diseases which affect the kidneys and have certain characteristics in common. One of the best and most comprehensive descriptions of nephritis and nephritic retinitis was published by Elwyn[7] who classified the individual disease entities as follows:

A. Glomerulonephritis, in which the principal pathology is inflammation of the glomeruli, with secondary changes in the tubules. This is divided into (1) focal glomerulonephritis and (2) diffuse glomerulonephritis. The former, in which only a fraction of the glomeruli are involved, is also divided into (a) embolic and (b) nonembolic. Diffuse glomerulonephritis may occur as an acute form in which all the glomeruli are uniformly involved and which either subsides or passes into subacute diffuse, subchronic, or the chronic diffuse variety.

B. Nephrosis or tubular degenerative nephritis. This group includes: (1) The nephrosis of pregnancy. (2) Lipoid nephrosis. (3) The nephrosis of amyloid kidney. (4) The nephrosis of mercuric chloride poisoning.

C. The arteriosclerotic diseases of the kidney. These include: (1) Arteriosclerosis of the renal artery and its larger branches. (2) Renal arteriosclerosis without renal insufficiency with the clinical syndrome of benign hypertension. (3) Renal arteriosclerosis with renal insufficiency, the malignant form of arteriosclerosis or the malignant form of hypertension.

At the outset it should be stated that two factors are stressed as essential for the presence of retinal changes as manifestations of any of the diseases mentioned. These factors are (1) a generalized arterial constriction, and (2) an increase in the blood pressure. Therefore, since these two determining conditions are absent in some of these diseases of the kidney, a retinitis does not occur. This is true in particular of the embolic and nonembolic glomerulonephritis, the lipoid nephrosis, amyloid nephrosis, the nephrosis of mercuric chloride poisoning, and arteriosclerosis of the retinal artery and its larger branches. The other diseases named are of importance from the standpoint of eye manifestations, since most of them are accompanied at some time in their course by generalized arterial constriction and increased blood pressure. Retinal arteriosclerosis and its complications are not a part of the typical picture of nephritic retinitis but occur only in certain forms of nephritis where it is present as a complication.

Eye Manifestations.—Following the description of Elwyn,[7] the changes in the fundus which occur in the course of a recent case of progressive diffuse glomerulonephritis will be found chiefly in the optic disc, retinal vessels, and in the retina itself. These changes will vary according to the severity and duration of the nephritis. Ordinarily the optic disc is congested with its margins somewhat blurred and poorly outlined. The arteries on the disc may be slightly narrowed or unaffected, while the veins are normal or somewhat dilated.

The caliber of the retinal arteries is definitely narrow, especially in the smaller branches. The arteries are attenuated and thinned so that the smaller branches may disappear from view, while the veins may show no changes.

The changes which occur in the retina usually take place near the disc and extend out into the periphery for several disc diameters. They include the following: (a) retinal edema, (b) retinal hemorrhages, (c) cotton-wool patches, (d) white spots with sharp outlines, (e) white spots which are glistening in appearance and a star-shaped figure around the macula.

The edema of the retina is usually more pronounced close to the disc which it surrounds and may extend out into the periphery for several disc diameters. The retina around the disc has a grayish, striated appearance. When the disease is mild in character, the retinal edema may be only slight and even absent around the disc. The edema is due to an exudation of plasma into the optic nerve head and retina. This produces varying degrees of papilledema and a swelling of the inner layers especially in the retina. The elements of the various layers and the fibers in the nerve fiber layer are separated by the fluid which exudes from the capillaries. Cystlike spaces may form as the result of the dense accumulation of fluid between the separated elements.

The hemorrhages in the retina may vary in their sizes and shapes. They are usually seen near the vessels and are linear, streaked or flame-shaped. They may also be seen lying close to the cotton-wool patches or around the patches. They occur in the nerve fiber layer where they lie in the direction of nerve fibers. Other hemorrhages may be small and round and occur in the deeper layers of the retina.

The cotton-wool patches are located in the superficial layers and are white in color with irregular outline and shape. Their edges are fluffy and their size varies from slightly smaller than that of a pea to nearly the size of the disc. Hemorrhages are often found at their margin and the retinal vessels are sometimes covered in part by the patches. The cotton-wool patches may be present only with narrowed arteries in a mild nephritis. They result from the more dense accumulation of fluid with fibrin in the inner layers of the retina.

The opaque, white, shiny spots are irregular in shape and size varying from that of a pinhead to about one-half the size of the disc. They have a sharp outline and are usually seen lying near the disc in the deeper layers of the retina. They are scattered about between the disc and macula and tend to coalesce to form groups. They may be seen early in association with the edema around the disc but are more commonly visible later when the edema has subsided. They may be present for a long time after the cotton-wool patches have disappeared.

The glistening white spots are usually found around the temporal side of the disc and macula. They are dirty-white in color and discrete, although they may coalesce and gravitate toward the fovea, leaving the latter unaffected. They mostly group themselves in radiating lines around the fovea forming the star-shaped figure typical of this condition. This is due to the fact that they collect between the fibers of Henle. Sometimes the figure may be only partly formed. Histologically, these spots consist of deposits of fat and lipoids. The presence of the star-shaped figure, as well as the sharply outlined round spots, indicates the chronic nature of the disease.

When the condition is observed later in its course, the edema and cotton-wool patches in the retina will no longer be seen. They are indicative of the acuteness of the process. The same is true of swelling of the disc which might be observed to a degree of several diopters of choking. The papilledema usually occurs with the other lesions described although it may recede later in the disease. Choroidal and retinal arteriosclerosis may be present as complications. Retinal arteriosclerosis, in particular, may occur in older patients who develop nephritic retinitis. As a result the additional vascular changes will also be found. These are characterized by marked tortuosity of the vessels, alterations in the caliber of their lumina and areas of thickening of the vessel walls. The veins may be irregular and show marked tortuosity with compression at the point of arterial crossing. Occlusion of the smaller branches of the arteries or veins may occur in advanced cases. Thrombosis of the central vein with the presence of extensive retinal hemorrhages may also occur. Vitreous hemorrhages and detachment of the retina are rare complications.

Considerable confusion still exists concerning the nature and production of the various forms of glomerulonephritis, especially in the chronic form. This was pointed out in a review by Wagener[8] who concluded that it is very difficult to attribute the occurrence of retinopathies in glomerulonephritis to any single mechanism. Although some authors feel that the eye changes are primarily renal while others consider them hypertensive, it does seem that there is considerable agreement in the thought that they are basically nutritional regardless of whether these retinal changes in chronic glomerulonephritis are designated as "angiospastic," "hypertensive," "ischemic," "anoxemic" or "arteriosclerotic." While there is some uniformity in the understanding and interpretation of the basic factors concerned in cardiovascular disease and the retinal complications, there is an obvious need for more uniform nomenclature and criteria for diagnosis.

Acute Diffuse Nephritis.—This disease is caused chiefly by scarlet fever and streptococcic infections, usually as a sequela. It is characterized by the presence of urinary changes, edema, increased blood pressure and renal insufficiency in severe cases. The increased blood pressure is accompanied by generalized constriction of the arteries and arterioles which produces the pallor of the skin and the retinal changes seen in these cases. The arterial constriction may be sudden in its appearance and varies in the arterioles of the retina causing the edema, cotton-wool patches and other retinal lesions resulting from impaired nutrition. The acute diffuse nephritis may subside leaving no serious signs of

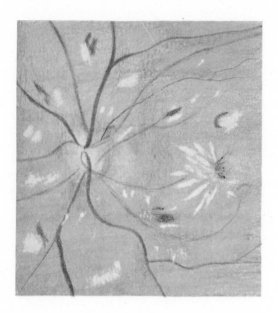

Fig. 190.—Drawing showing retinal changes in nephritis. Swelling of the disc as shown by blurred and indistinct margins. Numerous hemorrhages and white cotton-wood exudates with star-shaped figure around the macula. (From Tassman: Medical World, October, 1936.)

its former presence other than traces of lipoid deposits, or some proliferation of glial tissue and white perivascular sheaths. In other cases it fails to subside and becomes subacute, or it changes to one of the chronic forms.

Subchronic and Chronic Diffuse Glomerulonephritis.—These forms of the disease may progress over a number of years with periods of remission which are later followed by further progress. When the blood pressure is not increased and generalized arterial constriction is absent, nephritic retinitis is also absent. In most instances, however, arterial constriction, both general and in the retinal vessels, is present, so that the corresponding retinal changes are also found. When the increased blood pressure and arterial constriction persist, the picture of nephritic retinitis is presented. After a period of years added signs of arteriosclerosis develop, especially in the heart and brain. Here again will be found the tortuosity and thickening of the vessels, irregularities in the lumen, irregularities in the light streak, and, at times, the complications of arteriosclerosis, such as obstruction of arterial or venous branches with the accompanying changes. When the arterial constriction is relaxed in chronic nephritis, the retinal changes regress. As a rule, however, the condition progresses with continued hypertension until just before death. The persistent presence of nephritic retinitis is significant of maximal contraction of all the small arteries of the body and a terminal uremic state.

Nephrosis.—From the standpoint of manifestations in the eye, the nephrosis of pregnancy is the only disease of importance in this group. This will receive further discussion in a later chapter, but it should be stated here that generalized constriction of the arteries and a persistent elevation in blood pressure are prominent characteristics. As a result, a retinitis may develop in this disease. In the others there is an absence of these two factors, so that a retinitis does not occur as a rule. The changes here are degenerative and affect chiefly the tubules, whereas in glomerulonephritis the changes are inflammatory in character and occur chiefly in the glomeruli. The nephrosis of pregnancy resembles very much the picture seen in an acute diffuse nephritis. The retinal manifestations include narrowing of the arteries, early edema about the optic discs, and the appearance of cotton-wool patches. The other spots and deposits in the retina are rarely seen here, however, and arteriosclerosis does not occur.

Arteriosclerotic Diseases of the Kidney.—In the senile type of arteriosclerosis of the renal artery, typical eye manifestations are absent because the disease is not characterized by a generalized arterial constriction and an increase in the blood pressure.

The second disease in this group is the arteriosclerosis of the kidney which occurs without impairment of the renal function (essential hypertension). Here, arterial changes in the kidneys are always found and these cases may change to the malignant form. This disease is characterized early by temporary elevations in the blood pressure in patients about 50 years of age and older. As time passes, the increase in blood pressure tends to remain higher, and although all other symptoms may be absent, later changes of arteriosclerosis are superimposed with the appearance of the corresponding symptoms. These may refer to involvement of the heart, brain, and coronaries with signs of obstruction, aneurysm, and hemorrhage. Signs of retinal arteriosclerosis are found when the cerebral arteriosclerosis develops. Prior to this and in the stage of hypertension alone no characteristic changes are present in the retina. In essential hypertension alone there are none of the signs of retinitis such as edema of the disc and retina, exudates, cotton-wool patches and a star-shaped figure in the macula. This is due to the absence of a generalized arterial constriction in this condition. When changes in the retinal vessels are present, they are the result of arteriosclerosis in older patients who did not suffer a persistent hypertension. In others early arteriosclerotic changes in the retina would indicate the presence of essential hypertension which is persistent. These cases usually die of cardiac or cerebral disease or some intercurrent condition.

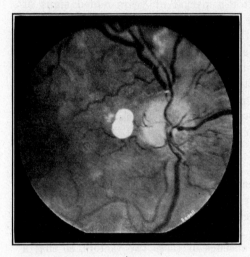 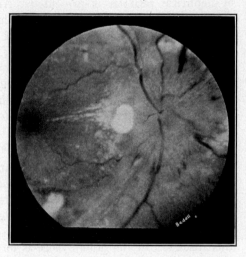

A.   B.

Fig. 191.—*A,* Malignant hypertension nephrosclerosis of right eye in man aged 44, who had had hyperpiesia for years, and who died of uremia four weeks after photograph was taken; extreme artery changes with sclerosis, irregular caliber and stiff walls indenting full veins, retinal edema and hemorrhages, new vessels on disc. *B,* Chronic nephritis in a 34-year-old male. Vision 20/20. Marked neuroretinitis with macular star. (Courtesy of Dr. Arthur J. Bedell.)

When at times, a rather sudden generalized constriction of the arteries of the body develops in these cases, the disease becomes one of malignant renal sclerosis or malignant hypertension. The vessels of the kidney, brain, and retina now show signs and symptoms of acute arterial constriction superimposed on those of arteriosclerosis. The blood pressure ranges from 200 to 300 systolic and 140 to 190 mm. diastolic. Symptoms of kidney disease and insufficiency develop.

The retinal changes observed on ophthalmoscopic examination in this disease include irregular tortuosity and narrowing of the arteries with occasional obliteration of some smaller branches, marked tortuosity of the veins, venous compression at points of crossing, edema of the optic disc and retina, white spots and the glistening white spots in the deeper layer, hemorrhages of various sizes and shapes, cotton-wool patches, and a star-shaped figure in the macula. The edema and swelling of the optic disc may be quite severe, and the choking may measure 5 to 6 diopters. Both eyes are affected, although the condition may be more severe in one than in the other. The vision becomes seriously impaired and the prognosis is very grave. These patients usually die from uremia.

SUMMARY OF RENAL DISEASES, WITH AND WITHOUT RETINITIS (BASED ON DESCRIPTION BY ELWYN)

I. Glomerulonephritis
Inflammation of the glomerule is the principal pathologic process with secondary changes in the tubules.

(a) Focal (only a fraction of the glomeruli are involved)

- Embolic — No generalized arterial constriction.
- Nonembolic — Absence of increased blood pressure. Absence of nephritic retinitis.

(b) Diffuse

- Acute / Subacute — Etiologic factors: scarlet fever, streptococcic infections, etc. Generalized arterial constriction throughout body to varying degree. Increased blood pressure—renal insufficiency—narrowing of arterioles of retina with retinitis—arterial constriction in brain with edema and cerebral symptoms. May recede or become chronic.

- Subchronic / Chronic — Results from acute and subacute. Long duration and recurs. Retinal changes correspond to amount of arterial constriction and increase in blood pressure. Edema and albuminuria without retinitis in absence of hypertension occurs in a few, but retinitis with persistent hypertension and constricted arteries in most. Continuous increased blood pressure leads to arteriosclerosis especially in heart and brain. Added changes in retinal arterioles. Usually progressive and complicated by obstruction, etc. Persistent renal retinitis indicates maximal contraction of the small arteries of body and presages uremic termination.

II. Nephrosis
Tubular degenerative nephritis and absence of inflammatory changes in glomeruli.

(a) Nephrosis of Pregnancy: The only one associated with generalized arterial constriction, persistent hypertension and retinitis.

(b) Lipoid Nephrosis — No increase in blood pressure or generalized arterial constriction. Therefore, no retinitis.

(c) Amyloid Kidney — Symptoms of chronic diffuse nephritis, only rare, and retinitis, only occasional.

(d) Mercuric Chloride Poisoning: Increased blood pressure occasional and mild. No nephritic retinitis.

III. The Arteriosclerotic Diseases of the Kidney

(a) Arteriosclerosis of renal artery and larger branches has no increased blood pressure or generalized arterial constriction. Therefore, no nephritic retinitis.

(b) Renal Arteriosclerosis without insufficiency (essential hypertension): Common type of hypertension in advanced age (50 to 70). May be the only symptom. Produces arteriosclerotic changes in time (cardiac, coronary, aneurysm, brain hemorrhage and edema). Death from cardiac failure and apoplexy. Generalized arterial constriction absent and constriction of retinal arteries absent. No retinitis present.

(c) Renal Arteriosclerosis with renal insufficiency (malignant renal sclerosis or malignant hypertension). Arteriosclerosis becomes malignant. Changes more marked. Other organs show arterial changes. Added generalized arterial constriction over entire body. Marked hypertension (200-300 systolic and 140-190 diastolic) Marked arteriosclerosis of brain and retina. Renal symptoms and renal insufficiency develop—Cerebral symptoms. Added retinal changes of diffuse glomerulonephritis. Death from uremia, cardiac or cerebral disease.

References

1. Dienst, Eva C., and Gartner, Samuel: Pathologic Changes in the Eye Associated With Subacute Bacterial Endocarditis. Report of Five Cases With Autopsy, Arch. Ophth. **31:** 198, 1944.
2. Cohen, Martin: Choroidal Sclerosis in Coronary Arteriosclerosis, Arch. Ophth. **19:** 487, 1938.
3. Goldstein, I., and Wexler, D.: The Ocular Pathology of Periarteritis Nodosa, Arch. Ophth. **2:** 288, 1929.
4. Goldstein, I., and Wexler, D.: Bilateral Atrophy of the Optic Nerve in Periarteritis Nodosa, Arch. Ophth. **18:** 767, 1937.
5. Dunphy, E. B.: Tr. Am. Ophth. Soc. **30:** 420, 1932.
6. Anderson, R. G., and Gray, E. B.: Spasm of the Central Artery in Raynaud's Disease, Arch. Ophth. **17:** 622, 1937.
7. Elwyn, H.: Nephritic Retinitis, Arch. Ophth. **11:** 300, 1934.
8. Wagener, H. P.: Retinopathy in Glomerulonephritis, Am. J. M. Sc. **209:** 257, 1945.

CHAPTER XVI

DISEASES OF THE BLOOD

The diseases of the blood are the result chiefly of changes which take place in its constituents, such as the red blood corpuscles, white blood corpuscles, hemoglobin, and the blood platelets. These changes may occur in the number or form of the various constituents and are characterized by the presence of a marked anemia and also by alterations in other organs with their accompanying signs and symptoms. The eye may participate prominently in the manifestations of an anemia and, especially in the more severe cases, will present characteristic evidences. It should never be omitted, therefore, in the examination of a patient who suffers with a disease of the blood.

Secondary anemia occurs as the result of other acute and chronic disease but more important here is the form of hypochromic anemia which results from the sudden and profuse loss of blood with hemorrhage and recurrent hemorrhages in the presence of other internal disease. These may produce an ischemia and accompanying manifestations of the decrease in the amount of blood in the organ or structure. Such manifestations may be observed in the eye in some cases on ophthalmoscopic examination.

The anemias as a group include a large number of diseases of the blood, some of which have been described in other chapters. According to the classification of Ottenberg,[1] they are caused by a variety of etiologic factors. From an ophthalmologic standpoint, the most important of these would be the anemias which result from: 1. Deficiencies—(A) iron deficiency (loss of blood and hypochromic anemia); (B) deficiency of antianemic principles (pernicious anemia, pregnancy pernicious anemia, etc.). 2. Injury to the blood-making organs—(A) osteosclerosis, leucemias, and Hodgkin's disease, Gaucher's disease, Niemann-Pick disease, Schüller-Christian disease, and others with lipoid deposits in bone marrow; (B) interference with regeneration of blood, diseases of the spleen (Banti's syndrome).

Most of the chronic forms of disease with disturbances or alteration in the hemopoietic system may exhibit a marked progressive anemia, accompanied by enlargement of the liver and spleen and a distinctive blood picture. The variety and extent of the eye changes may be said to depend in general on the type and involvement of the other structures, particularly those of the blood and the blood-forming tissues.

The eye changes in the anemias include chiefly: 1. Changes in the appearance and size of the retinal vessels. 2. Changes in the retina itself (principally pallor, hemorrhages, and edema). 3. Edema and swelling of the optic discs. 4. Exophthalmos. The first three are characteristic especially of those which are considered as primary and secondary anemias, i.e., pernicious anemia, sudden loss of blood, purpura, the leucemias, and splenic anemia. Exophthalmos and displacement of the eyeball occurs chiefly with lymphoma, i.e., lymphatic leucemia, Hodgkin's disease, lymphosarcoma, chloroma, and also the diseases involving the bone marrow with lipoid deposits in the bones of the orbit, as in Schüller-Christian disease. In others such as Gaucher's disease and Niemann-Pick disease, which may be accompanied by a mild hypochromic anemia, the eye changes are produced by the characteristic deposits in other structures.

Pernicious Anemia

Pernicious anemia is a severe macrocytic anemia in which there is a lack of secretion in the stomach of an adequate amount of substance essential to the nutrition of the red blood cells in the bone marrow. It is characterized by a marked reduction in the number of red blood corpuscles, a reduction in hemoglobin, hyperplasia of the bone marrow, the appearance of megalocytes, achlorhydria, and degenerative changes in the posterior and lateral columns.

The etiology of pernicious anemia is not known, but it occurs most commonly between the ages of 40 and 60 years, affects both sexes equally and a familial tendency is not uncommon. The cardinal pathologic changes present an atrophic gastritis, megaloblastic hyperplasia of bone marrow, widespread degeneration of parenchymatous viscera and muscles, free iron in various organs, and focal degeneration in the white matter of the spinal cord.

Symptoms.—The general characteristics include an insidious onset, great weakness, marked pallor and slight wasting.

The symptoms resulting from the anemia are: weakness, faintness, swelling of the ankles, dyspnea, palpitation, and commonly amenorrhea.

The gastrointestinal symptoms are associated with achylia and atrophic gastritis. The tongue is red in the early stages and becomes sore. Later it is smooth and atrophic. There is flatulence, dyspnea, vomiting, and diarrhea.

The nervous symptoms include paresthesia of the extremities, tingling and numbness which are common and occur early, occasional mental symptoms, spasticity of the lower extremities, ataxia, loss of bladder and sphincter control.

The patient on general examination may appear fairly well nourished, with a lemon-yellow tint of the skin, wide-set eyes, and low blood pressure. A rapid pulse, soft systolic hemic murmurs, and probable cardiac dilatation may be found. The liver and spleen are palpable in some cases. The abdomen is frequently distended, edema may be present and a hemorrhagic tendency occurs occasionally. The spinal cord involvement is characterized by loss of vibratory sense and sense of motion, spastic paraplegia, exaggerated knee reflex, and a bilateral positive Babinski.

The examination of the blood presents certain distinct characteristics as follows: (1) A great reduction of erythrocytes. The count may be as low as 500,000 per cu. mm., although it is more often between 1,500,000 and 2,000,000. During remissions it may be as high as 3,000,000 to 4,000,000. (2) The reduction in hemoglobin is not as great and therefore relatively high. This leads to a (3) high color index, (4) increase in the mean corpuscular volume, (5) leucopenia during a relapse, (6) reduction in platelets, and myeloid or granulocytic leucocytes, (7) increase in macrocytes and immature cells. (8) The presence of a hyperbilirubinemia as shown by the indirect van den Bergh. This parallels the intensity of the lemon tint of the skin and conjunctiva which is probably due to a deposition of this type of bilirubin in the tissues. (9) Low cholesterol content. (10) Reticulocytes increased.

The gastric analysis is important. There is a characteristic achlorhydria, which is unchanged after the use of histamines.

The urinalysis may reveal an increased urobilin and traces of albumin.

Eye Manifestations.—Manifestations of pernicious anemia may be found in the eyes when the erythrocytes and hemoglobin have been reduced in amount sufficient to impair the integrity of the structures supplied. This corresponds to an average of about 1,500,000 red blood cells and about 40 per cent hemoglobin. As previously mentioned, the conjunctiva is likely to show the same yellow tint of the skin. The changes in the fundus of the eye are due chiefly to the impaired nutrition resulting from the altered condition of the blood. This alteration is revealed in the capillaries of the optic nerve and the arteries of the retina. The former are very pale in color and as a result they impart a pale color to the nerve head, the margins of which may be blurred. The retinal arteries are narrow, pale in appearance, and suffer a fatty degeneration of their walls. As a result the entire retina has a much paler appearance than normal, and hemorrhages occur from rupture of the vessels. These are usually flame shaped, superficial, and occur in the nerve fiber layer around the disc and in the periphery. The smaller vessels may reveal small dilatations and points of occlusion. The retinal veins are tortuous and greatly distended. Large round hemorrhages may occur in the deeper layers of the retina and preretinal hemorrhages may also be present. The vision of the eye is affected to a greater extent when the hemorrhages occur in or around the macular region.

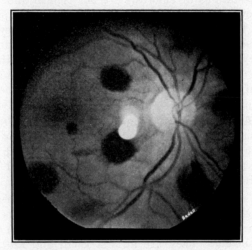

Fig. 192.—Retinitis in pernicious anemia in the right eye of a woman aged 47 who was seriously ill. The rounded thick retinal hemorrhages are most suggestive of the blood state. (From Bedell: J. A. M. A., March 18, 1939.)

A characteristic of the hemorrhages seen in this condition, but one which also occurs in leucemia, is the presence of a white spot in the center of the hemorrhage. They are considered to be due to the collection of leucocytes which group themselves in this location.

The optic nerve rarely shows much change early in the disease, except that it is paler in color and may reveal the hazy margins previously mentioned. Later, however, there may be an edema about the disc and retina. The vision is reduced to some extent and if the disease is of long standing, the optic nerve becomes atrophic.

Hypochromic Anemia

There are several forms of hypochromic anemia which include ordinary chlorosis, idiopathic hypochromic anemia, the hypochromic anemia of pregnancy, the acute or chronic anemia due to loss of blood, and that which results from the presence of hookworm disease. The eye manifestations of the menstrual disorders and pregnancy with which anemia may be associated will be described in the following chapter.

Chlorosis.—This is a term which may be employed to include the hypochromic anemia occurring in young adolescent girls and the idiopathic hypochromic anemia which is sometimes called chronic chlorosis. It is common in women between the ages of 25 and 45 but rarely occurs after the menopause. The symptoms of both are almost identical and include pallor, fatigue, dyspnea, and weakness. Gastrointestinal symptoms, such as dyspepsia, nausea, vomiting and constipation, may be present. In chronic chlorosis, achlorhydria is more common than in ordinary chlorosis, but is not a constant finding. The skin of the patient is pale with a greenish tinge which leads to the designation "green sickness."

The characteristic blood findings are a decided reduction in the hemoglobin and a low color index. The erythrocytes number from 3,000,000 to 5,000,000.

The eye manifestations of chlorosis are not typical and not very frequent in occurrence. However, the conjunctiva is found to be pale and reveals a bluish-green tint. There may be a moderate edema of the eyelids. The retina and the retinal vessels are pale in color. The veins are tortuous and congested. There is a tendency to venous thrombosis, and neuroretinitis may be present. The optic disc, in marked cases, is blurred in outline and there may be a moderate amount of swelling of the disc. Hemorrhages in the retina are few in number and infrequent.

Ankylostoma Americanum.—An anemia results with infestation from *ankylostoma americanum* and *duodenale*. Additional factors present here are a low iron intake, chronic gastrointestinal disturbances, achlorhydria, decreased iron utilization, and in some cases a further aggravation by an apparent atrophy of the gastrointestinal mucosa.

In this form of hypochromic anemia the eye manifestations are characterized by blurred vision, nystagmus, diplopia, and contraction of the visual fields. Hemorrhages occur in the retina which may resemble those found in the primary form of anemia. They are at first small and are found principally around the optic disc. The latter is pale in color.

Anemia From Hemorrhage.—One of the most frequent causes of hypochromic anemia among all classes of people is the loss of blood such as occurs in ulcerating conditions of the gastrointestinal tract, chronic bleeding from peptic ulcer, hemorrhoids, menorrhagia, metrorrhagia, and chronic ulceration of the colon. Profuse bleeding may occur with a marked reduction of the hemoglobin.

When hemorrhage is sudden and profuse, an acute anemia is produced which causes a circulatory impairment and which affects the optic nerve and retina. An acute edema of the optic nerve and retina occurs quickly and is characterized by the presence of irregularly scattered large white areas about the retinal vessels. They may be present only for a short period and gradually disappear. The retinal arteries are narrow, but hemorrhages in the retina are not found. The color of the vessels and the entire retina is pale. The optic disc itself may show evidences of a probable optic neuritis with slightly blurred margins and later a pallor of the disc. These changes are accompanied by sub-

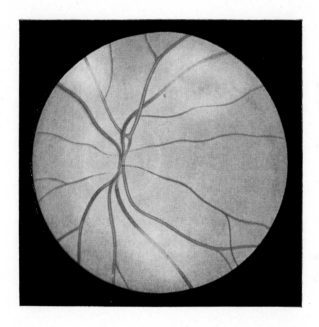

Fig. 193.—Retinosis from loss of blood. (After Koellner, from Troncoso: Internal Diseases of the Eye and Atlas of Ophthalmoscopy, F. A. Davis Co.)

jective symptoms, chief of which is sudden reduction and impairment of vision. This is not necessarily a permanent condition, however, and in many the vision may improve after a while.

A case of amblyopia resulting from distant hemorrhage in which the patient suffered a crushed chest was reported by Cox.[2] Three days later, both fundi were found to be ischemic with no discrimination between the vessels, disc and macula. The vision gradually cleared; six months after the accident, the visual fields had improved sufficiently for the patient to go about without aid, but there remained an absolute central scotoma in each eye.

Purpura Hemorrhagica (Thrombocytopenia).—Idiopathic thrombocytopenic purpura or Werlhof's disease is characterized by purpura which occurs in repeated crops and which varies in size from that of a pin point to larger areas. The cause is unknown. The blood is affected by a decrease in the blood platelets, delayed bleeding time, and nonretractile clot. Another variety is the secondary thrombocytopenic purpura which is associated with aplastic anemia, benzol poisoning, and excessive irradiation.

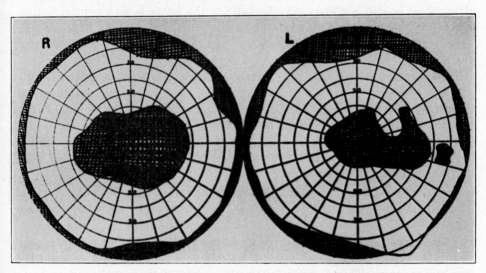

Fig. 194.—Visual fields showing absolute central scotoma in both eyes following hemorrhage after chest injury. (From Cox: Arch. Ophth., November, 1944.)

The eye manifestations consist principally of the presence of hemorrhages in the retina. They are small and are found near the optic disc while larger ones may occur in the periphery. The former are superficial while the latter occur in the deeper retinal layers. Preretinal hemorrhage may also occur. Occasionally the hemorrhages may be accompanied by hyperemia and edema of the optic disc, optic neuritis with definite blurring of the disc margins, and papilledema. The vision of the patient may become seriously impaired.

Cases of thrombocytopenia purpura have been reported in which cerebral symptoms occurred together with choked discs. In some of these hemorrhages were said to have occurred into the meninges, optic pathways, subdural space and the ventricles. Watkins, Wagener, and Brown[3] reviewed the literature of these cases and reported three patients with thrombocytopenic purpura in whom bilateral choked discs were present without demonstrable evidence of intracranial injury. A fourth case of choked disc occurred in the presence of severe hemorrhage from a gastric ulcer but without pathologic evidence of an intracranial lesion at autopsy.

These authors concluded that the loss of vision in these patients resulted from anoxemia. The reduction of oxygen in the blood which results from an acute or chronic loss of blood might lead to anoxemia of the tissues of the optic nerve and retina which in turn would produce papilledema. Edema of the brain arising from the same cause might be a factor in the production of the papilledema and also of the paralysis of the lateral rectus muscles which also occurs at times in such cases.

Purtscher's Disease.—This condition originally described by Purtscher has also been variously designated in the past as retinal teletraumatism, traumatic angiopathy and, most recently by Spaeth,[4] as traumatic liporrhagia retinalis (Verhoeff). Traumatism is the etiologic factor. The patient sustains an injury, usually to the chest, thorax or head, in which fractures may occur, although it is still not clear whether or not the latter is an essential factor. The injury, however, in most of the cases is of a crushing variety which results in a venous congestion with secondary manifestations in the cranium and changes in the retina of the eye.

The eye manifestations are characterized by a retinal angiopathy, the principal features of which are enlargements of the retinal vessels, retinal hemorrhages and the presence of edema and white spots in the retina. Papilledema, papillitis and preretinal hemorrhages have also been said to occur. Both eyes are usually involved. The retinal changes may not cause a marked impairment in vision unless the macula is involved. The lesions often heal, leaving no trace of their presence.

The retinal hemorrhages may be numerous and are usually of the striate, punctate or petechial variety. They may lie contiguous to the vessels but are apparently not connected with, or related to, the white spots.

The white spots are the prominent feature of this condition. They appear as bright white specks which occur predominantly in the region between the disc and macula. They usually follow the course of the vessels and may extend into the periphery of the retina. They frequently obscure the veins to which they show a close relationship. Although their size may vary, they have been described in outline and appearance as "scattered snowflakes." Their margins are indistinct and split into fine striations. They regress rapidly, diminish in number and density and dissolve into fine silvery bright punctae and striae.

The cause of these white spots has been variously described. In some of the earlier cases, it was considered that the condition results from thrombosis of the intracranial vascular sinuses or that a sudden increase of intracranial pressure occurs with cerebrospinal fluid being forced along the vaginal sheath to account for the retinal changes. Purtscher originally postulated that the condition resulted from pathologic changes in the venules alone. In one of two cases reported by Spaeth, the retinal lesions were both arterial and venous.

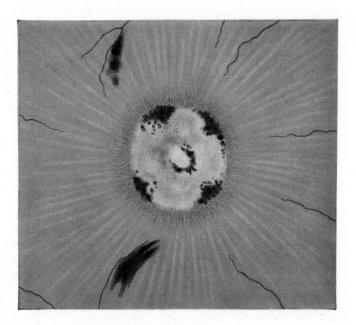

Fig. 195.—Traumatic liporrhagia retinalis. (Purtscher's Disease.) (From Spaeth, Arch. Ophth., March, 1944.) Showing central macular lesion as seen with red free light. Flame-shaped hemorrhage to left below is in proximity to an arteriole. The one above is near a venule. A corona of droplet hemorrhages is seen around the central lesion which had a yellow-ish tint best seen with green illumination.

The hemorrhages were mostly venous and usually involved the smaller veins. Two arteries, however, also showed hemorrhages. The patient had sustained a chest injury in a collision by being thrown against the front of a street car which he was operating when it became derailed. The fundi showed venous tortuosities, edema, with massive "exudates" into each macula, extensive perimacular edema, and infiltration with radiating lines about the right macula. There were many fine hemorrhages into each macula and larger extramacular, flame-shaped hemorrhages. White spots were scattered about, all in close proximity to the retinal vessels. At least one of these spots lay on a terminal arteriole, overlying and almost ensheathing it. Another smaller lesion with indistinct outline corresponded exactly to Purtscher's original description. It followed the course of the retinal nerve fibers.

Spaeth agreed with Verhoeff who suggested that the designation "traumatic liporrhagia retinalis" adequately describes this condition. He concluded that there occurs a somewhat generalized diffusion of fat droplets in the fundus of the eye, the picture being modified by a generalized hemorrhagic situation in the retina or brain, or both, due to factors other than the emboli themselves. This is probably a severe disturbance in the venous circulation of the retina, brain and brain stem. Spaeth quoted Verhoeff as follows:

"The white spots characteristic of Purtscher's retinosis never occur in ordinary cases of increased intracranial pressure, even when this is extremely high. They also never appear after thrombosis of the cavernous sinus or complete obstruction of the central vein. Hence, they must have some other cause. They occur only in cases in which there have been fracture and obstruction of the retinal veins. Their appearance strongly suggests the presence of fat. Simple obstruction or embolism of a retinal vessel never produces them; therefore, fat emboli would not do so. Most likely they are due to venous obstruction associated with traumatic hyperlipemia. Distention of the small vessels might permit the fat to pass into the tissues, either by diapadesis or through small breaks in the distended vessels. Usually some blood is extravasated with the fat."

Leucemia

Leucemia is a fatal disease of the blood-forming tissues and is characterized especially by the presence in the circulating blood of precursors of the normal leucocytes in predominating proportions. Several types of leucemia are differentiated by the type of leucocyte present in each. The two main varieties of the disease are the lymphatic and myeloid leucemia. Both may be either acute or chronic. The acute lymphatic and myelogenous leucemias are difficult in most instances to differentiate since both run practically the same course. Many of the signs and symptoms in the two chronic forms are also alike. In addition to these there is also an acute monocytic leucemia and an aleucemic leucemia. The acute monocytic leucemia is characterized by a monocytosis. Aleucemic leucemia is probably a chronic form of leucemia in which the leucocytes in the circulating blood have been reduced in number to normal or subnormal, but the pathologic cells such as myeloblasts, myelocytes, and lymphoblasts are still found.

Acute Leucemia.—The acute lymphatic type is more common than the myelogenous. The onset is usually sudden, and the disease is often preceded by an acute infection. The lymphatic glands of the neck become greatly enlarged and painful while the overlying skin apears to be indurated and ready to rupture. The spleen is enlarged and hemorrhages may occur in the skin and nasal mucous membranes with epistaxis.

The blood reveals a rapid and marked anemia with the number of erythrocytes decreasing to a million or less. The hemoglobin is reduced to about 20 per cent, and there is a leucocytosis of from 15,000 to 40,000. The red cells may be well formed or there may be some immature red cells present, but the white cells show large numbers of immature forms. In the lymphoid variety the predominant cell is a small lymphocyte, while in the myeloblastic form, the predominant cell is a myeloblast. The platelets may also be rapidly diminished in number and, together with increased capillary permeability, account for the hemorrhagic tendency. The course of the disease is usually rapid and terminates fatally.

Chronic Leucemia.—The onset of both chronic lymphatic and chronic myelogenous leucemia is insidious and the disease may be present for some time before it is recognized. The symptoms in general include fatigue and weakness, dyspnea, palpitation and pallor. The anemia becomes a striking feature and dominates the picture as the disease progresses. Other signs are tachycardia, increased metabolic rate, loss of weight, exacerbations of fever accompanied by excessive sweating.

In myelogenous leucemia the spleen is generally greatly enlarged while in lymphatic leucemia, the lymph glands are the site of adenopathy. They may become very large and firm but are painless. The spleen may also enlarge slightly but not to the same extent as in the myelogenous variety.

The blood picture in the myelogenous variety shows an increase in the number of granulocytes while in the lymphatic variety, there are large numbers of leucocytes which resemble the normal small lymphocyte. The granulocytes may number from 20,000 to 1,000,000. As the anemia progresses, the normoblasts and erythrocytes show stippling and basophilia. In the late stages the platelets are reduced in number. In the lymphatic variety the granulocytes are not especially increased, but the leucocytes may total over 10,000 per cu. mm. The predominant feature is the enormous number of lymphocytes. The hemorrhages into the skin and mucous membranes which occur when the anemia is marked are probably due to the reduced number of platelets.

The course in both forms of the disease is very chronic, and it eventually terminates fatally from either an intercurrent infection, severe anemia, hemorrhage, or some form of visceral thrombosis.

Eye Manifestations.—Both forms of leucemia are accompanied by eye changes, although they may be somewhat more common in the myelogenous variety. In addition to some manifestations in the external eye such as conjunctivitis and scleritis, the principal changes affect the retinal vessels and retina. The characteristic ophthalmoscopic picture is often designated as leucemic retinitis.

In the analysis of the various types of leucemia at Johns Hopkins Hospital by Goldbach,[5] forty-five cases of acute lymphatic leucemia revealed positive eye findings in twenty-five cases, or 55 per cent. Of forty-two cases of chronic lymphatic leucemia, positive eye findings were present in twenty-eight, or 62 per cent. In nine cases of acute myeloid leucemia, eight, or 90 per cent, showed positive eye findings, while in 143 cases of chronic myeloid leucemia, positive eye findings were present in eighty-two, or 60 per cent.

In addition to the fundus changes, Goldbach reported the occurrence of sluggish pupillary reactions, anisocoria, mydriasis, blepharitis, conjunctivitis, scleritis, and nystagmus.

Cohen[6] reported the occurrence of an orbital lymphatic tumor growth in a case of chronic lymphatic leucemia in a man 65 years of age. He explained the presence of a leucemic nodule in the orbit as originating from lymphatic spaces around the adipose tissue or from perivascular lymphatic spaces as a result of the abnormal state of the blood.

The fundus changes occur in both eyes and are characterized, in some cases, by a change in color. This may not be typical. The condition of the blood produces a yellowish or grayish-yellow color in mild cases. Later and in more severe conditions the fundus is darker in color.

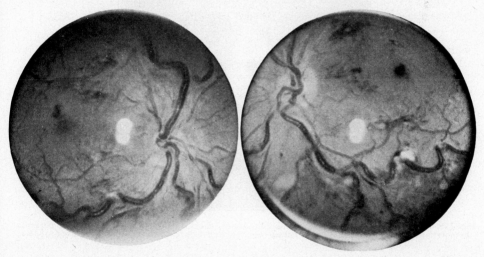

Fig. 196.—Retinal changes in leucemia. Edema and pallor of discs, veins dark, full, and tortuous; arteries normal; numerous hemorrhages. (From Gibson: Arch. Ophth., September, 1938.)

The retinal and choroidal vessels are pale and the retinal veins show an increase in caliber with marked distention. The optic disc may be hazy or blurred in outline, a few irregular white spots may be seen in the area of the macula, and whitish exudates resembling those seen in nephritis may be present.

The changes in the caliber and the tortuosity of the veins are significant of the altered blood picture in leucemia. The flow of blood in the capillaries and veins is impaired so that a seepage of the blood elements occurs in the capillaries and causes a pressure on the perivascular lymph sheaths. This results in a secondary edema of the retina which may be further aggravated by the location and character of the hemorrhages (Goldbach). The hemorrhages and enormous distention of the veins, which are the characteristic findings, are also accounted for by the stasis in the circulation of the capillaries and diapedesis. The distention of the veins may be so great in severe cases that they become very tortuous and sausage-shaped. The hemorrhages in leucemia are striking in that they contain a white center. This has been variously attributed to a collection of leucocytes, serum, and debris, but Goldstein and Wexler[7] found that they presented little indication of their presence histologically. They described dilatation of the retinal vessels, increase in the number of leucocytes in their lumen, and slight edema of the disc as almost constant features. The retinal veins may show prominent perivascular sheaths due to infiltration of leucocytes.

The hemorrhages may occur in large numbers and in almost any size or shape. Gibson[8] in a study of twenty-two cases of leucemia, pointed out a close parallelism between the degree of anemia and the extent of retinal hemorrhage. He found that the number of hemorrhages increased with a corresponding decrease in the red cells. There was no relation between the white cell count and the amount of retinal hemorrhage.

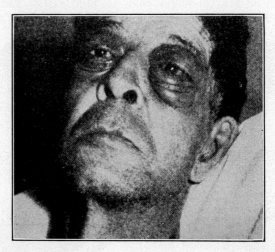

Fig. 199.—Monocytic chloroma showing exophthalmos, chemosis, and edema of lids and petechial hemorrhages on the thorax. (From Gump, Hester, and Lohr: Arch. Ophth., December, 1936.)

Monocytic Leucemia.—The occurrence of monocytic leucemia is not common. It probably affects males more frequently than females, and chiefly the young. It runs a rapid course and is characterized by the presence of hemorrhages in the skin and mucous membranes. The patient shows pallor, anemia, exhaustion and an elevation of temperature. The liver, spleen, and lymph nodes may be enlarged, and tumors occur in the viscera and skin. The white cell count is greatly increased and may number over 1,000,000. The average is about 45,000 to 50,000. The hemoglobin and number of platelets are decreased. The predominant cell is the monocyte, the origin of which is not definitely known.

The disease is comparatively rare, but the eye manifestations were described by Gump, Hester and Lohr,[9] who reported a case in a white man 55 years of age. Both eyes were involved. There was an orbital tumor in the left eye, exophthalmos in both eyes, limitation of ocular rotation in both eyes, bilateral papilledema, concentric contraction of the visual fields with enlarged blind spot in both. The orbital infiltration continued to increase until both

Fig. 197.

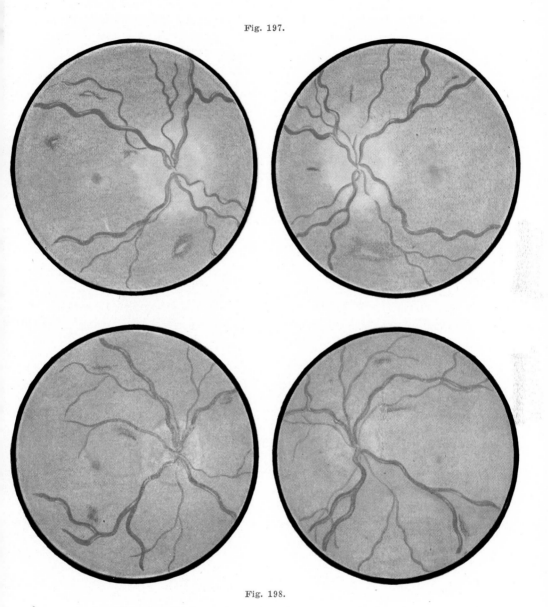

Fig. 198.

Fig. 197.—Fundi in chronic myelogenous leucemia.
Fig. 198.—Fundi in subacute lymphatic leucemia.

eyes were equally proptosed. There was a marked edema about the orbits with increasing chemosis of the conjunctiva. The papilledema was persistent to the extent of about 3 diopters. Exudates and small flame-shaped hemorrhages appeared about the optic disc. The vision in both eyes became greatly diminished.

The eye manifestations were accompanied by diminished hearing with otitis, moist râles at the base of the left lung, enlargement of the spleen and palpable cervical, axillary, and inguinal lymph nodes. The white cell count showed 43 per cent adult monocytes. Petechia developed over the abdomen, flanks, and lower lumbar region. The patient was treated by orbital and abdominal roentgen irradiation without result. A bilateral lobar pneumonia developed which terminated fatally.

Gump and associates[9] suggested for this case the name of monocytic chloroma. The autopsy revealed a diffuse neoplastic infiltration which conformed in distribution to that of chloroma. The pathologic diagnosis was reticulocystoblastoma.

Chloroma.—This condition is characterized by the presence of a rapidly growing malignant tumor which involves the hematopoietic system, with a characteristic tendency for the tumor, which is green in color, to localize in the orbit, producing exophthalmos. The exophthalmos may be the first symptom present. The disease affects children most commonly and usually has a fatal termination.

Frost[10] who reported a case of chloroma in a 4-year-old boy, emphasized the fact that the underlying pathology reveals the disease to be a particular type or unusual form of myelogenous leucemia. The presence of localized growths of myeloid elements and myelogenous leucemia which progresses rapidly to a fatal termination are the outstanding features. Frost stated that the tumor must be green in color in order to designate the condition as chloroma. In this, he was opposed to the statement of Gump and associates, that the tumors may not be green. The cause of the green color has not been definitely determined, but it has been variously attributed to the presence of porphyrin in the tumor, lipochrome, blood pigment and phagocytosis of the blood in obstructed capillaries by endothelial cells.[11]

The chief pathologic changes in the disease include a primary hyperplasia of the bone marrow, producing masses of immature white blood cells below or in the periosteum of the flat bones with metastasis to other structures through the blood stream. The hyperplasia in the areas of the bone marrow increases in size with rarefaction of the bony trabeculae. If they break through, greenish flat tumors are produced over the inner surface of the skull, vertebrae and ribs.

The blood picture and the presence of the greenish tumor mass which contains embryonic myeloid cells are important in making the diagnosis of the condition. In the aleucemic stage of the condition, the saliva cell count has also been said to be of aid. The test for Bence-Jones protein in the urine is also employed to differentiate this condition from myeloma, in which it occurs more commonly. The tumors also are said to lack the green color in myeloma, and a tendency to spontaneous fracture is said to be common in the latter condition.

In addition to exophthalmos, other ocular manifestations in chloroma include keratitis from exposure of the cornea, anisocoria, sluggish pupils, mydriasis, conjunctivitis, cataract, optic neuritis and retinitis.

Treatment of the condition is principally by roentgen therapy and transfusions. The irradiation usually relieves pain and causes a reduction in the size of the tumor. Transfusions aid in relieving the symptoms and reducing the number of abnormal cells in the blood. Surgical removal of the tumor is attempted only for biopsy.

Banti's Syndrome or Splenic Anemia.—This condition is characterized by enlargement of the spleen, a tendency toward gastric hemorrhages, epistaxis, cirrhosis of the liver with ascites, especially in the later stages, and a progressive anemia. The etiology of the condition is obscure, but it is known that a venous congestion of the spleen takes place associated with cellular proliferation. The cause of the anemia is also unexplained except by direct loss of blood from hemorrhage. The early anemia of the disease may be due to splenic dysfunction, without evidence of a direct destructive action by the spleen or of any definite toxic or hemolytic agent. A hypochlorhydria or achlorhydria usually occurs.

Eye Manifestations: Any changes which would occur in the eyes of a patient with Banti's syndrome could not be considered as typical of a disease, since this condition is not considered to be a distinct clinical entity. As a matter of fact, no such cases have been found with a description of any eye changes. However, I had the opportunity to examine a patient with Banti's syndrome and observed marked changes on ophthalmoscopic examination of the eyes. The blood examinations revealed a hemoglobin of from 48 to 32 per cent and a red blood count of 2,000,000. There was a marked prothrombin deficiency, 28 per cent.

On ophthalmoscopic examination, the optic discs were blurred in outline and revealed a considerable amount of edema. The retinal arteries were pale and the retinal veins were greatly distended. There was also a marked pallor and moderate edema present in both retinae. A number of round and linear superficial hemorrhages were seen in the retina of both eyes close to the discs and also in the periphery. Many of these hemorrhages surrounded a white center and were similar to those which occur in leucemic retinitis. There was also a number of small yellowish-white areas of infiltration near the macula in the left eye.

Since there is no specific pathology in this condition which can identify a definite disease, the changes which are found in the optic nerves, retinae, and retinal vessels in such a case can be attributed to the marked anemia and blood changes which are present.

Polycythemia (Erythremia)

Polycythemia is a rare disease of unknown origin characterized by an increase in the red blood cells and the hemoglobin content, symptoms of which are those referable largely to the nervous system, splenomegaly and cyanosis. Two types of the disease are described. A primary form known as polycythemia vera, which has no definite etiology and typical symptoms and blood picture, is found among all groups, usually between the ages of 40 and 60 years. A sec-

Fig. 200.

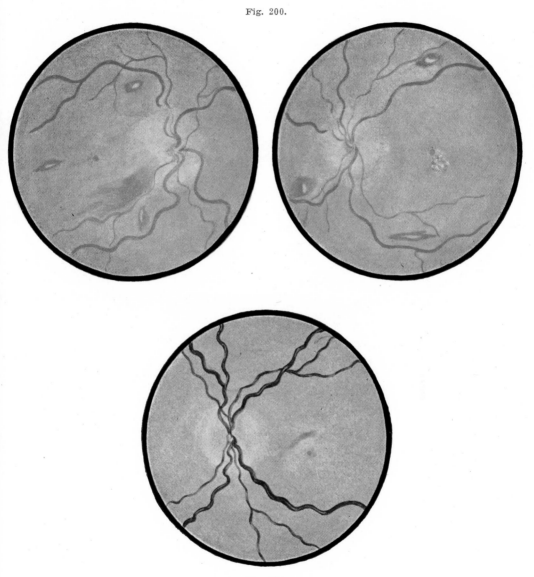

Fig. 201.

Fig. 200.—Banti's syndrome with severe anemia.

Fig. 201.—Fundus in secondary polycythemia.

ondary form known as erythrocytosis occurs in high altitudes among patients with congenital heart disease and also as a result of moderate, temporary toxemia. The symptoms and signs are alike in both forms, but the cyanosis is usually more pronounced in the secondary form.

The pathologic process affects the bone marrow which is increased due to a hyperplasia of the red blood cell elements.

The symptoms include headaches, dizziness, and fainting attacks. There is an inability to concentrate, loss of memory, nervousness, irritability, tinnitus, blurred vision, diplopia and paresthesia. Pain may be complained of in the abdomen and epistaxis and slight hemorrhages occur.

The main physical signs observed are (1) general congestion and dilatation of the vessels, (2) a plum-colored cyanosis, (3) enlarged spleen and palpable liver, (4) cardiac hypertrophy and increased blood pressure.

The blood changes consist of an increased volume which is often double the normal. The red blood cells are normal in appearance but are increased greatly in number and may total from 7 to 12 million. The hemoglobin content is also increased and may be as high as 120 per cent, or higher. The color index is reduced. A leucocytosis of 15,000 to 20,000 may be present and includes mainly polymorphonuclears. The platelets are increased, and the uric acid content is high.

The disease usually runs a long course with intermissions. There is no specific form of treatment available, but phenylhydrazine and venesection are usually employed. Death generally occurs from cardiac failure or thrombosis.

Eye Manifestations.—Both forms of polycythemia may be associated with ocular manifestations which are either mild or severe. The lesion affects the fundus of the eye in particular, and the degree depends on the severity of the general disease, that is, the number of the red cell count and the hemoglobin content. The principal sign is the unusual distention and engorgement of the retinal veins, which is due mainly to the increase in the volume. The veins themselves have a purple color and their walls are thin. The retina has a cyanotic appearance. The engorgement of the veins is apparent in the smaller branches as well as the larger vessels, and in severe cases the crossing of the arteries gives the distended veins the appearance of being sausage shaped.

The arteries are usually normal in size, or only slightly larger. There is, therefore, a marked disproportion between the size of the veins and arteries. The optic disc may show a slight edema and occasionally a few small hemorrhages may be present in the retina. The vision in most of these cases is not seriously impaired. Visual disturbances of different degrees have been described, however, even in the absence of serious retinal changes. These range from photophobia and hazy vision to retrobulbar neuritis and marked loss of vision.

In a report of seven cases of polycythemia, Cohen[12] called attention to cyanosis retinae which is associated with many diseases and suggested that the term should not be applied exclusively to the condition associated with congenital heart disease but to polycythemia as well, with which it is also associated. Five of his cases were of the primary type and revealed the distention and purplish color of the retinal veins while the arteries were normal in color and caliber. He attributed the change in color to excessive replacement of oxygen by carbon dioxide and the ocular lesion to the resultant venous stasis. The vision was normal in all except one case. Two cases of the secondary type revealed a marked distention and bluish color of the retinal veins, while the retinal arteries were only slightly distended and presented a purplish color. They revealed no fundus complications and the vision was unaffected in both.

I found a case of erythrocytosis in a man who first complained of loss of vision in the left eye. On ophthalmoscopic examination he was found to have a small hemorrhage above the macula of the left eye with an area of edema extending down toward the macula. The retinal veins in both eyes were distended and presented a bluish-purple color. There was a small paracentral scotoma in the visual field of the left eye, but the ocular examination was practically negative otherwise.

The patient was employed in a zinc refining plant and on examination of the blood, the red blood count was found to be 6,000,000 and the hemoglobin, 130 per cent. The liver was moderately enlarged but complete general physical examination revealed no other abnormalities. The patient discontinued his occupation temporarily and in a short time the blood count returned to normal and the hemorrhage and edema near the macula completely cleared. The vision also returned to normal. There has been no recurrence of the condition to date. The polycythemia was temporary in duration and together with the ocular lesion was probably due to a chemical intoxication which was mild in character.

Hodgkin's Disease

Hodgkin's disease, or lymphogranuloma, was first described by Hodgkin in 1832. At present it is considered to be a disease which is characterized chiefly by an enlargement of the superficial lymph glands, the specific cause of which is unknown. The adenopathy is generalized, but the cervical lymph nodes are usually the first involved. It begins on one side but soon becomes bilateral. The glands are hard and freely movable. They do not become attached to the surrounding tissues. Their enlargement is accompanied by weakness, loss of weight, remittent temperature, and anemia. The blood examination reveals a leucocytosis with eosinophilia and granulocytes. There is usually an absolute monocytosis. The myeloblastic and erythrocytic tissue in the bone marrow may be crowded out by a great increase of the cells typical of the disease which causes an anemia of the Addisonian type and bronzing of the skin.

Histologically, there are many large pale cells with a vesicular nucleus which later develop into giant cells with several nuclei (Dorothy Reid cells). Eosinophiles are abundant and later there is an extensive diffuse fibrosis. The spleen is often enlarged from hyperplasia. Although the exact cause is not known, the condition has been variously considered to be an atypical form of tuberculosis, a specific infection of unknown etiology, a true tumor formation, and a condition intermediate between infectious granulomas and tumor. Craver, in describing the treatment of blood disorders,[13] stated that the tendency is to regard the disease, especially in its early and intermediate stages, "as an inflammatory process, probably caused by various stimuli of the lymph node system, chief among which is possibly tuberculosis. There is certainly much clinical evidence, though perhaps not so much laboratory evidence, that tuberculosis may play a large part in the etiology of Hodgkin's disease."

The disease must be differentiated from tuberculosis, leucemia and aleucemic leucemia, and lymphosarcoma. In the latter condition the tumor is not as hard in consistency, and in Hodgkin's disease there is no tendency to invade and infiltrate the surrounding tissues. Lymphosarcoma also occurs more frequently later in life. In tuberculosis the clinical course of the glandular involvement differs from that in Hodgkin's disease which is steadily progressive and leads to a fatal termination. In leucemia there is a high lymphocyte count, and in aleucemic leucemia, the giant cells and eosinophiles are not found in the histologic sections. Hodgkin's disease may continue for years and go on to become Hodgkin's lymphosarcoma.

Eye Manifestations.—Involvement of the eye in Hodgkin's disease is comparatively rare. This was pointed out by Kravitz,[14] who reported a case which occurred in a woman 82 years of age. This is a much older age for the disease to occur than usual. A small cystic tumor was present at the left superior orbital border near the inner angle. The tumor increased in size and a ptosis developed. On removal and dissection of the tumor, it was found to have a firm consistency and was contained in a thick white capsule. The remaining tissue later increased in size and two new growths appeared along the upper border of the left orbit. Histologic examination showed the tumor to have all the features of Hodgkin's disease. The patient had a mild anemia, but otherwise the chest revealed no masses or enlarged nodes. There was no enlargement of the cervical or other lymph glands at this time, but there was a history of previous bilateral parotitis which subsided on treatment by roentgen irradiation. Later some small lymph nodes of the superficial cervical glands were observed. Signs of pressure developed in the chest which were found on roentgen examination to be due to large masses of glands. The case was not terminated at the time of the report.

Treatment of the condition consists mainly in irradiation of the enlarged glands which is followed by their rapid disappearance, especially early in the disease. The swellings may return, however. Craver stated that the general practice in giving local irradiation is to use a fairly small dose at a time, not over 100 or 200 roentgens, and that the treatment should be individualized.

Other forms of treatment include the use of arsenicals, iron, fresh air, rest, sunshine, and a nutritious diet.

References

1. Ottenberg, Reuben: Reclassification of the Anemias, J. A. M. A. **100:** 1303-1311, 1933.
2. Cox, R. A.: Amblyopia Resulting From Hemorrhage, Arch. Ophth. **32:** 368, 1944.
3. Watkins, Charles H., Wagener, Henry P., and Brown, Robert W.: Cerebral Symptoms Accompanied by Choked Optic Discs in Types of Blood Dyscrasia, Am. J. Ophth. **24:** 1374, 1941.
4. Spaeth, Edmund B.: Traumatic Liporrhagia Retinalis (Verhoeff): Purtscher's Disease, Arch. Ophth. **31:** 191, 1944.
5. Goldbach, L. J.: Leukemic Retinitis, Arch. Ophth. **10:** 808, 1933.
6. Cohen, M.: Orbital Lymphoma in Chronic Lymphatic Leukemia, Arch. Ophth. **11:** 617, 1934.
7. Goldstein, I., and Wexler, D.: Histologic Observations on the Fundus in Leukemia, Arch. Ophth. **13:** 26, 1935.
8. Gibson, G. G.: Clinical Significance of the Retinal Changes in Leukemia, Arch. Ophth. **20:** 364, 1938.
9. Gump, M. E., Hester, E. G., and Lohr, O. W.: Monocytic Chloroma, Arch. Ophth. **16:** 931, 1936.
10. Frost, Albert D.: Chloroma: Report of a Case With Hematologic Study, Tr. Am. Acad. Ophth. **42:** 123, 1937.
11. Terry, T. L., and Dvorak-Theobald, Georgianna: In discussion of Frost's case.
12. Cohen, M.: Lesions of the Fundus in Polycythemia, Arch. Ophth. **17:** 811, 1937.
13. Craver, L. F.: The Treatment of Blood Diseases, J. A. M. A. **115:** 297, 1940.
14. Kravitz, D.: Hodgkin's Disease of the Lid, Arch. Ophth. **21:** 844, 1939.

CHAPTER XVII

DISORDERS OF MENSTRUATION AND PREGNANCY

The numerous and complex possibilities concerned with the normal and altered function of the female generative organs obviates any detailed discussion of the subject in this instance. Moreover, the possible connection between their normal function and the function of some of the ductless glands might justify this consideration in the chapter dealing with that subject. But with the little knowledge at hand and the lack of any definite clinical pattern at the present time, the question of cause and relationship is still open in many of these disorders.

Menstruation.—The period of menstruation is frequently accompanied by eye manifestations of a disturbing nature in women who appear to be normal in all other respects. In other instances the eye manifestations may occur with abnormal conditions of menstruation due to pathologic changes such as occur in pituitary disease.

In the first group menstruation is frequently accompanied by headache and visual disturbances which are severe enough to cause the patient to request an eye examination. The ocular symptoms are best described as being of a reflex nature and ophthalmoscopic examination invariably reveals a normal fundus. The refractive state of the eyes may also be normal as is often true when these patients are examined. When corrective lenses are found necessary, their use might relieve the complaints to some degree, since an uncorrected refractive state of the eyes may aggravate the condition. Reading and the performance of close work is accompanied by asthenopia and severe headache.

Edema of the eyelids and blue rings are often present at the time of menstruation. These usually clear up later. The degree of anemia present in these patients is also a factor concerned with the type and severity of the ocular symptoms.

After studying a large number of subjects by a technique advocated for angioscotometry, Evans[1] demonstrated a scotoma apparently associated with the menstrual period. This defect is wedge shaped, with its apex at the blind spot and its base located peripherally. It responds to the influence of gravity, and transient fluctuations may be produced as by digital pressure on the eyeball. Most of the scotoma occupies the upper field over 10 degrees above the fixation point. The size and shape may change with various phases of the menstrual cycle. It is modified by the inhalation of oxygen and is absent during some or all stages of uncomplicated pregnancy. Evans felt that this defect is consistently present and that it is reasonable to designate the defect as "the scotoma of menstruation."

Other visual field defects such as enlargement of the blind spots and temporary reduction in the peripheral fields have also been shown by others to occur during menstruation.

Amenorrhea.—Suppression of the menses may be accompanied by a sensation of fullness and heaviness about the eyes. The eyelids may be slightly puffed and the conjunctiva injected. A hyperemia may be present in the retinal vessels and optic disc. Small retinal hemorrhages and an acute retrobulbar neuritis may occur occasionally.

Ocular hemorrhages have been recorded in a number of instances in women who suddenly began to menstruate. Subconjunctival hemorrhage as vicarious menstruation of the conjunctiva was reported by Poos.[2] In one case a patient 22 years of age suffered with amenorrhea with general disturbances for several years. Subcutaneous injection of a pituitary preparation on two consecutive days was followed by slight menstruation and bilateral hemorrhages in the conjunctiva from the limbus down to the fornix. Another woman, aged 29, began to menstruate after strenuous close work. On the following morning she noticed an extensive hemorrhage near the temporal canthus of the right eye.

Three cases of recurring hemorrhages in the vitreous associated with menstruation were reported by Satanowsky.[3] Improvement after treatment with calcium occurred in one.

Metrorrhagia.—Reflex ocular symptoms characterized by the presence of headache and asthenopia occur with metrorrhagia. Attacks which are similar to migraine and transient periods of amaurosis are also complained of.

When metrorrhagia or menorrhagia results from disease of the pituitary, it may be accompanied by more pronounced eye manifestations because of pressure on the optic chiasm. This would produce a bitemporal hemianopia and various degrees of optic atrophy.

Diseases of the Uterus.—The abnormalities of the uterus to be considered here include displacement, infection, and hemorrhage.

Displacement of the uterus may result only in the manifestation of reflex ocular symptoms. Pain in and about the eyes and refractive asthenopia are present. Reflex headache is often an accompanying symptom.

Infections of the uterus and uterine appendages may be the source of a septic iritis, iridocyclitis, and metastatic ophthalmia.

Uterine Hemorrhage.—Hemorrhage from the uterus, especially when prolonged or profuse enough to cause an anemia, may be accompanied by visual disturbances. These cases might be included in the group of hypochloremic anemia resulting from hemorrhage.

Ocular manifestations may appear, usually in both eyes, which are characterized by sudden loss of vision and the presence chiefly of an optic neuritis or neuroretinitis. The optic nerve head is swollen with blurred margins and surrounded by an area of edema which may extend out beyond the macular region. The swelling of the nerve heads may measure as much as four diopters and the visual fields may reveal defects, a type of which has been described in these cases as an impure nasal hemianopia.[4]

The prognosis in these cases is usually good for the ultimate recovery of vision on cessation of the hemorrhage. However, serious loss of vision and even blindness may result. A case of amaurosis following uterine hemorrhage, occurring in spells over a period of two years, was reported by Langdon.[5] The vision was reduced to the ability to count fingers at two feet and the optic discs were covered with a white, fluffy material which completely blurred the margins. The blood count revealed a hemoglobin of 45 per cent, red cells 1,880,000, and white cells 22,000. After treatment by transfusions, the general condition of the patient improved. A hysterectomy was performed later which was followed by improvement of the vision to practically normal in each eye, with only some disturbance of light sense remaining after a period of four months. Langdon attributed the loss of vision in such cases solely to the anemia. Zentmayer,[6] who also described two cases of this type which were complicated by other diseases, felt that the systemic condition was a contributing cause of the amaurosis.

Transient hemiplegia with loss of vision in one eye was reported by Thomson[7] in a pregnant woman who suffered with a moderate uterine hemorrhage. The left eye was blind and she had lost the power of her right arm and leg. She recovered from the hemiplegia in two days, but the visual loss persisted. The ophthalmoscopic examination showed evidences of closure of the central retinal artery. Atrophy of the optic nerve developed. The author felt that the symptoms were due to thrombosis of the internal carotid artery which led to necrosis of the pituitary gland, as suggested by other symptoms of pituitary disturbance such as abnormal feelings of coldness and the absence of mammary reaction. The transient hemiplegia was attributed to arterial spasm.

Pregnancy.—The ordinary pregnancy, otherwise uncomplicated before delivery, is rarely accompanied by serious ocular manifestations. Pigmentation of the skin of the eyelids without other manifestations is an example. Increase in the intraocular tension has been observed in the course of pregnancy in the absence of any other manifestation, but this is also a rare occurrence. A case of this kind reported by Dubois[8] coexisted with the pregnancy during the early months and disappeared in the fourth month following spontaneous delivery. The visual acuity was unimpaired but decreased the day preceding the miscarriage. The increase in ocular tension was attributed to the pregnancy.

Changes in the optic nerve and visual fields are recognized manifestations of enlargement of the pituitary gland in pregnancy. The exact relationship between the pituitary and the visual defects noted in these cases is not always clearly understood. It is usually considered that during pregnancy the pituitary undergoes a physiologic enlargement which produces the optic nerve affection and visual field defect by pressure on the chiasm. The optic nerve may be found to have blurred margins and show some degree of swelling. The optic neuritis which occurs has been attributed also to the effect of toxins. The typical visual field defect is the presence of a bitemporal hemianopia. Retrobulbar neuritis which was accompanied by the chiasmal syndrome of Cushing was reported by Hagedoorn[9] in which the condition improved after delivery but recurred during the succeeding pregnancy and led to the diagnosis of suprasellar meningioma. When the bitemporal field defect is due to physiologic enlargement of the pituitary of short duration, the vision and vision fields of the patient may return to normal after recovery. This does not always occur, however, and in some cases the optic nerve manifestation is seen in the presence of other complicating disease such as disseminated sclerosis.

Papilledema in the absence of the typical retinitis of pregnancy is rare, but it has been observed with increased intracranial pressure. Schaeffer[10] described two cases of this kind with headache, vomiting, choked disc, and increased intraspinal pressure. The pathogenesis was not explained. Recovery took place in both cases after delivery. The one pregnancy continued to full term with birth of a living child following treatment by lumbar puncture. The second received radiotherapy and injection of mercury cyanide which resulted in premature labor and birth of a dead child.

Vomiting of Pregnancy.—Two cases of hemorrhagic retinitis which occurred with severe vomiting of pregnancy were reported by Stander,[11] who considered it probable that the ocular condition was caused by a change in the permeability of the capillary walls. He also pointed out that necrosis in the anterior lobe of the hypophysis is sometimes seen in fatal cases of vomiting in pregnancy. The appearance of hemorrhagic retinitis with severe vomiting of pregnancy is significant of a bad prognosis and an indication for therapeutic abortion.

Ballantyne,[12] in a report of six cases of pernicious vomiting in pregnancy and a review of the literature, stated that edema of the papilla and retinal hemorrhages are late ocular evidences. The earliest eye manifestation was found to be a defect in the central vision resulting from a retrobulbar neuritis. The diagnosis is difficult to make at this time and it is emphasized that it is important to examine the eyes as soon as impaired vision is complained of in these patients. The final stage is a well-defined papilledema with flame-shaped peripapillary hemorrhages radiating from the disc. There are no exudates and no changes in the blood vessels. The eye signs differ from those in diabetes, hypertension and nephritis because of the marked loss of vision.

The treatment recommended is vitamins B and C if the diagnosis can be made early. If the persistent vomiting in pregnancy does not respond readily and the advanced ocular manifestations are present, a termination of the pregnancy is indicated.

Toxemia of Pregnancy.—The toxemia of pregnancy usually occurs between the third and ninth month. The greater number probably occur during the later period or during the last month. It is divided clinically into the preeclamptic and eclamptic stages. In all cases it is characterized by the presence of hypertension, the severity of which may in a general way be said to serve as a guide to the presence and extent of the retinal manifestations. Toxemia of pregnancy does not, however, depend on the presence of previous hypertension or nephritis. Since most of these women are young, hypertension before pregnancy is rarely present, although nephritis may occur more often. When either of these conditions should be present before the pregnancy, they will serve to intensify the toxemia. The onset of the condition is usually sudden, and the clinical picture which ushers in the pre-eclamptic stage is characterized by moderate hypertension, very little edema, and a slight albuminuria. If these symptoms do not increase, the delivery may take place normally, after which the condition subsides. They may become more severe, however, with a further increase in blood pressure, more severe urinary changes as increased albuminuria, and casts, edema, and also retinal changes as indicated by the presence of vasospasm. This now constitutes the pre-eclamptic stage, and the symptoms are very similar to those of acute diffuse glomerulonephritis. The renal function is unimpaired, however, and the blood changes of renal insufficiency are absent. The onset of convulsions with a sudden rise in blood pressure ushers in the stage of eclampsia. The sudden increase in blood pressure is the first manifestation and is followed by the convulsions. This also occurs in the absence of renal insufficiency although there may be a slight increase in the urea and total non-protein nitrogen of the blood. In all other respects the eclamptic stage resembles also the picture of acute diffuse nephritis with the convulsions and cerebral symptoms as complications. The clinical symptoms were all explained by Elwyn on the basis of the generalized arterial constriction which is present.

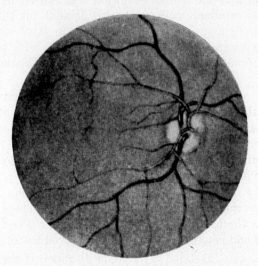

Fig. 202.—Attenuation of retinal arterioles in the preorganic stage. Hypertensive toxemia of pregnancy. (From Gibson: Am. J. Ophth., January, 1938.)

The presence of such symptoms as anemia, edema, hypertension, arteriosclerosis, and others in a patient during the early period of pregnancy, would indicate the presence of nephritis and are not due to the toxemia of pregnancy. A knowledge of their presence should even serve as a contraindication to pregnancy in such patients. Once the toxemia of pregnancy has developed, most of the patients will later show evidences of arteriosclerotic nephritis, or glomerulonephritis and hypertension following the more severe forms. It is, therefore, important that the condition be recognized early in order to determine the procedure to be followed during the pregnancy, and also to prevent the possibility of permanent kidney and vascular disease later, by interrupting the pregnancy at the time indicated.

Retinal Manifestations.—The retinal changes serve as one of the best indications of the state of the toxemia and are of utmost importance from a diagnostic and prognostic standpoint in this condition. These changes are ordinarily designated as the retinitis of pregnancy or the retinitis of toxemia of pregnancy.

As pointed out by Duggan and Chitnis[13] among others, the retinitis of pregnancy is separate and distinct from that which is due to nephritis and whenever chronic nephritis complicates pregnancy, the visual disturbances are due to the nephritis rather than pre-eclamptic toxemia. Numerous studies by various investigators during recent years have led to a better understanding and correlation of the retinal changes with those of toxemia as well as with those of hypertension and nephritis.

The retinal manifestations of the toxemia of pregnancy are divided into two main groups: (1) those which belong to the preorganic stage and (2) those of the organic stage. The recognition of the importance of the former especially has led to a decided increase in the number of cases of this group. If the condition remains after the pregnancy, the period of the first years which follow are designated as the latent stage. The routine ophthalmoscopic examination of all such cases is of the utmost importance.

Gibson,[14] who reported the results of the examination of thirty-nine cases in which only five revealed a normal fundus, described the four changes which occur. The earliest visible sign of the disease is attenuation of the retinal arterioles which usually occurs first in those of the nasal periphery. This is characterized by a reduction in their width. The attenuation is usually noted about the time the diastolic blood pressure reaches 95 mm. Hg.

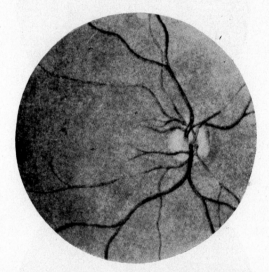

Fig. 203.—Retinal arteriolar spasm with localized marked constriction as seen in severe vasospastic preorganic disease. (From Gibson: Am. J. Ophth., January, 1938.)

When the narrowing of the vessel becomes marked, areas of angiospasm occur in which the column of blood can no longer be distinguished. The angiospasm may affect one or more arterioles completely. The surrounding retina supplied by the angiospastic vessels may show signs of edema. When the edema covers a portion of the vessel it may resemble in appearance the angiospasm itself. The exact cause of the vascular response is not known but, in discussing vasospasm in eclampsia, Smith et al.[15] call attention to a disturbance in water balance as one of the most certain premonitory signs of approaching toxemia, and that the vasospasm itself is responsible for the retinitis.

The changes of attenuation and angiospasm thus far described constitute the preorganic stage of the disease. With the proper management and treatment many of the cases progress no further and more serious damage is averted. On the other hand, when the condition is persistent over a long period of time, it leads to the presence of sclerosis, and introduction of the organic stage of the disease. The length of time in which this occurs depends on variable factors in the blood pressure and its effect on the particular individual. The sclerosis is characterized by a thickening of the vessel wall which encroaches on its lumen and which results in its narrowing. The condition of the walls of the arterioles and the calibre of their lumen, with regard to the degree of sclerosis manifested, should be carefully studied on ophthalmoscopic examination.

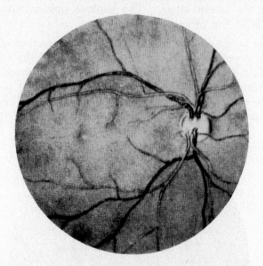

Fig. 204.—Retinal arteriolar sclerosis, hypertensive type. Hypertensive toxemia of pregnancy. (From Gibson: Am. J. Ophth., January, 1938.)

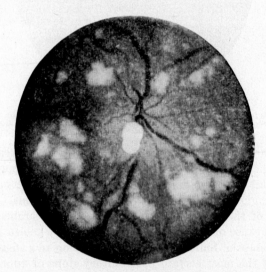

Fig. 205.—Hypertensive toxemia of pregnancy. Angiospastic retinitis. (From Gibson: Am. J. Ophth., January, 1938.)

When the sclerosis is followed by the appearance of hemorrhages, exudates, and edema in the retina, in the case of pregnancy with hypertension, the ophthalmoscopic picture then constitutes a retinitis of the toxemia of pregnancy.

If the sclerosis of the arterioles continues, for several years after delivery, the condition is in the latent stage. This persistent and prolonged sclerosis eventually leads to the terminal stage of the disease in which the retinitis resembles that seen with malignant hypertension. The clinical symptoms presented will depend then on the organs more seriously involved by the pathologic process affecting the vessels. The picture may be that of chronic nephritis, cerebral hypertension or malignant hypertension.

During the course of the pregnancy, the time at which the retinal changes appear, as observed on ophthalmoscopic examination, is of great importance in the prognosis and further progress of the case. If no signs other than attenuation of the retinal vessels are noted, the case remains in the preorganic stage and the normal delivery may be accomplished with a complete recovery of the retinal condition. If angiospasm occurs early, however, regular and repeated ophthalmoscopic examination is indicated, since further changes showing the presence of the organic stage with the appearance of sclerosis may be expected to follow. The exact transition from one stage to the next is very difficult to determine in many cases. However, the appearance of exudates, an early edema about the disc, or signs of retinitis are a serious complication, and even in the absence of clinical contraindications their presence is significant of continued manifestations of the disease, and termination of the pregnancy should be advised.

Detachment of the retina is a complication which occurs occasionally in the course of a case of toxemia of pregnancy. This does not usually result in any permanent impairment of vision, for the condition of the retina returns to normal after recovery from the toxemia.

Puerperal Septicemia.—The septicemia resulting from infection during the puerperium may result in the presence of a metastatic choroiditis or retinitis, and retinal hemorrhages. Papillitis and retrobulbar neuritis may also occur during the puerperium but these manifestations are rare.

Lactation.—About the seventh or eighth week in normal or prolonged lactation the vision may become impaired by the appearance of an optic neuritis. The condition usually affects both eyes and may continue for several months. It may be terminated, however, by weaning. The exact cause is unknown. The vision usually improves, although its recovery may be slow.

References

1. Evans, J. M.: A Scotoma Associated With Menstruation, Am. J. Ophth. 24: 507, 1941.
2. Poos, F.: Subconjunctival Hemorrhage as Vicarious Menstruation of the Conjunctiva, Klin. Monatsbl. f. Augenh. 91: 661, 1933.
3. Satanowsky, P.: Relapsing Hemorrhages in the Vitreous and Menstruation, Arch. de Oftal. de Buenos Aires 13: 173, 1938.
4. de Schweinitz, G. E.: In discussion of Langdon's Case, Arch. Ophth. 10: 99, 1933.
5. Langdon, H. Maxwell: Amaurosis After Uterine Hemorrhage, Arch. Ophth. 10: 99, 1933.
6. Zentmayer, W.: In Discussion of Langdon's Case, Arch. Ophth. 10: 99, 1933.
7. Thomson, A. M. Wright: Post-Partum Arterial Obstruction Associated With Hemiplegia, Brit. M. J. 1: 387, 1940.
8. Dubois, A.: Glaucoma or Ocular Hypertension in a Pregnant Woman; Disappearance of the Trouble After Spontaneous Miscarriage, Ann. d' ocul. 172: 142, 1935.
9. Hagedoorn, A.: The Chiasmal Syndrome and Retrobulbar Neuritis in Pregnancy, Am. J. Ophth. 20: 690, 1937.

10. Schaeffer, H.:   Choked Disc in Pregnancy With Syndrome of Increased Intracranial Pressure, Arch. d' Ophth. **49**: 325, 1932.
11. Stander, H. J.:   Hemorrhagic Retinitis in Vomiting of Pregnancy, Surg., Gynec. and Obst. **54**: 129, 1932.
12. Ballantyne, A. J.:   Ocular Complications in Hyperemesis Gravidarum, J. Obst. & Gynaec. Brit. Emp. **48**: 206, 1941.
13. Duggan, J. N., and Chitnis, V. K.:   Retinitis of Pregnancy, Brit. J. Ophth. **21**: 585, 1937.
14. Gibson, G. G.:   The Clinical Significance of the Retinal Changes in the Hypertensive Toxemia of Pregnancy, Am. J. Ophth. **21**: 29, 1938.
15. Smith, L. W., Weiss, E., Lillie, W. I., Konzelman, F. W., and Gault, E. G.:   Cardiovascular-Renal Disease, New York, 1940, D. Appleton-Century Co., Inc.

CHAPTER XVIII

DISEASES OF THE ENDOCRINE GLANDS AND METABOLISM

The disorders of the endocrine glands do not act as a simple cause and effect. From the many investigations made in recent years, one thing that has been established with regard to the endocrine glands is the fact that their function and dysfunction are closely connected with that of other systems and processes. The autonomic nervous system and certain biochemical reactions in the body, for example, have an effect in regulating the endocrine functions. Moreover, certain of the diseases of metabolism are produced by, or at least associated with, glandular dysfunction. And lastly, one gland may possess what appears to be a specific function of its own, but it may also, by separate action, have a regulating effect on the function of another. It is, therefore, not only difficult at times definitely to classify a particular disease, but it is often impossible to determine whether a certain disorder results from the hyperfunction of one gland, the hypofunction of another, or both.

The Autonomic Nervous System and the Eyes

The autonomic nervous system bears a close relationship to the function of the endocrine glands as well as to certain manifestations of endocrine disease and metabolism in the eye. This was pointed out by Lemoine,[1] who described the autonomic nervous system as one which is not independently controlled but as an "involuntary outflow from the cerebrospinal system with peripheral plexuses at the sites of distribution which are connected by neurons to the cerebrospinal system. These are divided into the sympathetic, parasympathetic, and visceral systems. The sympathetic comprises the thoracolumbar outflow, while the parasympathetic includes the cranial and sacral."

The parasympathetic controls the ciliary muscle, and with stimulation it produces a contraction of the pupil and increase in the accommodation of the eye in addition to other manifestations such as lacrimation, sweating, and salivation.

The structures in the eye which are governed by action of the sympathetic are the dilator pupillae muscle, the unstriped muscle fibers in the levator palpebrae superioris which elevates the upper lid, and the smooth muscle fibers (Müller's muscle) at the back of the eye, which are said to push the globe forward. Therefore, stimulation of the sympathetic produces a decreased lacrimation, dilatation of the pupil, retraction of the upper eyelid, and proptosis or exophthalmos. From this it can be understood how a destructive lesion of the sympathetic leads to constriction of the pupil by the now unopposed fibers of the sphincter pupillae, drooping or ptosis of the upper eyelid and sinking or retraction of the eye, enophthalmos. (See Horner's syndrome.)

Because of their pharmacologic action on the autonomic nervous system, certain drugs have been employed in recent years in a number of internal ocular diseases. This pharmacology was early investigated and elucidated by Velhagen, Alles, Gaddam and more recently Myerson and Thau.[2] The results of these early investigations led to the concept that the activity of any organ governed by autonomic stimulation is the result of a balanced action between acetylcholine in the parasympathetic system and sympathin which is supposed to exist in the sympathetic. The latter has not as yet been isolated, but acetylcholine is produced as the result of a reaction between choline and acetylchloride. This occurs in the interneuronic synapses of the parasympathetic and sympathetic systems and also at the junction of the parasympathetic and the organic cell. Acetylcholine, therefore, is responsible for stimulated activity of the parasympathetic. This action is said to occur in the presence of a choline esterase, which was found by Stedman to be present in the tissues. The esterase has the property of entering into chemical combination with acetylcholine and thereby inhibiting its action. In the sympathetic system, sympathin, which is similar to epinephrine, is supposed to be produced at the neurocellular junction.

Those drugs which act on the parasympathetic system, such as prostigmine, are synergistic in their action and are known as the cholinergic drugs. Whereas the effect of the esterase is to inhibit the action of acetylcholine, this is overcome when the synergist prostigmine is administered. In other words, it is thought that prostigmine will abolish the effect of the esterase and thereby enhance the effect of acetylcholine. The latter has been found to exist in the iris, ciliary body, aqueous and retina of the eye, and it has been experimentally found to activate the sphincter of the isolated iris, even after the use of atropine. It has also been suggested that an excessive accumulation of the choline esterase is a factor in the onset of presbyopia, since the quantity present is sufficient to overcome the action of the smaller amount of acetylcholine.

Clinically, cholinergic drugs acetylcholine and prostigmine can be employed in the eye in rather strong concentration without causing any general effect. They are apparently absorbed and destroyed locally without absorption and effect on the general circulation. Their effect is to constrict the pupil to the size of a pin point and increase the accommodation of the eye. The light reaction is not affected by their use. The palpebral fissure is narrowed and the intraocular tension is decreased. Mecholyl (acetylcholine) can be instilled into the conjunctival sac in concentrations up to 10 per cent or stronger without producing any general effect. The instillation of one drop of mecholyl, 1 per cent, followed by one drop of prostigmine, 1 per cent, in the conjunctival sac of an ordinary individual, will produce a marked miosis, reduction in intraocular tension, and an increased accommodation. Another important effect is a dilatation of the peripheral vessels and of the deeper vessels when administered subconjunctivally. Because of the effect in reducing the intraocular tension mecholyl and prostigmine in combination have been employed rather widely in cases of glaucoma. In cases of obstruction of the retinal arteries and in other eye conditions accompanied by abnormal constriction of the arteries, they are employed for the vasodilator effect. Prostigmine has also been used for vasodilatation in the treatment of other peripheral circulatory disturbances such as thromboangiitis obliterans, Raynaud's disease, and other cases of vascular occlusion.

The drugs which stimulate the sympathetic system are known as the adrenergic drugs and are sometimes spoken of as sympathomimetic drugs. They are naturally antagonistic to the cholinergic group and produce the opposite effects on the eye. They are synergists of atropine, however. By their action on the sympathetic, they produce a widening of the palpebral fissure with a tendency to protrusion of the eyeball, a dilatation of the pupil and even marked mydriasis, constriction of the peripheral vessels, and an impairment of the accommodation. Included in this group are adrenalin, ephedrine, cocaine, benzedrine, and paredrine. In addition to the action described they have a tendency to increase the intraocular tension when employed in the eye. This effect is rarely encountered in practice when the drugs are used alone in ordinary dosage. Glaucoma has been caused, however, by the repeated and regular intranasal use of ephedrine. Cocaine, in addition to its anesthetic effect, is often instilled into the eye like adrenalin and paredrine in order to produce mydriasis and the breaking up of early synechia of the iris. Very often they are used in combination with one another and with atropine. With the latter, they are often employed in order to produce paralysis of the accommodation for the purpose of refraction.

Disorders of the Autonomic Nervous System.—Overstimulation of the sympathetic system has been described as the cause of the ocular manifestations of hyperthyroidism, such as exophthalmos and its accompanying signs. Conversely, the opposite action in hypothyroidism has been said to cause the enophthalmos, conjunctivitis, decreased lacrimation and decreased blinking occurring in this condition. Other instances of overstimulation of either the parasympathetic or the sympathetic in association with disorders of the endocrine glands are numerous.

Certain disturbances of metabolic and emotional rhythm were described by Foster Kennedy[3] as the result of disturbances of the parasympathetic and sympathetic systems which are linked and perhaps activated by hormonal messengers, chiefly from the hypophysis, but stimulated and controlled through the subthalamus to the thalamus, and then to the prefrontal cortex. Some of the neuroses often show evidences of instability of the autonomic nervous system. Poorly sustained and subnormal accommodation of the eyes, migraine accompanied by disturbances of the ocular muscles and accommodation, may be produced by altered action of the parasympathetic and sympathetic systems.

Adie's Syndrome.—Excessive worry and emotional stress and strain are apparently a factor in disorders of the autonomic nervous system. Adie's syndrome may be found in patients of this kind. This is a pupillary phenomenon which was described first by Sanger and Strassburger separately in 1902, as one in which the patient showed a myotonic pupil with an absence of knee jerks and ankle jerks. It was later described by Adie in 1931 with a report of six cases, as a "pseudo-Argyll-Robertson pupil with absent tendon reflexes," benign in character but resembling tabes dorsalis. The pupils in Adie's cases failed to react or responded poorly to light and manifested a tonic slow reaction with convergence, followed later by an even slower dilatation. There was no evidence of syphilis or other neurologic symptoms present. Adie later reported an additional number of cases and described it as "a benign disorder *sui generis.*"

Foster Kennedy et al.[4] reported a series of five cases and gave the following description. The syndrome may present a complete or an incomplete form. In the former one or both pupils fail to react normally to light and have a tonic convergence reaction. There is an absence of one or more deep tendon reflexes. The incomplete form may present tonic pupillary reactions alone, atypical tonic reactions alone, atypical pupils with absent tendon reflexes, and absent tendon reflexes alone.

The phenomenon is differentiated from the Argyll-Robertson pupil which shows miosis, the normal accommodation or convergence reaction, the absence of light reaction, and poor reaction to mydriatics. The Argyll-Robertson pupil is also always bilateral. Adie's syndrome is usually unilateral and the involved pupil is usually larger than the other. After a short delay during accommodation, the pupil contracts to a greater degree than normal. It may remain small after convergence and then proceed to dilate at a slower rate than contraction. Direct and consensual light reflexes are completely or almost completely abolished. However, the pupil does dilate again after being in a dark room and with exposure to daylight it contracts very slowly again. The contraction may continue until the pupil becomes much smaller than it was before dilatation in the dark room. It then dilates again slowly to its original size. With mydriatics the pupil acts normally. About 80 per cent of the patients are young women.

In nearly all of the cases reported, there was a history of emotional disturbance. The syndrome has been reported also in cases with influenza, diabetes, and other diseases, but Adie restricted the occurrence to those who are otherwise in good health. Kennedy and associates stated also that this restriction should be followed in classifying the syndrome, but it is true that other evidences of vasomotor instability are frequently presented by these patients. It has also been noted with other sympathetic disorders.

Atypical cases of Adie's syndrome occur in which various degrees of the manifestation may be present. Some authors believe that it occurs with syphilis, but others are in agreement with Adie, that it is of sympathetic origin. Sheie,[5] however, studied six cases of Adie's syndrome and found that the affected pupils were all sensitized to mecholyl (acetylcholine). From this, he postulated the theory of the site of the lesion as a partial parasympathetic denervation peripheral to the ciliary ganglion.

Lowenstein and Friedman,[6] who studied a number of Adie and non-Adie pupils, concluded that Adie's syndrome is due to heredodegenerative disease localized in the autonomic centers of the diencephalon and their connections with the mesencephalon. It is characterized by pupillotonic reactions with irritative (not paralytic) sympathetic symptoms and the absence of tendon reflexes. They believed that in general it has no syphilitic etiologic factor but that it may be produced as a syndrome by so-called asymptomatic syphilis nervosa. They also felt that some cases may be due to congenital syphilis since the nervous manifestations of congenital syphilis are often localized in the sympathetic center. Physostigmine was found to contract the Adie pupil like the normal pupil; however, it restored the ability of the Adie pupil to react to light and to dilate to distant vision in from twelve to twenty minutes after instillation. It was felt that the physostigmine test will serve to differentiate Adie's syndrome from similar conditions due to acquired syphilitic infection.

Horner's Syndrome.—This is a syndrome described by Horner in 1869 and is characterized by sinking in of the eyeball (enophthalmos), ptosis or drooping of the upper eyelid, slight elevation of the lower lid, marked constriction of the pupil, narrowing of the palpebral fissure and changes in vasomotor and sudorific activity of the skin of the face.   The presence of enophthalmos as part of the syndrome is sometimes questioned.   Opinions differ somewhat concerning the exact cause of some of the elements of the symptom complex. Some of the factors of the typical syndrome are not present in all instances. This can be explained by the involvement of certain nerve fibers in some instances while in others these same fibers escape.   Paralysis of the cervical portion of the sympathetic occurs probably more frequently than that of others.

The most severe eye manifestations were found by Cobb and Scarlett[7] in eleven cases to be due to injuries of the seventh and eighth cervical and first dorsal nerve roots.   Injuries to the cervical portion of the sympathetic trunk cause less severe symptoms while injuries to the spinal cord present the least severe manifestations.

Horner's syndrome may occur after disease or injury to the brain stem, to the lower part of the cervical portion of the spinal cord, to the upper part of the dorsal portion, or to the superior cervical sympathetic ganglion or the postganglionic nerves as well as to some of the nerve roots.

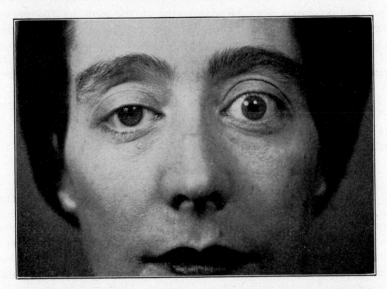

Fig. 206.—Horner's syndrome.   (I. S. Tassman, Wills Hospital.)

The most frequent causes of Horner's syndrome mentioned by De Jong[8] are spinal cord tumor and syringomyelia at the level of the seventh or eighth cervical or first thoracic portion of the spinal cord.   The syndrome may also be caused by cervical tumor, enlarged lymph nodes, cervical rib, aortic aneurysm, mediastinal tumor, disease of the esophagus, and traumatism.   Operations on the cervical portion of the sympathetic may result in the appearance of the syndrome.

Cogan[9] studied the differences in accommodation in the two eyes of a number of patients who had been operated on with removal of portions of the sympathetic on one side.   The patients all exhibited the oculopupillary syndrome on the affected side.   In all of them, the condition was only a partial manifestation because the superior cervical ganglion was not involved.   With a complete Horner's syndrome, the affected pupil fails to dilate after instillation of cocaine solution.   This serves as a diagnostic feature of the condition.   Adrenalin, on the other hand, will continue to affect the eye by dilatation of the pupil, even after removal of the cervical sympathetic ganglion.

Diseases of the Parathyroid Glands

There are four parathyroid glands which normally are found behind the lateral lobes of the thyroid.   They secrete a hormone which controls the calcium balance between the blood and the tissues.   Their function may be influenced to a slight extent by the pituitary.   The active principle of the parathyroid is called parathormone.   In the condition of hypoparathyroidism, the blood calcium drops from its normal level of 10 mg. per cent with an accompanying rise of phosphorus.   When the calcium level falls below 7 per cent, the syndrome known as tetany appears.

Tetany is a clinical syndrome which exhibits a state of increased irritability of the neuromuscular control.   Parathyroid tetany follows removal of the parathyroid glands which can occur accidentally with thyroidectomy.

Hypoparathyroidism may be manifested in the eyes by the presence of twitching movements of the eyelids, increased secretion of tears, blepharospasm, and ciliary spasm.   Deficient parathyroid function may also be the cause of cataract.   These cataracts are usually bilateral and do not improve with treatment other than surgical removal.   Their presence has been attributed to the decrease of calcium in the blood.   There seems to be no connection between this occurrence and the development of ordinary senile cataract.   The treatment of cataract with injections of parathormone by Kirby[10] failed to produce any improvement in vision or in the objective appearance of the cataract of these patients.

Diseases of the Thyroid Gland

The function of the thyroid gland is to manufacture the hormone thyroxin which is carried to the nucleated cells of the body by the circulation.   A sufficient amount of iodine is necessary for its formation.   The total tissue content of thyroxin is about 16 mg.   With a decrease in function of the thyroid, the oxygen consumption or basal metabolic rate falls to about minus 40 per cent.

Increased action of the thyroid gland or hyperfunction is characterized by the presence of goiter and hyperthyroidism.   Goiters may be divided into the adolescent type of colloid goiter, nontoxic colloid or adenomatous, and toxic, which are either simple (colloid, cystic, and adenomatous) or exophthalmic goiter (Graves' disease).   They are nearly all characterized by the symptoms of hyperthyroidism.

Exophthalmic Goiter (Graves' Disease; Basedow's Disease).—Exophthalmic goiter is a disease characterized by a state of accelerated tissue oxidation and increased activity of the autonomic nervous system occurring in both sexes, but more frequently among females.   The cause is unknown but it apparently exists outside of the thyroid gland.   Some cases seem to be related to focal infection while a prolonged strain or marked nervous shock precedes the onset of others.   It has been thought that the sympathetic nervous system might in some way cause the hyperfunction but no satisfactory explanation of the initial origin has been offered.   The fact that thyroidectomy does not cure the disease is evidence that exophthalmic goiter is not a primary disease of the thyroid gland. Although many of the symptoms may disappear, and the basal metabolic rate may return to normal, a nervous instability usually persists. Moreover, a regeneration with the formation of new hyperplastic tissue and hyperfunction may occur after partial removal.

The disease is characterized by the presence of irritability, tremor, nervousness, and palpitation. These symptoms are referable to the active state of the sympathetic nervous system. The patient is usually an anxious, restless individual with a staring expression and a warm moist skin. There is a fine tremor of the extended hands which is an important and constant sign in this condition. The pulse is rapid and regular with the rate being in proportion to the degree of toxicity. The diastolic pressure is low and the pulse pressure is high. The gland is usually enlarged bilaterally. A thrill may be present on palpation. At times, the thyroid is not enlarged in conditions of hyperthyroidism.

The basal metabolic rate is increased in proportion to the degree of hyperthyroidism. The hyperthyroidism is considered to be moderate in degree with a metabolic rate of 25 to 50 per cent, while above 50 per cent it is considered to be severe. In severe cases the pulse rate may be increased to 140 or higher, while the basal metabolic rate may be increased to 75 and 100 per cent. A glycosuria and hyperglycemia are present during the digestive period but the fasting blood sugar is normal. A hyperthyroidism of long standing causes a strain on the heart and dilatation or auricular fibrillation may occur.

The treatment of exophthalmic goiter is both medical and surgical. The former includes physical and mental rest, attention to the nutrition with increase of the calcium intake and water, sedation by the use of phenobarbital and sodium bromide when required. Surgical treatment consists of removal of the thyroid gland and the administration of iodine. Subtotal thyroidectomy is usually not a cure but a means of controlling the disease.

Eye Manifestations.—The most frequent and most pronounced ocular manifestations are probably caused by alterations in the function of the thyroid gland. The internal secretion of the thyroid is concerned with stimulation of the sympathetic system and exerts an influence on metabolism as well as on the function of other glands, such as the pancreas, pituitary, and the gonads.

Exophthalmos is the most prominent eye manifestation of hyperthyroidism. It is usually bilateral and may be present in varying degrees. This may occasionally be very slight and questionable. The degree of exophthalmos can be measured by means of an exophthalmometer (Hertl). This consists of a metal frame with a small mirror on either side, which reflects the image of the cornea of each eye. The exophthalmometer is placed in front of the patient's eyes with each side of the instrument resting at the external corner of the orbit. The examiner can observe the anterior portion of each eyeball in the mirror of the instrument and can measure the degree of protrusion on a scale below the mirror. The results of such measurements are of value in determining and following the progress of the exophthalmos.

Edema of the conjunctiva is nearly always associated with or follows a case of marked exophthalmos, while in mild cases the conjunctiva is pale and moist. The skin of the eyelids is often pale and taut. When the exophthalmos is marked, the eyes protrude so far that it is very difficult for the eyelids to cover the eyeball. This is accompanied by an edema, congestion, and chemosis of the bulbar conjunctiva. Exposure of the cornea may result from the inability to close the lids. This requires a protective covering for the eyeballs in these cases, in the form of an eye pad or in maintaining closure by the application of adhesive strips from the upper to the lower eyelids. Continued exposure in cases of marked exophthalmos may otherwise result in ulceration of the cornea and ulcerative keratitis. Perforation and infection with loss of the eyeball may follow.

Some of the classical ocular signs of hyperthyroidism have been attributed to stimulation of the sympathetic system and the anterior displacement of the eyeball. These include: (1) von Graefe's sign, which is characterized by a lag or failure of the upper eyelid in following the rotation of the eyeball from above downward; (2) Stellwag's sign which is a decrease in the frequency of blinking; (3) Moebius' sign is a weakness of convergence; (4) Dalrymple's sign is the widening of the palpebral fissure accompanied by the staring expression; (5) Gifford's sign is the difficulty in everting the upper eyelid and the presence of a transverse ridge due to spasm of the orbicularis muscle.

In addition to the edema and chemosis of the conjunctiva in marked cases of exophthalmos, the eyeball becomes fixed and paralysis of the ocular muscles and diplopia may occur.

The presence of exophthalmos has been explained in various ways, but the true explanation is still lacking. It was for a long time considered to be due to the presence of an increased amount of fat in the orbit, but this is not generally accepted at the present time. An absorption of water has been said to occur with an increase in mass of the tissues. The muscles become thickened and in many cases are inflamed. The marked protrusion of the eyeballs in severe cases may show little variation from day to day or week to week, even though the patient is under treatment and shows improvement in the metabolic rate, pulse rate, and nervous symptoms. The chemosis and edema are also persistent and may be troublesome because of the attendant irritation and lacrimation. Optic neuritis may also occur but this is a rare complication.

Occasionally, exophthalmos may occur in cases of hyperthyroidism following thyroidectomy, when it was absent or only mild in character prior to the operation. Such cases may become quite marked and persist in the absence of some of the severe general symptoms. A satisfactory explanation for the occurrence has not been offered. The results obtained from experiments on laboratory animals would seem to indicate that progressive exophthalmos following thyroidectomy can be caused by an increased secretion of the thyrotropic hormone of the anterior pituitary.

Treatment.—The treatment of exophthalmos occurring with hyperthyroidism depends principally on the treatment of the primary disease. Local treatment is only symptomatic in the average case. In mild cases the cornea should receive constant attention and protection from any possible exposure. This can be accomplished by the instillation of liquid petrolatum to cover the cornea, or by the application of an eye pad or strips of adhesive to approximate the eyelids. This should always be done in more severe cases and especially during sleep. When the exophthalmos is very marked and it is not possible to bring the eyelids together, a canthotomy or even more radical surgery, such as removal of a portion of the roof of the orbit (Naffzinger operation), may be necessary.

If the cornea showed signs of oncoming keratitis as evidenced by clouding or even when ulceration has occurred, atropine sulfate, 1 per cent solution, should be instilled and hot compresses should be regularly applied.

Hypothyroidism.—Defective secretion of the thyroid gland results in a lowered content of thyroxin in the cells which may be far reaching in its secondary effects. A primary deficiency in function in adults may lead to the development of myxedema. This disease may result from a primary atrophy of the gland or it may occur secondary to thyroidectomy or thyroiditis. Occasionally it may follow after a toxic exophthalmic goiter which has gradually recovered with a fibrosis of the gland accompanied by sufficient destruction of tissue to cause myxedema.

This condition is much more common among the female sex and is attended by symptoms which are characteristic of and which parallel the lowering of the metabolic rate. These include headaches, backache, fatigue, and a dry skin. The metabolic rate may range from minus 30 to 40 per cent and is accompanied by a slowing of speech and mentality. The facies of the patient are rather characteristic. There is an absence of expression and an almost "mask-like" appearance. The weight is increased, and there is a puffiness of the skin of the face. The respirations and pulse are slowed, the latter averaging 50 to 60 per minute. After several years the heart may become greatly dilated and weakened. Hypercholesteremia associated with vascular sclerosis and hypertension may develop.

When defective thyroid function has its onset in fetal life or in infancy, it is characterized by the development of cretinism. This results in impaired physical and mental development. The patient may show signs of idiocy, and the physical appearance presents a short, "pot-bellied" child without expression, thick tongue, and enlarged buttocks.

The treatment of hypothyroidism in an adult consists in the administration of thyroid extract or thyroxin which usually produces gratifying results. The mental and physical condition of the patient improves, and the metabolic rate increases. This should be brought about gradually, however, since sudden increase in the metabolism may result in cardiac embarrassment.

Eye Manifestations.—The manifestations of hypothyroidism which occur in the eyes are usually characteristic of hypofunction of the sympathetic nervous system and lowering of the metabolic rate. The eyes appear to be set farther apart especially in the condition of myxedema or cretinism. Enophthalmos may be present. The other manifestations are not as pronounced as those which occur with hyperthyroidism. The skin of the eyelids is pale and may become puffed and edematous. The conjunctiva is dry, pale and conjunctivitis or marginal blepharitis may be present. Lacrimation is decreased while blinking is increased, and the eyelashes and eyebrows become thin. Strabismus is frequently associated with hypothyroidism, and chalazia, myopia, or opacities of the lens are not uncommon.

Lemoine[1] found the incidence of hyperthyroidism to be high in cases of cortical cataract, and he also called attention to edema of the retina around the disc and macula as an ocular sign associated with hypothyroidism. The edema may extend into the periphery of the retina for a distance of 4 or 5 disc diameters, and the disc itself may be elvated as much as 3 diopters with an accompanying decrease in the vision.

Diseases of the Pituitary Gland

The pituitary gland develops embryologically by an upward growth of epithelial cells from the roof of the pharynx. These cells come into contact with an extension downward from the diencephalic floor. The anterior lobe is formed by epithelial cells of ectodermal origin, while the posterior lobe is composed of glial cells of diencephalic origin which are attached to the midbrain by the infundibular stalk. In the upward passage of the epithelial cells from the pharynx, a tube of cells is formed which usually disappears after the contact is made with the downward diencephalic growth. It is important to recall this in connection with the formation of craniopharyngiomas, which develop because of a persistence of these cells.

The pituitary gland rests in a bony fossa, the sella turcica, and is connected with the midbrain by its infundibular stalk which pierces the diaphragm of the sella. The gland measures normally about 6 by 10 by 14 mm.

The hormones of the anterior lobe of the pituitary include a growth hormone which regulates the growth and development of bones and viscera; a gonadotropic hormone, which controls estrin production and the menstrual cycle in the female, spermatogenesis in the male, and other sexual characteristics in both male and female; a thyrotropic hormone which influences the function of the thyroid; an adrenotropic hormone which acts on the cortex of the adrenal and when deficient, causes atrophy of the adrenal cortex; a lactogenic hormone (prolactin) which influences the secretion of milk.

The posterior lobe extracts have a marked pressor action on the blood pressure which is considered to be produced by an intermediary action of the adrenal gland. An oxytocic action influences the intestinal tone, peristalsis, and the uterus in pregnancy. Another action is an antidiuretic effect which is employed therapeutically in the treatment of diabetes insipidus.

Hyperpituitary Function.—Hyperfunction of the anterior lobe of the pituitary results in gigantism. This is caused by a diffuse hyperplasia or tumor development of the eosinophilic cells of the anterior lobe. The growth hormone is produced in excess. The condition usually starts about the time of puberty, and the skeletal growth is extremely rapid in the next few years. Headaches may be complained of if a tumor is the cause, and if other pressure symptoms should be noted, an x-ray examination of the skull is indicated. The excessive production of the growth hormone is usually associated with a deficient gonad factor. This results in sexual immaturity of the patient. With persistence of the hyperfunction after growth has ceased, acromegaly is superimposed on the gigantism.

Acromegaly is the disease syndrome which results from hyperfunction with excessive production of the growth hormone after the epiphyses of the long bones have united. In many cases an adenoma is found which is composed of eosinophilic cells. The degree of acromegaly is directly proportional to the number of eosinophilic cells in the gland. When degeneration later occurs, the condition becomes one of pituitary insufficiency and hypofunction.

Eye Manifestations.—The physiologic enlargement of the pituitary which occurs during pregnancy and produces a bitemporal contraction of the visual fields has been referred to previously. The ocular manifestations of hyperfunction are caused by the increased stimulation of the sympathetic system and by pressure of varying degrees on the chiasm by enlargement of the pituitary gland. As a result of the latter, the typical visual field defect is bitemporal hemianopia, but in a number of cases the visual field defects may be atypical.

DeSchweinitz in the Bowman lecture, 1923, described the variations in the position of the optic chiasm with relation to the sella and pituitary. He showed that in the average case, the chiasm is placed over the diaphragm sella and under the pituitary; in 5 per cent, the chiasm is just anterior to the pituitary, while in 4 per cent it is just behind the pituitary. From this it can be seen that the result of enlargement of the pituitary with reference to the effect on the chiasm will depend on the anatomic group to which the case belongs.

When only the mesial portion of the chiasm is involved, the decussating fibers that come from the nasal portion of the retina are destroyed with a bitemporal hemianopia. When the external portions of the decussation are destroyed, it results in a binasal hemianopia. This is a rare occurrence but it may result from a lateral enlargement of the hypophysis. When the lesion is anterior or on the lateral side of the decussation, blindness in one eye and temporal hemianopia can result. Lesions which affect the posterolateral side of the chiasm will produce partial or complete homonymous defects in the visual field.

The changes in the pituitary are associated with other ocular manifestations, such as diminished vision, pallor of the disc, optic atrophy in advanced cases, and the changes in the pupillary reflex. Other symptoms are headache, either frontal or temporal, increased weight, increased sugar tolerance, lowered metabolic rate, polydipsia and polyuria, and cessation of menses. Mild cases may be characterized by only transient disturbances of the vision and visual fields.

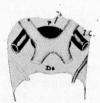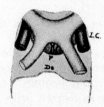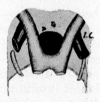

Fig. 207.—Variations in position of the optic chiasm with relation to the pituitary body P, the tuberculum sella Ts, the dorsum sella Ds, and the internal carotid I.C. (From Duke-Elder: Text-Book of Ophthalmology.)

In acromegaly and hyperfunction opacities of the lens may be found. When the posterior lobe of the pituitary lobe is affected, angioneurotic edema and diabetes insipidus sometimes occur.

Hypopituitary Function.—Hypofunction of the pituitary may manifest itself in any one of several ways. A deficiency of both lobes of the pituitary is said to result in the condition known as Fröhlich's syndrome. This is characterized by a girdle type of obesity and sexual underdevelopment. The latter is due to deficiency of the gonadotropic factor. The metabolic rate is somewhat decreased, and there is an increased carbohydrate tolerance. The Fröhlich type of obesity, when present with retinitis pigmentosa in patients who exhibit a lowered mentality, constitutes the Laurence-Moon-Biedl syndrome. The retinitis pigmentosa in this condition has also been said to be due to hypofunction of the pituitary.

Another manifestation of hypopituitarism is known as Simmond's disease which is described as a progressive form of cachexia in adults due to deficiency of the anterior lobe of the pituitary. As a result all of the functions of this lobe are restricted. The body shrinks with a progressive emaciation and asthenia. Amenorrhea in the female occurs. There is a progressive loss of weight which may continue for years. The condition may be caused by the presence of a craniopharyngioma.

Hypofunction of the posterior lobe of the pituitary may result in night blindness, blepharitis, heavy shaggy eyebrows, and changes in the eyelashes.

Diseases of the Pancreas

The internal secretion of the pancreas, which is considered to be insulin, is concerned with the control of carbohydrate metabolism. Variations in the quantity of insulin result in changes in the concentration of blood sugar, and when these changes occur suddenly, pyogenic infections, changes in the lens, and refractive changes may occur in the eyes. Opacities may occur in the lens and result in the formation of cataract which may progress to maturity. Variations in the amount of insulin which result in changes in the concentration of blood sugar may also lead to the presence of hemorrhages in the retina and in the vitreous of the eye.

The normal body is constantly receiving a supply of insulin from the pancreas which is carried to the cells of the tissues by the blood stream. It is there concerned with the storage of glucose as glycogen and oxidation of the latter. In its absence oxidation of glucose in the muscles is reduced almost to zero. The hormones of some of the other endocrine glands, such as pituitrin, thyroxin, and adrenalin, may directly or indirectly have an antagonistic action to insulin and tend to balance the blood sugar level.

Diabetes Mellitus.—Diabetes mellitus is a disease of metabolism which is characterized by a failure of the tissues of the body to oxidize carbohydrate at the normal rate. This failure is due to a lack of insulin. In addition there is a defective storage of glycogen and hyperglycemia with resulting glycosuria, and secondary disorders of fat and protein metabolism occur. The reduced production of insulin may vary in degree, with various degrees of severity in the resulting clinical diabetes.

The subject of diabetes is very vast, the various features of the disease and its complications covering a wide field, so that its description here need be presented only in capsule form.

In the etiology of diabetes, heredity, obesity, and racial susceptibility are important predisposing factors. It is a common disease among all groups of people but especially in those who have previously been overweight and among the members of the Jewish race.

There is also a relationship to the action of some of the other glands. A number of patients with acromegaly and eosinophilic adenomas of the anterior lobe of the pituitary have hyperglycemia with glycosuria. Hyperfunction of the pituitary may inhibit the action of insulin enough to produce a hyperglycemia. This is not, however, associated with a decrease in the production of insulin in the pancreas, as in diabetes mellitus. Hyperthyroidism may also be associated with hyperglycemia and glycosuria. Thyroxin and epinephrine seem to produce a tendency for increase in the blood sugar.

Arteriosclerosis is very commonly associated with diabetes but it is very doubtful that it has any importance as a causative factor Diabetes is a disease chiefly of middle life and therefore occurs at an age when arteriosclerosis also becomes manifest. The importance of nervous strain or sudden severe nervous shock is also doubted as an etiologic factor, but many patients show signs of an unstable nervous mechanism.

The blood sugar in the veins normally ranges from 80 to 120 per cent. It is lowest before breakfast in the morning and temporarily rises after each meal. In mild cases of diabetes the fasting blood sugar may be normal and will become higher as the diabetic condition becomes more severe. When the blood sugar rises to 150 mg. per cent, it can be safely regarded as evidence of the presence of diabetes.

Since the ability to oxidize carbohydrate is impaired, the protein supply is called upon to supply necessary calories. This is more pronounced in severe cases and results in ketosis, especially if fat oxidation is incomplete. Tissue destruction occurs, the degree of which can be determined by the nitrogen content of urine and feces. The destruction of tissue is accompanied by a rapid loss of weight.

Clinically, the symptoms of diabetes mellitus are thirst, increased urinary frequency, and loss of weight. These are dependent on the presence of hyperglycemia and glycosuria. The shift of water from the cells to the body fluids results in dehydration and thirst. Polyuria is another early and common symptom. The volume of urine secreted by the kidneys is large and has a high specific gravity. Other symptoms sometimes present are increased appetite, pruritus vulvae, weakness, and constipation. They are due chiefly to the glycosuria.

Complications of diabetes occur in the form of cardiovascular disease, infections, and acidosis (ketosis). The cardiovascular disease occurs principally in the form of arteriosclerosis of unknown etiology. When it was not present previously, it develops earlier in a diabetic patient than otherwise. There appears to be an excess lipoid in the blood. The excess lipoid is also contained in the intima of the larger arteries. There is apparently little difference fundamentally between the arteriosclerosis in diabetes and that which occurs without diabetes.

Infections are said to be common in diabetes because of the hyperglycemia. If the circulation is good in controlled diabetics, the susceptibility to infection is probably not increased and the healing of surgical wounds is not delayed. Infections are common in the skin and occur in the form of abscess and carbuncles. The diabetic is also more susceptible to active tuberculosis than the nondiabetic, especially in the uncontrolled case and among younger patients.

The acidosis which occurs in diabetes is due to the incomplete oxidation of fatty acids. The symptoms in severe cases are hunger, dry skin, and a flushed appearance. The pulse is rapid, tongue dry, and there may be vomiting with epigastric pain. When the CO_2 capacity is below 16 volumes per cent, it is usually associated with unconsciousness. The breath of the patient has an odor of fruit which is partly due to acetone. Hyperglycemia and ketonemia are present, while glucose and acetone are present in the urine. In children, a leucocytosis is usually marked, but this returns to normal with improvement of the condition.

Treatment.—The treatment of diabetes can briefly be said to require a systematic plan which should be outlined by a physician experienced and familiar with the management of these cases. An active cooperation on the part of the patient is also necessary. The system of treatment should include the management of the diet, use of insulin when necessary, and the treatment of complications.

The aim of treatment in general is to control the diabetic state completely, which means that the diet should provide sufficient calories to maintain weight but not overweight, while in those under fifty who are obese, diet and exercise should be prescribed to reduce the weight. The blood sugar should not exceed 150 mg. per cent at any time in the day and glycosuria should be absent.

The use of insulin is an aid and not a cure in the treatment. It is indicated when suitable regulation of the diet of the patient is not sufficient to control the diabetic state and also in the treatment of acidosis or other emergencies. The treatment of the other complications of diabetes will depend on their nature and the conditions under which they are presented.

Eye Manifestations.—Diabetes may reveal or be accompanied by manifestations in almost any of the structures of the eye. The most striking and important changes, however, are probably those which occur in the retina. Those which can be said to be due to diabetes alone are also probably second in frequency only to those which occur in the lens in the form of cataract. Because of the very common association of retinal arteriosclerosis, however, in cases of diabetes, the number of cases with retinal lesions far surpasses those which reveal other manifestations. Thus, in a series of 2,360 cases of diabetes mellitus personally examined by McKee,[11] 476 patients presented retinal lesions.

It is interesting to consider here the degree of the relationship of some of the eye manifestations to the age of the patient, the use of insulin, and the blood sugar concentration.

It has been frequently observed that the incidence of ocular lesions in young patients is not as great as in older patients and in those cases of long standing. McKee stated that diabetes is often more severe during the first three decades, the values for blood sugar may be higher and the insulin requirements usually higher than at any other time in life. Of ninety-six consecutive patients between the age of 6 and 31 years, he found the fundus normal in all but four. Hemorrhages in the retina increase in number as the diabetes grows milder with each increasing decade and "with increased duration of the diabetes, the incidence of deep retinal hemorrhages is out of proportion to the accompanying increased age of the patient, as reflected in the average age group." The role of insulin in the production of hemorrhages in diabetics has long been suspected and discussed but there does not appear to be any correlation between the use of insulin and the occurrence of lesions. The absence of many of the characteristic ocular manifestations in young patients with diabetes is probably due to the fact that the disease is so far of shorter duration than that which is seen in older patients, and ocular lesions have not had sufficient time to become manifest.

The blood sugar level at any one time also bears no definite relationship to the occurrence of eye lesions. Sudden changes in the blood sugar, however, and pronounced changes occurring over a period of time may be a factor in the production of some of the ocular manifestations.

Changes in the Refraction.—Changes in the refraction of the eye in a patient with diabetes are not uncommon. Such a change is usually observed in older patients who are known diabetics. This may be characterized by a sudden decrease in the vision which had previously been normal or it might take the form of repeated smaller changes in the vision over comparatively short periods of time and necessitate unusually frequent refraction and change of glasses. The cause of such change is not definitely known, but it is considered to be due to the effect of the sugar concentration on the refractive index of the crystalline lens. An increase in blood sugar is supposed to be accompanied by an increase in myopia, whereas a decrease in blood sugar is accompanied by a decrease in refraction manifested by an increase in hyperopia.

The Accommodation and Ocular Muscles.—The ability to use the eyes for close work may become impaired in some patients with diabetes because of a weakened condition of the accommodation. In these cases the accommodation is persistently below normal, and attempts to read or perform close work for any length of time are followed by headache, blurred vision, and even vertigo. The condition may improve to some extent with improvement in the general condition, but it is invariably necessary to prescribe a stronger lens than usual for reading and close work in these cases.

Occasional cases of paralysis of an extraocular muscle are also encountered. Although it is customary to refer to this as the result of a toxic condition, there is no exact explanation available. The sixth nerve is the one most frequently affected, with an impaired action of the external rectus muscle resulting. The muscle of only one eye is usually involved and is unable to rotate externally much beyond the midline. Attempts to do so result in diplopia. The condition may persist for a long time but may improve to some extent with improvement in the general condition.

Diabetic Changes in the Iris.—The most frequent manifestations of diabetes in the iris occur in the pigment epithelium and are characterized by edema, swelling, and degeneration of the epithelium with the liberation of free pigment. The stroma is not ordinarily affected but in some instances this may also become edematous and atrophic. An atrophic iris is not infrequently observed in cases of long standing, on direct examination, and can be studied in detail on slit lamp examination.

In rare cases a proliferation of newly formed blood vessels may be seen on the surface of the iris in the form of a ring around the pupillary border. The condition which is noninflammatory is known as diabetic rubeosis. It is also associated with glaucoma.

Diabetic iritis is not very common; McKee listed only eleven in his series of 2,360 patients. Iritis may occur in a diabetic, however, as the result of some intercurrent condition in which case it might be severe. Occasionally an old iritis may recur following an operation on the eye of a diabetic patient.

Cataract in Diabetics.—The occurrence of cataract in patients suffering with diabetes is very common. This is especially true of the cases found among older patients. The reason for the high incidence of this manifestation is not definitely known. Most of the patients who are under observation and treatment for diabetes are within the age limits when ordinary senile cataract may be found without the presence of diabetes. Many also are known to have arteriosclerosis. Moreover, cataract is observed with comparatively less frequency in children who are diabetics. The relationship of hyperglycemia to the development of cataract in these cases has been considered. As a result of the study of 238 patients with senile cataract, O'Brien[12] found that the normal sugar level was disturbed in about half the cases. In those patients with a low dextrose tolerance, there occurred repeatedly a hyperglycemia, and the lens was subjected to higher concentration of sugar in the surrounding fluids. O'Brien felt that this condition may have an effect on the lens when prolonged over a period of years.

The development of cataract in diabetes bears a closer relationship to the duration than to the severity of the disease. The characteristic type of cataract in diabetes is said to differ from the ordinary type of senile cataract by its subcapsular involvement. According to O'Brien, Molsberry, and Allen,[13] it usually occurs in younger patients and children and is more rare among adults. It affects both eyes and develops very rapidly. The appearance is rather characteristic with the presence of a large number of white, flake-like opacities spread out over a wide subcapsular network of vacuoles. The opacities become more diffuse and progress to the stage of complete and uniform clouding of the lens. The cataractous lens in diabetes reveals practically no difference in chemistry or in other respects from ordinary senile cataract.

When the stage of maturity has been reached, operation for the removal of the cataract can be performed. The presence of diabetes is no contraindication, but the diabetic state of the patient should be controlled. In addition the presence of advanced arteriosclerosis and especially vascular hypertension in these patients should receive attention before operation is resorted to. The danger from postoperative intraocular hemorrhage is greater in such cases.

Diabetic Retinosis (Retinitis).—The description of the retinal changes occurring in diabetes as a "retinosis" rather than a retinitis was recommended by Troncoso with the explanation that the process is one of a degenerative nature in the retina rather than inflammatory. Many authors, however, continue to employ the less accurate designation of "retinitis," probably because it is difficult to discard a term which has become more or less fixed by long and repeated use.

The appearance of the most pronounced manifestations of diabetes in the eye are to be seen in the retina on ophthalmoscopic examination. Both eyes are nearly always affected but not necessarily to the same extent. Since diabetes is a disease more common in middle life, arteriosclerosis of the retinal vessels is also present in most cases with the accompanying changes. In the acute or early stages of diabetes and in children, arteriosclerosis is usually absent. It is therefore possible to observe cases of diabetic retinosis in association with advanced sclerosis of the vessels with little or no evidence of retinal involvement. In the 476 persons with retinal changes in McKee's series of cases,[9] he found arteriosclerosis of the retinal vessels present in 205, diabetic "retinitis" in 41, diabetic "retinitis" with arteriosclerosis in 28, and the "retinitis" of arteriosclerosis in 26. The arteriosclerosis was graded as beginning, moderate, and severe.

Elwyn[14] referred to 3,893 diabetic patients in whom the vessels were graded in the various age groups by Waite and Beetham. Sclerosis was absent in 1,042, or 62 per cent, as follows:

AGE GROUP	NUMBER OF PATIENTS	NUMBER OF PATIENTS WITHOUT SCLEROSIS	PER CENT
under 10	130	130	100
between 10 and 19	464	451	97
between 20 and 29	274	253	92
between 30 and 39	315	153	48
between 40 and 49	512	49	9
between 50 and 59	1,001	6	0.6

From this it can be readily seen how the percentage of cases with arterio-sclerosis steadily increases from none in those under 10 years to nearly all but 0.6 per cent in those between 50 and 59 years.

The characteristic lesions in the retina in diabetic retinosis are observed on examination with the ophthalmoscope and consist of hemorrhages and white spots which are commonly spoken of as exudates. These spots or patches are

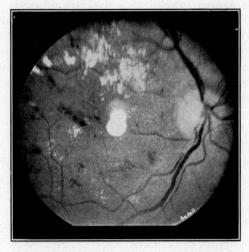

A.

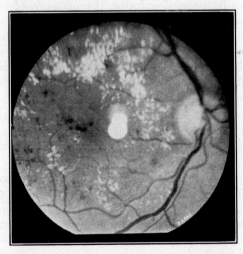

B.

Fig. 208.—*A*, Retinitis in diabetes in a woman aged 62; blood sugar content, 157 mg.; extensive glistening yellow-white exudates; many retinal hemorrhages. *B*, Retinitis in diabetes. Photograph taken five months later shows the extension of the retinal change even when the diabetes was seemingly under control. (Courtesy of Dr. Arthur J. Bedell.)

found principally at the posterior pole of the fundus and are less numerous in the anterior periphery. At first they appear to be white but soon take on a somewhat glistening, yellow or waxy appearance. Their edges are well outlined and differ in this respect from the whiter cotton-wool patches of retinitis, which have a fluffy or striated outline. They have a tendency to arrange themselves around the region of the macula in the form of a circle or part of a circle. The presence of the patches is considered to be a degeneration with deposits of hyaline and lipoid material in the retina. They are not the manifestation of an inflammatory process.

The hemorrhages which occur in association with these patches, present a picture which is almost typical of a diabetic retinosis. The characteristic hemorrhages are small, round, or oval, and have rather sharp edges. They are situated in the deeper layers of the retina under the retinal vessels and occur in greater numbers in older patients. In some, however, there may be very few. When arteriosclerosis or hypertension is present in the same patient, hemorrhages may be present which are more superficial and are flame shaped or streaked. These are due to the hypertension and are not characteristic of diabetes.

The cause of the retinosis in diabetes has received a great deal of attention and discussion. This seems to lead to the opinion that it results from a local circulatory disturbance in the retina which causes an impairment of the nutrition and production of the lesions. Elwyn[14] explained the process on the basis of a peristasis or prestasis which takes place in the terminal vessels. This causes a dilatation of the terminal vessels with the occurrence of hemorrhages by diapedesis. Persistence of the dilatation leads to a chronic state of deficient nutrition and deficient oxygen supply which is followed by secondary changes. This then becomes manifest in the deposit of fats and lipoids.

It should again be pointed out that the presence of these retinal changes does not depend on the severity of the disease, but rather on the prolonged duration of a hyperglycemia even in mild cases. Elwyn believes that there is a "loss of stability in the mechanism" which ordinarily maintains the blood sugar at a normal level. The increased sugar level, after a time, causes the dilatation of the terminal vessels which results in the condition of prestasis with the appearance of hemorrhages and deposits in the retina.

Others believe that arteriosclerosis is the important factor in the production of the lesions, and there is also another group which believes that the hemorrhages and yellowish spots are the results of toxic or biochemical changes which occur in diabetes.

The vision in diabetic retinosis may not be greatly impaired. This depends mostly on the location of the lesions in the retina. Many patients continue on for years with only a gradual and slight loss of vision, unless the hemorrhages occur in the macula. In that case there would be a decided impairment of vision. The optic nerve is rarely involved, and the same is true of the choroid.

When arteriosclerosis is predominant, the retinal vessels will reveal more pronounced manifestations of this condition, and cardiac, renal, or cerebral changes may also be present. The retinal arteries become tortuous, and in advanced cases they may present the "corkscrew appearance." The veins are dilated at their distal extremities and may be very tortuous and beaded. Hemorrhages of various sizes and shapes may then occur and in these cases the optic nerve later becomes atrophic. Hemorrhages may occur into the vitreous with a resulting proliferative retinitis. In some few cases proliferative retinitis may be present without hemorrhages in the vitreous.

Eye manifestations in young patients with diabetes are probably not as rare as generally supposed. This was demonstrated by O'Brien and Allen,[15] who found pathologic changes in the retina due to diabetes in twenty-three patients of a series of 555 under 31 years of age. Two additional young patients with diabetes also showed evidences in the retina of advanced hypertension and nephritis. In the twenty-three patients with retinopathy, most of the lesions were hemorrhages and areas of degeneration similar to those which occur among adults. The hemorrhages were located principally in the area around the macula or in the temporal area and were both small puctate and striate in variety. Ten of the patients showed areas of hard, waxy degeneration in the central part of the fundus which were small and yellowish white in color. In seven of the patients, cotton-wool patches were present along the course of the temporal vessels. Lipemia retinalis was observed in an 11-year-old girl. A 14-year-old girl whose diabetes had never been well controlled showed retinal hemorrhages and edema of the nerve heads. The fundi improved and appeared normal, however, after three months of rigid control.

Since the retinal changes observed in these younger patients were found to be the same as those seen in older patients, it would indicate that the pathology is due to the diabetes only. Moreover, it seems that control of the diabetes is followed by an improved unit in the retinopathy. The same does not seem to occur in the older patients who come under observation and treatment.

The same authors studied another group of 260 patients under 21 years of age with diabetes, in which they found changes in the lens in thirty-six. The cataracts were extracted in three of these. In ten of the others, the visual acuity was impaired to some degree. The diabetes in each of these patients had been uncontrolled for a period of months or years previously. After one or two years, six of the patients in whom the lens was formerly clear developed opacities. After they were placed under control, the opacities failed to show any further increase after six months. In five patients with strict control, the opacities were said to have shown an arrested development after six months, while in seven patients with insufficient control, the opacities were found to continue to increase. These results of control of the diabetes are also lacking in older patients with diabetic cataracts.

The refraction was studied in twelve patients between the ages of 8 and 28 who were previously untreated. Daily refraction under scopolamine for a period of from ten to fourteen days following the use of insulin therapy showed a relative hyperopia of 1 to 3D. which developed in from three to five days after treatment started. This disappeared in from seven to ten days.

Bloch[16] reported two patients with juvenile diabetes who came under his observation with changes of the fundus, neither of whom had renal pathologic change or abnormal blood pressure. One of these patients was 37 years of age and probably a borderline case of juvenile diabetes, as Bloch stated. The other patient was a 26-year-old woman with a number of small hemorrhages in the retina of each eye above and below the macular region. Two irregular white areas were also visible in the right eye above the superior macular vein. This author also felt that diabetic changes in the fundus show marked differences from those occurring in arteriosclerosis and in hypertension, especially with reference to the optic nerve and macular region.

Lipemia Retinalis.—Lipemia is a complication of diabetes which occurs chiefly in young patients when the lipoid content of the blood rises above 5 per cent. It is characterized by a cloudiness and milky condition of the plasma. Acidosis is apparently a factor in the production. The fat content of the blood may increase without the presence of lipemia. The condition of the fat may, therefore, also be a factor.

Lipemia retinalis is comparatively rare and usually occurs in younger patients, the average age being about 25. It is usually present when the blood fat is increased above 8 per cent and is more likely to occur with acidosis or after recovery from acidosis. The pathogenesis of the condition has not been explained.

On examination with the ophthalmoscope the color of the retinal arteries and veins is found to be changed. Their color may vary from a pale salmon-pink to a chocolate or creamy appearance, depending probably on the degree of lipemia present. The earliest changes are found in the terminal vessels and those in the periphery appear more pale. The arteries and veins are wider and resemble flat strips of ribbon. The condition is always found with diabetes but one case was found by Wagener to occur in a patient with lymphatic leucemia.

Jaffe and Schonfeld[17] reported a case in a 30-year-old white man with diabetes. In a search of the literature they found only forty cases which had been previously reported. In their case the total lipoid content of the blood was 21.7 per cent and the ophthalmoscopic description was typical. The retinal arteries and veins were pale salmon in color, which later became darker. They were slightly wider than normal, and the veins and arteries could only be differentiated from each other with difficulty, although the veins were a little wider and faintly purplish. The vessels were flat and light reflexes were absent. The optic nerves were normal in appearance and the vision was unaffected.

Lipemia may also occur in a number of other conditions such as pneumonia, alcoholism, asphyxia, phosphorus poisoning, malnutrition, pregnancy, tuberculosis, xanthomatosis.

McKee and associates[18] reported a case associated with a moderate acidosis, xanthomas and carotenemia. Another unusual case reported by Falls[19] occurred in a patient over 60 years of age. The patient presented a complication of diseases including severe emaciation, starvation, pneumonia, diabetes mellitus, infarct of the kidney, pulmonary abscesses and xanthomatosis, any of which could contribute to the lipemia. The level of blood lipid fell from 6.2 to 2.52 Gm. per 100 c.c. before death. This was thought to be the sixty-second case to be reported and the second oldest patient. The author suggested that for lipemia retinalis to occur in an elderly patient with mild diabetes, it is necessary for severe systemic complications to be associated such as those present in this case.

The prognosis in lipemia retinalis is usually good. With a diet containing a low fat content and adequate treatment with insulin, the condition readily improves.

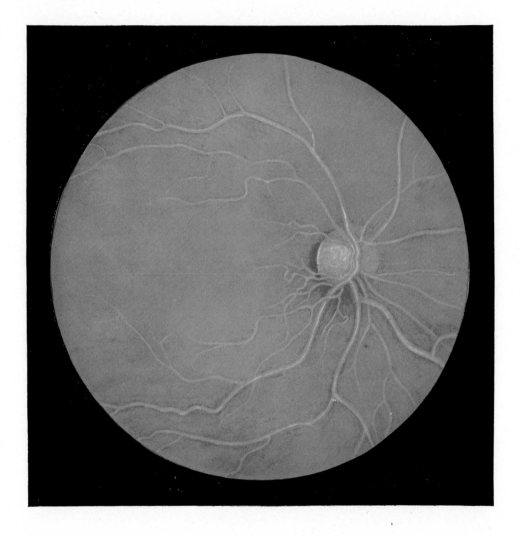

Fig. 209.—Lipemia retinalis. (After Muskat, from Troncoso: Internal Diseases of the Eye and Atlas of Ophthalmoscopy, F. A. Davis Co.)

Hypotony.—Hypotony may occur in diabetic coma with a decrease in the intraocular tension. The resulting condition of the eyeball is known as ophthalmalacia and, although quite rare, it is characteristic of the more severe forms of diabetic coma. The etiology is not known but it has been said to be due to changes in the molecular concentration of the blood and also to acidosis. Hypotony does not occur in acidosis without coma, however. With modern improvement in the general management and treatment of diabetes, the condition has been very rare.

Gout

Gout is a disorder of the metabolism of purine bodies resulting in an excess of uric acid salts in the blood. It is characterized by remissions and exacerbations of swollen, painful, tender joints accompanied by fever and general malaise. The exact etiology is unknown. It occurs most frequently between the ages of 35 and 50 years, is predominant in males of the upper class, and has a hereditary tendency.

Premonitory symptoms of malaise, depression, and indigestion are followed in a day or two by pain in a joint. This is usually the metatarso-phalangeal joint of the great toe which is hot, swollen, bluish-red in color, and very tender. Although only one joint is usually involved, the condition may be polyarticular. Those of the hand, knee, shoulder, and vertebrae may be involved. Chills, moderate fever, and a leucocytosis may also characterize the attack. The inflammatory process usually subsides gradually after two or three days and clears up in a week or two. Successive attacks may occur which result in chronic disturbances such as tophi, arthritis, and nephritis.

Eye Manifestations.—The eye manifestations of gout are the result of a disease in which the elimination of waste products is deficient because of a disorder of metabolism of proteins. This is characterized in the eye by the presence of what has always been designated as a gouty iritis.

Both gout itself and its manifestations in the eye are far less common today than in years past. This is probably due to the fact that more attention is paid to diet and greater discretion is exercised in the choice and quantity of foods consumed by an individual.

Gouty Conjunctivitis.—Although the iritis and uveitis are thought of in connection with gout and gouty diathesis, the conjunctiva and sclera are also involved. The conjunctiva shows a characteristic hyperemia with distention of the capillaries and larger vessels. The condition is usually chronic in form, and a slight amount of serum sometimes exudes from the dilated vessels and the lids become thick and pasty. Recurrent hemorrhages of various sizes may also occur.

The patient complains of difficulty in opening the eyelids in the morning, and the lids feel heavy and stiff. There is a sensation of a foreign body being present with a "scratchy" feeling of the eye. These symptoms are often complained of in the absence of any marked congestion in the eye in mild cases. They are exaggerated during bad weather and by cold and dampness.

In many instances the patient complains of the ocular irritation during periods of remission of other symptoms. Although the examination of the external eye may reveal no marked signs, the possibility of gouty diathesis should not be overlooked and inquiry made to eliminate this cause.

The treatment should be directed principally toward the primary condition and correction of the diet. Local treatment is limited and should consist chiefly in the use of a mild alkaline wash and avoiding strong irritating solutions.

Scleritis and Tenonitis.—The association of scleritis and tenonitis with gout is probably rare and in most cases vague. Many of these cases are considered to be due to "rheumatism" and "gouty conditions," but the connection is rarely established. However, when gout is definitely known to be present, the associated scleritis or tenonitis may be very troublesome and severe. Crystalline deposits have been found in the sclera with gout.

The condition may be very painful especially on attempting to rotate the eyeball. The bulbar conjunctiva of both eyes is edematous when tenonitis is present. The condition may last for a few days or continue for several weeks before it subsides.

The treatment is here also directed toward correction of the primary gouty diathesis and the administration of salicylates. Locally, mild warm alkaline solutions can be employed two or three times daily.

Gouty Iritis.—Gouty or uratic iritis is at present comparatively rare. A number of cases are attributed to this condition when the etiology is uncertain or undetermined. The true iritis of gout is usually associated in the early stages with conjunctivitis and scleritis. It usually follows errors of diet and may or may not be associated with the joint involvement. The onset is usually sudden and is characterized by marked pain, redness of the conjunctiva, and some haziness of the cornea. The deeper vessels may be markedly injected and purplish in color. The cornea may show some precipitates and a low-grade exudation may be seen in the anterior chamber. Occasionally opacities may be present in the vitreous. The condition may be acute for several days and subside in about ten days to two weeks. Recurrent attacks are common and may result in deposits on the anterior lens. Subsequent attacks may prove more troublesome and result in additional lesions with corresponding impairment of vision.

The treatment here also consists of general therapeutics with the administration of salicylates or colchicum and careful attention to correction of the faulty diet. Locally, hot compresses soaked in an alkaline solution, applied to the eye for a period of fifteen minutes, three times daily, will afford relief. One drop of atropine sulfate, 1 per cent solution, should be instilled into the affected eye three times daily. The use of the eyes should be restricted, and they should be protected from strong light by the use of dark glasses.

Diseases of the Suprarenal Glands

There are two suprarenal glands which are composed of a cortex and a medulla. The cells of the former arise from the genital ridge. The cells of the medulla are chromaffin and arise from the embryonic sympathetic nervous system. The origin of the cortical cells is the same as that of the interstitial cells of the testes.

The function of the two types of cells, as well as the function of the cortex and medulla, is unrelated and separate. The medulla produces adrenalin which has a marked vasoconstrictor action and increases the blood pressure. It also stimulates the sympathetic nervous system. The cortex of the suprarenal is stimulated by the adrenotropic factor of the pituitary, and atrophy of the suprarenal cortex results from removal of the pituitary.

Hypersuprarenal Function.—Hyperfunction of the suprarenal glands is usually associated with tumors of either the cortex or the medulla, and they may arise from the cells of both. They produce different results, however.

Tumors of the cortex result in hyperfunction of the cortical cells which produces a syndrome of the genitals, with alteration in the organs and sexual characteristics in both male and female.

Tumors of the medulla are of three types. These are neuroblastomas, ganglioneuromas, and paragangliomas. The neuroblastomas are malignant and metastasize early. The cells of paragangliomas may secrete adrenalin with increase in blood pressure which might resemble malignant hypertension.

Hyperfunction of the medulla might be manifested in the eye by pallor of the conjunctiva, enlargement of the pupil, and constriction of the vessels, and occasionally exophthalmos.

Hyposuprarenal Function.—Adrenal insufficiency or relative hypoadrenalemia produces the exhaustion syndrome which is characterized by a low blood pressure, a decrease in plasma sodium with dehydration, and a slight decrease in the basal metabolic rate.

Another manifestation of deficiency of the cortex and medulla of both adrenal glands occurs in the form of Addison's disease. One of the striking characteristics is the bronzed pigmentation of the skin which may affect the skin of the eyelids.

Deficiency of the adrenal cortex may be manifested in the eye by enophthalmos while deficiency of the medulla causes a smaller pupil than normal and a moderate congestion of the vessels. The cortical extract has been said to have an effect in reducing the intraocular tension especially in cases of glaucoma, but this has not been consistently observed.

The Gonads

The function of the gonads is regulated chiefly by the anterior lobe of the pituitary and is stimulated by the adrenal cortex.

Hyperfunction of the gonads may result in either primary or secondary precocious sexual development, or it may occur itself as part of a general overdevelopment as seen in pituitary hyperfunction and acromegaly.

The gonads act on the sympathetic system and deficiency results in symptoms of overaction of the parasympathetic. Lemoine[1] described hypogonadism in patients who showed signs of hyperstimulation of the parasympathetic or vagotonia. The patients complained of blurred vision and discomfort in the eye, constant headache, and discomfort with use of the eyes. Relief was obtained by the administration of anterior pituitary extract.

References

1. Lemoine, A. N.: Ocular Manifestations of Endocrine Disturbance, Arch. Ophth. **19:** 184, 1938.
2. Myerson, A., and Thau, W.: Human Autonomic Pharmacology, Arch. Ophth. **18:** 9, 1937; J. A. M. A. **110:** 101, 1938.
3. Kennedy, Foster: The Hypothalamus, J. A. M. A. **114:** 2092, 1940.
4. Kennedy, Foster, et al.: Adie's Syndrome, Report of Cases, Arch. Ophth. **19:** 68, 1938.
5. Sheie, Harold G.: Site of Disturbance in Adie's Syndrome, Arch. Ophth. **24:** 225, 1940.
6. Lowenstein, Otto, and Friedman, E. D.: Adie's Syndrome (Pupillotonic Pseudotabes), Arch. Ophth. **28:** 1042, 1942.

7. Cobb, S., and Scarlett, H.: A Report of Eleven Cases of Cervical Sympathetic Nerve Injury, Causing the Oculopupillary Syndrome, Arch. Neurol. and Psychiat. 3: 636, 1920.
8. De Jong, R. N.: Horner's Syndrome, Arch. Neurol. and Psychiat. 34: 734, 1935.
9. Cogan, D. G.: Accommodation and the Autonomic Nervous System, Arch. Ophth. 18: 739, 1937.
10. Kirby, D. B.: Senile Cataract. Use of Parathyroid Extract, Arch. Ophth. 5: 754, 1931.
11. McKee, H.: Fundus Oculi in Diabetes Mellitus. A Clinical Analysis of the Appearance of the Fundus in 2,360 Cases, Arch. Ophth. 25: 773, 1941.
12. O'Brien, C. S.: Hyperglycemia in Persons With Advanced Senile Cataract, Arch. Ophth. 6: 806, 1931.
13. O'Brien, C. S., Molsberry, J. M., and Allen, J. H.: Diabetic Cataract: Incidence and Morphology in 126 Young Diabetic Patients, J. A. M. A. 103: 892, 1934.
14. Elwyn, Herman: Problem of Diabetic Retinitis, Arch. Ophth. 25: 139, 1941.
15. O'Brien, C. S., and Allen, J. H.: Ocular Changes in Young Diabetic Patients, J. A. M. A. 120: 190, 1942.
16. Bloch, Fritz J.: Retinopathy in Juvenile Diabetes Mellitus, Arch. Ophth. 28: 891, 1942.
17. Jaffe, M., and Schonfeld, W. A.: Lipemia Retinalis Due to Diabetes Mellitus, Arch. Ophth. 9: 531, 1933.
18. McKee, S. H., Wilson, D. R., Fowler, A. F., and Wilen, B.: Lipemia Retinalis, Am. J. Ophth. 25: 513, 1942.
19. Falls, Harold F.: Lipemia Retinalis: Report of a Case, Arch. Ophth. 30: 358, 1943.

CHAPTER XIX

AVITAMINOSIS AND DISEASES OF NUTRITION

The Vitamins

Many advances in the study of nutrition during the past decade have apparently established the fact that certain of the vitamins are essential to an adequate diet and that a marked deficiency of these vitamins will result in the production of definite pathologic tissue changes and the occurrence of certain known diseases. The exact manner in which these changes are produced is still unexplained, but with the constant and increasing amount of clinical evidence, it is now generally accepted that certain diseases in man are associated with the deficiency or absence of a particular vitamin or vitamins from the diet. For example, vitamin A has long been designated as the "ophthalmic vitamin" because of its effect in preventing xerophthalmia. Vitamin B is considered to have a particular effect on the nervous system, and its presence in the diet will prevent beriberi. Vitamin G is concerned with the prevention of pellagra.

Considerable experimental evidence has been produced to prove the occurrence of ocular manifestations in certain vitamin deficiencies. Pronounced clinical manifestations, however, which compare with the results of investigations on laboratory animals are not so common, because the diet of the average patient is probably never restricted to the same extent and with the same exactness as to produce the results obtained with experimental animals. On the other hand, it is a fact that many people will subsist for long periods on a diet which is uniform and at the same time deficient to a certain extent in the factors essential to a well-balanced diet. Although economic conditions and habitat are often the chief factors which determine the nature of a diet, the habits and personal tastes of an individual will frequently lead one to follow a uniform and unchanging diet for years, without any consideration of its nutritive value. Should such a diet be deficient in an essential vitamin, it could reasonably explain the clinical presence of certain ocular manifestations, which, although apparently not of a serious nature at first, become recurrent and progressive with the lapse of time. Such patients may suffer from a partial deficiency, or what has been described as a subclinical state of deficiency. In patients who are on a restricted diet for a long period of time for the treatment of some general disease, the danger of producing symptoms of a vitamin deficiency is, of course, obvious. Moreover, a mild deficiency may frequently occur as a direct complication of another disease, while in some instances, a patient may suffer with the manifestation of several deficiencies simultaneously. Lastly, the importance of the vitamins to the physician is concerned not only with their relation to the cause of certain well-defined diseases, such as pellagra, scurvy, beriberi, and rickets, but also with the fact that a chronic vitamin deficiency is considered to be responsible for the production of many vague, ill-defined, and borderline subjective symptoms and states of ill health which might puzzle the physician and greatly disturb the patient. These are equal in importance to those of the more clearly defined deficiency diseases

Vitamin A Deficiency

Vitamin A is a fat-soluble, thermostable substance found abundantly in: (1) Fats and oils (butter, cream, cod-liver oil, peanut oil, and nut butters, mutton and beef fat); (2) Meats (liver, kidney, heart, brains, and sweetbreads); (3) Milk (cow's whole milk, raw, dried whole milk, sweetened condensed milk, whole milk cheese); (4) Eggs, fresh or dried; (5) Vegetables (fresh raw carrots, fresh cabbage, lettuce, dried spinach); (6) Fish (salmon, herring, and roes); (7) Bananas and nuts.

The method of absorption and disposition is a subject concerning which little is known. Although vitamin A is present in the feces, its exact fate after ingestion is still undetermined. Rountree[1] showed that it is not excreted through the urine of young children and infants, even when generous amounts are fed. If there is a limit to the capacity to store vitamin A, it is not indicated by alimentary vitaminurea. A marked fecal loss was found to occur, but it was felt that this was not entirely dependent on the intake. The loss of vitamin A in infants seems to run parallel with the loss of fat.

In addition to being the cause of xerophthalmia, vitamin A deficiency has been described as lowering the resistance to infection, especially in the respiratory tract, as an alleged factor in the formation of urinary calculi, as a cause of skin lesions, and lesions of the nervous system.

The skin lesions resulting are said to be striking with the production of several varieties of dermatitis. A common manifestation is the occurrence of papules which vary in size and are distributed especially over the thighs, arms, and shoulders.

Eye Manifestations.—The manifestations of vitamin A deficiency as it affects the ocular structures were demonstrated experimentally in animals many times. Wolbach and Howe, in 1925, reported the specific tissue changes in conjunctiva, meibomian gland ducts, lacrimal glands, and cornea and showed a replacement of the columnar epithelium by a stratified, squamous, keratinizing type. This was in general confirmed by numerous other investigators. It is generally accepted that lesions of the eye are most frequent as the result of avitaminosis A.

Hemeralopia (Night Blindness).—One of the first subjective and perhaps one of the most discussed symptoms of clinical vitamin A deficiency is hemeralopia, or night blindness. In many instances this may occur only partially. Various means for measurement of the dark adaptation have been applied, all of which involve a common principle, i.e., the measurement of the ability of the eyes to adapt themselves to poor illumination. In some cases the patients are maximally adapted to the dark and the light threshold measured immediately afterward is taken as a criterion of dark adaptation. In other cases the patients are adapted to a moderately bright illumination either with or without preliminary dark adaptation, and measurements of light threshold are made at intervals in darkness following this. All of the present methods of measuring the dark adaptation are beset with certain difficulties and have certain limitations.

One of the most apparent results, however, indicates that the highest incidence of night blindness is found in families of the lowest income classes. Subnormal visual adaptation was also reported as occurring in 50 per cent of pregnant women examined by Edmund and Clemmesen.[2]

That a close relationship exists between the normal function of the retina and the presence of vitamin A has been demonstrated experimentally several times. It has long been known that the visual purple of the retina is slow to regenerate with vitamin A deficiency, when the eyes have been exposed to strong sunlight. Moreover, it has also been shown that vitamin A is plentiful in the normal retina.

Night blindness was found to occur among the natives of the Philippine Islands owing to the lack of vitamin A. It has also been said to occur among the fishermen of Labrador who were exposed to the strong sunlight at sea.

Xerophthalmia.—This is probably the characteristic manifestation of vitamin A deficiency and may present a variety of appearances. It has been produced experimentally in animals and described by many different investigators. Clinically, it was described by Bloch in 1917, when it occurred among the children of Denmark because of the lack of butter among the population.

Perhaps the most detailed clinical description of this condition was given by Pillat[3] who studied a great many of these cases among the soldiers of Southern China. He divided the disease into several stages. First, night blindness, which occurs as one of the early symptoms and is not accompanied by ophthalmoscopic findings. It may occur either alone or in association with other ocular symptoms. The second stage is xerosis epithelialis conjunctiva, which is described as a dryness of the conjunctiva of the eyeball, and which appears in four clinical forms: Bitot's spots, irregular xerosis of the bulbar conjunctiva, loss of luster of the bulbar conjunctiva, and wrinkling of the bulbar conjunctiva. Bitot's spots are triangular spots resembling a dense foam and occurring in the region of the palpebral fissure, with the base of the triangular area at the limbus and the apex toward the angle. The next stage of the condition is xerosis of the corneal epithelium, which is often associated with xerosis of the conjunctiva, but it may occur alone in rare cases. The final stage of the condition is keratomalacia, which had been hitherto described as occurring only in infants.

Pigmentation of the conjunctiva may also occur. This is light brown in color and is most marked in the semilunar fold and caruncle, extending from the first into the fornices, and then to the bulbar and lid conjunctiva. Such pigmentation may occur in the mildest and severest cases of vitamin A deficiency and is often the last symptom to disappear. It may be associated with night blindness, or it may occur alone.

Other Ocular Manifestations.—Meibomitis is of frequent occurrence. This has been said to be caused primarily by inactivity of the meibomian glands and is not of inflammatory origin. This inactivity causes the fatty content of the glands to be kept in the excretion ducts, irritating the gland itself and the margin of the lids. This permits germs to enter the glands and gives rise to a secondary inflammation.

Blepharitis and hordeolum are quite common in cases of vitamin A deficiency, being caused by the prevalence of bacteria in all parts of the eye and by the decrease of lacrimal fluid which occurs in cases mostly of long standing.

Among children, chronic conjunctivitis, phlyctenular conjunctivitis, or keratoconjunctivitis, recurring chalazion, and hordeolum, especially in the absence of any other cause, should lead to an investigation of the diet and the suspicion of vitamin A deficiency. The same is true of older patients who suffer with episcleritis and many cases of otherwise unexplained ulcers of the cornea.

Treatment.—In all cases in which a vitamin A deficiency in the diet is strongly suspected, the treatment should be directed toward correction of the diet and supplementing this with a sufficient quantity of vitamin A. The former might not always be possible, but the latter can always be supplied, at least in the form of cod-liver oil and carotin. It has been shown that cod-liver oil contains from ten to twenty times as much vitamin A as butter fat. Raw carrots can be added to the daily diet.

A consideration of the vitamin A intake daily requires an analysis of the patient's diet. According to Booher[4] the following recommendations for vitamin A intake are presented:

"The daily requirement for vitamin A just sufficient for the prevention of night blindness in a normal adult would appear to be on the order of from 20 to 30 U.S.P. units per kilogram of body weight, or a total of about 1400 to 2000 units daily for an adult weighing 70 kg. Allowing for a margin of safety and for the maintenance of a moderate storage of vitamin A in the body, a total of around 3000 units of vitamin A daily is suggested for the normal adult. Milk, butter, eggs, and green leafy vegetables should be used in quantities to provide a large proportion of this vitamin A allowance.

"For the growing child, about 6000 to 8000 units of vitamin A daily would presumably be adequate to take care of any extra needs associated with growth and development and to provide for a moderate bodily storage of vitamin A. A small supplement of some fish liver oil, in addition to liberal quantities of whole milk, butter, eggs, and green leafy vegetables are excellent for supplying vitamin A. Infants and especially premature or artificially fed infants should be supplied with liberal quantities since infants are born with very meager stores of vitamin A in the liver.

"The recommended allowance of vitamin A for pregnant and nursing women has been set around 5000 units or more daily, with a further suggestion that this allowance be supplied mainly by liberal amounts of milk, butter, cheese, eggs, green leafy vegetables, and some small addition of fish liver oil."

The local treatment of such manifestations as blepharitis, conjunctivitis, ulcers, hordeola, meibomitis, etc., should consist of mild washes and of avoiding additional irritation from the use of strong antiseptic solutions and ointments. Keeping the eyes and lids clean by bathing with tepid boric acid solution may suffice. If the cornea is involved, one drop of 0.5 per cent atropine sulfate solution should be instilled into the eyes once or twice daily and dark glasses should be worn to protect against strong light.

Vitamin B₁ Deficiency (Beriberi)

Vitamin B_1 (thiamine, aneurin, caterulin) and nicotinic acid are the components of vitamin B complex which are known to be of significance in maintaining normal neurologic function. It is a water soluble vitamin, and a large amount of it is lost when the water in which the foods are cooked is thrown away. The incidence of B_1 deficiency is high among patients suffering with chronic debilitating diseases and increased metabolism, alcoholism, pellagra, sprue, anemia, colitis, diabetes, tuberculosis, senility, malignancy, and other diseases which interfere with the nutrition.

Thiamine deficiency, or beriberi, commonly manifests itself as polyneuritis and frequently occurs in association with pellagra and other vitamin deficiency. It is characterized by subjective complaints, such as loss of appetite, weight, and strength, cramps, palpitation, shortness of breath, and diarrhea. As the peripheral neuritis develops, burning, numbness, and tingling of the extremities are complained of. As the condition progresses, these symptoms become more pronounced, and the gastrointestinal, peripheral nervous, and cardiovascular systems all may become involved. Anorexia, nausea, and vomiting may occur.

The peripheral nervous system is affected by a myelin degeneration of the peripheral nerves which leads to burning, tingling, and numbness. This may affect the soles of the feet, calves of the legs, and leads to weakness and degeneration. The tendon reflexes may be overactive early in the disease, but later are diminished or absent. In a few instances the disease is accompanied by edema and serous effusions. In these cases it is said to be due to changes in the heart, the peripheral vascular system, or the intercellular and intracellular fluids. The edema usually begins in the lower extremities and extends upward, being associated with hydrothorax, ascites, or pericardial effusion. In children the disease presents a more acute form, rapid in onset and without prodromal symptoms. All of the other symptoms may be present, however, and the disease may terminate fatally. No laboratory or other tests are at present available, and the diagnosis must be made from the symptoms with the aid of a therapeutic test.

Chronic alcoholism has been said to be a predisposing factor in cases of vitamin B$_1$ deficiency. It was explained by Fantus[5] as providing non-fat calories which increase the need for the thiamine and that "alcoholic neuritis" has been definitely shown to be a manifestation of thiamine deficiency.

Thiamine deficiency has also been found in association with diabetes in a number of instances.

Eye Manifestations.—Spies, Vilter, and Ashe[8] observed visual disturbances in more than 70 per cent of the patients who have frequent recurrences of beriberi, pellagra, or flavin deficiency. Some of the symptoms resemble those of vitamin A deficiency, and many of the patients have poor vision, dry burning of the eyes, and on examination show a marked conjunctivitis, particularly in the conjunctiva of the lower lid. The pupils in a great number of patients, especially children, are dilated.

Pronounced ocular manifestations of this deficiency alone are not often encountered. However, when it exists in association with diabetes or with alcoholism, advanced cases, especially, might show paralyses involving the third and sixth nerves. Wernicke's syndrome, which is observed in chronic alcoholism and in which bilateral ophthalmoplegia and ptosis may develop with optic nerve involvements, is said to be due to thiamine deficiency.

Tobacco-alcohol amblyopia which is characterized by a loss of vision, whitening of the optic disc, and the presence of a cecocentral scotoma on examination of the visual fields is found also in association with thiamine deficiency. This has been proved by the therapeutic test.

The optic nerve head has also been affected by optic neuritis. In 1929, Shastid[18] reported two cases of optic neuritis of unknown origin. In both the condition was cleared up by the administration of yeast with no treatment of any other kind.

Treatment.—The treatment of beriberi must be started in some cases when the diagnosis of the condition is only suspected and not yet confirmed. This constitutes the therapeutic test. The local treatment depends on the type of the ocular manifestation and in the presence of any external signs, only mild and symptomatic measures are required. These manifestations will improve and respond favorably to the general treatment if they are caused by the deficiency of B_1. According to Fantus[5] the response to an adequate dose of thiamine hydrochloride administered parenterally is usually prompt in alleviating the symptoms of vitamin B_1 deficiency. Symptoms of other origin will not be affected. The parenteral route is imperative in a therapeutic test to insure absorption. When more gradual utilization is desired, it is injected subcutaneously. Intravenous injection results in more rapid excretion and is no more effective than the intramuscular or intravenous route. Fantus found that a subcutaneous injection of 10 mg. daily is usually adequate, although 30 mg. daily may be required in more severe cases. This dose was recommended for ten days as a therapeutic test, the first signs of improvement being a disappearance of edema, decrease of paresthesia and tenderness in the calves. A characteristic sign is an increased feeling of well-being in mild cases. Alleviation of any of the characteristic signs and symptoms is confirmation of the diagnosis.

When no improvement occurs in severe cases after ten injections of 30 mg. of thiamine chloride, curative results are not to be expected. If the therapeutic test is favorable, the underlying cause of the deficiency should be discovered and corrected, if possible. The injections of sufficient thiamine chloride should be continued until the patient is cured. A high level of vitamin B_1 intake should also be continued after a cure is obtained by including in the diet wheat germ, yeast, rice polishings, or their extracts, liver, whole wheat bread and cereals, eggs, nuts, lean pork, and legumes. The diet should also be supplemented by the addition of other vitamins, since it has often been pointed out that one deficiency rarely occurs without another, and B_1 especially appears to be closely related to the other components of B complex.

If the patient is a chronic alcoholic and shows signs of pellagra in association, nicotinic acid should be administered in addition to thiamine hydrochloride and, of course, the use of alcohol should be prohibited.

Aring et al.[6] stated that the neuritides of beriberi (alcoholic and nonalcoholic neuritis) as well as those of pellagra, tuberculosis, pernicious anemia and pregnancy, respond promptly to large doses of B_1. They recommended intravenous injections of 50 mg. twice daily for one week, which were followed by a rapid alleviation of symptoms.

For optic neuritis or alcoholic amblyopia 10 mg. of synthetic thiamine hydrochloride by mouth, once daily for three or four weeks, will result in improvement of the condition, as indicated by improvement of vision and the visual fields. When the synthetic thiamine hydrochloride is not available to the patient, brewer's yeast may be employed in doses of two teaspoonfuls twice daily before meals.

Vitamin B_2 Deficiency (Pellagra)

Vitamin B_2 or G is the second fraction or component of the B complex. A deficiency or absence of this fraction in the diet is the cause of pellagra. Vitamin B_2, however, has also been found to consist of several factors, the most important of which are nicotinic acid and riboflavin. A deficiency of both of these factors is considered to be responsible for the occurrence of pellagra, and both have been employed separately and together for the treatment of the condition. However, pellagra as a dermatitic condition, or what has been designated by Sydenstricker et al.[7] as the syndrome of glossitis and dermatitis, with or without psychic symptoms and diarrhea, appears to be due to the deficiency of nicotinic acid and responds to the administration of the specific factor. Signs and symptoms of B_2 deficiency other than these, and including especially the eye manifestations, are considered as the result of riboflavin deficiency and are commonly designated by the term "ariboflavinosis." The administration of nicotinic acid effects the symptoms resulting from deficiency of that particular factor, but not those of ariboflavinosis, and the administration of riboflavin for the treatment of this deficiency will affect its cure, but will have no effect on any of the symptoms of the related deficiency which might be present. In other words, these substances are specific for their own clinical syndrome.

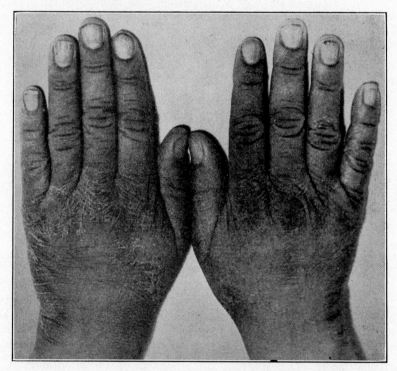

Fig. 210.—Lesions on dorsa of the hands in "alcohol pellagra and polyneuritis." (From Carroll: Arch. Ophth., December, 1936.)

Pellagra may, therefore, be considered as a syndrome affecting the skin, alimentary tract, and the central nervous system. It has been described by Spies et al.[8] as a disease attacking all classes of society, all races, and both sexes. In the United States it is most common in the Southern States. It may begin early in childhood and can be diagnosed clinically by the characteristic glossitis and dermatitis. The skin is rough, red, desquamating, cracked, and sharply separated from the healthy skin. The lesions occur bilaterally on the back of the hands, elbows, knees, ankles, neck, axilla, and perineal region. They are symmetrical, but change in appearance, becoming more highly pigmented with age.

The alimentary tract symptoms usually appear first. Anorexia, burning of the tongue, and abdominal pain occur as prodromes and are followed by glossitis, stomatitis, gingivitis, pharyngitis, gastritis, and enteritis. The lips are red, swollen, and cracked, and the tongue becomes fiery red, swollen, and smooth. The gums become red and ulcerated. Vincent's angina may be superimposed. Fiery red ulcers have been found on gastroscopic examination. The gastric analysis showed an achylia in 60 per cent. Diarrhea is watery and severe, accompanied by abdominal pain and distention. The genitourinary tract may also be affected with the urethra or vagina commonly affected. Vincent's organisms are found in abundance.

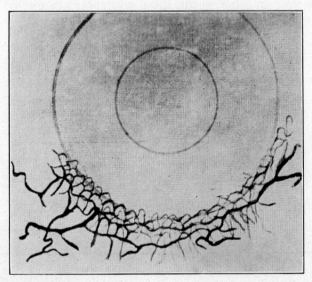

Fig. 211.—Diagram showing congestion and proliferation of limbic plexus which was found to be the earliest sign of ariboflavinosis. (From Sydenstricker, Sebrell, Cleckley, and Kruse: J. A. M. A., June 22, 1940.)

Symptoms of central nervous system affection are also very common. In the late stages of the disease the patients have hallucinations, delusions, and depression. They may also become maniacal and delirious. On the administration of nicotinic acid in proper doses, the patient will show immediate improvement.

Ariboflavinosis.—Deficiency of the riboflavin factor of vitamin B$_2$ seems to be the one more responsible for the occurrence of the eye manifestations in this disease. The importance of riboflavin in the human diet has been demonstrated a number of times. A detailed description of riboflavin is given by Johnson and Eckardt,[9] who state that it is an intensely yellow, water-soluble pigment which exhibits a distinct green fluorescence under ultraviolet rays. It has been isolated from milk, liver, egg white, and other foods. It is destroyed by visible light and by ultraviolet rays in both alkaline and acid solutions. At the present writing it is believed that practically all animal cells contain an enzyme which is used in the oxidation of carbohydrate by the cell. This is known as "Warburg's yellow enzyme." Johnson and Eckardt stated that the need for riboflavin in the diet is believed to be due to the fact that it is an essential constituent of the oxidation system of the yellow enzyme, and since the cells are incapable of synthesizing riboflavin, it must be continuously supplied from outside sources, to replace that lost in the excretions. Riboflavin is also essential for proper growth. In experiments on albino rats it has been shown that the yellow fluorescent pigment formed by the tubercle bacillus is identical with riboflavin, and this bacterial riboflavin can be isolated from dry tubercle bacilli.[10]

Eye Manifestations.—The ocular symptoms of the deficiency syndrome of ariboflavinosis have been described by a number of investigators.[7, 8, 9, 11, 12, 13]

These manifestations include the subjective complaints of photophobia, dimness of vision not caused by refractive errors. Twilight blindness occurring with leiodystonia and sprue was found to improve on administration of riboflavin by Pock-Steen.[14] Burning sensation of the eyes and roughness of the eyelids are troublesome.

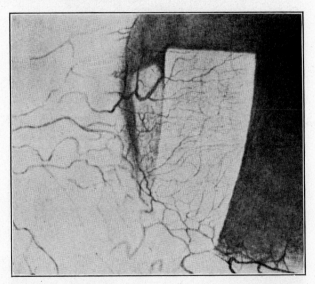

Fig. 212.—Advanced dietary keratitis. Drawing indicating degree of vascularization of the cornea in spontaneous ariboflavinosis of long duration. (From Sydenstricker, Sebrell, Cleckley, and Kruse: J. A. M. A., June 22, 1940.)

The Conjunctiva.—Among the early and more common objective signs is circumcorneal injection, which can frequently be seen with direct illumination. This is usually accompanied by a conjunctivitis characterized by injection of the conjunctival vessels. A seborrheic conjunctivitis may affect the margins of the eyelids.

The Cornea: (Rosacea Keratitis).—The cornea seems to become involved in ariboflavinosis by the occurrence of vascularization. The earliest change observed with the slit lamp has been described as a marked proliferation and engorgement of the limbic plexus with the production of very narrow capillary loops which outline the extreme margins of the scleral digitations and obliterate the narrow avascular zone between the plexus and the sclerocorneal junction. Sydenstricker et al.[7] stated that this condition can be definitely considered abnormal and possibly specific. It was observed to progress to vascularization of the cornea within a week in the absence of treatment and to regress rapidly during the administration of riboflavin. In the early invasion of the cornea the capillaries are seen to lie just beneath the epithelium and soon anastomose to

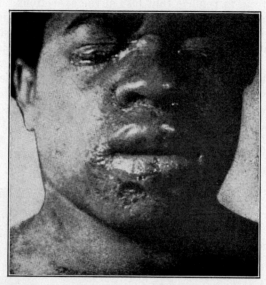

Fig. 213.—Severe ariboflavinosis showing cheilosis and photophobia with blepharospasm. (From Sydenstricker, Sebrell, Cleckley, and Kruse: J. A. M. A., June 22, 1940.)

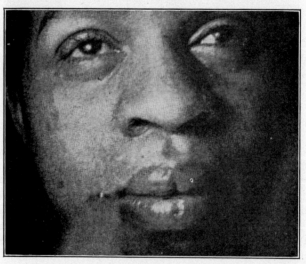

Fig. 214.—Same patient after ten days' treatment with riboflavin. Keratitis, facial lesions, and cheilosis cured. (From Sydenstricker, Sebrell, Cleckley, and Kruse: J. A. M. A., June 22, 1940.)

form a row of loops from which additional capillaries arise. This progress of anastomosis of capillaries continues until an extensive vascularization is produced. The cornea in general may appear slightly steamy or reveal the presence of an early nebula. Other vessels also may invade the substantia propia and are found at varying depths in the cornea. Late in the condition a deep plexus of vessels may be seen to develop. In chronic relapsing ariboflavinosis universal vascularization and extensive superficial and interstitial opacities may occur. In this disease the vascularization and keratitis differ from the interstitial keratitis of syphilis in that the superficial plexus and superficial cornea have already been more extensively involved than the posterior.

This form of keratitis which was described previously as rosacea keratitis occurring in ariboflavinosis (Johnson and Eckardt) was designated by Sydenstricker et al. as "dietary keratitis." It is accompanied by other signs of ariboflavinosis, such as redness of the buccal surface of the lips, maceration and fissures of the lips, seborrhea of the nasolabial folds, alae nasi, eyelids, and ears. A common manifestation has been described as so-called "shark skin" eruption which is characterized by seborrhea and follicular keratosis of the forehead, malar prominences, and chin. Acne vulgaris and telangiectasis may be present.

Cosgrove and Day[15] reported twenty-eight patients with corneal disease treated with riboflavin with varying results. It was found that patients with interstitial keratitis associated with hereditary syphilis responded more rapidly with the use of riboflavin than when antisyphilitic treatment was employed alone. Patients with various corneal diseases recovered more rapidly with riboflavin treatment, while those with allergy and linear keratitis showed no improvement.

Connors and co-workers[16] found that rosacea keratitis, marginal ulcers and catarrhal corneal infiltrates all respond immediately to the parenteral injection of riboflavin. These conditions were believed to result from an actual or relative insufficiency of the flavoprotein enzymes. These authors encountered only one patient with typical superficial vascularization and superficial marginal infiltrates in the arcus senilis area who did not respond satisfactorily to the intravenous use of riboflavin and the oral use of vitamin B complex. This patient's lesions did heal promptly when riboflavin and whole blood were given. Connors and associates felt that the whole blood supplied some factor or initialed some process necessary for the metabolism of riboflavin. They postulated also that in addition to dietary deficiency, disorders in the metabolism of riboflavin enzymes may be responsible for the development of corneal disease.

The Iris.—The pupil in ariboflavinosis is usually found to be dilated. Iritis is present in a number of cases. The iris has been described as revealing an abnormal accumulation of pigment on its anterior surface. Evidence of congestion of the iris plexus has been observed in all cases of excessive pigmentation.

The Lens (Cataract).—Cataracts have been produced by Day, Langston, and O'Brien[17] in young albino rats which receive a diet deficient in vitamin G. Other manifestations found included lacrimation, conjunctivitis, keratitis, a pasty condition of the eyelids and alopecia of the eyelids. All of these changes cleared up when the rats were again fed autoclaved yeast, which is rich in vitamin G. It has since been argued, however, that it is improbable that patients are ever deficient in riboflavin to an extent sufficient to produce cataract. No specific changes in the human lens have as yet been described as "ariboflavinosis opacities" (Johnson and Eckardt).

Optic Nerve (Optic Neuritis).—A few cases of optic neuritis have been reported of unknown origin but which cleared upon the administration of yeast. Two such cases were reported by Shastid,[18] who suggested the connection of vitamin B deficiency with the cause of the optic neuritis in his patients, since the condition cleared up without other treatment.

A case of optic neuritis due to pellagra was also reported by Levine.[11] The optic neuritis began to subside in three days with gradual improvement in the vision on the administration of vitamin B_2.

Treatment.—The treatment of the eye manifestations of riboflavin deficiency consists in the specific treatment of the dietary deficiency. As soon as the diagnosis has been made, a well-balanced diet should be immediately administered. The local treatment is of minor importance.

Specific treatment will bring about a remission of the symptoms and signs characteristic of the disease. It must be remembered, however, that riboflavin is changed when exposed to light. In addition to being inactivated by light, it is also destroyed when the hydrogen-ion concentration is not on the acid side. The natural source of riboflavin is food, but in addition to supplying a satisfactory diet including the essential vitamins, riboflavin can be prescribed in synthetic form. The usual dosage is about 5 mg. a day by oral administration. Relief of ocular symptoms is usually obtained in from two to seven days. Brewer's yeast can also be prescribed. The use of alcohol and tobacco should be eliminated, although cures have been reported by the administration of riboflavin even though the use of alcohol was not entirely eliminated.

The foods which have a tendency to prevent pellagra with ariboflavinosis include buttermilk, wheat germ, tomato juice, fresh beef, dried yeast, canned turnips, salmon, eggs, green cabbages, peas, and beans. The treatment should, of course, be prescribed according to the individual requirements of the patient. Severe cases should be hospitalized and any coexistent conditions should receive treatment. In patients with a mixed deficiency, brewer's yeast powder, in from 50 to 75 Gm. daily by mouth, is beneficial. Liver extract, 75 to 100 Gm. or wheat germ, 150 Gm., may also be employed. Yeast and wheat germ are considered helpful because, in addition to riboflavin, they also supply B_6, B_1 and nicotinic acid, as well as proteins, minerals, enzymes, and other essentials. It should also be remembered that withdrawal of riboflavin from the diet causes a recurrence of the condition with the eye manifestations being among the first to reappear. The general hygiene of the patient should receive attention, and he should be protected from strong light and sunlight.

Vitamin C Deficiency

Vitamin C (cevitamic acid) is very unstable and is destroyed by heat and neutral or alkaline solutions, drying and ageing. It does resist cooking, however, and if air is excluded, it is unaffected by canning. It is present in the milk of cows fed on green foods, especially in fresh fruit juices, such as orange juice, lemon juice, and tomato juice. It is destroyed by boiling of milk.

The reserves of vitamin C in newborn infants are depleted early, so that a deficiency might occur which will lead to the production of scurvy. This is first manifested by irritation, restlessness, lack of resistance to infection, and impaired growth. The disease has been shown to result from a defect in the cement substance of the endothelial cells of the blood vessels caused by a lack

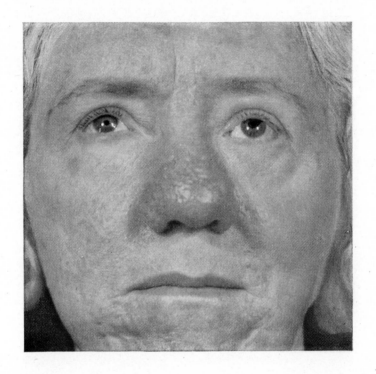

Fig. 215.—Patient with typical rosacea keratitis accompanied by flushed skin, telangiectasia, rhinophyma. (From Johnson and Eckardt: Arch. Ophth., May, 1940.)

of vitamin C in the diet. The increase in the permeability of the blood vessel walls which occurs is important in the cause of the hemorrhages and is responsible for many of the symptoms present. Although more common among infants between the ages of 10 months and 2 years, scurvy may occur at any age. In addition to the tendency to hemorrhage, it is characterized by swelling and sponginess of the gums, anemia, and pathologic bone changes. In the adult scurvy usually manifests itself first by a loss of physical tone. Frequently, pains in the joints and muscles are complained of, and as the disease progresses, the gums become swollen, sore, and bleed on the slightest trauma. Hemorrhages occur elsewhere on the body, as petechia, or even as ecchymosis in the muscles. Epistaxis, bloody diarrhea, or hematuria may be severe and even fatal. Death may result from shock or secondary infection.

Eye Manifestations.—The eye manifestations of vitamin C deficiency are not numerous or pronounced. Those which occur are undoubtedly the result of hemorrhage in patients with scurvy. A partial or subclinical deficiency will scarcely produce any clinical manifestations in the eyes.

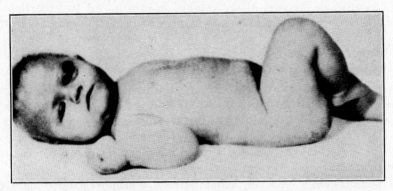

Fig. 216.—Exophthalmos with marked hematoma of the lid in infantile scurvy. (From Dunnington: Arch. Ophth., November, 1931.)

Exophthalmos.—Although hemorrhages in scurvy may occur from any vessels of the eye (lids, conjunctiva, anterior chamber, retina), the most prominent are evidently those which occur in the orbit and result in exophthalmos. Probably the best description of this condition was given by Dunnington[19] in reporting a case of infantile scurvy with exophthalmos. The exophthalmos may appear suddenly because of its hemorrhagic origin and may be very pronounced. The direction of the proptosis is usually forward, downward, and outward. This is due to the fact that the exophthalmos is caused by subperiosteal hemorrhages which, in most cases, occur along the orbital plate of the frontal bone. It has been explained that this is a favored site for the occurrence of subperiosteal hemorrhage in infantile scurvy because of the rapid increase in the size of the orbit in infants between 1 and 1½ years of age. The absorption of these hemorrhages is rather slow in the absence of antiscorbutic treatment. In early cases of scurvy the exophthalmos may be very slight with the edema of the eyelids being the prominent symptom. The latter is a rather frequent finding in infantile scurvy. In other instances, the exophthalmos may be extreme. The exophthalmos may be accompanied by a swelling of the lid due to ecchymosis, which might also occur to a marked degree.

Exophthalmos in scurvy occurs mostly in infants and may be unilateral or bilateral. In the latter cases, however, one eye is usually affected more than the other. The left eye has been found to be more frequently involved. The motility of the eye is at first only slightly impaired, but this impairment increases in older cases. There is no pulsation present, and the exophthalmos cannot be reduced. A possible complication of extreme exophthalmos is involvement of the cornea. Because of the inability to close the eyelids, the cornea in these cases is exposed and is liable to suffer with keratitis and ulceration. An early sign of this is oncoming haziness with loss of luster.

Vitamin C and Cataract.—The relation of vitamin C to the production of cataract has been studied experimentally in animals, but there is little, if any, knowledge concerning the clinical relationship. Cataract does not occur as a clinical manifestation of scurvy. However, vitamin C does seem to have some function in the metabolism of the lens. Bellows[20] found that the cevitamic acid concentration in the blood plasma of patients with cataract was lower than that in normal subjects and also that a larger quantity of vitamin C was required to cause an increase in the content in cataractous patients than in the normal. Since vitamin C is known to be present in certain amounts in the normal aqueous and lens, these findings led to the conclusion that a diminution of this substance in the aqueous and lens of cataractous eyes precedes the development of opacities and is not secondary to it.

Treatment.—The treatment of ocular manifestations of vitamin C deficiency is specific. As soon as the diagnosis is established, the patient should be placed on a proper diet and sufficient vitamin C. This can be easily supplied in the form of orange juice or by any of the synthetic preparations of ascorbic acid. Unless the antiscorbutic diet and supply of vitamin C is continued, relapses are apt to occur.

In Dunnington's case the exophthalmos, which was quite marked, was reduced, and the eye appeared practically normal after the administration of 3 ounces of orange juice daily for four days. The child left the hospital in excellent condition in a week.

The intravenous and oral administration of vitamin C has been found to be beneficial in cases of hemorrhagic diathesis.

Yudkin[21] has treated patients with various types of hemorrhagic retinitis with cevitamic acid. The time required for repair to take place in these cases was found to be shortened. Retinal and vitreous hemorrhages were found to respond better to treatment with lemon juice than with synthetic vitamin C, as evidenced by the more rapid clearing of the extravasation of blood and edema. The juice of at least four or five lemons daily can be prescribed.

In patients with oncoming cataract, the diet may also be regulated and maintained at an adequate level. Lemon juice and orange juice should be prescribed for daily use, and the general condition of the patient, with particular reference to the cardiovascular system and the gastrointestinal system, should receive the proper attention. The proper diet, including the essential vitamin, and the general management of the patient with oncoming cataracts cannot be expected to arrest the condition, but rather to improve the general physical state of the patient.

Vitamin D and E Deficiency

It is not possible at the present time to describe any distinct manifestations of vitamin D and E as such. The lack of vitamin D in the diet is apparently associated with the deficiency of vitamin A and the occurrence of manifestations of xerophthalmia. It is also considered to be in some way associated with the formation of opacities in the lens, although there is no direct clinical evidence of this.

Vitamin K Deficiency

Vitamin K, which is also known as the "antihemorrhagic vitamin," appears to be an essential for the normal amount of prothrombin. The latter is a necessary constituent of the blood to ensure normal clotting. A hypothrombinemia or deficiency of blood prothrombin would result in a prolonged clotting time.

Although there is no evidence of the direct effect of a deficiency of blood prothrombin on the condition of the eyes, it is possible that continued or recurrent intraocular hemorrhage might to some extent be controlled by the administration of vitamin K. Of course, the prothrombin clotting time is usually taken as a measure of the level of vitamin K in the body. Although a real nutritional deficiency of vitamin K is rare, cases may occur as the result of improper absorption and assimilation rather than from inadequate intake. In some older patients, who are to undergo operation for senile cataract or for glaucoma, it might be well as a routine procedure to administer vitamin K both preoperatively and postoperatively. Since hemorrhage is frequently an undesirable and disturbing complication in these cases, the vitamin K may serve to decrease the seriousness of this occurrence. It can be administered orally or intramuscularly in doses of 1 or 2 mg. daily.

Botulism

Botulism is a type of food poisoning caused by the toxins of the anaerobic saprophytic organism, *Clostridium botulinum*. It is characterized by cranial motor nerve involvement and other nervous symptoms. The organism grows in a great variety of canned protein-containing foods, both plant and animal. The incubation period ranges usually from eighteen to thirty-six hours. The first symptoms in most cases are fatigue, headache, dizziness, and weakness. There may be at the onset considerable gastric distress with nausea, vomiting, and diarrhea, which is followed by obstinate constipation. The main features of the disease are dimness of vision, diplopia, ptosis, dilatation of pupils, difficulty in articulation, and in swallowing. Muscular weakness is progressive and there is incoordination. Blindness may occur, and death is most frequently due to respiratory paralysis.

Eye Manifestations.—Disturbances in vision appear early in botulism. Vision becomes dim due to the failure of the ciliary muscles which is much more marked when hypermetropia is present. The other early visual symptoms and signs are ptosis, diplopia, dilated pupils, and, sometimes, complete external and internal ophthalmoplegia. Barbel[22] described a case of optic nerve involvement in which paresis of both sixth nerves, diplopia, nystagmus, and choked disc were found on examination of the eyes. Perimetry revealed a paracentral scotoma and enlargement of the blind spot in the right eye and a large central scotoma in the left eye. During the eight months of observation the choked discs began to reveal an optic atrophy.

References

1. Rountree, J. I.: Absorption and Retention of Vitamin A in Young Children, J. Nutrition 3: 265, 1930.
2. Edmund, C., and Clemmesen, S.: On a Deficiency of A Vitamin and Visual Adaptation, London, Oxford University Press, 1936.
3. Pillat, Arnold: The Main Symptoms of the Eye in Vitamin A Deficiency in Adults, Nat. M. J. China 15: 585 and 614, 1929.
4. Booher, Lela E.: Vitamin A Requirements and Practical Recommendations for Vitamin A Intake, J. A. M. A. 110: 1920, 1938.
5. Fantus, Bernard: The Therapy of Subvitaminosis B₁, J. A. M. A. 115: 450, 1940.
6. Aring, Charles D., Evans, Joseph P., and Spies, Tom D.: Some Clinical Neurologic Aspects of Vitamin B Deficiencies, J. A. M. A. 113: 2105, 1939.
7. Sydenstricker, V. P., Sebrell, W. H., Cleckley, H. M., and Kruse, H. D.: The Ocular Manifestations of Ariboflavinosis, J. A. M. A. 114: 2437, 1940.
8. Spies, Tom D., Vilter, Richard W., and Ashe, William F.: Pellagra, Beriberi, and Riboflavin Deficiency in Human Beings, J. A. M. A. 113: 931, 1939.
9. Johnson, Lorand V., and Eckardt, Robert E.: Rosacea Keratitis and Conditions With Vascularization of Cornea Treated With Riboflavin, Arch. Ophth. 23: 899, 1940.
10. Current Comment: Riboflavin in the Tubercle Bacillus, J. A. M. A. 115: 1550, 1940.
11. Levine, Joseph: Pellagra as a Cause of Optic Neuritis, Arch. Ophth. 12: 902, 1934.
12. Spies, Tom D., Hightower, D. P., and Hubbard, L. H.: Some Recent Advances in Vitamin Therapy, J. A. M. A. 115: 292, 1940.
13. Johnson, Lorand V., and Eckardt, Robert E.: Ocular Conditions Associated With Clinical Riboflavin Deficiency, Arch. Ophth. 24: 1001, 1940.
14. Pock-Steen, P. H.: Eye Symptoms in Patients With Leiodystoma and Sprue: Twilight Blindness, Geneesk. tijdschr. v. Nedirl Indië 79: 1986, 1939.
15. Cosgrove, K. W., and Day, Paul L.: The Use of Riboflavin in the Treatment of Corneal Diseases, Am. J. Ophth. 25: 544, 1942.
16. Conners, C. A., Eckardt, R. E., and Johnson, L. V.: Riboflavin for Rosacea Keratitis, Marginal Corneal Ulcers and Catarrhal Corneal Infiltrates, Arch. Ophth. 29: 956, 1943.
17. Day, P. L., Langston, W. C., and O'Brien, C. S.: Cataract and Other Ocular Changes in Vitamin G Deficiency, Am. J. Ophth. 14: 1005, 1931.
18. Shastid, T. H.: Optic Neuritis and Vitamin B, Am. J. Ophth. 12: 903, 1928.
19. Dunnington, John Hughes: Exophthalmos in Infantile Scurvy, Arch. Ophth. 6: 731, 1931.
20. Bellows, John: Biochemistry of the Lens: Cevitamic Acid Content of the Blood and Urine of Subjects With Senile Cataract, Arch. Ophth. 15: 78, 1936.
21. Yudkin, Arthur M.: Vitamins in Treatment and Prevention of Ocular Diseases, Arch. Ophth. 19: 366, 1938.
22. Barbel, J. E.: The Disease of the Optic Nerve in Botulism, Russk, Arch. Oftal. 8: 591, 1932.

CHAPTER XX

DISEASES OF THE NERVOUS SYSTEM

Neurosyphilis

Neurosyphilis is one of the commonest organic disorders of the nervous system. Involvement may occur fairly early in the course of infection, even in the first year. In the secondary stage of syphilis more than half of the patients manifest meningeal involvement with the presence of a positive spinal fluid.

Syphilitic Meningitis.—Meningeal involvement is a common occurrence in the course of the disease and the meninges may be widely or acutely affected, but early involvement may run a latent course. Symptoms of chronic diffuse syphilitic meningitis are often confusing because of the simultaneous occurrence of either tabes or general paresis. Ocular manifestations are frequent, partly because of involvement of the base of the brain by the pathologic process.

Oculomotor paralyses, especially of the third nerve, are seen often. Various forms of pupillary disturbance arise. These include inequality, irregular pupils and, more important, disturbances of the reflexes such as the Argyll-Robertson pupil (absence of light reaction with reaction to accommodation), and also absence of reaction to both light and accommodation.

Of even greater importance is the involvement of the optic nerve. The process may directly involve the sheath of the optic nerve producing, as a rule, some form of optic neuritis, retrobulbar neuritis, neuritis with papillitis and most commonly, optic atrophy. An early ophthalmoscopic finding is hyperemia of the optic disc which later appears as an optic neuritis.

The visual field examination may be of great aid in the diagnosis and prognosis. This may reveal an early concentric contraction of the peripheral field, a marked contraction of the red and green fields, and central defects of various types.

Involvement of the optic tract and chiasm is occasionally found with signs of homonymous or bitemporal hemianopia.

Involvement of the gasserian ganglion may give rise to various sensory disturbances. The entire trigeminal nerve or any of its divisions may be involved, producing paresthesia, hyperesthesia, or anesthesia. When corneal anesthesia occurs, a neuroparalytic keratitis may result.

According to Drake,[1] who analyzed fifty cases of acute syphilitic meningitis and meningo-encephalitis collected from the literature, paralysis of the cranial nerves is one of the most prominent symptoms. Papilledema was also an important sign, but it responds well to antisyphilitic treatment, leaving a postneuritic atrophy. Previous treatment in these cases, especially with arsphenamine, was not found to affect greatly the development of acute syphilitic meningitis.

Tabes Dorsalis.—Tabetic optic atrophy is considered as occurring in cases of spinal involvement, to differentiate it from chronic syphilitic meningitis.

The primary atrophy of this type is usually unremittingly progressive and, fortunately, is fairly rare, occurring in 6 to 8 per cent of tabetics. Serologic studies of both the blood and cerebrospinal fluid may be completely negative.

The pathologic process occurs in the nerve close to the eyeball; it consists of a chronic inflammation of both the interstitial and parenchymatous tissues of the nerve with an exudate of lymphocytes and plasma cells and a marked proliferation of connective tissue and neuroglia. Subsequently, sclerosis and obliteration of the vessels results, impairing the nutrition of the nerve fibers. The exudative process spreads from the brain to the optic nerve via the lymph sheaths of the vessels.

The fundamental clinical picture of tabes is based on the following signs and symptoms: (1) pupillary changes, (2) lightning pains, (3) absence of deep reflexes, (4) visceral disturbance, (5) disturbances of sensibility, (6) lymphocytosis of the cerebrospinal fluid, and (7) usually a positive Wassermann reaction of blood or cerebrospinal fluid, or both. In the early stage of the disease there may be no ataxia; however, it may appear later on.

Eye Manifestations.—Some impairment of the pupillary reaction is found in the great majority of cases of tabes. The Argyll-Robertson pupil, which consists of loss of the pupillary reaction to light but which is present on accommodation-convergence, is the most valuable single sign of tabes and occurs in over 70 per cent of tabetics. In about 15 per cent pupils are inactive both to light and accommodation. The Argyll-Robertson pupil may exist for years without any other obvious sign of tabes or general paresis. As a rule, the pupils are unequal on the two sides and often irregular.

Paralyses of external ocular muscles occur quite commonly in tabes. Any muscle may be affected, but the external rectus suffers most frequently. This may be either transient or permanent. Ptosis may also be present.

Optic atrophy which has been previously described (See Syphilis) occurs in 6 to 8 per cent of tabetics and is a very early symptom of the condition. So much so that the initial complaint by the patient is failing vision; in addition, foggy vision and difficulty in recognizing colors are complaints which point to loss of central vision. Fleeting diplopias are frequently mentioned. These patients see better in dimmed rather than in strong light. They also show signs of defective adaptation.

The study of visual fields shows that they are extremely variable, inasmuch as Leslie Paton suggests that the pathology is also variable in its mechanism for producing visual loss. Commonly and early there is a depression of the whole field with concentric contraction of the peripheral field for white and red and green, while central acuity is well preserved. Later, diminished visual acuity with sector cuts may occur, rarely, central scotoma and hemianopic defects.

One eye is usually affected some time before the other, or both may be involved simultaneously. Onset and course may be slowly progressive, but the progress of tabetic atrophy is relentless in eventually leading to blindness.

On ophthalmoscopic examination the marked pallor of the disc is striking, with the color being either white or gray. The grayish tint is due to the lamina cribrosa which is distinctly seen. The pallor is due to the local anemia of the nerve head, and the degree is not in direct proportion to the extent of the atrophy. It may be noted very early with loss of adaptation but without actual loss of vision. The physiologic excavation is clearly seen if present, and the blood vessels are usually normal except for slight reduction in caliber.

Treatment.—The course of primary tabetic optic atrophy is progressive and in most cases eventually terminates in blindness. The treatment of the condition has been discussed previously. (See Syphilis.) This can only serve to check the progress, if the case is seen early enough, and includes the use of iodides, mercury, and bismuth. Regular ophthalmoscopic examination should be made to observe the appearance of the disc during the course of treatment. This should also be accompanied by regular visual field studies.

Fever therapy produced with use of the Kettering hypertherm, injections of typhoid and malaria, and attempts to improve the circulation and nutritional state of the optic nerve by retrobulbar injections of vasodilators, are also employed.

Tuberculosis of the Nervous System

Tuberculous intracranial lesions are not of great importance or frequency in the production of eye manifestations. They may be considered here as occurring in the form of tuberculous meningitis and tuberculoma.

Tuberculous Meningitis.—In tuberculous meningitis, papilledema is found in about 20 per cent of the cases, and optic neuritis in about 30 per cent (Uthoff). In many of these cases it is impossible to make a diagnosis of the ocular manifestations and, especially, to differentiate between the presence of optic neuritis and papilledema. The general condition of the patient is usually such as to preclude the possibility of satisfactory examination and an examination of the visual fields is mostly impossible. Increased intracranial pressure is often present, however, with resulting papilledema.

In many of these cases, the choroid of the eye reveals the presence of miliary and discrete tubercles, either near the disc or in the periphery of the fundus. (See Tuberculosis.)

Paralysis of the oculomotor nerves occurs and conjugate movements of the eyes may be impaired.

Tuberculoma.—Tuberculoma is extremely rare in occurrence, and following the general rule, it affects chiefly children and young adults, and males more than females. Tuberculomas are often multiple and are found subtentorial; an associated meningitis or meningeal tuberculosis is found as a rule. The pathology is that of tuberculous tissue elsewhere. Miliary tubercles tend to be disseminated throughout the brain and spinal cord by the spinal fluid. The brain is swollen and covered with a gelatinous exudate, especially at the base.

Clinically, tuberculomas are considered as intracranial tumors; however, they have important differences which aid in a differential diagnosis. These are: (1) The patient with a tuberculoma will show a general infection and (2) papilledema, when present, is a late manifestation, since the tuberculoma increases in size chiefly at the expense of brain tissue and produces signs of pressure only in a late stage.

Operative treatment is sometimes attempted in cases of tuberculoma, because the condition is considered to be an intraocular tumor. Such an attempt is attended by the danger of dissemination of the tuberculous process and the development of tuberculous meningitis.

Epidemic Encephalitis

Epidemic encephalitis is a disseminated infection of the brain stem marked by symptoms which vary greatly. Of all the virus diseases, epidemic encephalitis is of singular interest to ophthalmologists because of the prominence of oculomotor symptoms in the different epidemics.

The onset of the disease is insidious, while the acute stage shows a characteristic neurologic picture. There is usually some disturbance of sleep (hypersomnia, insomnia), hyperkinesis and akinesis, paralysis of ocular muscles, particularly of conjugate movements, nystagmus (either vertical or horizontal), paralysis of convergence, paralysis of accommodation and pupillary disturbances. Optic neuritis has been reported with bitemporal and homonymous hemianopia, also papilledema which arises from a complication, e.g., basal meningitis with an increased spinal pressure. Transient diplopia is a most frequent, single diagnostic feature of the acute stage (Foster Kennedy). The symptoms of the acute stage vary within the course of a few days. They are not permanent and the disease passes eventually into a chronic stage when signs of Parkinsonism become evident.

In the chronic stage the permanent symptoms are principally oculomotor. All possible types of palsies may occur. Ptosis of the eyelids is a frequent symptom associated with paresis or paralysis of both external recti. Disturbances of associated movements are common, as diminution or loss of conjugate movements up or down, but not so frequently lateral (described as syndrome of Parinaud). The latter is due to the predilection of the infection for the quadrigeminal plate. There is also insufficiency of convergence, paralysis of divergence (Ward Holden), paresis of accommodation which is bilateral in contrast to that of syphilis which is unilateral, and nystagmus either vertical or horizontal.

Pupillary disturbances are fairly common. These include a sluggish reaction to light and accommodation, and the Argyll-Robertson pupil which is not infrequently seen. Many involuntary movements such as blepharospasm and stammering occur in the disease. Rhythmic muscle spasms of extrinsic eye muscles, spasmodic attacks of ocular deviation, and the oculogyric crises are also prominent.

Epidemic Meningitis

Meningitis occurring in epidemic form is caused by the meningococcus. The disease was formerly fatal in more than one-third of the cases, but since the use of sulfa drugs, this has been greatly reduced. The onset is characterized by the presence of a nasopharyngitis and, in some cases, simultaneous conjunctivitis. The infection spreads by way of the blood stream with the rather sudden appearance of evidences of septicemia.

Early in the disease there may be involvement of almost any of the organs, including the brain, spinal cord, heart, lungs, skin, and kidneys. Various manifestations may be present such as petechia, arthritis, myocarditis, otitis, lymphadenitis, and ocular complications. Neurologic complications and sequelae cover a wide range of conditions which include encephalitis, hemiplegia, tremors, vasomotor changes, facial palsies, cerebellar ataxia, muscular atrophy, emotional instability, gait disturbances, and changes in personality. Labyrinthine disease and deafness, either partial or complete, result in a fair number of cases.

Epidemics of the disease occur at intervals in various localities. These are usually followed by a period of quiescence during which only isolated cases occur. This may be followed after a time by a fresh outbreak.

Kernig's sign and rigidity of the neck are characteristic, but definite diagnosis can be made by recovery of the organisms from the cerebrospinal fluid.

Eye Manifestations.—Ocular manifestations and complications in epidemic meningitis have been reported to occur in from 10 per cent to as many as 45 per cent of cases. These have probably decreased in recent years because of the use of the specific serum earlier in the course of the disease.

In a study of ninety-three cases of epidemic meningitis, Heath[2] listed 16.1 per cent with ocular conditions which he described as "ocular residue." These included pupillary changes (dilated pupils and anisocoria), muscle disturbances (convergent squint, divergent squint, convergence weakness, nystagmus, and paralysis of superior rectus with head tilt), optic neuritis and neuroretinitis, and endophthalmitis. In all of the reports paralysis of the extraocular muscles, metastatic ophthalmia, and endophthalmitis seem to be the most common complications. Optic neuritis is probably next in frequency, followed in order by anomalies of the pupils, conjunctivitis, corneal involvement, and lastly optic atrophy.

Lazar[3] in a study of cases between the years 1933 and 1935 found the two major ocular complications to be endophthalmitis and paresis of the external recti muscles. He stated also that microscopic examination of the eyes in these cases of endophthalmitis showed nothing to distinguish the condition from that produced by other blood-borne infections.

Dunphy[4] described the ocular manifestations in each of the structures of the eye in detail.

The conjunctiva was involved in a fair number of cases by meningococcic conjunctivitis. Although the meningococcus has been isolated from the secretion of the conjunctiva in patients suffering with epidemic meningitis, it has also been cultivated from the eyes of those who did not have the disease.

The pupillary changes found to be present are a dilatation of the pupils and fixed pupils. These usually become normal after recovery from the disease. Inequality of the pupils may also occur, as well as absence of the light reaction.

The extraocular muscles are frequently involved and reveal transient forms of strabismus, either convergent or divergent. Paralysis of the external rectus muscle may become permanent. Nystagmus, either rotary or vertical, may occasionally be found.

The cornea is rarely involved. Parenchymatous keratitis and ulceration have been found to occur. Corneal ulceration may result from the presence of other complications.

Optic neuritis may begin as an early hyperemia of the optic nerve head. Papilledema rarely occurs. The acute cerebral amaurosis with temporary blindness may occur in infants.

Treatment.—The local treatment should include first, the protection of the eyes from light. Hot, wet compresses of boric acid should be applied in cases of corneal involvement, and one drop of atropine sulfate, 1 per cent solution, should be instilled twice daily. The conjunctival sac should be flushed regularly with boric acid solution. Antimeningococcus serum can also be instilled into the conjunctival sac and subconjunctival injections have been recommended for iritis and metastatic involvement. Intravenous and intraspinal injections are of value in the treatment of the ocular complications of central origin especially. Intraocular injection of meningococcus serum was recommended by Dunphy in cases of early ocular involvement. The dosage of meningococcus antitoxin as recommended by Lazar is 50,000 units in a 10 per cent solution of dextrose and sodium chloride by vein, for infants up to 2 years of age. This is repeated two or three times. For children over 6 years of age, the dosage is 100,000 units and sometimes 60,000 to 80,000, intravenously.

More recently, sulfadiazine, sulfamerazine, and penicillin have been employed with very good results.

Brain Abscess

Brain abscess may follow the spread of infection from pyogenic diseases of the middle ear, mastoids, nasal sinuses, and from abscess of the lung. The clinical history may indicate the possible source of the infection.

The clinical course of a brain abscess usually presents three stages (Macewen): (1) an initial stage during which constitutional symptoms of the infection, such as fever, rigor, vomiting, and pain in the head, predominate; (2) the second stage follows an intermediate quiescent period and is characterized by pain in the head, slow cerebration, apyrexia, slow pulse, oculomotor paralysis, and papilledema; (3) the third or terminal stage may resolve itself into a diffuse cerebral picture of fever, convulsions, and coma. The pus may spread into the ventricles, membranes, and may cover the brain; or encapsulation with localizing signs of the abscess may occur. The signs and symptoms are the same as those of other intracranial tumors.

Eye Manifestations.—Benedict,[5] in a symposium on brain abscess, described the manifestations from the standpoint of the ophthalmologist.

Choked disc or papilledema is the most prominent sign and is present in about 30 per cent of the cases. It is usually bilateral and the measurable swelling varies from 3 to 6 diopters. During the time the abscess develops, the amount of choking may fluctuate, but this becomes fixed when the abscess is encapsulated. Abscesses occurring in some locations may reveal little or no choked disc. Abscess of the frontal lobe, unless very large, ordinarily does not cause choked disc. Benedict, however, referred to Lillie who found choked disc of from 1 to 6 diopters in eight out of eleven cases of encapsulated abscess of the frontal lobe.

Abscess of the temporal lobe which nearly always results from disease of the middle ear is the most common location for the production of choked disc.

Visual field changes are also more common with temporal lobe abscess. Abscess of the frontal lobe rarely produces characteristic field changes except when they occur at the base of the brain. Hemianopia is the characteristic visual field manifestation and is common in temporal lobe and occipital lobe abscesses. It may be either a complete or incomplete homonymous hemianopia, and although it is prominently associated with chocked disc, it may occasionally occur alone.

Bilateral amaurosis, probably resulting from secondary optic atrophy, has been reported in abscess of the cerebellum and abscess of the occipital lobe.

Paralysis of the extraocular muscles is rare, although paralysis of the sixth nerve, with impaired motility of the external rectus of the involved side, may occur in frontal abscess. The third nerve may be partially involved in association with choked disc in temporal lobe abscess. This may be manifested by the presence of ptosis on the affected side, paralysis of accommodation and of the pupil. Horizontal, vertical, and rotary nystagmus is especially common in cerebellar abscess.

Treatment.—With regard to treatment, Benedict emphasized the importance of choosing the proper time for surgical intervention. If operation is performed before the abscess becomes encapsulated, the patient seldom recovers, whereas an encapsulated abscess of the brain can be drained or removed with very slight risk. Encapsulation of the abscess can be considered to be completed when the degree of choked disc becomes stationary and the clinical picture resembles that which occurs with a brain tumor in the same location.

The Demyelinating Diseases of the Nervous System

The demyelinating diseases of the central nervous system are considered to consist of four clinical types, namely disseminated sclerosis (multiple sclerosis), acute disseminated encephalomyelitis, neuromyelitis optica (Devic's disease), and encephalitis periaxialis diffusa (Schilder's disease). The etiology of this group is unknown, but it is generally suspected to be an infectious agent or a neurotropic virus. In a review of this subject, Berliner[6] stated that "it is not impossible that all these conditions are variations of one main entity, and that their clinical differences are due mainly to degrees of involvement or to predilection for special tissue."

Leslie Paton[7] described them as four virus infections, the exact nature of the virus being at present unknown, but the differences in clinical cases may be due to a variation in the virulence of the poison or in susceptibility of the affected structure.

All four of these infections have one characteristic in common, namely the liability to manifest early involvement of the optic nerve, with the myelin sheath being the first tissue attacked, either in the optic nerve, the centrum ovale or the spinal cord tracts.

Since they are all demyelinating diseases, they are characterized by a retrobulbar type of optic neuritis with characteristic pain and loss of function.

Paton also gave four main differentiating points which are important. These are: (1) The loss of sight precedes ophthalmoscopic changes. (2) The ophthalmoscopic changes are of short duration. (3) The discs show no change after the swelling subsides. (4) Recovery of the vision usually occurs when the swelling subsides.

Disseminated Sclerosis.—Disseminated (multiple) sclerosis is one of the commonest disorders of the central nervous system with the possible exception of neurosyphilis. It occurs frequently during the third and fourth decades of life and is characterized by a long protracted clinical course marked by spontaneous remissions.

The pathologic process is characterized by sclerotic patches found chiefly within the white matter of the central nervous system. The sclerotic patch, however, is the terminal stage of the process. The early lesion is a patch of perivascular infiltration consisting of lymphocytes, plasma cells, and compound granular cells. The myelin becomes swollen and undergoes dissolution. The axis cylinder is affected similarly but not to the same extent. When sclerosis occurs, it is capable of retaining or regaining function. There is finally a proliferation of fibrillary astrocytes which lend to the patch its sclerotic character. The optic nerve, chiasm, and tract show involvement in all cases, and scarcely any fibers remain unaffected in the entire course.

Clinically, the onset may be rather sudden, especially where the lesion has involved the optic nerve or oculomotor nerve, and blindness or diplopia is noticed. The history commonly begins with numbness or weakness of the extremities, slight fever, and rarely headache and vomiting. There are two recognized types with important differences from the standpoint of prognosis. The remitting type, which is the more common, shows acute exacerbations after long intervals of time, while the main course of the disease is quiescent. The fulminating type is more rare. It is characterized by a progressive course with rapid deterioration, no remissions, and continues on to a fatal termination.

The symptoms of disseminated sclerosis may be enumerated as follows: emotional instability with either euphoria or depression, blurred vision, diplopia, nystagmus, and scanning speech. Motor paralysis of the upper motor neuron type occurs which may be hemiplegic, paraplegic, or monoplegic in distribution. Intention tremors and ataxia may be present.

The deep reflexes are increased and the earliest sign of disseminated sclerosis is absence of abdominal and epigastric reflexes. Paresthesias, which are multiple and evanescent, are common; sphincter disturbances are transient early, becoming more troublesome later in the disease.

Eye Manifestations.—The first and most prominent ocular symptom of disseminated sclerosis is retrobular neuritis which is manifested by sudden loss of vision and ocular pain. The fundus may appear normal except for an ensuing temporal pallor. There is considerable difference of opinion as to the number of cases of optic neuritis and retrobulbar neuritis due to disseminated sclerosis. This is brought about by the fact that disseminated sclerosis may develop years after an attack of retrobulbar neuritis. It is often said, therefore, that a retrobulbar neuritis without any other known cause is a manifestation of disseminated sclerosis, even in the absence of other signs or symptoms of the disease.

Benedict[8] reviewed the records of 400 patients seen at the Mayo Clinic from 1920 to 1940 who were suffering from retrobulbar neuritis. It was intended to determine whether the inclusion of doubtful cases in the category of multiple sclerosis was justified. Multiple sclerosis was suspected in ninety of the patients by the elimination of other factors which might cause blindness. In forty-one of the ninety patients, further evidences of the disease appeared. In none of the patients in whom further symptoms of multiple sclerosis failed to appear was the retrobulbar neuritis and scotoma found to result from any other cause. It was possible to make a diagnosis of other causes such as arteriosclerosis, diabetes, encephalitis, arachnoiditis and exogenous toxemia in many patients at the time of the first episode of blindness. A tentative diagnosis such as alcohol-tobacco amblyopia was made in some of the obscure cases on the basis of history and clinical findings. In others, multiple sclerosis was also suspected on the basis of the history, ocular signs and general symptoms. Benedict concluded from this review that it would seem reasonable to presume that the condition is due to multiple sclerosis in the absence of signs or symptoms of other causes of retrobulbar neuritis, even though the etiology cannot be substantiated on any other basis.

In 500 cases of proved disseminated sclerosis studied by Lillie,[9] the visual disturbance was a primary manifestation in 15 per cent, and the second or third in 35 to 40 per cent. The condition usually affects one eye, although it may occur later in the other eye. The loss of vision is sudden and rapid, in the average case; the fundus reveals no pathology. In other acute cases, optic neuritis, papillitis with several diopters of swelling, and rarely even papilledema have been present on ophthalmoscopic examination. The lesion in these cases is considered to be located just behind the lamina cribrosa or in front of the entrance of the central vessels. The fact that this occurs more often than suspected has been pointed out by a number of investigators, including Paton and Berliner. In others, it is further removed from the globe and involves the papillomacular bundle of nerve fiber.

The changes in the visual fields are rather typical, being characterized by the presence of a central or paracentral scotoma. The peripheral field may show a slight contraction. This may be a little more pronounced when the condition subsides. A slight enlargement of the blind spot may also be found at that time.

Vibratory nystagmus may be present in some of the cases. This may be coarse or fine, bilateral, and more marked on looking to the side and in elevation and depression of the eyes.

The pupils are sometimes unequal, but they usually react to light unless optic atrophy has taken place.

In a fair percentage of cases transient paralysis of the ocular muscles is seen. Involvement of the sixth nerve is more common than that of the third.

The prognosis is good for recovery of vision when the attack subsides. This may occur after a few weeks in some cases, but in nearly all it clears up sooner or later. The disease itself however, may last for years and gradually progress to a fatal termination.

Acute Disseminated Encephalomyelitis.—Acute disseminated encephalomyelitis represents an acute febrile condition involving both the brain and spinal cord. It occurs as a sequel during convalescence from other acute illnesses as chicken pox, measles, or postvaccinal. Furthermore, it may arise epidemically without any discoverable preceding illness. Rapid and extensive demyelinization of the white matter throughout the central nervous system, perivascular infiltration with lymphocytes and plasma cells, and proliferation of histiocytes and fibrillary astrocytes characterize the pathologic picture. Also, a prominent feature of the pathologic process is the attack on the visual pathway, e.g., nerves, chiasma, tracts, and higher centers.

Clinically, the disease shows an indefinite incubation period with the exception of that form which arises postvaccinal where a period of seven to thirteen days is definite. The onset is acute with the presence of fever, headache, dizziness, and vomiting. The state of consciousness varies from apathy and drowsiness to coma. Within a few weeks evidences of rapid destruction are noted, with the occurrence of strabismus, facial and hypoglossal palsies, monoplegia, hemiplegia, ascending paralysis and sphincter disturbances. Spinal fluid examination may show a slight increase in pressure and lymphocytosis. Mortality rate is around 40 per cent.

Eye Manifestations.—The ocular lesions are obscured because of the severity of the clinical process and reports are scanty. Early, slight swelling and hyperemia of the disc and venous congestion of the retina may be observed. Far more characteristic is the occurrence of optic neuritis. If this is bilateral it should be regarded as very suspicious. The involvement may not be simultaneous, and hence frequent examinations are necessary. The optic tracts and visual centers may also be involved. The field defects where they can be secured show either central or paracentral scotomas.

Neuromyelitis Optica (Devic's Disease).—Neuromyelitis optica is an acute or subacute infection without a demonstrable cause, presenting symptoms of an ascending myelitis and bilateral optic neuritis which occur almost simultaneously. It is not limited to a specific age group, is very rare, and rapidly fatal. It may also become stationary, and then retrogressive. Demyelinization of the white matter, perivascular infiltration, and little or no gliosis are seen pathologically. The difference in the pathology of disseminated sclerosis and neuromyelitis optica is not marked. However, in the latter disease destruction of nerve fibers is far greater, and the demyelinated patches are not clearly demarcated but rather ill-defined. Clinically, the disease is marked by an ascending paralytic process beginning with weakness and pains or parasthesia in the legs, then cutaneous and visceral anesthesia, sphincter disturbances and paralyses of the trunk muscles, extremities, or of the respiratory muscles which prove fatal. Laboratory examination of the blood, cerebrospinal fluid, and urine is usually negative. The disease shows no mental symptoms.

Eye Manifestations.—Acute diminution of vision which may progress to total blindness is complained of frequently. Both eyes are usually involved and bilateral optic neuritis is seen early in the course of the disease. In most cases it precedes the symptoms of myelitis. The ocular findings do not differ then from those found in disseminated sclerosis except for the bilateral involvement in neuromyelitis optica. The occurrence of optic neuritis in this condition has been attributed to the lesion being present near the lamina cribrosa. A clinicopathologic study of a case by Noran and Polan[10] showed the changes in the optic nerves, the chiasm or tracts to be the same as those found in the spinal cord.

Fluctuations in the acuity of vision occur, and recovery has been reported in some cases.

Encephalitis Periaxialis Diffusa (Schilder's Disease).—Encephalitis periaxialis diffusa was described by Schilder in 1912 while attempting to differentiate it from a group known as diffuse cerebral sclerosis. It is a demyelinating disease found during infancy and childhood, affecting chiefly the white matter in the cerebral and cerebellar hemispheres, with marked destruction of myelin sheaths and gliosis. It follows a prolonged course and usually terminates fatally. Clinically, there is an acute onset with gastrointestinal disturbances, after which the picture is dominated by cerebral symptoms, such as apathy, convulsions, paralyses, deafness, and amaurosis.

Eye Manifestations.—Paton[7] states his belief that Schilder's disease, of all the forms of optic neuritis, must be recognized as a distinct entity, because the disease can be distinguished both clinically and pathologically. In the other forms described, the differences are obscure and doubtful, often appearing to be variations in degree of disseminated sclerosis. More than one-third of the cases reveal the presence of optic neuritis. In Berliner's report of about thirty-five cases in the literature,[6] blindness, either complete or incomplete, was found in 60 per cent. It was a late symptom in 75 per cent of the cases. Bilateral optic atrophy was noticed before death in 90 per cent.

Cerebral blindness may be an early symptom in this disease because of the marked tendency for the severe cerebral changes to occur around the posterior horns of the lateral ventricles. At the same time the optic discs and pupillary reactions may be unaffected.

Myasthenia Gravis

Myasthenia gravis is a disease of unknown etiology which is characterized clinically by abnormal muscular fatigue, limited earlier to the bulbar group of muscles and later involving the muscles of the extremities. It is probably commoner among females and occurs between the ages of 20 and 50 years. Symptomatically, the conspicuous feature is rapid fatigability of the muscles when in action and a quick return of function on relaxation. The Jolly reaction is an electrical reaction employed to elicit the muscular exhaustibility. By this test the motor nerves fail to respond to stimulation with the faradic current, while stimulation with the galvanic current produces a normal response. It has not been uniformly accepted, however, as a diagnostic test in myasthenia gravis.

Periods of remission may occur in the course of the disease which may last for several years. In some it may become stationary, while in others it follows a prolonged course with increased weakness of nearly all of the muscles.

Little has been learned regarding the pathology of the condition. The site of the lesion is not definitely known. Lymphorrhages occurring in the muscles and an enlargement of the thymus gland in a large number of cases are factors most prominently mentioned. Because of this lack of knowledge concerning the pathology and cause, the treatment of the condition has been conducted mostly along experimental lines.

It is generally considered, however, that the condition is characterized by a disturbance of muscle metabolism. Some interference with the normal action of acetylcholine probably occurs in these patients. This drug occurs normally in the interneuronic synapses and at the myoneural junctions in the presence of a choline esterase which inhibits the parasympathetic action of acetylcholine. If there is an excessive amount of the esterase present, the action of the acetylcholine is reduced. Prostigmine has been found to be of great benefit in these cases because it is pharmacologically synergistic with acetylcholine, enhancing its action probably by overcoming the inhibitory effect of the choline esterase.

Eye Manifestations.—The eyes play an important part in the manifestation of myasthenia gravis, since the bulbar muscles are commonly affected. Ptosis of the eyelids is one of the most important signs. It was found by Uthoff and Bielschowsky in 80 per cent of the patients. One or both eyes may be affected, and the ptosis may be present very early. For this reason, the case may first come to the attention of the ophthalmologist.

Weakness of the ocular muscles and diplopia also occur. Constans and Radl[11] found diplopia to be the first symptom complained of in 80 per cent of their series of eleven patients. Neuromotor dysfunction was considered to be the cause. The weakness and ptosis are usually more pronounced late in the day. The ocular rotations may be limited in certain directions. The pupillary reactions may be unaffected, but convergence and accommodation power is sometimes weakened. This is characterized by inability to read very long without tiring and the necessity for holding reading matter at a greater distance from the eye than usual in order to see clearly.

In sixty-three proved cases of myasthenia gravis studied at Johns Hopkins Hospital by Walsh,[12] approximately 25 per cent of the patients sought the attention of an ophthalmologist first. Moreover, there was not a single patient observed in whom there was no evidence of ocular involvement, and in a large majority the ocular signs and symptoms occurred early. In some cases the disease seemed to affect only the ocular muscles for long periods. These were designated by Walsh as purely "ocular" myasthenia.

Ptosis of the lids of either one or both eyes is nearly always present sometime during the course of the disease. This finding is usually more pronounced when the patient is tired. The ptosis is often associated also with limitation of the ocular rotations in one or both eyes. Improvement or disappearance of the ptosis nearly always follows the administration of prostigmine.

Edema of the eyelids may also occur infrequently as an early symptom, while retraction of the upper lids has also been noted. In one of the cases described by Walsh, the patient had retraction of the lid on one side and ptosis on the opposite. The retraction occurred after a previous ptosis. This was said to point to the abnormality being peripheral in myasthenia gravis.

Weakness of the orbicularis oculi is very common and often associated with bilateral facial weakness. In addition to the weakness of the eyelids, there is often difficulty in the speech and in swallowing. Walsh found changes in the accommodation in only one case. Although the occurrence of myasthenia gravis in young children has always been questioned, it is worthy of note that Walsh observed five cases in children below the age of 10 years and that cases have been found to begin between the ages of 1 and 2 years and as late as 75 to 80 years.

Tests of muscle power have been attempted from time to time for the purpose of noting the effects of various forms of treatment. The ocular muscles were employed in this respect by Abraham,[13] who employed the maddox rod to test the phorias and prisms to test the duction power of the muscles. He found that the muscles stimulated do not tire. They contract on stimulation but fail to relax promptly or completely and remain in a prolonged state of contraction. He concluded that myasthenia gravis is, therefore, not a true myasthenia.

Schlezinger[14] felt that the greatest difficulty is encountered with muscles innervated by the cranial nerves in the choice of satisfactory procedures, since measurements are unreliable because of excessive variability of reaction. He found protrusion of the tongue to be the only satisfactory method of testing the strength of the muscles.

Treatment.—The results obtained from pharmacologic tests with the drugs found to be of some benefit in this disease seem to indicate that there is an obstruction to normal conduct of an impulse from the nerve to the muscle. This obstruction could be present at the myoneural junction and may involve the normal action of acetylcholine. This was demonstrated by the use of prostigmine with remarkable effect in the treatment of the condition. The results were so pronounced that in doubtful cases prostigmine has come to be used as a diagnostic test. Remissions may occur, however, when the drug is

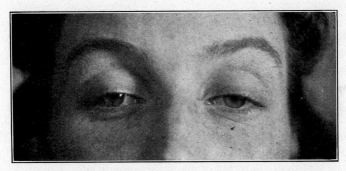

Fig. 217.—Myasthenia gravis. Bilateral ptosis before using prostigmine. (Clinic of Dr. L. B. Lehrfeld, Wills Hospital.)

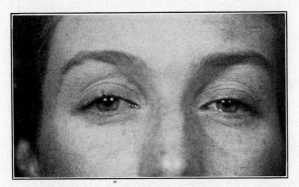

Fig. 218.—Myasthenia gravis. Showing wider palpebral fissure after use of prostigmine. (Clinic of Dr. L. B. Lehrfeld, Wills Hospital.)

discontinued, since it does not cure the disease. The effect of prostigmine is clearly demonstrated on the ptosis, since the lids are found to be elevated soon after the administration. Prostigmine bromide can be given orally in 15 mg. tablets, up to sixteen or eighteen daily. Prostigmine methylsulfate may be administered subcutaneously or intramuscularly in ampoules of 1.6 mg. (1/40 gr.) combined with atropine sulfate, 0.6 mg. (1/100 gr.), in sterile water. The atropine is added to overcome any abdominal discomfort caused by parasympathetic stimulation of the intestines by prostigmine.

It was found also that the effect of prostigmine is augmented when used in association with one of the sympathomimetic drugs. Thorner and Yaskin[15] employed ephedrine and prostigmine but found benzedrine even more satis-factory. Schlezinger[14] found ephedrine beneficial when used with aminoacetic acid, but he felt that the oral administration of combined prostigmine and ephedrine provided the most satisfactory form of therapy.

Bennett and Cash[16] felt that there was some evidence that a primary muscle disorder other than a neuromuscular block might occur in certain stages of this disease. They found that the patient with myasthenia exhibits a pro-nounced sensitivity to curare. One-tenth the ordinary physiologic dose of curare will produce an exacerbation of the symptoms and generalized curariza-tion will add new symptoms of myasthenia. They believed, therefore, that these phenomena suggested a specific test. Injection of one-tenth the usual physiologic dose followed by the administration of prostigmine methylsulfate was considered to be a safe procedure. They presented five patients with different phases of the condition who showed a specific response to this test with curare.

The management and general treatment of myasthenia gravis belongs to the neurologist. The ocular manifestations, however, should remain under the observation of the ophthalmologist. Transient relief and remissions may be obtained in the diplopia complained of and also in the ptosis. The use of prisms to overcome the diplopia is not of much benefit in most of the patients because of the transient character of the muscle condition. The use of a celluloid or plastic clip to fit over one lens of the glasses worn by such a patient will act as an occluder and provide relief in a troublesome case. The ptosis may be improved in a marked case by the use of a pair of spectacles with a metal bar which serves as a crutch to fit over the upper lid under the supraorbital rim to elevate the eyelid.

Progressive Lenticular Degeneration (Wilson's Disease)

Wilson's disease, or hepatolenticular degeneration, is a disease of unknown origin which is characterized by involuntary movements, rigidity, degeneration of the lenticular nuclei and cirrhosis of the liver. It has been considered to be familial but is not hereditary or congenital. It usually occurs between the ages of 20 and 30 years and may follow an acute or chronic course. Rigidity, contractures, tremors, and choreic movements are present. There is impair-ment of voluntary motion and emotional disturbances with some deterioration later. Pathologically, there is a degeneration in the lenticular and caudate nuclei. A mixed type of cirrhosis of the liver is marked. The disease may terminate fatally in a short time in acute cases, while other patients may live for years.

Eye Manifestations.—One prominent eye manifestation is considered to be characteristic of this disease, when present. In some cases a typical greenish-brown pigmentation ring occurs in the cornea. This pigmentation was first described by Kayser in a case considered to be disseminated sclerosis. Later it was seen by Fleischer in a case of Wilson's disease and has since been called the Kayser-Fleischer ring. The ring of pigment is found around the circum-ference of the cornea about 1 mm. inside the limbus, and in some cases, it can actually be observed with direct illumination and the aid of a loupe. The writer only recently studied a case in which the ring could be seen in this way. The corneal slit lamp should be employed, however, for examination in all cases. This will eliminate the possibility of overlooking the condition and also affords opportunity for detailed study. The color of the pigmentation has been variously described as brown and various combinations of brown, green, blue, gray, and olive. These different tints are mixed in with brown so that on examination with the slit lamp it has the appearance of a band in which the colors are seen to blend with one another from one border to the other. The pigmentation occurs in the deeper layers of the cornea and Descemet's membrane, where it is found on microscopic examination to be caused by the presence of granules or nodules, the exact nature of which is not determined.

A number of spectroscopic examinations have been made in the past and the various results reported the pigment to be due to copper, silver, urobilin and derivatives of hemoglobin. Eckardt and co-workers,[17] in a recent report of the spectrographic analysis of two cases, found zinc, copper and iron in the ashed corneas. The cornea of one patient showed the presence of silver and aluminum in addition. They felt that the pigment deposits in the cornea in Wilson's disease may vary from case to case and that this pigment may be more complex than previously supposed, even though it shows certain similarities in each.

Pigment has also been found in the center of the anterior capsule of the lens. The lens itself, however, is not opaque. Because of its appearance, this pigmentation has been described as "sunflower cataract." Gartner[18] reported six cases of Kayser-Fleisher ring in which the lens also showed this pigmentation. In one case the condition was bilateral, and under slit-camp examination it appeared as an extremely thin layer of pigment on the anterior capsule tinted a delicate blue. The surface was granular and the edges fuzzy. Most of the patients described by Gartner had an attack of hepatitis before the age of 10 and atrophic cirrhosis of the liver developed later. There was mental deterioration in all and extensive degeneration of the brain in addition to lenticular degeneration. Hypogonadism was present in four, and six of the patients came from three families. The parents in each were first cousins, and there were two sets of identical twins among the persons affected.

Syringomyelia

This is a chronic disease of the spinal cord characterized by the formation of cavities which might extend into the medulla. It is manifested by the presence of sensory signs referable to the portion involved. The cause of the disease is unknown, but segments of the cord are said to undergo degeneration and cavitation as the result of glial proliferation near the central canal.

The condition may occur early in life and is more common in males than females. It usually affects the lower cervical and upper thoracic cord and may extend up and down, or transversely. It is slowly progressive with remissions for indefinite periods which may prolong the disease for years.

Eye Manifestations.—The extent and the type of the eye manifestation depend on the degree of extension of the proliferative process. Ocular signs are more common when the involvement is above the cervical segment. Syringobulbia from extension into the medulla may cause paralyses of the cranial nerves affecting chiefly the fifth and seventh. This is characterized by pain in the side of the face and impaired action of the orbicularis muscle, resulting in incomplete closure of the eyelid. The third and sixth nerves may also be involved.

Vasomotor disturbances may be produced as a result of involvement of the lateral horns of gray matter. This may cause sympathetic disturbances which are manifested in the pupils especially. Horner's syndrome may also be present. (See Horner's syndrome.)

Usually the pupils are unequal in size or both are contracted. The palpebral fissure may be slightly narrowed and enophthalmos may be noted.

The ophthalmoscopic evidences of the disease, when present, are confined chiefly to the optic disc which may present either a papilledema or optic atrophy. The papilledema is said to be due to internal hydrocephalus.

Amyotrophic Lateral Sclerosis

This disease is characterized by the presence of a progressive muscular atrophy which may involve the muscles of the head, neck, shoulders, and extremities. The cause is unknown, and it is more common among the male sex. The age of onset is about 35 years, and the disease is slowly progressive with a poor prognosis for recovery.

Eye Manifestations.—The eyes rarely show manifestations of the condition, but with involvement of the medulla and bulbar paralysis, the ocular muscles may be affected with signs of fibrillary twitching, wasting, and impaired action of the lids. There is an associated involvement of the facial muscles which is characterized by impairment of mastication, swallowing, and phonation.

Epilepsy

Epilepsy is not a disease entity but a state or condition in which recurrent paroxysms of convulsive movements, either with or without loss of consciousness, result from many different causes. The condition may be present in an individual without apparent cause. This is sometimes spoken of as idiopathic epilepsy. It may occur in patients with brain tumors, cicatrices of the brain following injury, and other diseases of the nervous system. Epileptic attacks may be associated with altered conditions in other organs and the circulatory system.

Epileptic attacks may occur at any time of life but usually begin early in childhood. The traumatic type may come on shortly after the time of injury. Attacks of the ordinary variety without focal lesion are usually designated as either grand mal or petit mal. The latter is milder, less frequent in occurrence, and may even be unrecognized. Severe attacks are usually accompanied by convulsive movements and loss of consciousness. They are preceded by prodromal symptoms, such as nervousness, irritability, and trembling which is accompanied by a sensation of warning, or aura. The aura may assume one of several different forms. The attack itself is characterized by involuntary movements and gestures, such as frothing, biting the tongue, clenching the teeth, and rigidity of the body.

Eye Manifestations.—The eye manifestations of epilepsy are not characteristic. Jacksonian epilepsy, for example, and others due to focal conditions as cerebral tumors and scars, may show protrusion of the eyeballs, extreme rotation of the eyes to the side, lacrimation, and dilatation of the pupils.

In nonfocal epilepsy the most pronounced eye manifestation occurs in connection with the aura, which is often characterized by visual sensations. Epileptic attacks have also been produced by light stimulus. In an examination of ninety-six cases of epilepsy, including functional and organic types, by Mayer,[19] visual auras were found in twenty-one. These included "blurred vision"; "half vision"; "seeing flashes or dots of light"; "seeing definite objects"; "light passing across the eyes" and "complete blindness." Auras, such as diplopia and oculogyric movements, occurred in some cases. In none of the cases were the attacks excited by light. The auras characterized by the presence of visual sensations are frequent. They may assume various forms and patterns as described in Mayer's cases.

Errors of refraction are common and include hyperopia and myopia with astigmatism. Their presence is probably only coincidental, although it is still considered by some that a direct relationship exists between the presence of refractive states of the eye and epilepsy.

Most of the other ocular conditions found in patients with epilepsy are probably also coincidental. These include inequalities of the pupils, Argyll-Robertson pupil, nystagmus, anomalies of the extraocular muscles with the exception of diplopia as an aura, and fundus changes. Among the latter, changes have been described in the retina and optic nerve. Hyperemia, optic neuritis and optic atrophy have all been found, but it cannot be said that these fundus changes are in any way directly related to the epilepsy, but rather as a manifestation of some coexisting organic condition.

The visual field studies reveal various types, with peripheral contractions and tubular fields perhaps most common. Mayer found this variety in fourteen patients, one bizarre field in a functional case and a spiral field in an organic case. In testing the fields with flashes of light he found no contraction in any of the cases. The results of visual field studies in these cases must be interpreted with consideration for the inaccuracies introduced by early exhaustion and the mental state of the patient.

King and Walsh[20] explained the temporary amaurosis and hemianopsia occurring in epilepsy on the basis of temporary exhaustion of the visual cortex due to the epileptic discharge. They also drew attention to a case described in which the amaurosis seemed to be caused by spasm of the retinal vessels.

Migraine

Migraine, or hemicrania, is characterized by attacks of paroxysmal headache occurring on one side of the head. It is often accompanied by nausea, vomiting, and visual disturbances.

The etiology of the condition is not known, but it is sometimes considered to be associated with arterial spasm. It is also thought by some that the condition has a relationship with epilepsy. It is common among women, and it often occurs at the time of the menstruation.

Eye Manifestations.—To describe the eye manifestations, it is necessary to describe the attack. This may be preceded by a prodrome with the occurrence of one-sided headache, which is severe and throbbing in character. It may be accompanied by nausea and vomiting which in some cases bring relief from the attack. The visual disturbances assume a variety of forms. These can be grouped as visual hallucinations, such as seeing flashes of light, scintillations, zigzag lines, and brightly colored spectra; visual field disturbances, such as hemianopia or quadranopia and the presence of central and scintillating scotomas; photophobia, blurring and the sensation of seeing moving objects. In ordinary cases the fundi are found to be normal on ophthalmoscopic examination. The attack may subside only to be followed by another after an interval of a week or longer. There is a tendency for attacks to become less frequent later in life, and in some instances the condition takes on the form of epilepsy.

Migraine has been variously associated with a state of spasm of the cerebral vessels, refractive errors, oculomotor disturbances, and allergy. Various forms of treatment include regulation of the diet, ergotamine tartrate, foreign proteins, and also decompression in severe and persistent cases.

Ophthalmoplegic Migraine

Ophthalmoplegic migraine must be separated from the migraine previously described. This is a special form which is associated with ocular paralysis. The paralysis may last for some time after the attack. The migraine is not localized or confined to any special part of the head. Any of the muscles of the eye may be paralyzed, the third nerve being most commonly affected. This is characterized by the presence of either ptosis, mydriasis, paralysis of the sphincter of the iris and accommodation, or a combination of all of those mentioned. Intervals between the attacks are of indefinite duration. Recovery from paralysis may take place during intervals, but in time it becomes more or less permanent.

These cases have also been described as recurrent third nerve palsy due to the presence of focal lesions such as an inflammatory vascular changes with the presence of edema which involves the root of the third nerve. The function returns and paralysis disappears when the edema subsides.

Hemianopia has in some instances also been associated with the attack, especially among pregnant women. The hemianopia is usually of a transitory character but it may also be permanent.

Hysteria

Hysteria is a condition which is difficult to define without being led into the realm of psychology and a consideration of various theories advanced to explain the hysterical state or makeup. For our purpose, it is probably sufficient to state that definite subjective complaints and objective evidences of disease are presented by a patient without an organic basis. It is considered to represent a reaction to mental strain in one with a personality defect.

The symptoms cover a wide range of disorders and disabilities which may affect speech, movement, coordination, hearing, gastrointestinal tract, visual apparatus, and vasomotor derangement. Pain is a prominent subjective symptom and is out of proportion to the nature or severity of any cause. It may be relieved by a placebo as readily as by the administration of an anesthetic.

Eye Manifestations.—The ocular manifestations of hysteria occur infrequently and not as extensively as other manifestations. Riley[21] restricted the hysterical manifestations to those that can be produced by the higher centers alone, probably including in these the basal ganglions. The functional manifestations of oculomotor control are limited to unilateral and bilateral ptosis, cramps and deviations of conjugate gaze, paralysis of any form of conjugate gaze, or to complete bilateral immobility. The presence of a functional oculomotor disturbance depends on the recognition of other hysterical evidences and on the identification of a sufficient psychic mechanism.

Spaeth,[20] in a comprehensive review of the subject, described Head's outline as an index of the ocular manifestations. These include: (1) Disturbances of sensibility affecting the cornea and conjunctiva; photophobia and neuralgia. (2) Visual disturbances such as monocular and binocular diplopia, polyopia, erythropia, micropia and amaurosis, reduced retinal function of color and light sense as hemeralopia (Landolt), and visual disturbances. (3) Disturbances of motility including ptosis, blepharospasm, strabismus, spasm of accommodation causing myopia and astigmatism, cycloplegia, miosis and mydriasis, accommodative asthenopia, nystagmus, conjugate deviation, internal recti insufficiency, and external ophthalmoplegia. (4) Disturbances of secretion as epiphora, lacrimation and decreased secretion. (5) Patient's complaint of insomnia, dizziness, vertigo, and inability to concentrate caused by the eye condition.

Ophthalmoscopic examination in cases of hysteria reveals a normal fundus. The results of visual fields may reveal a marked contraction of the peripheral fields and the presence of spiral or tubular fields, often considered to be characteristic or pathognomonic of hysteria. Various forms of contractions and dyschromatopsia and color inversions have also been found.

A case of unilateral hysterical amblyopia was treated by the author in a young married woman who lost the vision in her left eye suddenly. A detailed history of her domestic life, absence of organic disease and absence of any pathologic evidences in the ophthalmoscopic examination of the affected eye suggested the diagnosis. This was confirmed when it was found that the patient had binocular single vision when she was tested with a major amblyoscope. The patient was assured that her vision would return and within two to three weeks she recovered.

Mahoney and Linhart[23] divided hysterical amblyopias into the three following groups: 1. Acute hysterical amblyopia occurring suddenly either alone or with other symptoms. 2. Chronic amblyopia resulting as a reaction in a psychobiologically underdeveloped individual. 3. Mixed hysterical amblyopia which occurs with some of the characteristics of psychoneurotic neurasthenia.

Narcolepsy

Narcolepsy was described by Levin[24] as a syndrome characterized by brief attacks of sleep and brief attacks of flaccid paralysis without loss of consciousness, usually following in response to some emotion such as either pleasant or unpleasant laughter or excitement. The paralysis occurring in response to emotion is called cataplexy. The syndrome is much more common in men and usually begins in the second or third decade. When it is once started it usually persists.

The attacks of sleep of narcolepsy occur with significant frequency under conditions duplicating those which elicited sleep and other manifestations of cerebral inhibition in Pavlov's experiments. From this and other evidence it was suggested that narcolepsy results from a disturbance in the cerebral cortex or elsewhere which renders the cortex unduly exhaustible or "inhibitable." The attacks of sleep arise from inhibition of the whole cortex and the flaccid paralysis from inhibition of the motor cortex plus, probably, certain subcortical motor centers.

Eye Manifestations.—The frequency of attacks of diplopia in narcolepsy has been described as occurring under a variety of conditions, and it was suggested by Levin that "they arise from transitory inhibition of a cortical mechanism for binocular vision." Sleep diplopia was designated as that which occurs when the patient sees double either just before he falls asleep or just after he awakes. Predormital diplopia is said to be common and a number of cases have been reported in which the patient has diplopia at the beginning of the sleep attack. These cases support the hypothesis, similar to Pavlov's experiments, that a center of mechanism for binocular vision exists which regulates the ocular movements to prevent diplopia. When the patient is in the process of falling asleep, the center is inhibited too soon, which results in predormital diplopia. If the center remains inhibited too long after he awakes, the patient has postdormital diplopia. This center for binocular vision would seem to be in the cortex rather than below, since the cortex contains centers for simple ocular movements as the response to light.

The center for uniocular vision is probably spread over a large part of the cortex, probably including parts of both occipital and both frontal lobes. The diplopia is said to come probably from inhibition of the anterior part of the center.

Diplopia occurring in a cataplectic attack is said to be due to probable emotional stimulus causing inhibition of motor centers. Diplopia occurring in reading is likewise said to be due to inhibition of the center for binocular vision.

Neurasthenia

Neurasthenia is a form of the psychoneuroses in which the patient has many subjective complaints characterized by sensory symptoms and functional changes. The state of health is always impaired and fatigue and inability to meet ordinary physical demands are common. Pain in various parts, pressure sensations in the head, and backache are usual complaints. In this condition as in hysteria, the complaints are also psychologic and have no physical or organic basis. Anxiety and unexplainable fear are often persistent. Symptoms and complaints may be numerous.

Eye Manifestations.—Most of the ocular complaints are subjective in character and might include a long list of such symptoms recited by the patient. A characteristic tendency of the neurasthenic patient with multiple complaints is to present a written list of symptoms in definite order. In other instances great anxiety might be exhibited with regard to some minor evidence on the external eye. The fear of ultimate blindness in the absence of any pathology in the eyes may be the chief complaint. The fear might be caused by the knowledge of blindness occurring from known cause in some friend or relative. The fear persists despite even professional advice to the contrary. Many such patients go from one ophthalmologist to another or from one hospital to another.

Fatigue is a disturbing factor in these patients and is often complained of with regard to ordinary use of the eyes. Pain and refractive asthenopia are common, even when the proper glasses are prescribed and worn. The patient is reluctant to admit any relief. The trouble is constantly present and is borne with an attitude of resignation, although attempts to obtain relief are always continued.

References

1. Drake, R. L.: Ocular Syphilis, Arch. Ophth. **9**: 234, 1933.
2. Heath, P.: Visual Sequelae From Epidemic Meningococcus Meningitis, Trans. Am. Acad. Ophth., p. 489, 1936.
3. Lazar, N. K.: Early Ocular Complications of Epidemic Meningitis, Arch. Ophth. **16**: 847, 1936.
4. Dunphy, E. B.: Ocular Complications of Cerebrospinal Meningitis, Arch. Ophth. **15**: 118, 1936.
5. Benedict, W. L.: Symposium "Brain Abscess." Abscess of the Brain From the Standpoint of the Ophthalmologist, Trans. Am. Acad. Ophth., p. 52, 1929.
6. Berliner, M. L.: Acute Optic Neuritis in Demyelinating Diseases of the Nervous System, Arch. Ophth. **13**: 83, 1935.
7. Paton, Leslie: Papilledema and Optic Neuritis, Arch. Ophth. **15**: 1, 1936.
8. Benedict, William L.: Multiple Sclerosis as an Etiologic Factor in Retrobulbar Neuritis, Arch. Ophth. **28**: 988, 1942.
9. Lillie, W. I.: Clinical Significance of Retrobulbar and Optic Neuritis, Am. J. Ophth. **17**: 110, 1934.
10. Noran, H. H., and Polan, C. G.: Devic's Disease (Ophthalmoneuromyelitis); A Clinicopathologic Study, Arch. Ophth. **27**: 707, 1942.
11. Constans, G. M., and Radl, R. B.: Myasthenia Gravis, Minnesota Med. **25**: 873-880, 1942.
12. Walsh, F. B.: Myasthenia Gravis and Its Ocular Signs, Am. J. Ophth. **28**: 13, 1945.
13. Abraham, S. V.: Myasthenia Gravis, Arch. Ophth. **7**: 700, 1932.
14. Schlezinger, N. S.: Evaluation of Therapy in Myasthenia Gravis, Arch. Int. Med. **65**: 60, 1940.
15. Thorner, M. W., and Yaskin, J. C.: The Treatment of Myasthenia Gravis, Am. J. M. Sc. **194**: 411, 1937.
16. Bennett, A., and Cash, P.: Myasthenia Gravis: Curare Sensitivity; A New Diagnostic Test and Approach to Causation, Arch. Neurol. & Psychiat. **49**: 537, 1943.
17. Eckardt, R. E., Stolzar, I. H., Adam, A. B., and Johnson, L. V.: The Pigment of the Kayser-Fleisher Ring, Am. J. Ophth. **26**: 151, 1943.
18. Gartner, Samuel: Kayser-Fleisher Ring Associated With Hepatolenticular Degeneration; Report of Six Cases, Arch. Ophth. **26**: 595, 1941.
19. Mayer, Leo L.: The Eye in Epilepsy, Arch. Ophth. **17**: 486, 1937.
20. King, Arthur, and Walsh, Frank B.: Temporary Amaurosis and Hemianopsia Due to Epilepsy, Am. J. Ophth. **25**: 398, 1942.
21. Riley, H. A.: The Central Nervous System Control of the Ocular Movements and the Disturbances of This Mechanism, Arch. Ophth. **4**: 885, 1930.
22. Spaeth, E. B.: The Differentiation of the Ocular Manifestations of Hysteria and of Malingering, Arch. Ophth. **4**: 911, 1930.
23. Mahoney, V. P., and Linhart, W. O.: Amblyopia in Hysteria, War Med. **3**: 503, 1943.
24. Levin, Max: Diplopia in Narcolepsy, Arch. Ophth. **29**: 942, 1943.

CHAPTER XXI

INTRACRANIAL TUMORS

Expanding lesions of the brain are manifest clinically by signs of increased intracranial pressure, namely headache, choked disc, and vomiting. However, not all of these are present or are necessary for a diagnosis of brain tumor. The occurrence of papilledema with intracranial pressure is grossly valuable for a diagnosis of tumor but not of great localizing value of the tumor with the exception of tumors of the posterior fossa or those near the third ventricle when the papilledema appears early and is of an excessive character. Of greater localizing value are the visual defects found in perimetric study when some part or parts of the optic pathway are encroached upon by the lesion. For a better understanding of the possible interruptions of the optic pathways, a short description of the latter, according to Abbott[1] follows:

Optic nerve fibers from the retina pass in the optic nerve to the chiasma where a partial decussation occurs, uncrossed fibers from the temporal retina persist in the optic tracts in the same order while fibers from the nasal retina are crossed in the chiasm; consequently, the right tract consists of fibers from the two right halves of the retinae and the left tract from the two left halves. The optic tract ends in the posterior part of the external geniculate body on the same side. The last neuron passes from the external geniculate body in the radiation of Gratiolet (lateral wall of the inferior horn of the lateral ventricle) and ends in the calcarine fissure in the occipital lobe (area striata).

Interruption of the optic nerve by a lesion proximal to the chiasm results in blindness and loss of pupillary reflex, if all the fibers are destroyed; in partial destruction, scotomas and contraction of visual fields are obtained by perimetry. A lesion in this region will also produce the Foster Kennedy syndrome of optic neuritis on the side of the lesion and contralateral papilledema in frontal lobe tumors.

Involvement of the mesial part of the chiasm as by a suprasellar tumor, hydrocephalus, suprasellar aneurysm or tumor of third ventricle will compress the decussating fibers from the nasal halves of the retinae and produce bitemporal hemianopic loss in the visual fields (in addition to the optic atrophy).

Involvement of the lateral portions of the chiasm by a tumor of the third ventricle, aneurysm of both carotid arteries, cyst of hypophysis, or symmetrical gummas would produce a binasal hemianopia which is exceedingly rare.

Involvement of the optic tract, primary visual centers, or Gratiolet's radiation produces homonymous hemianopia because either both the right or the left halves of the visual fields are involved. An important diagnostic aid to tract lesions is Wernicke's hemianopic pupillary reaction where a lesion proximal to the point at which reflex fibers to the Edinger-Westphal nucleus are given off produces pupillary inactivity to light when light is cast into the blinded halves of the retina while a lesion distal to the nucleus will not interrupt the light reflex for pupillary activity.

Bilateral lesions involving visual memory centers in the cortex produce conceptual blindness in which the patient can see an object on a flat surface but is unable to recognize it. Destruction of the cuneus in one hemisphere and destruction of the occipital convexity in another produces conceptual blindness with superimposition of a homonymous hemianopia.

Interruption of the optic pathways in association with certain specific neurologic signs and symptoms has led to description of syndromes or symptom complexes prominent among which are the following: (1) frontal lobe syndromes, (2) temporal, (3) occipital, (4) quadrigeminal plate, and (5) chiasmal syndrome.

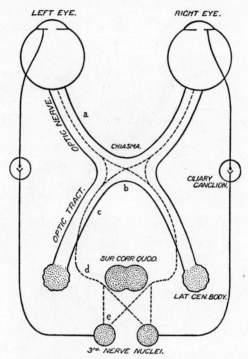

Fig. 219.—Scheme of the pupillary pathway. Lesion at left optic nerve *a* causes blindness of the left eye, abolition of direct light reaction of the left eye, with retention of consensual, and abolition of consensual of right eye with retention of direct. At chiasma *b*, bitemporal hemianopia, neither direct nor consensual reflex abolished. At left optic tract *c*, contralateral (right) homonymous hemianopia, Wernicke's hemianopic pupil reaction. At superior brachium on both sides *d*, Argyll-Robertson pupils. At both afferent fibers coming to left nucleus *e*, unilateral (left) Argyll-Robertson pupil. At *e* on both sides, bilateral Argyll-Robertson pupils. (From Wolff: The Anatomy of the Eye and Orbit, The Blakiston Co.)

Frontal Lobe Tumors.—The lesions of the frontal lobe more commonly encountered are gliomas, meningiomas, abscess and aneurysm, especially noted as causes of the Foster Kennedy syndrome. This syndrome is due to a space-taking lesion of the frontal lobe which, in addition to producing increased intracranial pressure, causes damage by pressure to the optic nerve and the olfactory tracts. Thus it is manifested as papilledema on the contralateral side of the tumor and optic neuritis or optic atrophy on the same side of the tumor. The ocular findings described above, together with other neurologic symptoms as unilateral (ipsilateral) anosmia, early character changes, aphasia (with a left-sided tumor) contralateral hemiparesis, contralateral facial nerve weakness, forced grasping and involuntary movements, render the diagnosis of frontal lobe lesions more precise and definite in view of the marked difficulty associated with the diagnosis of these tumors. The appearance of these localizing symptoms depends on the location of the tumor and its character. The differential diagnosis of gliomas and meningiomas can illustrate this since gliomas of the frontal lobe frequently produce no ocular symptoms while meningiomas of the lower surface of the lobe do manifest ocular signs. Again, meningiomas of the vault may show no ocular symptoms, whereas a meningioma arising from the lesser wing of the sphenoid shows exophthalmos, limitation of ocular movements, oculomotor paralysis, optic atrophy, fullness of the temporal fossa and

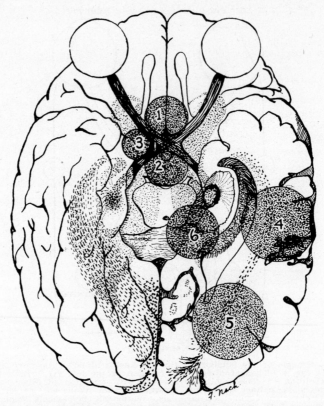

Fig. 220.—Drawing illustrating the optic pathways and the critical points which are common sites of tumors of the brain. *1, 2,* Chiasmal tumors. *3,* Tumors affecting the optic tracts. *4,* Tumors of the temporal lobe. *5,* Tumors of the occipital lobe. *6,* Tumors of the quadrigeminal plate. (From Globus: Arch. Ophth., May, 1933.)

dense orbital bone shadows on x-ray. Furthermore, anosmia and optic atrophy are liable to arise earlier with meningiomas than with gliomas, whereas frontal lobe symptoms and papilledema are liable to arise later with meningiomas than with gliomas.

Lillie[2] emphasized the importance of the perimetric fields in the exact localization of basal lesions of the frontal lobe. He described the characteristic sign in a unilateral lesion as a homolateral central or cecocentral scotoma, associated with either a normal, pale, atrophic or choked disc, with contralateral normal central vision and choked disc.

In a bilateral lesion, bicentral or cecocentral scotomas are associated with bilateral choked discs.

Temporal Lobe Tumors.—Tumors of the temporal lobe are usually localized when accompanied by such signs as uncinate seizures, speech disturbances (aphasia), generalized convulsions, contralateral hemiparesis, and increased intracranial pressure. The aphasia signifies a lesion on the left side and renders the diagnosis easier than with one on the right side where few if any localizing signs are discoverable. However, involvement of Meyer's loop which forms a part of the geniculo-calcarine tract produces a quadrantic type of hemianopic defect which aids in localizing a temporal lobe tumor. The ophthalmoscopic signs consist of bilateral papilledema, visual hallucinations and quadrant homonymous hemianopia.

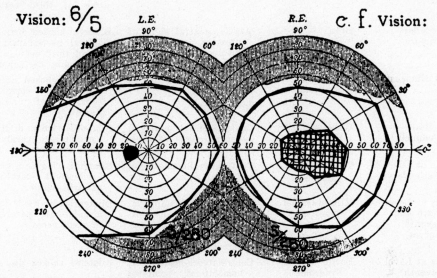

Fig. 221.—Visual fields in the case of glioma in the right frontal lobe. *R.E.,* Concentric contraction for form and colors; cecocentral scotoma. *L.E.,* Normal for form and colors; blind spot enlarged. Fundi: right eye, pallor of disc; left eye, choked disc, 3 diopters. (From Lillie: Tr. Sect. Ophth., A. M. A., May, 1927.)

Occipital Lobe Tumors.—A negative neurologic picture with homonymous hemianopia characterizes lesions of the occipital lobe. Bilateral papilledema appears early in this type of tumor and renders visual field studies difficult. Unformed visual hallucinations are more characteristic in occipital lobe lesions while formed visual hallucinations occur in temporal lobe lesions. Lesion of the left occipital lobe is further localized when, in addition to the hemianopia, aphasia and word blindness occur.

Quadrigeminal Plate Tumors.—According to Globus,[3] this syndrome is due principally to pinealomas producing an interruption of the association fibers between the lateral geniculate and anterior quadrigeminate body. The ocular symptoms are paralysis of upward gaze, skew deviation and Argyll-Robertson pupils. Diplopia, manifestations of disease of the midbrain, such as tremors and rigidities, pyramidal tract and cerebellar signs are also found. Because of the location of the tumor, the general signs caused by intracranial pressure may be marked. These include, chiefly, headache, vomiting, and papilledema. Some indirect signs which result from pressure on distal portions may also be presented. These include polyuria, polydipsia, anomalies of growth and secondary sex changes.

The various syndromes according to Abbott[1] are as follows:

LESIONS OF THE PONS, MIDBRAIN, CEREBELLUM, AND MEDULLA

	Type	*Neurologic*	*Ophthalmologic*
Pineal Gland	Frankl Hochwart	General signs of pressure, bilateral deafness, ataxia precocity; indirect hypopituitary signs due to pressure	Bilateral choked disc, limitation of upward gaze, normal or concentrically contracted fields
Third Nerve Nucleus	Nothnagel's Syndrome	Ataxia, general signs of pressure	Bilateral choked disc; bilateral partial paralysis of third nerve; normal fields
Cerebellar Tumor	Bruns' Syndrome	Ataxia, general signs of pressure, ataxia before involvement of third nerve	Bilateral choked disc, bilateral partial paralysis of third nerve, normal fields, nystagmus
Red Nucleus	Benedikt's Syndrome	Contralateral ataxia in incoordination	Bilateral choked disc, homolateral complete paralysis of third nerve
Cerebral Peduncle	Weber's Syndrome	Contralateral hemiplegia, general signs of pressure	Bilateral choked disc, homolateral paralysis of third nerve
Pons at Level of Sixth Nerve	deRaymond's Syndrome	Contralateral hemiplegia, general signs of pressure	Bilateral choked disc, homolateral paralysis of sixth nerve
Pons at Level of Sixth and Seventh Nerves	Millard-Gubler Syndrome	Contralateral hemiplegia, general signs of pressure, homolateral complete paralysis of seventh nerve	Bilateral choked disc, homolateral paralysis of sixth nerve
Pons at Level of Seventh Nerve	Foville's Syndrome	Contralateral hemiplegia, homolateral complete paralysis of seventh nerve, general signs of pressure	Bilateral choked disc
Cerebello-pontine Angle	Angle Syndrome	Homolateral deafness and tinnitus, homolateral paresthesia of fifth nerve; later motor paralysis of fifth nerve, homolateral complete paralysis of seventh nerve, ataxia, pressure	Bilateral choked disc, anesthetic cornea (homolateral), paralysis of sixth nerve (homolateral), nystagmus

TUMORS OF THE TEMPORAL, PARIETAL, AND OCCIPITAL LOBES AND THE BASAL GANGLION

Location			
Temporal	Tumor	Uncinate generalized convulsions; contralateral hemiparesis; general signs of pressure	Bilateral choked disc, quadrant homonymous hemianopsia, visual hallucinations
Parietal	Tumor	Incomplete sensory loss (contralateral), general signs of pressure	Bilateral choked disc, homonymous hemianopsia
Occipital	Tumor	Localized occipital headache; negative neurologic signs	Bilateral choked disc, homonymous hemianopsia

| Basal Ganglion | Tumor of Striate Body | Parkinsonian Syndrome | Bilateral c h o k e d disc, homonymous hemianopsia |
| | Tumor of Third Ventricle, pushing latter into thalamus and into capsule | Fluctuating symptoms, general signs of pressure, contralateral hemiplegia and hemianesthesia, deep or occasional convolutions | Normal pale or choked disc, homonymous hemianopsia; may have limitations of upward gaze |

Pituitary Tumors

Pituitary tumors may be divided into the intrasellar or those originating from the anterior lobe of the pituitary gland and suprasellar or tumors of the pituitary area which give rise to the chiasmal syndrome. (See Pituitary gland.)

Intrasellar tumors are adenomas of the anterior lobe and are classified according to the histologic cell type as: (1) eosinophile, (2) basophile, and (3) chromophobe. An eosinophile adenoma consists of eosinophilic cells and the tumor is of frequent occurrence while the basophile adenoma, or Cushing syndrome, is rarely seen, and, finally, the chromophobe adenomas made up of cells which do not take a specific dye are probably the most frequent in this group.

Eosinophile Adenoma.—These tumors are seen between the ages of 15 and 50 and most commonly during the third decade. The clinical picture is that of the hyperpituitary syndrome, either gigantism or acromegaly, depending on whether union of the epiphyses has taken place in the long bones. Acromegaly probably occurs with greater frequency than gigantism. Sexual impotence in the male and amenorrhea in the female arise due to disturbance of the sexual hormone in the anterior lobe. Persistent, severe headaches are prominent in the course of the expanding tumor but cease conspicuously when the tumor ruptures through the diaphragm sellae and becomes suprasellar. Compression of the mesial part of the chiasma (the decussating fibers) accounts for the principal ocular symptoms: (1) primary optic atrophy and (2) bitemporal hemianopia. Field defects begin in the superior temporal quadrants, rotating clockwise in the right field and anticlockwise in the left; irregular expansion of the tumor produces corresponding variations in the fields, e.g., pressure on an optic tract will show a homonymous hemianopia while forward extension shows exophthalmos and oculomotor paralyses. Visual loss precedes the appearance of optic atrophy by a considerable interval, hence, the unquestioned value of early and persistent perimetric study. Diagnosis depends chiefly on progression through the quadrants of the field changes and enlargement of the pituitary fossa as revealed by roentgen rays.

Basophile Adenoma.—This is characterized by a striking clinical picture described by Cushing. It consists of a painful obesity limited to face, neck, and trunk. Sexual dysfunction such as amenorrhea in females and loss of libido and impotence in males is especially prominent. Hypertrichosis of face and trunk is marked in females and preadolescent males, while the skin over the abdomen shows purple striae. These patients complain of fatigue, abdominal pains and backaches, while the blood pressure is elevated. The basophile adenoma is a fatal tumor and ocular symptoms are rarely noted, because of its small size, and because the condition is fatal before the tumor is large enough to involve the chiasm. The diagnosis is based on constitutional symptoms.

Chromophobe Adenomas.—Chromophobe adenomas of the pituitary body present a clinical picture of hypopituitary syndromes. Onset of tumor in the preadolescent is responsible for Froehlich's syndrome or dystrophia adiposo-genitalis. The patient presents an infantile shape and marked deficiency in

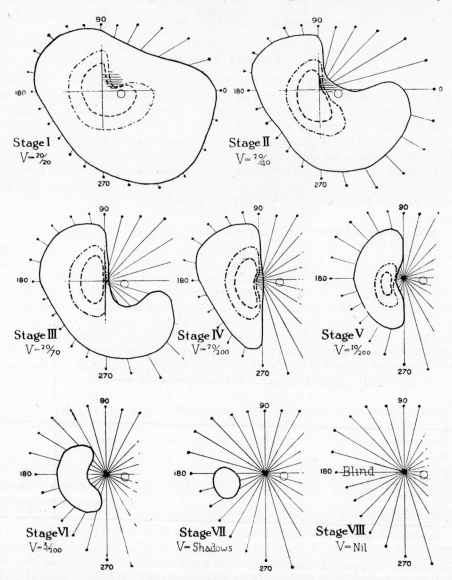

Fig. 222.—Showing the eight stages of a progressing right temporal defect in pituitary disease. (From Cushing and Walker: Brain, March, 1915.)

development with hypoplasia of the external genitalia, absence of secondary sexual characteristics, adiposity of trunk, while the extremities are graceful and thin. In the adult there is adiposity of the trunks, decreased basal metabolic rate, sexual disturbances as amenorrhea in females and impotence in males. The ocular symptoms do not differ essentially from those of the eosinophile group. These include, chiefly, optic atrophy and bitemporal hemianopia as well as scotomatous field defects indicative of rapid growth of the tumor. Roentgen appearance of sella (which is expanded) is of great diagnostic value when considered along with signs of hypopituitarism.

Suprasellar Tumors—The Chiasmal Syndrome

Suprasellar tumors produce the characteristic chiasmal syndrome. This consists of primary optic atrophy, bitemporal hemianopia and usually a normal sella turcica as revealed by x-ray examination, with an enlargement in primary pituitary tumors. The suprasellar group includes: (1) craniopharyngiomas, (2) adenomas, (3) meningiomas, (4) gliomas of the optic chiasm, (5) aneurysms, (6) parachiasmal arachnoiditis.

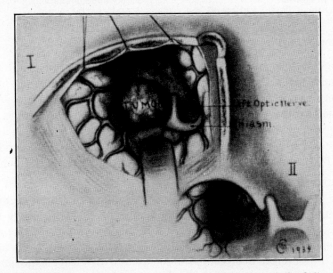

Fig. 223.—Meningioma of the sphenoid ridge, showing compression of the left optic nerve and displacement toward the midline. (From Elsberg and Dyke: Arch. Ophth., November, 1934.)

Craniopharyngiomas (Rathke Pouch Tumors).—These are tumors arising from epithelial rests along the craniopharyngeal duct. Being congenital, they are apt to cause symptoms rather early; however, they are not limited to any period and may occur at any age. The clinical picture varies with the differences in age; e.g., in childhood, headaches and vomiting, inhibition of growth and sexual development, adiposity of head and trunk, "cracked pot" sound on percussion of skull, dilated sutures (by x-ray) and papilledema, make up the picture; in the adult group, lack of sexual development as loss of libido or amenorrhea occur; also adiposity, papilledema, optic atrophy, and bitemporal hemianopia. The x-ray is an important aid in the diagnosis since calcification of the tumor appears as spotty suprasellar shadows seen on stereoscopic x-ray films. Damage to the tuber cinereum by these tumors is very frequent and clinically is manifested as diabetes insipidus. The ocular symptoms consist of primary optic atrophy and bitemporal hemianopia.

Wagener and Love[4] reported on twenty-three patients with craniopharyngioma and six with epidermoid tumor. Of those with craniopharyngioma, they found normal optic discs in five; choked disc in eight, pallor of the discs in four, and simple atrophy in six. Of the five craniopharyngiomas in patients with normal optic discs, two were anterior to the chiasm, one to the right of the right optic nerve, one to the left of the chiasm and left optic nerve and one posterior to the chiasm. The three remaining tumors which caused only pallor of the discs were all anterior to the chiasm; one showed suprasellar extension. The six cases with simple optic atrophy were anterior to the chiasm and one showed suprasellar extension.

The field defects listed in these twenty-three cases were as follows:

Bitemporal hemianopsia	2	Temporal anopsia with amaurosis of other eye	2
Bitemporal scotoma	1		
Bitemporal hemianopsia with unilateral central scotoma	3	Homonymous hemianopsia	2
		Homonymous hemianopsia with unilateral central scotoma	6
Bitemporal scotoma with unilateral central scotoma	1	Generalized contraction	2
Bitemporal hemianopsia with bilateral central scotoma	1	No defects	2
		Fields unobtainable	1

The primary presenting symptoms were headache in thirteen, loss of vision in sixteen and pituitary dysfunction in seven. The authors emphasized the fact that simple evacuation of the cyst is not sufficient, since it can refill and may cause damage to the optic nerve, chiasm or tracts by pressure. With impairment of vision or increased intracranial pressure, the capsule must be extensively resected and the operation should be done early. The method of choice seems to be by an extradural approach through the transfrontal bone flap.

Suprasellar Adenoma.—These tumors are rapid in their growth and take origin either from the sella turcica escaping through the diaphragma sellae or from the infundibulum. The expanding tumor produces pressure atrophy of the sella as visualized by roentgen rays and also symptoms of decreased pituitary function are manifest. The ocular symptoms are also primary optic atrophy and bitemporal hemianopia associated with either a normal sella (to x-ray) or an enlarged one in which case symptoms of hypopituitarism will appear.

Suprasellar Meningiomas.—These tumors take their origin from the meninges surrounding the pituitary diaphragm. These are slow growing, tough, fibrous and have a rough surface; pathologically, they are endotheliomas. The onset of tumor is manifested chiefly in middle age when the outstanding complaint is impairment of vision, often the only symptom. At this stage primary optic atrophy and bitemporal hemianopia and negative roentgen rays of the sella are the chief symptoms. Endocrine disturbances, such as diabetes insipidus, hypopituitarism, are not found when the tumor is still operable. The irregularity of the growth is manifested in the inequality of involvement of the two eyes and also in the asymmetric defects in the fields. Ophthalmoscopic examination reveals bluish-white discs with sharp edges and vessels of normal caliber. The diagnosis is based on primary optic atrophy, bitemporal hemianopia which may be asymmetric, of slow development, and negative roentgen rays. Finally, there is a negative endocrine picture.

Suprasellar Gliomas.—These are principally found in children between the ages of four to twelve. In Cushing's series of cases the average was at twelve

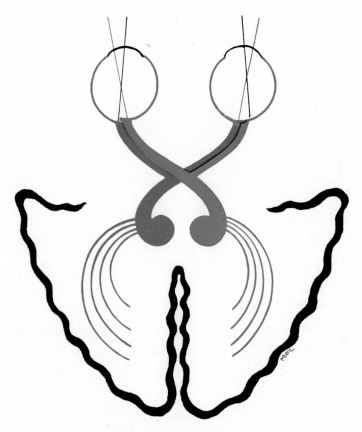

Fig. 224.—Drawing showing optic nerves crossing at chiasm. (Modified after Traquair.)

years of age. The tumors arise from the chiasm or adjacent wall of the third ventricle; however, the chiasm is not the site of election for gliomas since only 2 per cent are found in this region. The clinical picture consists of: (1) marked visual loss, (2) generalized neurofibromatosis (as frequent as 30 per cent), (3) development of hypothalamic symptoms, and (4) enlarged optic foramina as seen by roentgen rays. The visual fields show either homonymous or bitemporal loss; however, bizarreness and asymmetry seem to be characteristic in view of the infiltrative character of the lesion. The ophthalmoscopic findings are those of primary optic atrophy but superimposed papilledema may occur. Occasionally, the growth may extend to the disc and be noted as a measurable swelling.

Parachiasmal Arachnoiditis.—Arachnoiditis or pseudotumor or local serous meningitis is of recent description and is not of precise definition as yet. The arachnoid membrane of the chiasm is necessarily exposed to many, and various pathologic conditions and the etiologic possibilities are as diverse as syphilitic basal arachnoiditis, encephalitic processes, infections from the paranasal sinuses and middle ear, various blood-borne infections, and trauma. The concept and clinical diagnoses should be restricted to cases where the pathology is essentially that of chiasmal meningeal changes. Clinically, the picture consists of a negative neurologic examination and the chiasmal syndrome of primary optic atrophy and bitemporal hemianopia. These patients complain of headaches, loss of vision, somnolence, and fever. In syphilitic basal arachnoiditis where primary optic atrophy, bitemporal defects with a positive Wassermann are the only findings, recent reports indicate that surgical removal of the adhesions has improved visual acuity whereas preceding vigorous antisyphilitic treatment has been of no avail; i.e., we are describing a luetic condition where the chiasm alone is affected and which does not warrant a diagnosis of tabes on the eye findings alone. The visual fields, for operative cases, should favor a concentric restriction with bitemporal loss.

Ryan,[5] in reporting three cases of optochiasmic arachnoiditis, stated that any type of field defect or combination of defects might be found. The usual symptoms were headache and loss of vision, either unilateral or bilateral and more advanced in one eye than the other. The headache usually comes on in the afternoon, is localized in the frontal region and is aggravated by close work. Ryan described the syphilitic types in three groups: The first group included bilateral optic atrophy, heteronymous fields and visual defects, nearly complete blindness, a normal ventricular system and no evidence of internal hydrocephalus; the second group was characterized by secondary optic atrophy; and the third group was characterized by papilledema without hydrocephalus. He also advised vigorous antiluetic treatment before and after surgery. Surgery is performed in order to free the adhesions about the optic nerve and chiasm.

Goldsmith,[6] in reporting three cases of chiasmic arachnoiditis, described the adhesions as binding the optic nerves and chiasm to the brain, to one another, to the larger vessels and to the dorsum sella. Although the adhesions are often avascular, the vessels may be congested. Small calcareous plaques have also been described in advanced cases. In one of Goldsmith's patients, a cyst was present from a collection of fluid between adhesions. The optic nerves may become atrophic and edematous as a result of band constriction. The visual loss may result from meningeal changes, and the arachnoiditis may cause mechanical pressure by the adhesions or cysts. The loss of vision may be complained of early and progress gradually or it may suddenly increase and terminate in complete blindness. Other symptoms resulting from involvement of the infundibulum may also occur. These include polyuria, polydypsia, increased appetite and obesity.

Patients with arachnoiditis require examination and surgical intervention by the neurosurgeon.

Aneurysm of the Vessels of the Circle of Willis

The exact diagnosis of an intracranial aneurysm is difficult, but in the past decade cases in which a definite clinical diagnosis was made during life have been reported more frequently than previously. The diagnosis of some of these was confirmed at autopsy. In 1934 Garvey[7] reported four cases of intracranial aneurysm and the clinical findings in a fifth. In two of the cases the diagnosis was confirmed at autopsy, and in a detailed review of the subject, Garvey emphasized the clinical symptoms and signs which may lead to the diagnosis of the condition during life. Some idea of the incidence might be obtained from the fact that the four cases described were the total number encountered in a series of about 400 autopsies extending over a period of seven months.

Aneurysms of the carotid portion of the circle of Willis are said to be more common than those of the vertebral. The middle cerebral vessels are most frequently affected, while the internal carotid and basilar are next, followed by the anterior cerebral, posterior communicating, anterior communicating, vertebral, posterior cerebral and inferior cerebral. The location is usually at a point of junction of two arteries or at a branching point. They occur with almost equal frequency on either side with the left being perhaps slightly favored. Age is not a factor, since aneurysm may develop at any time of life and has been reported in young children as well as older patients. The ages of 30 to 50, however, are probably most common.

The weakness in a certain portion of a vessel wall which leads to the formation of an aneurysm at this point is, in most cases, due to the presence of arteriosclerosis. In fact, the rupture and hemorrhage as well as the formation of the aneurysm are attributed to the patchy pathologic processes resulting from arteriosclerosis of the cerebral vessels. Endocarditis, syphilis, and high blood pressure are common causes, while trauma may also be a factor.

The symptoms of an aneurysm depend principally on the location and result chiefly from mechanical pressure. Sudden leakage and the underlying disease which causes the aneurysm also contribute to the signs and symptoms. An aneurysm may be present for a long time without presenting any troublesome or definite signs.

Eye Manifestations.—These are divided into three main groups and include: (1) those which result from the presence of an aneurysm in the anterior group of vessels in the circle of Willis; (2) those resulting from aneurysm of the posterior group of vessels; (3) those which result from rupture or leakage of the aneurysm. The focal signs presented before a rupture occurs are similar to those resulting from a brain tumor. It has also been pointed out by a number of investigators that symptoms may be absent in the presence of cerebral aneurysm which does not rupture.

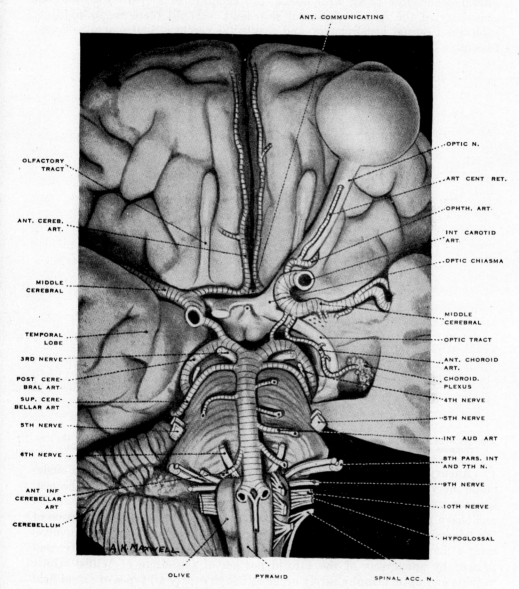

Fig. 225.—Blood supply of optic pathway and relation of vessels to optic tract and oculomotor nerve. (From Wolff: The Anatomy of the Eye and Orbit, The Blakiston Co.)

Aneurysms in the anterior group include those which arise from the intracranial portion of the carotid, the proximal portions of the middle cerebral artery and the circle of Willis at the point of bifurcation of these vessels. The clinical symptoms produced by these aneurysms are rather constant and uniform. Garvey, in quoting Cushing's description of the syndrome, stated: "Aneurysm should always be considered when an apoplectic attack or series of attacks of comparatively sudden onset is followed by symptoms pointing to the region of the internal carotid in its intracranial portion, namely, a unilateral oculomotor palsy with ptosis, and occipitofrontal pain with lowered sensitivity of the upper trigeminal skin field. Should there be, in addition, subhyaloid retinal hemorrhages, and should the cerebrospinal spaces be found to contain blood, a diagnosis is reasonably certain."

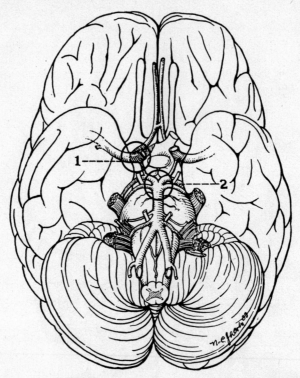

Fig. 226.—Drawing of the base of the brain and circle of Willis. The circles indicate the two common sites for aneurysmal formation. (From Garvey: Arch. Ophth., June, 1934.)

Aneurysm in the carotid portion of the circle of Willis involves the oculomotor nerve more frequently than any of the others. Paralysis of the oculomotor was described in all of Garvey's cases. Pain in the supraorbital region and sharp pain in the face are due to the involvement of the sensory portion of the trigeminal nerve. The optic nerve rarely reveals clinical signs of involvement although post-mortem examination has shown that it is frequently compressed by aneurysms of the carotid portion of the circle of Willis. Optic neuritis and optic atrophy rarely occur although nearly all types of visual field defects have been reported. These depend on the exact location and extent of enlargement of the aneurysm. When visual field defects are due to pressure, the optic nerve becomes atrophic, and the vision of the eye is impaired. I reported a striking case of fusiform aneurysm of both internal carotid arteries which resulted in pressure on both optic nerves.[8] The patient was a woman aged 32 who suffered pain over the eyes and loss of vision in the left eye first.

Other subjective signs and complaints were practically absent. Ocular examination revealed the presence of papilledema with good vision in the right eye and atrophy of the optic nerve with almost total loss of vision in the left eye (Foster Kennedy syndrome). The presence of a suprasellar lesion was suspected and a definite diagnosis was made at the time of operation. This revealed the presence of bilateral fusiform aneurysms of the internal carotid arteries, with the formation of anomalous loops in the course of the arteries and compression of the optic nerves. Because of the anomalous vascular condition found, it was felt that this case was one of congenital origin.

Weber's syndrome may result from aneurysm of the internal carotid and its branches. This is characterized by paralysis of the oculomotor nerve on the same side and a hemiplegia on the opposite side. The aneurysm causes compression of the cerebral peduncle and secondary pressure on the oculomotor nerve.

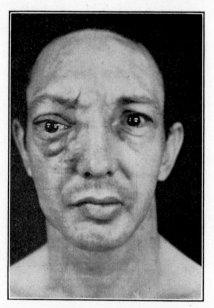

Fig. 227.—Photograph of patient, showing prominent displacement of right eye in case of traumatic carotid artery-cavernous sinus fistula. (From Browder: Arch. Ophth., July, 1937.)

Aneurysms of the vessels of the posterior group, as the basilar or vertebral and their branches, do not produce characteristic symptoms. Hemiplegia and paraplegia may occur from pressure on the pyramidal tracts. Pressure may also involve the cranial nerves (seventh, eighth, ninth, tenth, twelfth). An aneurysm at the bifurcation of the basilar artery will cause pressure on the oculomotor nerve.

Rupture and leakage of an aneurysm of the circle of Willis produces characteristic symptoms. Hemorrhage into the sheath of the optic nerve results in the presence of a large hemorrhage on the optic disc or alongside the disc, which is observed on ophthalmoscopic examination. The retinal veins are congested and other smaller hemorrhages, which have been attributed to obstruction, may be found elsewhere in the retina.

Prior to the occurrence of rupture other vague symptoms may be complained of. Sudden onset of more severe symptoms, such as paralysis and convulsions, may accompany the rupture. If the patient survives the accident, frontal headache, pain, blood in the spinal fluid, and signs of meningeal irritation may be present from subarachnoid hemorrhage. Paralysis of the oculomotor nerve may also result from pressure. The added symptoms of other diseases associated with the aneurysm or rupture, such as arteriosclerosis, syphilis, high blood pressure, and others, will also be observed.

References

1. Abbott, W. D.: Ocular Symptoms in the Diagnosis of Tumor of the Brain, Arch. Ophth. 6: 244, 1931.
2. Lillie, W. I.: Ocular Phenomena Produced by Basal Lesions of the Frontal Lobe, Pre-sessional Vol. Sect. in Ophth. A. M. A., Washington, D. C., May, 1927.
3. Globus, J. H.: Tumors of the Quadrigeminate Plate, Arch. Ophth. 5: 418, 1931.
4. Wagener, H. P., and Love, J. G.: Fields of Vision in Cases of Tumor of Rathke's Pouch, Arch. Ophth. 29: 873, 1943.
5. Ryan, E. R.: Optochiasmic Arachnoiditis; Report of Three Cases, Arch. Ophth. 29: 818, 1943.
6. Goldsmith, A. J. B.: Chiasmic Arachnoiditis, Proc. Roy. Soc. Med. 36: 163, 1943.
7. Garvey, P. H.: Aneurysms of the Circle of Willis, Arch. Ophth. 11: 1032, 1934.
8. Tassman, I. S.: Foster Kennedy Syndrome With Fusiform Aneurysm of Internal Carotid Arteries, Arch. Ophth. 32: 125, 1944.

CHAPTER XXII

DISEASES OF THE SKIN

The diseases of the skin in a number of instances appear to be associated with other disturbances and causes. For example, pellagra, as has been previously described, seems to be a condition closely identified with dietary deficiency and a disorder of nutrition. In the same way other dermatologic conditions have also at times been regarded as the result of gastric disturbances and faulty diet as well as faulty hygiene. Some cases are also considered to be closely associated with vasomotor disturbances.

One of the most common ocular manifestation of diseases of the skin is blepharitis which often results from a dermatitis of the eyelids. This condition was classified by Dowling[1] in four groups, according to the nature of the cause. The first includes those cases of eyelid dermatitis which belong to the infective variety; the second are those due to chemical irritants; the third are cases of seborrheic dermatitis, and the last are those with no known cause.

Lupus Erythematosus.—Lupus erythematosus is an exceedingly rare disease of the skin which is usually chronic and inflammatory in character. It is characterized by the presence of slightly marginated, red or violaceous patches of various sizes and occurring on the face more commonly than elsewhere. The patches are followed by areas of cicatricial atrophy.

Klauder and DeLong, who reported three cases,[2] described five clinical varieties: (1) a circumscribed or discoid form; (2) a chronic variety; (3) a diffuse or disseminated variety, which may be acute and terminate fatally; (4) a telangiectatic variety; (5) a nodular type.

Of these, the discoid form occurs most frequently and is located chiefly on the face and ears. It occurs less frequently on the scalp. The lesion is usually small at first and may vary in size from that of a pinhead to that of a pea. It appears as a slightly elevated spot with red color and a thin scaly covering. The spot gradually increases in size and may have a diameter of nearly a centimeter. The edges remain raised while the center later becomes depressed and atrophic, at the same time assuming a whitish appearance. Small, white scales adhere to the surface of the lesion which also contains dilated follicles. They usually occur on the cheeks and bridge of the nose with their margins sharply outlined. They may rarely occur on the scalp with loss of the hair follicles and result in the presence of round, bald areas. The lips and mucous membranes of the mouth may also be involved.

The etiology of the condition is not known, but tuberculosis, focal infection, and some undiscovered toxin have all been mentioned as a possible cause.

Eye Manifestations.—The eye disease is usually confined to the lids and conjunctiva and has the same clinical appearance as that on other parts of the skin. When the lid margins become involved, the condition may resemble blepharitis. Klauder and DeLong[2] pointed out the following differential features: the dry lid margins which are covered with fine adherent scales, the absence of inflammatory signs and redness seen in blepharitis, the violaceous color. There is no mottling of the eyelids, while the cilia are absent. The lid margins later become atrophic and have an irregular surface. The red or violaceous color disappears, and the cilia are destroyed. The atrophy does not produce any contraction so that ectropion or eversion of the lid margins does not occur.

Isolated lesions of the conjunctiva are not reported, but they might occur without being recognized. The diagnosis of lupus erythematosus of the lids can be made with certainty in the presence of typical lesions elsewhere in the skin. The condition is essentially the same in both.

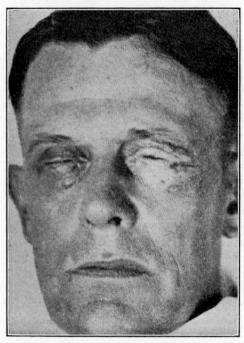

Fig. 228.—Lupus erythematosus of eyelids. (From Klauder and DeLong: Arch. Ophth., June, 1932.)

An interesting case of acute lupus erythematosus was reported by Abramowicz and Dulewicz,[3] occurring in a woman in the ninth month of pregnancy which was complicated by edema of the face and extremities. Fundus examination repeatedly revealed the presence of many small, oval spots in the region of the macula. The spots were the size of a pinhead, and brighter in color than the rest of the fundus. They had the appearance of flat cavities with shadowy areas in their depths. They decreased in number near the disc and had a rose color. The retinal vessels passed over the spots. The vision was unaffected. The eyes were not inflamed and showed little alteration. The edema of the face and extremities subsided after a caesarean operation. The diagnosis was made by the dermatologic clinic.

The case histories with the reports of the post-mortem examinations of four cases of acute and one of chronic lupus erythematosus disseminata were described by Maumenee.[4] The ophthalmoscopic and histologic findings in the eyes included cystoid bodies in the retina which appeared to be small fluffy white exudates on examination with the ophthalmoscope; small superficial retinal hemorrhages (seen in three cases); a slight papilledema found before death in three but in only two on histologic examination; a "septic choroiditis" manifested by slight round-cell infiltration of the choroid; on histological examination choroidal exudates and hemorrhages in only one. The cystoid bodies found in the retina on clinical and histologic examination in the five cases were considered to be a manifestation of a severe generalized reaction that accompanies the disease.

Treatment.—The recommendations for treatment include attention to the general health of the patient. An examination should be made for foci of infection and removal of any such foci is indicated when found. Of the various remedies employed in the treatment of this condition, the best results have been obtained with gold therapy. Even when successfully treated in this way, however, the disease may recur in some patients. This form of treatment is contraindicated in acute cases since the disease in these patients is aggravated. Severe systemic and skin reactions may follow.

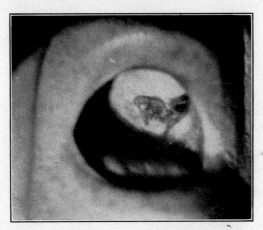

Fig. 229.—Oral pemphigus, showing lesion in mucous membrane of the mouth. Patient same as in Fig. 230. (Courtesy of Dr. J. V. Klauder, Wills Hospital.)

Klauder and DeLong recommended the use of gold and sodium thiosulfate in small doses of 10 mg. intravenously in the beginning. When the tolerance of the patient is determined, the dose is gradually increased up to a maximum of 100 mg. if no reaction occurs. The first few injections are usually followed by prompt improvement. The number of injections to be administered depends on the extent of involvement, the results obtained, and the tolerance of the patient. Most of the small patches disappear after a number of injections.

Pemphigus.—Pemphigus is a rare disease of the skin and mucous membranes characterized by the presence of round, oval blebs or bullae. These bullae may occur in groups over the skin or in the mucous membrane of the mouth as vesicles which rupture very soon after formation. On healing they may be followed by the formation of new vesicles which gives the mucosa the appearance of a rough, softened surface.

The etiology of the disease is unknown. It may be acute or chronic in its course and may be either benign or malignant in form. A gangrenous and a hemorrhagic variety have also been described clinically. It may occur in either sex and at any age. The prognosis is unfavorable and some cases are accompanied by severe systemic symptoms. Cutaneous pemphigus occurs in four varieties: (1) acute pemphigus which is rare and is characterized by the appearance of numerous bullae on the skin and mucous membranes accompanied by acute signs of toxemia; (2) chronic pemphigus vulgaris which runs a long course with remission and renewed attacks and without systemic symptoms; (3) pemphigus foliaceus which is another variety of the chronic form, extensive in character with large numbers of bullae resembling a generalized exfoliative dermatitis; (4) pemphigus vegetans in which the bullae rupture with a chronic discharge and septic absorption occurring. It affects principally the mucous membranes.

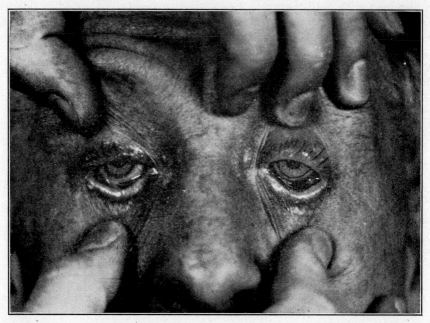

Fig. 230.—Ocular pemphigus. Same patient as in Fig. 229. (Courtesy of Dr. J. V. Klauder, Wills Hospital.)

The diagnosis is very often difficult since the appearance in the mouth, especially, may resemble that seen with syphilitic involvement, ulcerative stomatitis, Vincent's angina, and other forms of stomatitis. These conditions can usually be eliminated, however, by the history and by their response to specific treatment.

Eye Manifestations.—Ocular pemphigus is observed at the same time or after the appearance of the condition on other mucosa. It may only rarely appear before the formation of the lesions elsewhere or as an isolated condition.

The conjunctiva of the eye is the site of the affection. This is characterized by an essential shrinkage of the conjunctiva and the condition has been designated in this way. It occurs in both eyes although not necessarily at the same time. The chronic form is usually progressive over a long period of time. Remissions occur but are followed by renewed attacks and blindness may be the ultimate result. In milder cases the bullae eventually dry with crust formation and recovery.

The pathology of the disease is not clear. Martin,[5] in his report of an acute case in a 48-year-old negro, referred to Sattler who attributed the condition to a swelling of the connective tissue bundles and expansion of the interstices which become filled with fluid, and not by infiltration of the conjunctiva with lymphoid cells. On the other hand Smith, Myers, and Lamb[6] reported a case in a 61-year-old white woman who showed a general thickening of the bulbar conjunctiva resulting from dense infiltration with small lymphocytes and plasma cells, and edema near the limbus of the cornea. There was considerable newly formed connective tissue in the bulbar conjunctiva near the limbus. The observations of most investigators seemed to indicate that the process consists essentially of a deep invasion of the mucous membrane and the submucosa by the inflammatory process, followed by the formation of connective tissue and contraction of the membrane, rather than the formation of vesicles.

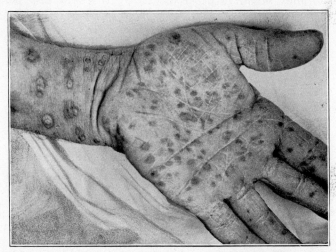

Fig. 231.—Erythema exudativum multiforme, showing typical involvement of the palms. (From Koke: Arch. Ophth., January, 1941.)

Klauder and Cowan,[7] in a comprehensive study of pemphigus with a report of eleven cases examined at Wills Hospital, divided this condition into three groups: (1) Cases of acute pemphigus which are characterized by a sudden onset, fever, and the presence of a widespread erythematous eruption of the skin. (They encountered none of this variety in their series.) (2) Chronic pemphigus, which may occur as an essential shrinking of the conjunctiva alone, or in association with pemphigus of the skin and mucosa of other parts. (Ten cases of the series belonged to this variety. In one patient the vision was still good after thirty years.) (3) A shrivelling process of the conjunctiva in association with several other diseases which are characterized by the presence of bullous eruptions in the skin and mucous membranes elsewhere. (Their series included one case of this variety.)

The symptoms include slight tenderness and soreness, itching, burning, and the presence of a discharge from the conjunctival sac. The conjunctiva shrinks and the formation of connective tissue results in distortion of the eyeball, contraction of the lids and retrotarsal folds with narrowing of the palpebral fissure. Symblepharon may occur later in the course of the disease. The cornea may become involved secondarily with the formation of vesicles and loss of epithelium. Ulceration of the cornea may follow. The ocular lesions of pemphigus may also rarely be combined with or form a part of certain other dermatoses.

Treatment of ocular pemphigus is chiefly symptomatic in the absence of any known effective therapy. Arsenic, radium, x-ray, high-frequency current, blood transfusions, sulfanilamide, arsphenamine, and neoarsphenamine have all been employed, but no satisfactory results or improvement of the condition have been obtained.

Erythema Exudativum Multiforme (Hebra).—As indicated by Klauder and Cowan,[7] lesions of the conjunctiva characterized by the presence of bullae and eventual shrinking may occur in association with lesions of the skin and mucous membranes found in other diseases. This was also pointed out by Cohen and Sulzberger.[9]

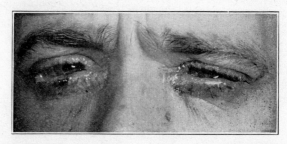

Fig. 232.—Erythema exudativum multiforme, showing conjunctivitis and vesicle formation on the right lower lid. (From Koke: Arch. Ophth., January, 1941.)

Such lesions of the conjunctiva and cornea occur in erythema exudativum multiforme. Originally described by Hebra, this disease is comparatively rare and of unknown etiology. It has been considered as a systemic condition of infectious origin. The acute onset is accompanied by fever, chills, headache, and pain in the joints. Marked inflammatory changes involve the cornea and conjunctiva which result in serious visual impairment and even in loss of the eye. The mucous membrane of the lips, mouth, tongue, palate, bronchi, and even vagina, may reveal the presence of an intense pseudomembranous inflammation while the skin reveals a widespread polymorphous eruption. The disease follows a rather long and chronic course but with the most serious results occurring in the eyes.

Eye Manifestations.—Bailey[8] reported three cases of erythema exudativum multiforme, with an excellent review of the subject. Pain in the eyes and photophobia are early complaints. The lids become swollen, and the margins are covered with pus which causes a matting of the cilia. The mucopurulent material accumulates in the conjunctival sac and has the appearance of a soft, fibrinous membrane. The palpebral conjunctiva is swollen, and the bulbar conjunctiva is injected. Follicles are prominent and necrotic patches may be present. These symptoms increase in severity with involvement of the cornea and ulceration and opacification taking place. The photophobia and irritation are constant and lead to marked blepharospasm. There may be a moderate or marked circumcorneal injection and the cornea itself loses its luster, and the involvement may extend through its entire thickness. The iris and anterior chamber may present exudative evidences of inflammation.

Scarring eventually takes place with the formation of fibrous bands which produce a narrowing of the palpebral fissure and obliteration of the fornix. Perforation of the cornea may not occur, but tenderness of the eyeball and photophobia persist and complete opacification of the cornea with loss of vision results.

The skin at the same time is covered with a diffuse macular and papular eruption which may also include a few hemorrhagic spots. The mucous membranes of the mouth, pharynx, tongue, and lips also reveal serious ulcerative, pseudomembranous and hemorrhagic areas. There is no direct relationship between the extent of skin and mucous membrane lesions. The conjunctival pathology may also vary from a simple hyperemia to a pseudomembranous condition. The disease may occasionally involve the mucous membrane of the mouth or the conjunctiva alone.

In the late stages the disease in the eyes may resemble trachoma, but the history and character of the discharge serve to differentiate the condition. Rupture of the bullae which is followed by scarring in chronic pemphigus may closely resemble this condition, but the chronic progressive course and character of the skin manifestations are important factors in the differential diagnosis.

In acute pemphigus the original lesion is bullous although the conjunctiva and mucous membranes may be covered with a pseudomembrane. Bailey stated that the diagnosis of acute pemphigus should not be made unless successive crops of blebs that rupture and become filled with pus or blood, or form dirty crusts, are present. These are the characteristic cutaneous lesions.

There is no satisfactory treatment available, but Bailey administered large doses of bacterial vaccines intravenously with some promise of success.

The treatment of the eyes is chiefly symptomatic and includes the use of warm, moist compresses, a mild eyewash, and the regular instillation of atropine sulfate, while the intraocular tension is observed. Local anesthetics, such as butyn or pontocaine, may be instilled for the pain, and the eyes should be protected from light by the use of black glasses.

Epidermolysis Bullosa Dystrophica.—This is a rare disease which may present several forms, i.e., a simple hereditary epidermolysis bullosa, hereditary epidermolysis dystrophica, and acquired epidermolysis bullosa dystrophica. This condition is also characterized by the presence of ocular and cutaneous lesions which are similar to those of pemphigus. The cutaneous lesions may resemble those seen in erythema multiforme or dermatitis herpetiformis. The etiology of the condition is unknown.

Eye Manifestations.—Ocular manifestations of epidermolysis bullosa dystrophica are rare. Cohen and Sulzberger,[9] who reported a case in a 7-year-old boy, found seven cases previously reported. They described their case as "atypical acquired bullosa dystrophica (toxica?)," and they also stated that identical ocular lesions may be combined or form part of certain other dermatoses, just as in pemphigus of the eye and skin.

The main eye manifestation in this condition is also an essential shrinking of the conjunctiva which involves both eyes, similar to that occurring in pemphigus.

The condition may begin with pain about the eyes, swelling of the lids, and the presence of a stringy mucous discharge. A pseudomembrane may be present and the conjunctiva becomes thickened. Vesicles appear on the cornea and ulceration may take place. Bands of fibrous tissue and symblepharon occur with contraction and obliteration of the conjunctival sac. The tarsal conjunctiva becomes white and atrophic.

In Cohen and Sulzberger's case the right eye was involved first and showed several early phlyctenules at the limbus of the cornea, and the condition resembled a phlyctenular keratoconjunctivitis. The left eye revealed only a mild blepharoconjunctivitis. In spite of all treatment the condition progressed with the formation of a necrotic ulcer and granuloma on the cornea of the right eye, shrinking and scarring of the conjunctiva, and symblepharon. The vision was reduced to light perception; the eyeball became soft and was finally enucleated. The entire cul-de-sac was obliterated. The left eye also grew progressively worse.

Histologic examination of the eye coincided with the histologic findings in the skin. The necrotic ulceration of the cornea was considered to result from the earlier condition in the conjunctiva or cornea itself.

Treatment seems to be of no avail. Only a mild eyewash and olive oil are recommended for use in the eye. Atropine should be instilled for the corneal involvement. Cohen and Sulzberger employed injections of neoarsphenamine in their case which seemed to check the progress of the cutaneous lesions and improve the general condition.

Both the ocular and cutaneous lesions were found to become exaggerated by the internal administration of iodides. They also called attention to the fact that hypersensitivity to iodine and arsenic has occasionally been reported in cases of epidermolysis bullosa.

Dermatitis Herpetiformis.—This is a rare dermatologic condition described by Duhring and is characterized by the presence of a multiform eruption which is widely distributed over the body and causes marked itching. General symptoms are absent. Erythematous areas over the skin are covered by vesicles which appear in successive crops. The eruption persists but may subside with a tendency to recur after a more or less prolonged interval.

Eye Manifestations.—The ocular involvement in dermatitis herpetiformis also occurs in the conjunctiva and presents a variety of lesions noted in other dermatologic diseases. These include principally the formation of vesicles and a pseudomembrane similar to that found in erythema multiforme. The conjunctiva becomes thickened, a discharge accumulates in the conjunctival sac, shrinking of the conjunctiva takes place, and finally fibrous bands and symblepharon occur. The cornea may become involved with opacification which may invade the entire structure with almost total loss of vision.

The treatment is here also chiefly symptomatic. A mild eyewash should be frequently employed and atropine instilled into the affected eye when the cornea is involved.

Erythema Nodosum.—This condition is characterized by the presence of large, nodular swellings in the skin which appear rather abruptly accompanied by fever, malaise, and pains in the joints. These nodules are dark red in color and occur mostly in children and young people. They appear in crops on the face and extremities and may subside after a period of time without recurrence. The condition has been said to be associated with rheumatism and tuberculosis.

Eye Manifestations.—The nodular swelling in erythema nodosum may occur in the eye under the conjunctiva. When present, it occurs simultaneously with the cutaneous lesion and also subsides at the same time. It may resemble a phlyctenule in appearance and can occur on the lid or under the bulbar and palpebral conjunctiva. The small nodules may be freely movable and are surrounded by a moderate amount of edema in the conjunctiva.

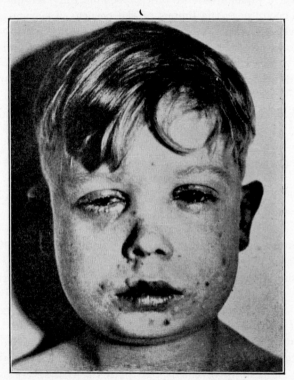

Fig. 233.—Essential shrinkage of conjunctiva in a case of epidermolysis bullosa dystrophica, showing cutaneous lesions on the face, bullae on left upper lid, and secretion covering the eyelids. (From Cohen and Sulzberger: Arch. Ophth., March, 1935.)

Xeroderma Pigmentosum.—This is a disease of the skin and mucous membranes which usually appears in children and early life and is characterized by the presence of pigmented lesions that occur principally on the skin of the face. It has been described as a hereditary disease, the transmission of which has recessive characteristics. Consanguinity has been noted in the parents of some patients.

The presence of the lesions seems to be activated by exposure to direct sunlight which at first produces an acute erythematous condition. Later, small, irregular spots of pigmentation appear which resemble freckles. In time these pigmentation spots become more pronounced; the skin may become dry while thinning, stretching and contraction takes place. Nodular growths may develop in the areas occupied by pigment. The condition later becomes actually malignant in character. The prognosis is poor and the patients usually succumb in early life to exhaustion, severe ulceration, hemorrhage or other complications.

Eye Manifestations.—Ocular lesions may occur on the eyelids, conjunctiva or cornea. The skin of the lower lids in particular may be the first to show the early pigmentation. Later, stretching and thinning of the skin may occur followed by ulceration and atrophy. Contraction may result in ectropion of the lid. The conjunctiva becomes injected and hyperemic. Small nodular growths which are pigmented and which resemble phlyctenules, granulomas, or angiomas may occur near the limbus of the cornea. Lacrimation, photophobia and serous discharge usually occur. The corneal epithelium becomes edematous and opacification follows invasion of the cornea. Ulceration and atrophy, which may also involve the iris, result. The cul-de-sac may become very shallow and even obliterated, while shrinkage of the lids, symblepharon and anklyloblepharon occur.

Reese and Wilber[10] recently reported four cases all of which occurred in small children, all girls. In at least two of the children the condition began after exposure to ordinary sunlight. They reported on the microscopic examination of one eye which developed an epithelioma of the cornea at the site of an exposure ulcer. Two of the patients died at the ages of 7 and 11 years, respectively, while the other two survived to the ages of 16 and 30 years. Three of the patients were siblings.

Treatment of the condition is of no avail in checking the process, which eventually assumes a malignant form. Symptomatic and palliative measures may afford relief. When the condition is recognized, sunlight should be avoided. The growths should be removed if possible by excision or irradiation and a mild ointment applied to the skin of the lids and conjunctiva. Reese and Wilber recommended fulgeration or small amounts of low voltage x-ray therapy for removal of keratoses. A mild warmed eye wash should be employed to flush the conjunctival sac regularly. Hot compresses can be employed and atropine sulfate, 1 per cent solution, is instilled in the eyes when the cornea begins to show signs of involvement. In patients with severe ocular complications, it may be necessary to enucleate the eye.

Hydroa.—This condition, also known as hydroa puerorum and summer prurigo, is a seasonal condition which affects the skin of exposed parts in the warm weather. It occurs among children and is characterized by the presence of very small elevations, each of which is covered with a small vesicle. Removal of the vesicle results in the formation of a blood-tinged crust. The condition is accompanied by very severe itching. It subsides with the onset of cold weather but recurs in the summer.

Eye Manifestations.—The conjunctiva is first involved and the appearance may resemble that seen in the bulbar type of vernal catarrh. The lids may contract with narrowing of the palpebral fissure. In others it may manifest itself as a severe conjunctivitis which may be accompanied by or followed by a keratitis. Small granulomatous and cystlike masses may also occur in the palpebral conjunctiva. These tissue masses may ulcerate and undergo necrosis and also involve the underlying sclera.

There is no satisfactory treatment available, but the patient should be protected from strong light since sensitivity to light is considered to be a factor. Symptomatic measures should be employed locally.

Psoriasis.—Psoriasis is a cutaneous affection which is characterized by the presence of small, round, and irregular red plaques on the skin of the neck, trunk, and the extremities. The lesions are slightly elevated and sharply outlined with a thin, white scaly covering which can be removed. They are not accompanied by pain but might produce slight itching at times. The cause is unknown and treatment which consists in the use of chrysarobin produces only relief and is not curative.

Eye Manifestations.—Ocular involvement is not common in psoriasis but lesions may occur on and near the eyelids. A chronic form of conjunctivitis is usually present. The conjunctiva may become involved by extension from the lids but such instances are infrequent. The manifestations of the condition may vary in different cases. Involvement of the cornea is rare, although such cases have been reported. Both eyes may be involved with small lesions near the limbus. They cause an opacity in the cornea with thickening of the epithelium, superficial vessel formation, and infiltration under Bowman's membrane. Ulceration and iritis may occur.

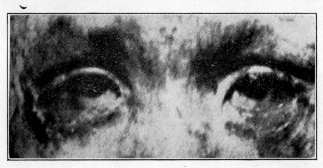

Fig. 234.—Xeroderma pigmentosa, showing usual skin lesions and atrophy of lower lids. (From Reese and Wilber: Am. J. Ophth., September, 1943.)

The treatment employed depends on the nature of the manifestation. A mild eye lotion should be used regularly and atropine instilled into the eye in cases where the cornea is involved.

Xanthalasma.—Xanthalasma is the name applied to discrete areas of discoloration which occur in the loose skin of the upper and lower eyelids. These areas are superficial and appear slightly thickened, occurring more frequently at the inner angles of the lids. They have a lemon-yellow color which gradually fades to a darker, waxy shade after a time. They are usually multiple and may occur on both eyes. As many as six areas might be found in a single case. A few smaller areas may be round or irregular in shape, but the larger ones are usually elongated. The latter may measure a centimeter in length and often curve in a direction parallel to the rim of the orbit.

The exact cause is unknown, but the condition is considered to be due to a fatty degeneration with the deposit of lipoid in the skin. The change is probably similar to that which occurs in other tissues such as atherosclerosis of the vessels, fatty deposits in the cornea, and other diseases associated with fatty metabolism.

Xanthalasma usually occurs in people of middle age or older and appears to be confined almost entirely to the female sex. Since arteriosclerosis is fairly common in patients of this age, the condition may result from lack of oxygen and the formation of cholesterol. Liver dysfunction has also been considered as an etiologic factor. Since many cases occur in women who have recently passed the stage of the menopause, the possibility of glandular changes as a determining factor.should be considered.

The familial tendency of xanthalasma can be demonstrated by a brother and sister with several well-marked patches on the lids of both eyes, under treatment in the clinic of Dr. L. B. Lehrfeld[11] at Wills Hospital. The paternal grandmother, father, and aunt of these patients were also known to present the same condition. The blood cholesterol in the woman was 298 and in the man 300 per cent.

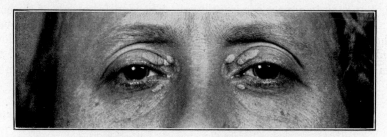

Fig. 235.—Xanthalasma in a woman.

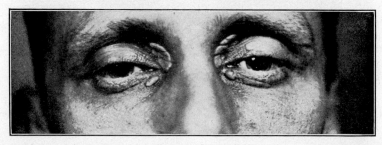

Fig. 236.—Brother of patient shown in Fig. 235. The paternal grandmother, father, and aunt all had the same condition. (Courtesy of Dr. L. B. Lehrfeld, Wills Hospital.)

The nature of the patches is not serious and causes no impairment, but they are usually prominent and sometimes unsightly. The patients often request their removal. They can be treated and usually successfully removed by the application of trichloro-acetic acid or by excision. Recurrences may occur, however.

Bowen's Disease (Intraepithelioma of the Cornea)

This disease was first described by Bowen in 1912[12] as a precancerous dyskeratosis which it was felt would eventually undergo malignant change. The lesions occurred in the skin and were regarded as a precancerous dermatosis. They are characterized by the presence of squamous or scablike patches or plaques in the skin. They may appear also to be wrinkled or papular. The histologic appearance is that of an epithelioma and is composed of dyskeratotic cells which occur intraepithelially. They eventually break through the basement membrane with infiltration into the surrounding tissues and metastasis. Metastasis has been said to occur also before the lesion becomes a true epithelioma.

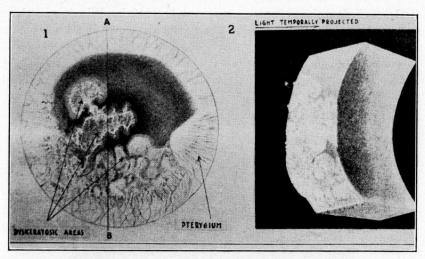

Fig. 237.—Bowen's disease of cornea. *1,* Drawing of lesion on right cornea, *AB* being the axis of a semischematic cut, a photograph of which, *2,* was obtained with the slit lamp. (From Weskamp: Arch. Ophth., April, 1944.)

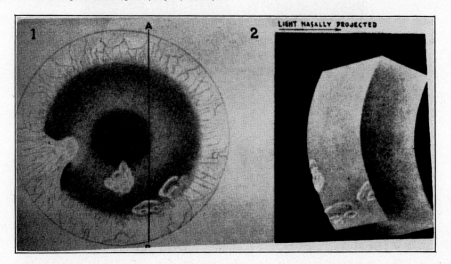

Fig. 238.—Bowen's disease of cornea. Appearance of lesion of left eye, *AB* being the axis of a semischematic cut, a photograph of which, *2,* was obtained with the slit lamp. (From Weskamp: Arch. Ophth., April, 1944.)

It is a chronic, slowly progressive disease which is perhaps slightly more common in females than males, although the percentage is nearly evenly divided. It occurs usually in patients past 50 years of age. The development of the disease may cover a period of many years. Although it is comparatively rare, a number of cases involving the skin and mucous membranes have been described. The symptoms are not marked and depend principally on the location. Diagnosis of the condition must be made by laboratory examination of a specimen taken for biopsy.

Eye Manifestations.—There are only about seven cases of Bowen's disease of the cornea on record to date. The first five cases were all reported in 1942 by McGavic.[13] Another case was reported in 1943 by Wise,[14] and the most recent to date was by Weskamp in 1944.[15] The diagnosis in all was confirmed by microscopic examination.

According to McGavic, the lesion must be differentiated clinically from pannus, filtering cicatrix of the cornea, Mooren's ulcer, epithelial proliferation, fatty degeneration of the cornea, and epithelial dystrophy of the cornea.

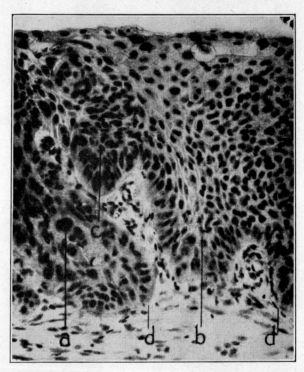

Fig. 239.—Photomicrograph showing proliferated rete pegs *a, b,* and *c* without violation of the basement membrane, *d.* Note the marked variation in cells and evidence of cellular unrest (poikilokarynosis). (From McGavic: Am. J. Ophth., February, 1942.)

The histopathologic picture of Bowen's disease of the skin as described by McGavic is as follows:

> The epithelium is thickened, and in the skin there are hyperplastic deranged pegs formed by the rete cells, giving a papillary appearance. Many of the epithelial cells show great variation in size, shape, and staining characteristics. Mitotic figures are of bizarre configuration with disordered polarity and may be more numerous than in cases of straightforward basal or squamous-cell epithelioma. Single nuclei may reach a tremendous size and are called "monster" cells. These may have single large nuclei or may be multinucleated

with the nuclei clumped together (clumping cells of Bowen). Division by amitosis may be demonstrable. The cytoplasm of the cells is often vacuolated. When extreme vacuolization occurs, the nucleus is completely surrounded, the two membranes giving a double-ringed appearance to the cell. These are the "corps rond" of Darier. Intercellular bridges may be shown, but intercellular fibrils are often not demonstrable. Surface cornification and parakeratosis with granule formation may be present. The basal cells may proliferate and lose

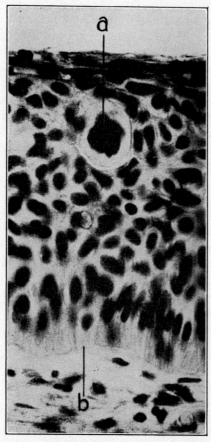

Fig. 240.—Photomicrograph (high power) showing a monster cell. *a,* With clumped nuclei in its center (clumping cell of Bowen). The marked variation in the proliferating cells is well demonstrated. Unviolated basement membrane, *b.* (From McGavic: Am. J. Ophth., February, 1942.)

their neat palisade arrangement, but there is no rupture of the basement membrane in this process. Infiltration by lymphocytes, plasma cells, and histiocytes is present beneath the epithelium as a rule. This, together with the increased vascularity, gives the lesion the false appearance of an inflammatory process. The cellular variation and unrest peculiar to Bowen's disease have been called "poikilokarynosis" by Darier; these features are necessary for the diagnosis of Bowen's disease.

The corneal involvement may follow the limbus or occur at different sites. The change from the normal epithelium to new growth is abrupt. Inflammatory reaction and new blood vessel formation can be seen between the tumor and the uninvolved Bowman's membrane. The new growth may remain localized without microscopic evidence of invasion or clinical signs of metastasis for as long as thirty years, but in 40 per cent of mucous membrane lesions and in 3 per cent of the skin lesions, malignant change was reported.

McGavic advised calling the lesion a Bowen epithelioma, to denote that the tumor is not only intraepithelial, but that it also shows the cellular changes regarded as necessary for differentiation from ordinary epithelioma in situ or Bowenoid epitheliomas. Other lesions which are said to be similar histologically are: 1. Ordinary early basal and squamous cell carcinomas; epitheliomas in situ may lack the cellular changes necessary for a diagnosis of Bowen epithelioma. 2. Arsenical keratosis, since arsenic was said to play a role in some cases of Bowen's disease. 3. Xeroderma pigmentosa. 4. Precancerous melanosis and diffuse malignant melanoma of the conjunctiva and skin. 5. Intraepidermal melanoma. 6. Senile keratosis. 7. Radiation dermatitis and carcinoma. 8. Leucoplakia. 9. Cancer in workers with paraffin. 10. So-called epithelial plaque or congenital benign epithelioma of the limbus.

Treatment.—The lesions should be removed by excision. This is not considered to be difficult and does not result in much scarring since they do not extend deeply. If the conjunctiva is also extensively involved by extension, it may require enucleation of the eye. Involvement of the palpebral conjunctiva may also require removal of part of the eyelids. The entire lesion is not necessarily removed at one sitting. Since it is slow in showing malignant changes, it is possible to remove the lesion in portions. The disease is, however, potentially a malignant neoplasm. Treatment by radiation or by the use of chemicals and actual cautery is contraindicated.

References

1. Dowling, G. B.: Dermatological Aspect of Affections of the Eye, Brit. M. J. 2: 794, 1937.
2. Klauder, J. V., and DeLong, P.: Lupus Erythematosus of the Conjunctiva, Eyelids and Lid Margins, Arch. Ophth. 7: 856, 1932.
3. Abramowicz, I., and Dulewicz, M.: The Fundus of the Eye in Acute Lupus Erythematosus (Erythema Perstans), Ann. d'ocul. 170: 599, 1933.
4. Maumenee, A. E.: Retinal Lesions in Lupus Erythematosus, Am. J. Ophth. 23: 971, 1940.
5. Martin, W. O.: Acute Ocular Pemphigus, Arch. Ophth. 3: 744, 1930.
6. Smith, R. C., Myers, E. A., and Lamb, H. D.: Ocular and Oral Pemphigus, Arch. Ophth. 11: 635, 1934.
7. Klauder, J. V., and Cowan, A.: Ocular Pemphigus and Its Relation to Pemphigus of the Skin and Mucous Membranes, Am. J. Ophth., June, 1942.
8. Bailey, J. H.: Lesions of the Cornea and Conjunctiva in Erythema Exudativum Multiforme (Hebra): Report of Three Cases With Grave Ocular Sequelae, Arch. Ophth. 6: 362, 1931.
9. Cohen, M., and Sulzberger, M. B.: Essential Shrinkage of Conjunctiva in a Case of Probable Epidermolysis Bullosa Dystrophica, Arch. Ophth. 13: 374, 1935.
10. Reese, A. B., and Wilber, I. E.: Eye Manifestations of Xeroderma Pigmentosa, Am. J. Ophth. 26: 901, 1943.
11. Lehrfeld, L.: Wills Hospital Clinic, Philadelphia, May, 1941. Personal communication.
12. Bowen, J. T.: Precancerous Dermatosis, J. Cutan. Dis. 30: 214, 1912.
13. McGavic, J. S.: Intraepithelial Epithelioma of the Cornea and Conjunctiva (Bowen's Disease), Am. J. Ophth. 25: 167, 1942.
14. Wise, George: A Case of Bowen's Disease of the Cornea, Am. J. Ophth. 26: 167, 1943.
15. Weskamp, Carlos: Bowen's Disease of the Cornea, Arch. Ophth. 31: 310, 1944.

CHAPTER XXIII

DISEASES OF BONES OF THE SKULL

Some confusion still exists among ophthalmologists with regard to the exact diagnosis or classification of the disease changes which occur in the bones of the skull to produce certain eye manifestations. The diseases to be considered from this standpoint are all characterized by a thickening which results in the formation of bony prominences. These are sometimes referred to as bony tumors, exostoses, hyperostoses, and bosses, which gradually increase in size and produce signs of pressure. The eye manifestations occur especially when such pressure is exerted because of the presence of the bony thickening or overgrowth in the walls of the orbital cavity or the adjacent cavities.

The diseases in which this condition occurs are designated chiefly as: (1) Paget's disease, (2) leontiasis ossea, and (3) orbital hyperostosis. Since the ocular manifestations may be very much alike in all of these, the difficulty arises in the classification of the bony change present, and in the exact diagnosis of the osseous disease. The differences are concerned principally with whether or not the bones of the skull are involved alone or in association with other bones of the skeleton, and also whether the bony prominences are only localized overgrowths in the orbit or part of a general thickening and broadening which affects all the bones of the skull. X-ray examination, the location and extent of the bony change, and the clinical findings are important aids in the diagnosis.

Paget's Disease

Paget's disease is considered to be a chronic disease of unknown etiology which affects the long and flat bones of the body. It usually occurs in middle life and older age, affecting males more frequently than females. It has been known to occur in more than one member of the same family, and it is nearly always accompanied by a generalized arteriosclerosis.

The disease is very slow and insidious in its onset, so that it may only be noticed at first in the enlargement of a single bone. The bones of the head show a gradual enlargement, while the bones of the extremities become thickened and bowed. X-ray of the skull shows a progressive thickening of the calvarium. The vertebrae and other bones all show the same enlargement and broadening. This anatomic change is chiefly a gradual absorption of one portion of the bone, while an ossification takes place in other parts, giving rise to the irregular enlargement which may take the shape of osseous hard tumor formations.

The disease may occasionally become arrested, but in most cases, it follows a chronic, progressive course which may lead to marked deformity, and death usually occurs as the result of some intercurrent disease. There is no known treatment which will improve the condition, and the therapy employed is ordinarily symptomatic.

Eye Manifestations.—The eye manifestations are usually produced as the result of the enlargement which occurs in the bones of the orbit in association with enlargement of the other bones of the skull. As a result a gradual de-

581

crease occurs in the cavity of the skull and the orbits, which might cause headaches, paralyses, visual impairment, and other symptoms.

The hard tumor formations commonly occur in the frontal bone and about
the orbit, and may be well localized and almost nodular in type. When such
nodular growths occur in the absence of other enlargement or thickening of
the rest of the bone, the condition is more likely to be a hyperostosis.

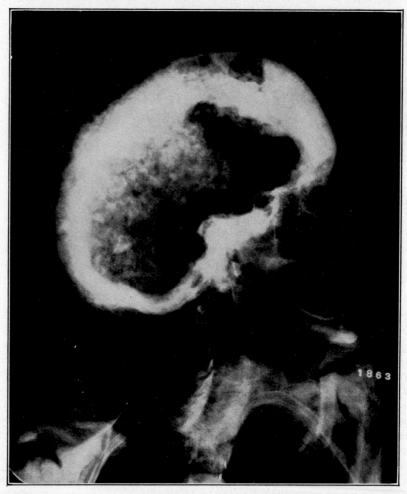

Fig. 241.—X-ray of skull in case of Paget's disease, showing characteristic areas of absorption
and calcification. Note the density of the base. (From Meakins: The Practice of Medicine.)

Exophthalmos.—As a result of the decrease in the orbital cavity, exophthalmos may result. This is probably present when the bony enlargement is well
advanced. It is perhaps not as commonly seen with Paget's disease as in the
other osseous diseases. The motility of the affected eye is impaired to a corresponding degree. In a case described by Ellis and McKeown[1] the left eye
showed marked exophthalmos in a 55-year-old colored man with vision of
20/200. The eyeball could be rotated freely. The exophthalmos was due to

an exostosis of the left orbit. The x-ray report suggesting an early Paget's disease was significant, but the orbital change was more probably a hyperostosis.

Fundus Changes.—The most common manifestation noted on ophthalmoscopic examination is optic atrophy. This is attributed in most cases to gradual pressure involving the optic nerve by the bony enlargement. This has been known to occur in cases especially affecting the bones of the orbit, resulting in a narrowing of the optic canal. In some instances the optic atrophy is probably due to arteriosclerosis and vascular changes which are also present.

Abeli[2] reported optic atrophy in a case in which the roentgen examination showed bony changes characteristic of Paget's disease. There was also an exophthalmos of the right eye with edema of the lids and conjunctiva and loss of motility. Vision was reduced to hand movements. The fundus also showed enlargement of the veins and contracted arteries. The nerve head of the left eye was also pale with vision 20/200 and a concentric contraction of the visual field.

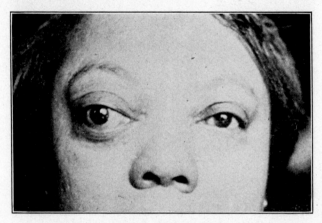

Fig. 242.—Unilateral exophthalmos. (Meningioma, sphenoidal ridge.) (I. S. Tassman, Graduate Hospital, University of Pennsylvania.)

In most of these cases concentric contraction of the visual fields is a common finding, due to the optic atrophy which is present, and probably also to the arteriosclerosis and vascular changes.

Angioid streaks of the retina were observed in two cases with Paget's disease by Lambert.[3] These patients also showed the presence of vascular changes in the retina.

Alternating squint, papillitis with beginning optic atrophy, contracted fields and enlarged blind spots were all found in a case reported as Paget's disease of the skull by Frey.[4]

Leontiasis Ossea

Leontiasis ossea is described as a hyperkeratosis of the skull which is characterized by an increase of all the bones, including those of the face. Other bones of the skeleton are rarely, if ever, involved. The condition occurs earlier in life than does Paget's disease; it affects females more frequently than males, and the cause is unknown.

Eye Manifestations.—The ocular involvements resulting from the presence of leontiasis ossea are very similar to those described for Paget's disease. The orbital cavity as well as the cranial and nasal cavities may be involved as the result of the more or less localized bony overgrowths. Exophthalmos, usually unilateral, impaired ocular motility, diplopia, and optic atrophy are the most common manifestations. They are also considered to be due to the pressure resulting from the bony enlargement. This may produce a narrowing of the optic canal with subsequent optic atrophy, here also.

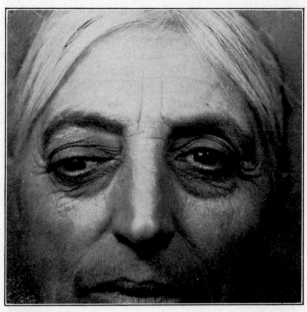

Fig. 243.—Exophthalmos and downward displacement of eye with tumor in roof of right orbit. (I. S. Tassman, Wills Hospital.)

Orbital Hyperostosis

The bony tumors of the orbit were divided by Benedict[10] into: 1. Osteomas; 2. Exostoses; and 3. Hyperostosis. The osteomas include those which are found principally on the superior and nasal walls and which arise from the ethmoid cells and frontal sinuses. It is sometimes difficult to determine the point of origin because of the lack of uniformity in the development of the tumor. The displacement of the eyeball does not always indicate the exact point of origin. They arise most commonly from the ethmoids, with the frontals and sphenoids next in order of frequency, and they may invade the orbit or cranial cavity from any of the bones containing these sinuses. They are diagnosed mainly by the history, symptoms, slow development, localization and visualization by stereoscopic roentgenography. The osteomas are usually removed surgically either by direct approach through the orbit or through the nose, depending on the structures involved.

The exostoses include the small projections of bone which arise from the margin of the orbit and which result from a chronic inflammatory process in the soft tissues. Patches or bands of newly formed bony tissue may encroach on the inner surface of the cranial cavity and result in pressure or irritation with circulatory disturbances in the prefrontal and frontal lobes at the base of the brain. Headache, asthenia, psychic changes, blindness, loss of the sense of smell and epileptiform seizures may occur.

Hyperplastic thickening of the posterior wall of the orbit may result from the presence of intracranial meningiomas which occur in the region of the sphenoidal ridge, and the anterior wall of the middle temporal fossa or temporofrontal region. The syndrome produced by these tumors was first described in 1922 by Cushing.[5]

Although cases of this kind are not common, subsequent reports have been made by Elsberg, Hare, and Dyke,[6] Alpers and Groff,[7] Cohen and Scarff,[8] and Knapp.[9] Knapp, in his report, described a case of meningioma in which the orbit was found to be filled with bony masses. The photomicrographs revealed meningioma typical of new bone formation in form and structure. This condition was at first believed to be circumscribed hyperostosis, and on attempting to remove the excess bone in the orbit by operation, it was found to be very hard and had to be chiseled and hammered off in parts. The diagnosis was made after a later operation by histologic examination. Therefore, in addition to the cases of hyperostosis circumscripta as a cause of thickening of the bony walls of the orbit, Knapp also emphasized the occurrence of the meningiomas, as described by Cushing.

Cohen and Scarff in their report of a case of meningioma of the left middle cranial fossa situated close to the sphenoidal ridge with unilateral exophthalmos gave an excellent description of the cardinal features of the syndrome.

The tumor is essentially fibroblastic and grossly resembles other fibroid tumors. Traversing the dura, it invades the contiguous bone causing a hyperplastic growth and thickening of the bone which is characteristic.

The clinical features which characterize these meningiomas include their tendency to arise from fixed points in the skull, to occur chiefly in adults, and to produce certain definite and constant clinical syndromes. The region of the sphenoid ridge, the temporofrontal region, and the posterior wall of the orbit are points of predilection. The tumor which is flat in shape, spreads out to involve a considerable surface of the bone, which has led to use of the term "enplaque" in designating the growth.

Eye Manifestations.—Unilateral exophthalmos and visual impairment are the prominent ocular manifestations of orbital hyperostoses resulting from this cause. The meningioma of the temporofrontal region was described by Knapp as occurring without associated neurologic symptoms and without increased intracranial pressure. It runs a characteristic slow course in this location, with exophthalmos as the chief ocular manifestation and absence of fundus changes until late in the course. In one of the cases reported there was a slight paresis of the external rectus muscle, exophthalmos, and no change in the optic nerve in the early stage. There was a unilateral bony deformity of the skull which on roentgen examination showed increased density and enlargement of the squamous portion of the temporal bone and of the large wing of the sphenoid with involvement of the outer and upper walls of the orbit. In another case there was thickening of the upper, outer orbital margin, and a definite tumor was palpated in the orbit behind the external canthus. The optic nerve was swollen and showed some neuritic atrophy. The roentgenogram revealed a bony tumor of the outer wall of the left orbit with increased density of the bone, especially of the greater wing of the sphenoid and outer surface of the frontal bone. The malar bone was also slightly involved, and the sella turcica was normal.

Cohen and Scarff pointed out that extension of the tumors along the sphenoidal ridge eventually involves the optic foramen and produces direct pressure on the optic nerve with resulting optic atrophy and blindness. Calcification on the apex of the orbit may cause constriction of the optic canal and diffuse thickening of bone in the region of the sella. The sphenoidal fissure may also be involved with an enlargement and change in shape causing paralysis of the nerves passing through and an interference with return of venous blood from the orbit. The clinical syndrome of middle cranial fossa meningioma, usually occurring in adults, is, therefore, slowly progressive exophthalmos with ophthalmoplegia, primary optic atrophy and thickening of the posterior orbital wall on the same side.

These patients may live for years because of the slow growth of the tumor, but marked visual impairment may result from continued progress of the condition.

Benedict pointed out that the same bony changes found in the roof of the orbit as a result of meningioma may also result from tumors within the orbit involving the periorbita. He enumerated the following as causes of hyperostosis of the walls of the orbit: hemangio-endothelioma, dermoid cyst, hemangioma with arteriovenous aneurysm, endothelioma of the brain, anomalous development of the sphenoidal ridge, squamous cell epithelioma of the nasopharynx, Mikulicz's disease, arteriovenous aneurysm in the brain, meningioma of the sphenoid ridge and neurofibroma of the orbit. The symptoms which could result are headaches, exophthalmos, diminished vision, visual field changes, impairment of ocular rotation, petit mal and grand mal. Roentgenograms of the orbit are important as an aid in their diagnosis. This will usually reveal any contiguous growth in the soft tissues by the presence of dense shadows and it will also reveal the extent of involvement or protrusion of the bone into the orbit by the location of the shadow.

The treatment consists in surgical excision of the bony tumor, when possible, although the condition may recur. Benedict stated that hyperostosis of the sphenoidal ridge or of the lesser wing of the sphenoid, when accompanied by visual disturbance or by exophthalmos, usually indicates a meningioma near the sella turcica. This is a favorable location for surgical removal by the transcranial route. When the vision can be improved, or when it is felt that the condition can be aided by surgery, the methods of approach must receive careful consideration.

Malignancy of Bones of the Orbit

The bones of the skull which enter into the formation of the orbit are occasionally involved by a malignant process which can result in pressure involving the ocular structures. Such a process may occur in one of the nasal accessory sinuses and extend to the sphenoid or ethmoid bones especially. The interior of the orbit or inner walls of the orbit are not necessarily involved. The lesser and greater wing of the sphenoid bone in particular may become involved by extension of a process arising within the sphenoid sinus. When the extension has progressed far enough to involve the sphenoidal fissure or optic canal, ocular symptoms will occur as the result of pressure on these structures.

Eye Manifestations.—Any neoplastic process which involves the structures passing through the sphenoidal fissure and optic canal may result in pressure on these structures and cause an ophthalmoplegia. The structures which pass through the sphenoidal fissure are the third, fourth, and sixth cranial nerves, the three branches of the ophthalmic division of the fifth nerve, the ophthalmic vein, the orbital branch of the middle meningeal artery (when it does not pass through the middle meningeal foramen), and the sympathetic fibers from the cavernous plexus, the sympathetic root of the ciliary ganglion, and (sometimes) the sensory root of the ciliary ganglion. The optic nerve, ophthalmic artery, branches of the sympathetic carotid plexus, and the orbital prolongations of the meninges which form the sheath of the optic nerve pass through the optic canal.

The ophthalmoplegia which results could be complete or incomplete, depending upon the extent of the involvement. The condition is nearly always unilateral, especially in the beginning, but may later become bilateral by further extension.

A few cases of this kind have been described in the literature as the orbital-apex sphenoid fissure syndrome, in which the condition was due to a traumatic, neoplastic, or inflammatory process. Most of these cases, however, presented incomplete eye signs with involvement of only some of the structures which pass through the sphenoidal fissure. When the malignant process involves both the sphenoidal fissure and the optic canal, the structures primarily involved are the second, third, fourth, and sixth cranial nerves, the ophthalmic division of the fifth nerve, sympathetic fibers, the ophthalmic vein, and the ophthalmic artery. This would constitute a syndrome which is characterized principally by complete ophthalmoplegia and loss of vision on the affected side, to which I have given the abbreviated name of S-O syndrome with complete ophthalmoplegia. (The letter S designates the sphenoidal fissure, while the letter O indicates the optic canal.) This appears to be a more accurate anatomical and descriptive name than the older orbital apex-sphenoid fissure syndrome. Moreover, the orbital apex may become involved by a pathological process without affecting any of the structures passing through either the sphenoidal fissure or optic canal.

The symptoms usually complained of are hyperesthesia or anesthesia of the upper lid, half of the forehead, and of the cornea; vasomotor disturbances; impairment of vision which, in many cases, results in blindness. Pain is fairly constant. It is localized behind the eyeball and radiates to the top of the head, to the forehead, and to the temples. The pain usually subsides when the ophthalmoplegia is at its height.

Other signs are diplopia, ophthalmoplegia of varying degree including ptosis, loss of accommodation, and an enlarged, fixed pupil. There may be only slight changes in the fundus, but involvement of the optic nerve occurs with optic atrophy late in the condition. Exophthalmos is not a typical finding and is only very slight when present. The syndrome may be bilateral but usually involves only one eye at a time. Months or years may elapse before the other eye becomes involved.

I have recently encountered two such cases, both of which were caused by carcinoma of the sphenoid and ethmoid sinuses. In the first case, the carcinoma was evidently primary in the sphenoid sinus, although the ethmoids on the affected side were also found to be involved at autopsy. The patient was a 58-year-old woman who suffered with headaches for quite some time. This was followed by epistaxis. The first signs of ocular involvement were sudden, complete ptosis of the right upper eyelid and loss of vision. When this first occurred, there was no pathology in the eyegrounds, but later, a gradual, progressive edema occurred around the optic nerve head and surrounding retina. Retinal hemorrhages also occurred late near the nerve head. There was complete immobility of the right eye and corneal anesthesia. The conjunctiva became edematous and congested, indicating obstruction to the circulation, but there was no exophthalmos. All of the structures passing through the sphenoidal fissure and optic canal were involved in this case. Exploration of the orbit revealed no involvement of the inner walls.

In the second patient, who is still under observation, the ptosis also appeared suddenly, and this was followed by complete immobility of the eye and loss of vision. In these cases of S-O syndrome, the ocular complications appear only after the pathological process has involved the sphenoid bone and progressed far enough to cause pressure on the structures which leave the cavernous sinus to enter the sphenoidal fissure and optic canal. In middle-aged or older patients especially, who are under observation for malignancy, the process may extend to the sinuses or sphenoid bone by metastasis or it may occur here primarily. The latter condition is more rare. However, the sudden appearance of ptosis or other ocular involvement in such patients should draw attention to the possibility of the S-O syndrome with ophthalmoplegia.

References

1. Ellis, Z. H., and McKeown, H. S.: Osseous Tumors of the Orbit, Arch. Ophth. 5: 449, 1931.
2. Abeli, R.: Optic Atrophy in Paget's Disease, Arch. Ophth. 4: 691, 1930.
3. Lambert, R. K.: Paget's Disease With Angioid Streaks of the Retina, Arch. Ophth. 22: 106, 1939.
4. Frey, W. G.: Paget's Disease of the Skull, Arch. Ophth. 18: 477, 1937.
5. Cushing, H.: The Cranial Hyperostosis Produced by Meningeal Endotheliomas, Arch. Neurol. and Psychiat. 8: 139, 1922.
6. Elsberg, C. A., Hare, C. C., and Dyke, C. G.: Unilateral Exophthalmos in Intracranial Tumors With Special Reference to Its Occurrence in the Meningiomata, Surg., Gynec. and Obst. 55: 681, 1932.
7. Alpers, B. J., and Groff, R. A.: Parasellar Tumors; Meningeal Fibroblastomas Arising From the Sphenoidal Ridge, Arch. Neurol. and Psychiat. 31: 713, 1934.
8. Cohen, M., and Scarff, J. E.: Unilateral Exophthalmos Produced by a Meningioma of the Middle Cranial Fossa, Arch. Ophth. 13: 771, 1935.
9. Knapp, A.: Orbital Hyperostosis: Its Occurrence in Two Cases of Meningioma of the Skull, Arch. Ophth. 20: 996, 1938.
10. Benedict, W. L.: Hyperostosis of the Orbit, Am. J. Ophth. 24: 1005, 1941.

INDEX